MW00331964

DRUGS AND NUTRIENTS

DRUGS AND THE PHARMACEUTICAL SCIENCES

A Series of Textbooks and Monographs

Edited by

James Swarbrick
School of Pharmacy
University of North Carolina
Chapel Hill, North Carolina

Volume 1. PHARMACOKINETICS, *Milo Gibaldi and Donald Perrier* (out of print)

Volume 2. GOOD MANUFACTURING PRACTICES FOR PHARMACEUTICALS: A PLAN FOR TOTAL QUALITY CONTROL, *Sidney H. Willig, Murray M. Tuckerman, and William S. Hitchings IV* (out of print)

Volume 3. MICROENCAPSULATION, *edited by J. R. Nixon*

Volume 4. DRUG METABOLISM: CHEMICAL AND BIOCHEMICAL ASPECTS, *Bernard Testa and Peter Jenner*

Volume 5. NEW DRUGS: DISCOVERY AND DEVELOPMENT, *edited by Alan A. Rubin*

Volume 6. SUSTAINED AND CONTROLLED RELEASE DRUG DELIVERY SYSTEMS, *edited by Joseph R. Robinson*

Volume 7. MODERN PHARMACEUTICS, *edited by Gilbert S. Banker and Christopher T. Rhodes*

Volume 8. PRESCRIPTION DRUGS IN SHORT SUPPLY: CASE HISTORIES, *Michael A. Schwartz*

Volume 9. ACTIVATED CHARCOAL: ANTIDOTAL AND OTHER MEDICAL USES, *David O. Cooney*

Volume 10. CONCEPTS IN DRUG METABOLISM (in two parts), *edited by Peter Jenner and Bernard Testa*

Volume 11. PHARMACEUTICAL ANALYSIS: MODERN METHODS (in two parts), *edited by James W. Munson*

Volume 12. TECHNIQUES OF SOLUBILIZATION OF DRUGS, edited by Samuel H. Yalkowsky

Volume 13. ORPHAN DRUGS, edited by Fred E. Karch

Volume 14. NOVEL DRUG DELIVERY SYSTEMS: FUNDAMENTALS, DEVELOPMENTAL CONCEPTS, BIOMEDICAL ASSESSMENTS, edited by Yie W. Chien

Volume 15. PHARMACOKINETICS, Second Edition, Revised and Expanded, Milo Gibaldi and Donald Perrier

Volume 16. GOOD MANUFACTURING PRACTICES FOR PHARMACEUTICALS: A PLAN FOR TOTAL QUALITY CONTROL, Second Edition, Revised and Expanded, Sidney H. Willig, Murray M. Tuckerman, and William S. Hitchings IV

Volume 17. FORMULATION OF VETERINARY DOSAGE FORMS, edited by Jack Blodinger

Volume 18. DERMATOLOGICAL FORMULATIONS: PERCUTANEOUS ABSORPTION, Brian W. Barry

Volume 19. THE CLINICAL RESEARCH PROCESS IN THE PHARMACEUTICAL INDUSTRY, edited by Gary M. Matoren

Volume 20. MICROENCAPSULATION AND RELATED DRUG PROCESSES, Patrick B. Deasy

Volume 21. DRUGS AND NUTRIENTS: THE INTERACTIVE EFFECTS, edited by Daphne A. Roe and T. Colin Campbell

Volume 22. BIOTECHNOLOGY OF INDUSTRIAL ANTIBIOTICS, Erick J. Vandamme

Volume 23. PHARMACEUTICAL PROCESS VALIDATION, edited by Bernard T. Loftus and Robert A. Nash

Other Volumes in Preparation

DRUGS AND NUTRIENTS

The Interactive Effects

edited by

Daphne A. Roe
T. Colin Campbell

Division of Nutritional Sciences
Cornell University
Ithaca, New York

MARCEL DEKKER, INC.   New York and Basel

Library of Congress Cataloging in Publication Data
Main entry under title:

Drugs and nutrients.

    (Drugs and the pharmaceutical sciences; v. 21)
    Includes bibliographies and indexes.
    1. Drug-nutrient interactions. I. Roe, Daphne A.
II. Campbell, T. Colin, [date]. III. Series.
[DNLM: 1. Drug interactions. 2. Drug therapy—Adverse
effects. 3. Drugs—Metabolism. 4. Nutrition—Drug
effects. 5. Nutrition disorders—Chemically induced.
W1 DR 893B v. 21 / QV 38 D79525]
RM302.4.D77 1984   615'.7045   83-27169
ISBN 0-8247-7054-4

MARCEL DEKKER, INC.
270 Madison Avenue, New York, New York 10016

Current printing (last digit):
10 9 8 7 6 5 4 3 2 1

PRINTED IN THE UNITED STATES OF AMERICA

Preface

This book was conceived in response to requests for a state-of-the-art text on drug—nutrient interactions. When we accepted the editorship of this volume, we decided that the book should be divided into two parts, with Part I being devoted to the effects of food and of nutrient intake on the disposition of foreign compounds and Part II having to do with effects of drugs on nutrition. We made an early decision to choose as our authors those scientists whose research is currently in these fields. Our authors were asked to stress methodological issues and to provide critical subject matter reviews. They have complied fully.

The book is intended for toxicologists who have the difficult task of interpreting serial or parallel studies of xenobiotics in experimental animals fed different diets. It is intended for oncologists who seek a better understanding of how nutrients affect chemical carcinogenesis. It is also aimed to meet the needs of nutritionists and clinical investigators concerned with interpretation of aberrant effects of therapeutic drugs which may be explained by food effects on drug disposition or drug effects on nutritional status.

Our thanks are due to the editorial staff of Marcel Dekker for guiding this book to publication. We are also indebted to our secretaries, Beverly Hastings and Joan McLain, who have communicated with our authors as well as our publishers and who have given us assistance in the many activities necessary to bring this book to completion.

Daphne A. Roe
T. Colin Campbell

Contents

Preface   *iii*

Contributors   *vii*

Introduction   *xi*

Part I   NUTRITIONAL EFFECTS ON DRUG AND FOREIGN
         COMPOUND ACTIVITIES

    1.   Methodologies Used for the Determination of
       Chemical Body Burdens   3
       J. Donoso

    2.   Plasma Binding, Distribution, and Elimination   21
       G. R. Wilkinson

    3.   Dietary Lipids and Foreign Compound
       (Carcinogen) Metabolism   51
       Bandaru S. Reddy and Peggy Smith-Barbaro

    4.   Retinoids and Drug-Metabolizing Enzymes   95
       Rajendra S. Chhabra

    5.   Availability of Cosubstrates as a Rate-Limiting
       Factor   119
       Gerard J. Mulder and Klaas R. Krijgsheld

6. Glutathione Conjugation Systems and
   Drug Disposition 179
   Donald J. Reed and Michael J. Meredith

7. Ascorbic Acid in Drug Metabolism 225
   David E. Holloway and Francis J. Peterson

Part II EFFECTS OF DRUGS ON NUTRITION

8. Drug–Nutrient Interactions in Teratogenesis 299
   Robert M. Hackman and Lucille S. Hurley

9. Human Milk: A Portal of Drugs from Mother
   to Infant 331
   Lynn Marie Janas and Mary Frances Picciano

10. Drugs, Appetite, and Body Weight 375
    David A. Levitsky

11. Anticonvulsant-Drug-Induced Mineral Disorders 409
    Theodore J. Hahn and Louis V. Avioli

12. Vitamin K and Vitamin K Antagonists 429
    Thorir D. Bjornsson

13. Drug-Induced Maldigestion and Malabsorption 475
    Philip G. Holtzapple and Sheldon E. Schwartz

14. Toxic Pancreatitis 487
    R. J. Laugier and H. Sarles

15. Risk Factors in Drug-Induced Nutritional
    Deficiencies 505
    Daphne A. Roe

Author Index 525
Subject Index 585

Contributors

Louis V. Avioli, M.D. *Division of Bone and Mineral Metabolism, The Jewish Hospital at Washington University, St. Louis, Missouri*

Thorir D. Bjornsson, M.D. *Division of Clinical Pharmacology, Duke University Medical Center, Durham, North Carolina*

Rajendra S. Chhabra, Ph.D. *Toxicology Research and Testing Program, National Institute of Environmental Health Sciences, Research Triangle Park, North Carolina*

J. Donoso† *Criteria and Evaluation Division, Environmental Protection Agency, Chemical Branch, Arlington, Virginia*

Robert M. Hackman, Ph.D.‡ *Department of Nutrition, University of California, Davis, California*

Theodore J. Hahn, M.D. *Department of Medicine, University of California at Los Angeles and the Wadsworth Medical Center, Los Angeles, California*

---

†Dr. Donoso is deceased.
‡*Present affiliation*: College of Human Development and Performance, University of Oregon, Eugene, Oregon

David E. Holloway, Ph.D.* *Division of Nutritional Sciences, Martha Van Rensselaer Hall, Cornell University, Ithaca, New York*

Philip G. Holtzapple, M.D. *Department of Medicine, Upstate Medical Center of the State University of New York, Syracuse, New York*

Lucille S. Hurley, Ph.D. *Department of Nutrition, University of California, Davis, California*

Lynn Marie Janas, M.S. *Department of Foods and Nutrition, Division of Nutritional Sciences, College of Agriculture, University of Illinois, Urbana, Illinois*

Klaas R. Krijgsheld, Ph.D. *Department of Pharmacology, State University of Groningen, Groningen, The Netherlands*

R. J. Laugier, M.D. *Department of Gastroenterology, Hôpital Sainte Marguerite, Marseilles, France*

David A. Levitsky, Ph.D. *Department of Psychology and Division of Nutritional Sciences, Savage Hall, Cornell University, Ithaca, New York*

Michael J. Meredith, Ph.D.† *Department of Biochemistry and Biophysics, Oregon State University, Corvallis, Oregon*

Gerard J. Mulder, Ph.D. *Department of Pharmacology, State University of Groningen, Groningen, The Netherlands*

Francis J. Peterson, Ph.D.‡ *Department of Poultry Science, Division of Nutritional Sciences, Cornell University, Ithaca, New York*

Mary Frances Picciano, Ph.D *Department of Foods and Nutrition, Division of Nutritional Sciences, College of Agriculture, University of Illinois, Urbana, Illinois*

Bandaru S. Reddy, Ph.D. *Naylor Dana Institute for Disease Prevention, American Health Foundation, Valhalla, New York*

Present affiliation: University of Miami School of Medicine, Miami, Florida
†*Present affiliation*: Department of Biochemistry, Vanderbilt University, Nashville, Tennessee
‡*Present affiliation*: James Ford Bell Technical Center, General Mills, Inc., Minneapolis, Minnesota

Donald J. Reed, Ph.D. *Department of Biochemistry and Biophysics, Oregon State University, Corvallis, Oregon*

Daphne A. Roe, M.D. *Division of Nutritional Sciences, Savage Hall, Cornell University, Ithaca, New York*

H. Sarles, M.D. *Department of Gastroenterology, Hôpital Sainte Marguerite, Marseilles, France*

Sheldon E. Schwartz, M.D. *Department of Medicine, Upstate Medical Center of the State University of New York, Syracuse, New York*

Peggy Smith-Barbaro, Ph.D.* *Naylor Dana Institute for Disease Prevention, American Health Foundation, Valhalla, New York*

G. R. Wilkinson, Ph.D. *Department of Pharmacology, Division of Clinical Pharmacology, Vanderbilt University School of Medicine, Nashville, Tennessee*

Present affiliation: Frito-Lay, Inc., Irving, Texas

Introduction

For many basic scientists and professionals in health-related disciplines, knowledge of drug—nutrient interactions has become a responsibility. We have been made aware of the dietary regulation of drug metabolism in animals and in man (Conney et al., 1977). Epidemiologists have provided evidence that differences in cancer incidence between and within populations may be diet-related. Toxicants naturally present in foods, trace substances produced in food by processing or cooking, intentional food additives, and food contaminants can initiate carcinogenesis. However, cancer development is also related to levels of food intake and particularly to levels of macro- and micronutrients consumed over time. McLean (1981) emphasized that short-term changes in food intake, insufficient to alter nutritional status to a presently detectable extent, may nevertheless alter response to environmental chemicals. Yet, in spite of our knowledge that diet and nutritional status can profoundly affect the outcome of chemically induced disease, toxicologists, chemical industries, and regulatory agencies have all been slow to control or to see the need to control the diets of their experimental animals. Newberne and McConnell (1980), based on their own extensive experience, concluded that natural-product and semipurified diets, because they vary in nutrient content, may bias interpretation of the results of toxicological testing. They recommended surveillance of both chemical contaminants and nutrients in the diets of animals used in all toxicological studies.

At the present time, we have a heightened awareness of the effects of diet on drug metabolism and, in a general sort of way, we know the potential outcomes. In Part 1 of this book, our aim is to take readers beyond this phase of knowledge and to present newer information on concepts and methodologies that will allow us to answer when, why, and how diet determines the effects of exposure to foreign chemicals. We have therefore assembled chapters from our most experienced colleagues on quantitation of the total body burden of foreign chemicals, measurement of the effects of plasma protein on drug disposition, and the determination of the effects of specific nutrients on drug metabolism. Two groups of authors have focused on interrelations between nutrition and drug conjugation, offering new conceptual and methodological information on diet-related substrates required for glucuronidation, methylation, sulfation, glutathione conjugation, and amino acid conjugation. A theme linking the chapters in Part 1 is the consideration of experimental protocols permitting us to explore drug–nutrient interactions.

New drug development and usage have been major factors that have broadened our knowledge of drug-induced malnutrition. This generalization has been upheld whether the drug has been newly synthesized to meet a therapeutic requirement or used for a new purpose. For example, knowledge of drug-induced vitamin B_6 deficiency was the result of widespread use of isoniazid as a tuberculostatic agent which began in the 1950s and the demonstration by Biehl and Vilter (1954a,b) that isoniazid toxicity resembles vitamin B_6 deficiency induced by deoxypyridoxine (Levy et al., 1967; Vilter et al., 1953).

On the other hand, realization that a drug can produce subclinical nutritional deficiencies was the result of advances in the biochemical assessment of nutritional status. Much of the information we have on the effects of anticonvulsants such as diphenylhydantoin on vitamin D and folate status is related to laboratory test findings not available until relatively recent years (Roe, 1981).

Advances in knowledge of drug-induced malabsorption were the result of independent observations that drugs of very different physical and chemical properties can reduce nutrient uptake. As early as 1927, it was shown that mineral oil could impair absorption of fat-soluble vitamins (Burrows and Farr, 1927). Later, Curtis and Ballmer (1939), in their studies on the effects of mineral oil on β-carotene absorption, laid the groundwork for the general concept that drugs can reduce the absorption of nutrients because of physicochemical events pertaining to the interaction of drugs and nutrients in the gastrointestinal tract. It was not until 30 years had passed that Faloon (1970) demonstrated that drugs could induce malabsorption, not only because of interaction with nutrients within the gastrointestinal tract but also because of mucosal damage, changes in the availability of bile salts, or impairment of the pancreatic exocrine function.

While significant expansion of knowledge of drug-induced malnutrition came about in the 1940s and 1950s, when drugs having antinutrient properties were developed, concurrent advances in knowledge relating to alcohol-associated nutritional disease can best be explained as an outcome of experience that alcoholics were the single population group most likely to have avitaminoses which could not be completely explained by dietary deficiencies. Riggs and Boles (1944-1945) proposed that Wernicke's syndrome was a form of thiamin deficiency occurring in alcoholics. Jolliffe (1940) was the first to point out that "any individual consuming an adequate diet may merely by the addition of alcohol calories, make the diet an inadequate one." In recent years, Jolliffe's theory has been amended because studies indicate that nutritional deficiencies in alcoholics and in alcohol-fed experimental animals are secondary to alcohol-induced impairment of nutrient absorption and utilization (Rogers et al., 1981).

We have now come of age in our understanding of effects of drugs on food intake, of drugs in food, and of changes in nutritional status attributable to drugs and alcohol. We have advanced in our knowledge of drug-induced cachexia, of drug-induced malabsorption, and of drugs as vitamin antagonists. In order to define future research needs in the field, it is necessary to have key investigators such as our contributors describe the state of the art.

Authors of chapters in Part 2 were called upon to discuss subject matters at the interface of nutrition and pharmacology. They were told to focus on recent advances, emphasize specific aims of research, describe methodology, and offer critical reviews of the literature concerning drug effects on nutritional status and intake of drugs with the diet. Specific topics covered include: drug-induced fetal malnutrition; drugs in breast milk; drug effects on appetite; anticonvulsants and rickets and osteomalacia; molecular events explaining the action of vitamin K antagonists (coumarin anticoagulants); drug-induced malabsorption; the role of macronutrients in the development of chronic pancreatitis; and the multifactorial etiology of drug-induced malnutrition.

Drug-induced malnutrition is preventable, but physicians and others involved in health care must acquire sufficient familiarity with the subject that prediction of risk becomes a reality. We therefore hope that this book will not only provide information that is critical to the assessment of the risk of diet manipulation on drug efficacy and safety but also to the assessment of the risk of drugs in the causation of nutritional disease.

REFERENCES

Biehl, J. P., and Vilter, R. W. (1954a). Effects of isoniazid on pyridoxine metabolism. *JAMA 156*:1549-1552.

Biehl, J. P., and Vilter, R. W. (1954b). Effect of isoniazid on vitamin B_6 metabolism: Its possible significance in producing isoniazid neuritis. *Proc. Soc. Exp. Biol. Med. 85*:389-392.

Burrows, M. T., and Farr, W. K. (1927). The action of mineral oil per os on the organism. *Proc. Soc. Exp. Biol. Med. 24*:719-723.

Conney, A. H., Pantuck, E. J., Hsiao, K.-C., Kuntzman, R., Alvares, A. P., and Kappas, A. (1977). Regulation of drug metabolism in man by environmental chemicals and diet. *Fed. Proc.* *36*:1647-1652.

Curtis, A. C., and Ballmer, R. S. (1959). The prevention of carotene absorption by liquid petrolatum. *JAMA* *113*:1785-1788.

Faloon, W. W. (1970). Drug production of intestinal malabsorption. *N.Y. State J. Med.* *70*:2189-2192.

Jolliffe, N. (1940). The influence of alcohol on the adequacy of the B vitamins in the American diet. *Quart. J. Stud. Alc.* *1*:74-84.

Levy, L., Higgins, L. J., and Burbridge, T. N. (1967). Isoniazid-induced vitamin B_6 deficiency. *Amer. Rev. Resp. Dis.* *96*:910-917.

McLean, A. E. M. (1981). Drug nutrient interactions from experiment to epidemiology. *Nutrition in Health and Disease and International Development, Symp. XII Internat. Congr.*, Alan R. Liss, Inc. New York, pp. 729-737.

Meltzer, H. J. (1956). Congenital anomalies due to attempted abortion with 4-aminopteroglutamic acid. *JAMA* *161*:1253.

Newberne, P. M., and McConnell, R. G. (1980). Dietary nutrients and contaminants in laboratory animal experimentation. *J. Exp. Pathol. Toxicol.* *4*:105-122.

Nichols, C. A., and Welch, A. D. (1950). On the mechanism of action of aminopterin. *Proc. Soc. Exp. Biol. Med.* *74*:403-411.

Riggs, H.E., and Boles, R. S. (1944-1945). Wernicke's disease. A clinical and pathological study of 42 cases. *Quart. J. Stud. Alc.* *5*:361-370.

Roe, D. A. (1981). Drug interference with the assessment of nutritional status. In *Clinics in Laboratory Medicine*, R. Labbe, Ed., Saunders, Philadelphia, pp. 647-664.

Rogers, A. E., Fox. J. G., and Murphy, J. C. (1981). Ethanol and diet interactions in male rhesus monkeys. *Drug-Nutrient Interactions* *1*:3-14.

Vilter, R. W., Mueller, J. F., Glazer, H. Z., Jarrold, T., Abraham, J., Thompson, C. and Hawkins, V. R. (1953). The effect of vitamin B_6 deficiency induced by desoxypyridoxine in human beings. *J. Lab. Clin. Med.* *42*:355-357.

DRUGS AND NUTRIENTS

Part I
NUTRITIONAL EFFECTS ON DRUG AND FOREIGN COMPOUND ACTIVITIES

1

Methodologies Used for the Determination of Chemical Body Burdens

J. Donoso[†]
Environmental Protection Agency, Chemical Branch,
Arlington, Virginia

I. INTRODUCTION

The body burden of a chemical (drug, pesticide, food additive, etc.) can be defined as the amount of that chemical present in the body at any one time as a result of its voluntary or involuntary exposure to that chemical. The concept of body storage is of particular interest in relation to those chemicals that show greater persistence in human tissues, and the ability of these chemicals to persist or accumulate in tissues is influenced by many factors, such as the physicochemical properties of the chemical itself; the intensity and duration of exposure or insult; the efficiency of absorption; the age, sex, and nutritional status of the exposed subject; and the integrity of some organs, especially the liver and the kidney.

Chemical body burden in the general population can also be augmented by chemical contamination of air, dust, water, and food, and the nature of the home and working environment. Thus differences in body burden levels distinguishing the general population from an occupationally exposed population may then be attributed to occupational exposure and to chemicals carried into the house on clothing and other items.

[†]Dr. Donoso is deceased.
The section on oral exposure was prepared by Daphne A. Roe, M. D., co-editor of this book, as Dr. Donoso died prior to the completion of the manuscript.

In our highly industrialized society, occupational health hazards routinely faced by workers include inhalation and oral and dermal exposure to toxic gases, liquids, or solids found in the working environment. A few examples may help to illustrate this statement. In the course of reduction of aluminum by the Hall process, variable amounts of fluoride are generated. These arise during the electrolyses of Al_2O_3 in the presence of cryolite (Na_3AlF_6), which acts as the electrolyte. During the electrolysis process, particulates (e.g., Na_3AlF_6) and gaseous (e.g., HF) fluorides are emitted to the working environment. Under these conditions, absorption of fluoride via inhalation or ingestion by workers, or both, may occur. Similarly, a wide variety of industrial situations and many opportunities for exposure to metallic lead or its compounds in the house and elsewhere may lead to the ingestion or inhalation of quantities of lead over and above those that occur naturally.

In the agriculture field, studies by Wolfe (1973) on several hundred pesticide applicators showed that over 97% of the pesticides to which the body is subjected in the course of most exposure situations are deposited on the skin. Although people differ in their tolerances and responses to different chemicals, it is essential to have methodology by which the body burden of sensitive as well as intoxicated populations can be determined.

Within the last two decades, a number of methods have been developed for the measurement of human exposure to chemical or biological agents. These methods can be divided conveniently into two groups:

1. *Direct methods*: These methods involve the use of some device to trap the chemical as it comes in contact with the individual during the exposure period. Then the amount of the chemical as determined by chemical analyses or any other method constitutes a direct measure of the particular exposure to the chemical under consideration.
2. *Indirect methods:* These methods involve the detection of either the chemical or its metabolites(s) in body tissues or excreta, or the measurement of some pharmacological effect of the chemical on the exposed individual.

II. DIRECT METHODS

The determination of exposure using direct methods requires the consideration of three routes of exposure: respiratory, dermal, and oral.

A. Respiratory Exposure

Respiratory or inhalation exposure, which results from the absorption of chemicals across the alveolar respiratory membrane, can be determined from measurements of the amount of chemical in the air expressed as either parts per million (ppm) or weight of chemical per cubic meter (m^3) of air and the actual tidal volume and respiratory rate measured under the working conditions being studied. It must be pointed out that in considering this approach, two problems immediately arise.

1. The minute alveolar ventilation is not constant; respiratory rates and the amount of air per breath (tidal volume) can change many times depending on the level of physical exertion and tissue oxygen demand. In practice, the average values for lung ventilation in humans as given by Spengler (1957) have been used; these values are 7.4 liters/min during rest, 29 liters/min during light work, and 60 liters/min during heavy work.

2. If the physical state of the chemical in the air is a particulate form, the larger particles (those greater than 10 μm in diameter) are either filtered out by the turbinates of the nose or are retained on the mucous membranes of the upper respiratory tract; if absorbed through these membranes or swallowed, oral exposure occurs in addition to inhalation exposure. However, smaller particles and vapors reach the deep parts of the lung, where they are absorbed into the blood or lymph and subsequently translocated to other parts of the body.

B. Dermal Exposure

Dermal exposure, which results from the absorption of chemicals across the skin surface, can be determined by (1) estimating the concentration of the chemical in the air impinging a unit surface area of exposed skin at different wind velocities; (2) using the pad or patch techniques, consisting of gauze, cellulose, or perhaps other absorbing or dust-retaining material; and (3) using swabs or liquid rinses of those areas exposed to the chemical under consideration.

Once the concentration of the chemical as determined by any of the aforementioned techniques has been established, the dermal exposure is calculated by assuming that the exposed subject wore a predetermined amount of clothing and that this clothing gave complete protection of the areas covered. Then the surface area of the usually unclothed body parts is measured using Berkow's (1931) values for surface area, and the total dermal exposure is calculated by multiplying the concentration of the chemical per unit area times the total surface area of the unclothed body parts.

Although the method used for the determination of dermal exposure appears to be quite accurate, there is probably greater disparity between exposure and absorption for the dermal than for any other route of exposure. This disparity arises from the fact that penetration of the chemical through the skin not only differs in respect to the chemical per se, but also in regard to the portion of the body with which the chemicals come in contact. Thus Feldmann and Maibach (1974), working with several pesticides, have shown that in the case of parathion, for instance, the extent of skin penetration is directly proportional to the amount of chemical reaching the skin, whereas in the case of lindane, with increasing concentration there is a relative decrease in the percentage that penetrates the skin. The effect of the region of the body on penetration of topical application of parathion showed enormous differences between sites. The skin penetration of this chemical varied; the forearm allowed the least (8%) penetration and the scrotum the greatest (above 100%).

C. Oral Exposure

Chemicals that gain access to the body via the mouth may be ingested in food, in alcoholic or nonalcoholic beverages, and in water, in which the chemicals may be nutrients or nonnutrients, including natural toxicants, contaminants, and the intentional food additives. Oral exposure to foreign chemicals also derives from smoking, from toothpaste, cosmetics, mouthwashes, drugs used for local effect in the mouth, sublingual drug preparations, industrial compounds accidentally ingested in the work place or in the home, and intake of therapeutic drugs intended for systematic effect after absorption.

In developing methods for determination of chemicals entering the body by this route, investigators have focused on specific aims: quantitating all sources of the chemical of concern, identification of extreme consumers, and measurement of change in health status that can be attributed to oral exposure. A further methodological concern has been to estimate that portion of the total body burden of the chemical of concern derived from each specific source, as for example, drinking water (Toxicity of Selected Drinking Water Contaminants, 1980).

With respect to food components, particular methodological concerns include: the concentration of the component, additive, or contaminant in each dietary item in which it occurs; the amount consumed for each suspect item; and the frequency with which each of these items is consumed. Methods in use include market-basket studies (Park et al., 1981), weighed food records (Disselduff et al., 1979), and adaptations of the British "Total Diet" study method to estimate level of consumption of the chemical of concern by extreme consumers (Coomes et al., 1982).

Appropriate use and constraints on the use of these various methods have been discussed by Tulinius (1982) and by James et al. (1982).

In monitoring intake of food contaminants it has been emphasized that there is a need to obtain information on food habits, method of food preparation, and the origin of foods consumed (Santodonato et al., 1981).

III. INDIRECT METHODS

A. Blood and Adipose Tissues as Indices

According to Durham and Wolfe (1962), "Any measure of drug absorption or its necessary sequela constitute an indirect method of exposure." It is not often convenient to measure absorption itself, but measurements of a compound or its biodegradation products in the blood tissue or excreta give information on minimal absorption. The technological advancements in the field of analytical biochemistry, combined with the development of new pharmacokinetic principles applicable to the study of the distribution and the mode of action of foreign compounds in the human body, have made this method an attractive procedure for the determination of body burdens of those intentionally or occupationally exposed to drugs, pesticides, or food additives.

To justify the use of tissues or excreta as indices of body burden, one must try to elucidate (1) what (if any) the relationship is between the dose or exposure to the chemical and its concentration in the tissues and excreta, (2) what the relationship is between the concentration of the chemical within the different tissues and excreta, and (3) if possible, what the relationship is between the concentration of the chemical in the different tissues and the length of exposure or insult.

As early as 1948, Howell (1948) found DDT-derived materials in a fat sample of a man with 4 years of occupational exposure and a history of eating foods known to bear appreciable residues. In 1950, Laug et al. (1951) reported DDT residues in the fat of 75 persons with no special occupation exposure. Studying the relationship between the concentrations of aldrin (HEOD) and DDT in blood and depot fat of 44 persons with no known occupational exposure, Robinson and Hunter (1966) found that the ratio of the mean concentration of HEOD in whole blood and depot fat was 159 (confidence limits 153–213), whereas the corresponding ratio for DDT was 306 (confidence limits 319–410). Although these two ratios were significantly different, they seemed to indicate that the portion of the total body burden of HEOD present in the blood was greater than that for DDT-type compounds.

Radomski et al. (1971) used four male and four female subjects in order to follow the diurnal variation in the concentration of lindane, BHC, dieldrin, p,p'-DDT, and p,p'-DDE in whole blood and plasma. In general, and regardless of the pesticides under consideration, the concentration of these compounds in either whole blood or plasma remained remarkably constant throughout the day; however, there was a minor but significant elevation in the plasma concentration of p,p'-DDT and p,p'-DDE after the lunch meal. It was also found that the daily concentration of the pesticides in whole blood or plasma did not change within a week if the blood samples were taken each day at the same time interval. Furthermore, in 20 random autopsy cases, good correlation was obtained between the blood and fat concentrations of dieldrin (r = 0.84), BHC (r = 0.87), and p,p'-DDE (r = 0.95).

The relative consistency in the concentration of pesticides in blood and its good correlation with that in fat suggested that the distribution of these compounds within the organism is compatible with the concepts of compartmental modeling, since it is more realistic to conceive of pesticide concentration in blood or plasma as primarily a reflection of their presence in other tissues (i.e., at any point in time, an equilibrium has been reached among the different compartments and the concentration of pesticide within each compartment remains constant rather than been purposefully transported from intake to storage site or storage site to excretion site, etc.).

All the data accumulated with respect to the consistency of whole blood and plasma concentration and the correlation with body fat concentrations indicate that these determinations constitute an excellent procedure for the evaluation of the pesticide body burden and previous exposure. Thus Hunter and Robinson (1967) conducted a feeding study where 13 subjects (no history of occupational exposure to pesticides) were randomly allocated to three groups (of three each) and intentionally fed with 0.01, 0.05, and 0.21 mg of HEOD (in gelatin capsules), respectively. A group of four subjects was used as control. The experiment lasted 18 months and during this time, samples of mixed venous blood and subcutaneous fat were obtained. A comparison of the concentration of HEOD in the adipose tissue and blood with the intentional oral exposure showed a positive correlation. An examination of the concentration of HEOD in the samples of blood and adipose tissues collected from the subjects at various times showed that there was a general tendency for them to correlate, and individual regression lines for five of the nine experimental subjects with oral exposure to HEOD were significant.

Hunter and Robinson (1967) use the concentration of HEOD in the two tissues at the end of the fifteenth month in the three groups of subjects given either 10, 50, or 211 µg of HEOD per day in order to assess the equivalent oral intake of HEOD by the general population. Two regression lines for concentration in the adipose tissue in relation to daily dosage and for concentration in the blood in relation to daily dosage, respectively, were calculated and both relationships were highly significant ($P < 0.001$). The two relationships were as follows:

Concentration of HEOD
in adipose tissue   = 0.26 + 0.65 × (measured daily dose
                           µg/kg BW per day)   (1)

Concentration of HEOD
in blood   = 0.0024 + 0.004 × (measured daily dose
                           µg/kg BW per day)   (2)

Equations (1) and (2) were also represented as

$$y_i = a_i + b_i x_i \qquad (3)$$

where

  y_i = concentration of HEOD in the ith tissue
  x_i = measured dosage (expressed in terms of μg or μg/kg BW
    per day)
  a_i and b_i = constants for the regression equation

By algebraic manipulation of equation (3), the estimated adventitious exposure of the general population (expressed as equivalent oral intake) was given by

$$x_i = \frac{y_i}{b_i}$$

where y_i is the average concentration of HEOD in the ith tissue of the general population.

From the average value for HEOD in the blood and adipose tissues of people in the United Kingdom, Hunter and Robinson (1967) calculated the mean equivalent oral intake of HEOD as 0.35 and 0.32 μg/kg body weight per day, respectively. These values compared favorably with the corresponding estimated average daily intake of 0.26 μg/kg body weight per day, based on analysis of whole-cooked meals consumed by the people surveyed.

B. Hair as an Indicator of Exposure to Heavy Metals

Hair samples are useful in providing a record of human exposure to some heavy metals (Kello and Kostial, 1978; Birke and Johnels, 1972; Giovanoli-Jakubczak and Berg, 1974). Hair appears to be an excellent indicator of mercury intoxication. The accepted theory which explains the relationship between dietary mercury and mercury in hair assumes that the concentration in the newly grown hair is a uniform function of the concentration in blood. Tsubaki (1971) showed that the variation of mercury concentration in hair with time appeared to parallel the variation in the blood in spite of the fact that the ratio of mercury concentration in hair to that of blood was about 500:1.

Several attempts have been made to correlate the daily intake of mercury with its concentration in blood and hair. Clarkson and Shapiro (1971) plotted the blood concentration of mercury against the daily intake of mercury from several sources and a straight line was obtained with a slope of 1.4 μg of mercury per gram of red blood corpuscles.

Al-Shahristani et al. (1976) measured the mercury concentration in the hair of 184 patients admitted to a hospital as a result of their exposure to mercury-contaminated wheat. The ratio of the mercury concentration in hair to the average body concentration was calculated for 30 of the patients whose mercury ingestion records were properly documented. The ratio ranged from 87:1 to 268:1, with an average value of 137:1. Using this ratio, the body burden of the remaining 154 patients was calculated and then the 184 patients were classified into four diagnostic categories according to the severity of their symptoms. Two peak mercury concentrations in hair of the people who ingested treated grain but showed no symptoms of methyl mercury intoxication ranged from a normal background value of $1-300$ µg/g, corresponding to a body burden of 10 µg-2.2 mg of mercury per kilogram of body weight. On the other hand, people with severe symptoms had peak hair concentrations for mercury of $400-1600$ µg/g, corresponding to an average body burden of $3-12$ mg of mercury per kilogram of body weight.

C. Use of Mathematical Models for the Determination of Body Burden

Knowledge gained from pharmacokinetic investigations with various drugs was made for a better understanding of their pharmacology and consequently for their more efficient use (Anderson et al., 1977; Bischoff et al., 1971; Dedrick et al., 1970). Similar studies of environmental contaminants whose exposure patterns are in many cases low level and long lasting have also led to a better understanding of their potential hazard (Anderson et al., 1977; Bungay et al., 1979; Lutz et al., 1977; Howell, 1948). Environmental contaminants such as lead and fluoride appear to be stored primarily in bone. It is not yet known with certainty what portion of the bone pool of lead can be mobilized later in life (e.g., by nutritional calcium deficiency, osteoporosis, bone fracture, hyperthermia, and many other causes). At the range of fluoride exposure in the industrial environment, approximately 50% of the absorbed fluoride is taken up by bone and essentially 50% of the absorbed dose is promptly excreted in urine (i.e., within 24 hrs) (National Academy of Sciences, 1971). The chemicodynamic principles governing fluoride deposition in bone are well described by Newman and Newman (1958).

Many halogenated hydrocarbons are excreted slowly by humans and animals and thus may persist in the tissues for years. The assumption is that these chemicals are inextricably deposited in adipose tissue. This assumption is based primarily on evidence of their limited biotransformation (minimal urinary excretion) and high lipid solubility (relatively low blood-fat partition). Exceptions to this general theory have been identified; in fact chlordecone (Kepone), unlike most polychlorinated hydrocarbons, is found in blood at levels 20 times higher than would be expected based solely on the total lipid content of blood

(Egle et al., 1978). However, when the details of the intake and output of a chemical are investigated, there does not appear to be a fixed or definite relation between the amount of the chemical absorbed during one time period and the amount excreted during the succeeding time period.

According to Sterling et al. (1964), the major intervening processes that have to be dealt with in the analysis of experimental data are three:

1. All physiological reactions to a chemical within the organism depend upon the amount of the chemical actually absorbed into the tissues. This amount varies but it is not identical to the amount of the chemical in the environment, in the ingested food or in the inhaled air.
2. The body may be regarded as a reservoir into which are added the variable amounts of the chemical and from which excretion proceeds.
3. From the point of view of experimentation, the properties of the tissue reservoir raise many problems, the most important of which, however, is that no single time lag exists between the absorption of some increment of the chemical and the increase of its excretion from the body.

Although the physiological processes interposed between the intake and output of chemicals are not open to direct observation, they are known and understood to the extent that their workings can be incorporated in a rigorous model. A pharmacological model is a means of expressing in an operational way a working hypothesis for the mechanism of drug or pesticide distribution and deposition; furthermore, it is a simplified representation of a real physical system derived from experimental observations, previous knowledge, and a number of assumptions (Jacquez, 1972; Anderson et al., 1977; Marcus, 1979; Lutz et al., 1977; Egle, 1978).

In formulating physiologically based models of the body, a mass conservation equation is written for each important recognized subdivision or compartment (Bungay et al., 1979). Importance relates to whether the compartment is a target tissue (for the chemical under consideration), a site of toxicity, or significantly influences the kinetics. Each compartment is assumed to be sufficiently homogeneous that it can be considered well mixed with respect to the internal distribution of the chemical.

According to Bungay et al. (1979), the essence of the modeling approach is to compute, by means of simultaneous solution of the set of mass balance equations, the variation over time in the amount of the substance or equivalently its concentration in each compartment. In this way, a number of substances can be followed. A study by Lavy et al. (1980) provided urinary excretion data from which estimates were made of the amount of 2,4,5-T absorbed by forestry workers during the application of the propylene glycol butyl ester of 2,4,5-T by four different methods: helicopter (both raindrop nozzle and microfoil boom), backpack spraying, and tractor-mounted mist blowers.

To establish an adequate pharmacokinetic model for the absorption and excretion of 2,4,5-T, Ramsey et al. (1979) considered the following data:

1. Oral administration of 5 mg/kg 2,4,5-T to humans (Gehring et al., 1973) or rats (Piper et al., 1973) as well as intravenous administration (Sauerhoff et al., 1976) or dermal application (Young et al., 1979) of 5 mg/kg 2,4,5-T to rats showed that this chemical was quickly absorbed and excreted unchanged in the urine.

2. Urinary excretion of 2,4,5-T by humans and rats occurred by an apparent first-order process with a half-life of 23.1 hr in case of oral administration to humans and 13.6, 10.7, and 24 hr for oral, intravenous, and dermal administration to rat, respectively. The excretion process was essentially independent of the route of administration, although the dermal absorption process in rats may have been slow in relation to the urinary excretion of 2,4,5-T.

Ramsey's pharmacokinetic model for the absorption, retention, and urinary excretion of 2,4,5-T or its esters is shown in Figure 1. The differential equations and initial conditions (time = 0) describing the dynamics of the pharmacokinetic model were

$$\frac{dS(t)}{dt} = - K_{ol}S(t) \quad \text{initial conditions } S(0) = D_0 \tag{4}$$

$$\frac{dB(t)}{dt} = - K_{ol}S(t) - K_{ie}B(t) \quad \text{initial conditions } B(0) = 0 \tag{5}$$

$$\frac{dE(t)}{dt} = K_{ie}B(t) \quad \text{initial conditions } E(0) = 0 \tag{6}$$

The value of $S(t)$ at zero time represents the dose D_0, which is the total quantity of 2,4,5-T absorbed. K_{ie} was calculated from the half-life for urinary excretion of 2,4,5-T in humans as reported by Gehring et al. (1973) [i.e., 23.1 hr = 0.96 day, which corresponds to 0.72 day^{-1} (0.96 = 0.693/K_{ie})].

To estimate the actual amount of 2,4,5-T absorbed (calculated as milligrams of 2,4,5-T) during each application, the following three methods were used.

Method A. Based on a pharmacokinetic parameter estimation technique in which the best parameter estimates are considered to be those that yield the closest fit of the calculated data to the observed data (using the least-squares criterion). In this case parameter estimates

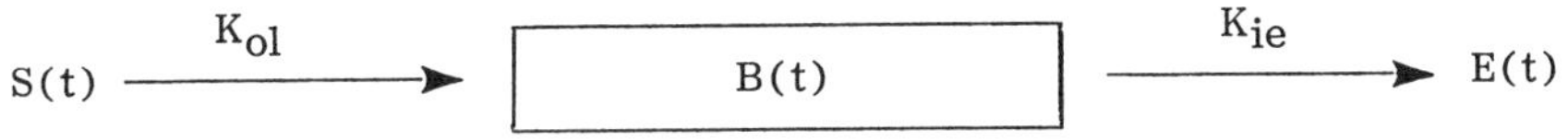

$$S(t) \xrightarrow{\quad K_{ol} \quad} \boxed{\quad B(t) \quad} \xrightarrow{\quad K_{ie} \quad} E(t)$$

where

$S(t)$ = amount of 2,4,5-T remaining to be absorbed at time t
$B(t)$ = amount of 2,4,5-T in the body at time t
$E(t)$ = amount of 2,4,5-T excreted in the urine at time t
K_{ol} and K_{ie} = first-order rate constants for the absorption and excretion of 2,4,5-T, respectively

Figure 1 Ramsey's pharmacokinetic model for the absorption, retention, and urinary excretion of 2,4,5-T or its esters.

were desired for absorption rate (K_{ol}) and for the total absorbed dose of 2,4,5-T (D_0). The excretion rate constant (K_{ie}) was set as 0.72 day^{-1} and the observed data consisted of milligrams of 2,4,5-T excreted in the urine per day.

Urinary excretion values for 10 workers in which there were no missing data points were plotted on semilogarithmic graph paper. The time course of urinary excretion of 2,4,5-T followed a kinetically consistent pattern with that of the model shown in Figure 1. The pharmacokinetic parameters for these data sets were obtained by using a digital computer and, as expected, the estimated amounts of D_0 varied considerably between individuals. However, the apparent first-order absorption rate constant K_{ol} was reasonably constant between individuals, the average value being 0.91 day^{-1} with a standard deviation of 0.2 day^{-1}. The foregoing analysis thus provided an estimate of the absorbed dose of 2,4,5-T or the body burden for 12 of the 41 exposures comprising Lavy's study.

Method B. Integration of the differential equations (4) to (6), and resolution for the total amount of 2,4,5-T excreted in the urine t days following exposure, designated at $E(t)$, resulted in equation (7).

$$E(t) = D_0 \left[1 - \frac{K_{ie} e^{-K_{ol}t}}{K_{ie} - K_{ol}} \frac{K_{oe} e^{-K_{ie}t}}{K_{ol} - K_{ie}} \right] \tag{7}$$

Solution of equation (7) using previously determined values of K_{ol} and K_{ie} at successive values of t reveals the cumulative fraction of the absorbed dose of 2,4,5-T that was excreted in the urine following exposure. The absorbed doses D_0 or body burdens at any one time during the exposure period were calculated by dividing the cumulative quantity of 2,4,5-T excreted in the urine by the appropriate fraction at that time.

Method C. By using the integrated form of the equation for the cumulative quantity of a chemical excreted as a function of time, an equation
was derived with which the absorbed dose was calculated based on the
interval (in this case daily) amount of 2,4,5-T excreted using the previously established values for $K_{oe} = 0.72$ day^{-1} and $K_{ol} = 0.92$ day^{-10}.
The calculation of D_0 or body burden by this method was independent
of the total (cumulative) quantity of urine collected. [For more details
on the study, the reader is referred to Ramsey et al. (1979).]

IV. BODY BURDEN MEASUREMENTS IN THE NUCLEAR ENVIRONMENT

Research and industrial operations in the field of nuclear energy are
carried out in almost every corner of the world. These operations
range from prospecting and mining to processing of radioactive minerals and fuel fabrication, and from the operation of research and power
reactors to the reprocessing of spent fuels. There is also an extensive
use of radioisotopes in agriculture, industry, medicine, and scientific
research.

A considerable amount of information on occupational and accidental
exposure to radiation has been amassed by measurements of blood,
urine, and feces (Lawrence, 1978; Kamath et al., 1964), by internal
organ counting and postmortem tissue analyses (Ross et al., 1981;
Spencer et al., 1966; Molla, 1975; Pohl and Pohl-Ruling, 1977), and
by whole-body counting (Gonzales, 1977; Eisenbud et al., 1969; Newton, 1977). It is not our intention to undertake an extensive review of
the methodology used in the assessment of body burden within the field
of nuclear energy but only to point out some of the circumstances under
which some of these methods can be best used.

Although modern techniques in radiation research call for the utmost
care and protection of the people engaged in such activities, the possibilities of internal radiation hazards present in facilities where radioactive materials are handled cannot be overlooked. The kind and extent of radiation hazards depend on the type of decay, the energy and
intensity of the radiation, and the selective localization of radionuclides
in specific body organs and/or tissues. Thus pure alpha emitters such
as ^{210}Pa and radionuclides such as ^{3}H, ^{14}C, and ^{35}S which emit low-
energy beta rays cannot be detected directly by in vivo counting methods and one must have resource to indirect methods (e.g., urine analysis). On the other hand, radionuclides such as ^{239}Pu, ^{90}Sr $+ ^{90}$Y,
and ^{32}P may be detected directly by means of low-energy x-ray or
bremsstrahlung, which are produced during nuclear transformation or
by interaction of high-energy beta rays with the tissues of the body.

The direct and indirect methods used in the assessment of internal
contamination are held to be complementary and it is usually recom-

mended that when possible, both methods be used together. This is particularly true in cases of accidental exposure. However, the choice of methods is dictated by the type of radionuclide in question.

A. Indirect Methods

Among the indirect methods of analysis, urine analysis is one of the most widely used for the routine measurements. The reason for this choice resides in the fact that urine is a regular output and explains the endemic activity available for deposition. In cases where insoluble compounds such as ThO_2, U_3O_3, and Co_2O_3 are concerned, fecal analysis was used because it was once thought that these compounds did not enter the bloodstream. Insoluble or practically insoluble compounds are almost completely excreted through the feces, providing higher activity for its measurement, consequently an increase in sensitivity.

B. Direct Methods

Simple whole-body radioactivity monitors designated as "shielded chair" and "shadow shield" counters are available for the assessment of body burdens of gamma-emitting radionuclides acquired in routine operations or in radiation emergency. The shielded chair counter is similar to the Argone tilting-chair arrangement described by Miller (1964). The operating philosophy of the counter is based on integral counting with an upper limit on the count rate being set to decide the internal contamination status of an individual. Vennart (1967) discussed the sensitivity requirements of whole-body counters for routine monitoring analysis. However, this system suffers from two drawbacks: (1) due to its geometry, the counting sensitivity changes appreciably due to redistribution of the radionuclide inside the body; and (2) its design does not permit one to obtain any information about localization of the radioisotope to conduct any redistribution studies.

Integral counting is of considerable value in a radiation emergency, where a large number of persons may have to be "screened" for internal contamination. The shadow shield moving counter described in detail by Hukkoo and Katoch (1971) was developed to circumvent some of the problems encountered with the shielded chair counter. Thus for uniformly distributed isotopes in the body, counts are collected in the proven and supine positions of the subject in the scanning mode of counting. For studies of localization and transmigration of radionuclides, the total body is compartmentalized into various sections and counts are collected by discrete position counting at each of the sections, thereby achieving a single-crystal multiple-position counting geometry (Miller, 1964).

REFERENCES

Al-Šhahristani, H., Shihab, K., and Al-Haddad, I. K. (1976). Mercury in hair as indicator of body burden. *Bull. WHO 53*, Suppl.

Anderson, M. W., Eling, T. E., Lutz, R. J., Dedrick, R. L., and Matthews, H. B. (1977). The construction of pharmacokinetic mode for disposition of polychlorinated biphenyls in the rat. *Clin. Pharmacol. Ther. 22*(5):765-773.

Berkow, S. G. (1931). Values of surface area proportions in the prognosis of cutaneous burns. *Amer. J. Surg. 11*:315.

Birke, G., and Johnels, A. G. (1972). Studies on humans exposed to methyl mercury through fish consumption. *Arch. Environ. Health 25*:77-91.

Bischoff, K. B., Dedrick, R. L., Zaharko, D. S., and Longstreth, J. A. (1971). Methrotrexate pharmacokinetics. *J. Pharm. Sci. 60*:1128-1133.

Bungay, P. M., Dedrick, R. L., and Matthews, H. B. (1979). Pharmacokinetics of halogenated hydrocarbons. *Ann. N. Y. Acad. Sci. 320*:257-270.

Clarkson, T. W., and Shapiro, R. E. (1971). The absorption of mercury from food, its significance and new methods of removing mercury from the body. *Proc. Symp. Mercury Man's Environ.*, Ottawa, Royal Society of Canada, pp. 124-130.

Coomes, T. J., Sherlock, J. C., and Walters, B. (1982). Studies of dietary intake and extreme food consumption. *Roy. Soc. Health J. 102*:119-123.

Dedrick, R. L., Bischoff, K. B., and Zaharko, D. S. (1970). Interspecies correlation of plasma concentrations. History of Methotrexate (NSC-740). *Cancer Chemother. Rep. 54*:95-101.

Disselduff, M. M., Try, G. P., and Berry, W. T. C. (1979). Possible use of dietary surveys to assess intake of food additives. *Food Cosmet. Toxicol. 17*:391-396.

Durham, W. F., and Wolfe, H. R. (1962). Measurement to the exposure of workers to pesticides. *Bull. WHO 26*:75-91.

Egle, J. L., Jr., Fernandez, S. B., Guzelian, P. S., and Borzelleca, J. F. (1978). Distribution and excretion of chlordecone (Kepone) in the rat. *Drug Metab. Dispos. 6*:91-95.

Eisenbud, M. C., Laurer, R., Rosen, J. E., Cohen, N., and Thomas, J. (1969). In vivo measurements of lead-20 as an indicator of cumulative radon daughter exposure in uranium miners. *Health Phys. 16*:637-646.

Feldmann, R. J., and Maibach, H. I. (1974). Percutaneous penetration of some pesticides and herbicides in man. *Toxicol. Appl. Pharmacol. 28*:126-132.

Gehring, P. J., Kramer, C. G., Schwetz, B. A., Rose, J. Q., and Row, V. K. (1973). Fate of 2,4,5-trichlorophenoxyacetic acid

(2,4,5-T) following oral administration to man. *Toxicol. Appl. Pharmacol. 26*:352-361.

Giovanoli-Jakubczak, and Berg, G. (1974). Measurements of mercury in hair. *Arch. Environ. Health 28*:139-144.

Gonzales, D. E. (1977). A general phantom procedure for calibrating inhaled Pb-212. Body burdens. *Health Phys. 32*(6):493-503.

Howell, D. D. (1948). A case of DDT storage in human fat. *Proc. Okla. Acad. Sci. 29*:31-32.

Hukkoo, R. K., and Katoch, D. S. (1971). Whole Body Counting on Radiation Workers. *BARC Rep. 54-8.*

Hunter, C. G., and Robinson, J. (1967). Pharmacodynamics of dieldrin (HEOD). I. Ingestion by human subjects for 18 months. *Arch. Environ. Health 15*:614-626.

Jacquez, J. A. (1972). *Compartmental Analysis in Biology and Medicine: Kinetics of Distribution of Tracer-Labeled Materials.* Elsevier, Amsterdam, Chap. 1.

James, W. P. T., Bingham, S. A., and Cole, T. J. (1982). Epidemiological assessment of dietary intake. *Nutrition Cancer 2*:203-211.

Kamath, P. R., Bath, I. S., Kamala, R., Tyenger, M. A. R., Koshy, E., Waingankar, U. S., and Kanolkar, V. S. (1964). Recent Radiochemical Procedures for Bioassay Studies at Trombay. *Assessment of Radioactivity in Man* (Proc. Symp. Heidelberg, 1964), IAEA, Vienna.

Kello, D., and Kostial, K. (1978). Lead and cadmium in hair as an indicator of body burden in rats of different age. *Bull. Environ. Contam. Toxicol. 20*:618-623.

Laug, E. P., Kunze, F. M., and Prickett, C. S. (1951). Occurrence of DDT in human fat and milk. *AMA Arch. Ind. Hyg. Occup. Med. 3*:245-246.

Lavy, T. L., Shepard, J. S., and Mattice, J. D. (1980). Exposure measurements of applicators spraying 2,4,5-trichlorophenoxyacetic acid in the forest. *J. Agric. Food Chem. 28*(3)626-630.

Lawrence, J. N. P. (1978). A history of PUQFUA. Plutonium body burden (Q) from urine analysis. *Rep. ISS LA-7403H.*

Lutz, R. J., Dedrick, R. L., Matthews, H. B., Eling, T. E., and Anderson, M. W. (1977). A preliminary pharmacokinetic model for several chlorinated biphenyls in the rat. *Dokl. Akad. Nauk. SSSR 5*:386-396.

Marcus, A. H. (1979). The body burden of lead: comparison of mathematical models for accumulation. *Environ. Res. 19*:79-90.

Miller, C. E. (1964). Low intensity spectrometry of the gamma radiation emitted by human beings. *Conf. Peaceful Uses Atomic Energy* (Proc. Conf. Geneva, 1978), 23 U. N., New York, p. 113.

Molla, M. A. R. (1975). Radionuclides in the autopsy samples from thorotrast patients. *Health Phys. 28*:295-297.

National Academy of Sciences (1971). *Biological Effects of Atmospheric Pollutants, Fluorides*, Washington, D. C.

Newman, W. F., and Newman, M. W. (1958). *The Chemical Dynamics of Bone Mineral*. University of Chicago Press, Chicago, p. 209.

Newton, D. (1977). Clearance of radioactive tantalum from the human lung after accidental inhalation. *Am. J. Roentgenol.* *129*:327-328.

Park, Y. K., Harland, B. F., Vanderveen, J. E., Shank, F. R., and Prosky, L. (1981). Estimation of dietary iodine intake of Americans in recent years. *J. Amer. Dietet. Assoc.* 79:17-23.

Piper, W. N., Rose, J. Q., Leng, M. L., and Gehring, P. J. (1973). The fate of 2,4,5-trichlorophenoxyacetic acid following oral administration to rats and dogs. *Toxicol. Appl. Pharmacol.* *26*: 339-351.

Pohl, E., and Pohl-Ruling, J. (1977). Dose calculation due to the inhalation of Rn-222, Rn-220 and their daughters. *Health Phys.* *32*:552-555.

Radomski, J. L., Deichmann, W. B., Rey, A. A., and Merkin, T. (1971). Human pesticide blood levels as a measure of body burden and pesticide exposure. *Toxicol. Appl. Pharmacol.* *20*: 175-181.

Ramsey, J. D., Lavy, T. L., and Braun, W. H., (1979). Exposure of forestworker to 2,4,5-T calculated dose levels. Toxicology Laboratory, Dow Chemical Company, Midland, Mich.

Robinson, J., and Hunter, C. G. (1966). Organochlorine insecticide: concentration in human blood and adipose tissue. *Arch. Environ. Health* *13*:558-563.

Ross, J. F., Ebaugh, F. G., Talbot, T. R., Santodonato, J., Howard, P., and Basu, D. (1981). Health and ecological assessment of polynuclear aromatic hydrocarbons. *J. Environ. Pathol. Toxicol.* 5:164-166.

Santodonato, J., Howard, P., and Basu, D. (1981). Health and ecological assessment of polynuclear aromatic hydrocarbons. *J. Environ. Pathol. Toxicol.* 5:1-364.

Sauerhoff, M. W., Braun, W. H., Blau, G. E., and Gehring, P. J. (1976). The dose dependent pharmacokinetic profile of 2,4,5-trichlorophenoxyacetic acid following intravenous administration to rats. *Toxicol. Appl. Pharmacol.* *36*:491-501.

Spencer, H., Rosoff, B., Lewin, I., and Samachson, J. (1966). Studies of Zinc-65 Metabolism in Man. In *Zinc Metabolism*, A. S. Prasad, Ed., Charles C Thomas, Springfield, Ill., p. 339-362.

Spengler, F. (1957). Interferometrische Bestimmung des Residualluftvolumens der Lunge mit der Stick Stoff Serien Methode in Geschlossenen Kreislaufsystem. *Klin. Wchnschr.* *37*:612.

Sterling, T. D., Kehoe, R. A., and Rustage, J. S. (1964). Mathematical analysis of lead. *Arch. Environ. Health* *8*:44-51.

Toxicity of Selected Drinking Water Contaminants (1980). In *Drinking Water and Health*, Vol. 3. Safe Drinking Water Committee, NAS. National Academy Press, Washington, D. C.

Tsubaki, T. (1971). Clinical and epidemiological aspects of organic mercury intoxication. *Proc. Symp. Mercury Man's Environ.*, Ottawa, Royal Society of Canada, pp. 131-136.

Tulinius, H. (1982). Choice of methods for gathering nutrition information. *Nutrition Cancer* 2:200-202.

Vennart, J. (1967). Whole body counters in routine monitoring. *Health Phys.* 13:61-72.

Wolfe, H. R. (1973). Workers should be protected from pesticides exposure. *Weeds, Trees, Turf*.

Young, J. D., Ramsey, J. C., and Braun, W. H. (1977). Pharmacokinetics of 2,4,5-PGBE ester applied dermally to rats. Dow Chemical Company, Midland, Mich., manuscript in preparation.

2

Plasma Binding, Distribution, and Elimination

G. R. Wilkinson
Vanderbilt University School of Medicine, Nashville, Tennessee

I. INTRODUCTION

It is well recognized that many substances of both endogenous and exogenous origin are present in the bloodstream as complexes with certain plasma macromolecules. Such binding is generally reversible, and therefore it serves as a carrier mechanism for the functionally active unbound ligand. Additionally, the distribution and elimination of a compound may be limited by plasma binding, and thus the interaction often functions to maintain the presence of the ligand within the body. The extent of binding is dependent not only on the concentration of the ligand, but also the amount of macromolecule to which binding occurs and its affinity, and the presence of competitive binding substances. Nutritional status, together with disease states and other factors, may, therefore, affect plasma binding by changing any of the latter three determinants.

A number of excellent reviews have been published on various aspects of small-molecule binding interactions (1--4). Accordingly, this chapter will address only some of the recent findings in the general area of plasma binding and its effects on the body's handling of the ligand. Major focus will be placed on the binding of drugs in humans, but the factors and principles involved are relevant to other species and ligands of more direct nutritional interest, such as hormones, vitamins, pigments, and certain ions.

II. NATURE OF PLASMA BINDING SITES

The plasma is a complex solution of many different proteins with a wide
range of concentrations which often exhibit considerable interindividual
variability. Serum differs from plasma in not containing fibrinogen
and other clotting factors. The investigation of the in vivo binding
of drugs is usually limited to plasma, whereas in vitro studies directed
toward kinetic and mechanistic aspects of the interaction frequently
use proteins isolated from serum. It is generally assumed that plasma
and serum binding are equivalent, but few studies have actually compared the interaction in both fluids. Plasma proteins important in the
binding of drugs and nutrients include albumin, α_1-acid glycoprotein,
lipoproteins, and a variety of globulins which transport specific biologically important compounds such as hormones, vitamins, and ions.
In general, small molecule binding interactions occur as a result of
hydrophobic binding due initially to electrostatic attraction reinforced
by hydrogen bonds and van der Waals forces. The concerted effect of
these different types of bonds frequently yields stable yet reversible
complexes. Covalent binding plays no role in the reversible binding of
drugs, hormones, and nutrients within the plasma.

A. Albumin

Albumin is the most abundant protein in the plasma, constituting 58 ±
4% of the total proteins. The normal concentration in men is 42 ± 3.5
g/liter, whereas women have an approximately 9% lower level, 38 ± 4
g/liter. The concentration is reduced in infants, 35 ± 3 g/liter, but
albumin increases within 3-4 months after birth. Aging leads to a decrease in albumin such that in the elderly the concentration may be as
much as 10−20% lower than that in young adults. A variety of diseases
lead to a reduction in the albumin plasma concentration, which is usually accompanied by an increase in the globulin levels. This may result
from the effect of the disease on the synthesis of albumin in the liver,
as occurs in cirrhosis, viral hepatitis, and cholera, and/or an increase
in catabolism as in the nephrotic syndrome, the trauma of surgery, and
major accidents, such as burns. Impaired synthesis may also occur because of a reduction in the pool of amino acids available due to malnutrition. Hypoalbuminemia may be profound in the case of kwashiorkor,
but even more modest malnutrition due to prolonged illness may markedly reduce the albumin level.

The human liver synthesizes about 14−17 g of albumin daily, which is
used as a source of amino acids to form other more specialized proteins
in the extravascular tissues. The latter distribution is possible despite
albumin's large molecular size (MW 66,248). Only about 40% of the
body's pool of about 310 g is retained within the vasculature, and
about 5% per hour leaves and is recycled via the thoracic duct over 2−3

days. Although albumin is present in urine, sweat, and other excretions, such loss is normally negligible and the catabolic half-life, as determined by [^{131}I]albumin studies, is 17 ± 5 days. Human albumin consists of a single polypeptide chain of 584 amino acid residues coiled to form a globular molecule. Approximately half of the molecule is arranged as an α-helix, about 15% is in the β-pleated sheet form, and the remainder is wound up to form an ellipsoid. Bovine albumin, and that of the rat, have similar but slightly different primary structures. Often, pronounced species differences exist in the binding characteristics of a ligand to albumin (5).

As indicated previously, albumin serves as a source of amino acids and protein in cellular metabolism. A second physiological function is the maintenance of the colloid osmotic pressure of the plasma; a significant decrease in the albumin level usually leads to edema of the tissues. The other major role of the plasma albumin is as a transport protein, especially for free fatty acids. In fact, albumin is the main carrier of these substances in the plasma, and purification of the protein from fatty acids is difficult, so that many commercially available forms of crystalline albumin are contaminated to a varying extent. Additionally, albumin binds various anions, cations, steroids, bilirubin, and a wide spectrum of drugs, especially those with acidic and neutral characteristics.

Because of the wide spectrum of divergent chemical structures which exhibit binding to albumin, it has generally been considered that the process is nonspecific and mainly dependent on the compound's lipophilicity. However, it now appears that only a few high-affinity sites and a variable number of different low-affinity binding sites are specifically involved. Based on fluorescent probe studies, the existence of two distinct and independent binding sites with quite different specificities on human albumin were postulated (6,7). Subsequently, a variety of other techniques have confirmed and further characterized these and other sites. The binding of several coumarin anticoagulants and their enantiomers, such as warfarin and phenprocoumon, involves a high-affinity site and one or two low-affinity sites. The primary binding is identical to the originally postulated site I (6,7) and it is the same as the major binding site for bilirubin (8). It also appears to be a major important site of interaction for many drugs (e.g., sulfonamide and penicillin derivatives, and certain analgesics) (9). The lone tryptophan residue of human albumin located at position 213 in loop 4 of the protein's secondary structure is essentially involved in this high affinity warfarin binding site (10).

Distinct from the warfarin site and exhibiting a greater degree of specificity is the diazepam binding site [site II (6,7)]. A number of benzodiazepines interact at this site, as does L-tryptophan, certain antihypoglycemic agents, antibiotics, and analgesics (8,11,12). Less is known of the molecular structure and location of this site compared to the warfarin site. Only one of the 18 tyrosine residues appears to be specifically involved, and there is evidence that histidine-46, arginine-145, and possibly lysine-194 are also important (12). This would locate the binding site in loop 3 of the secondary structure. In addition to these well established sites, two further specific binding loci have been recently described. The first of these appears to be quite specific for digitoxin and acetyldigitoxin (8), whereas tamoxifen is the only known ligand, so far, of the fourth site (13).

The binding of free fatty acids involves two high-affinity sites and several with considerably lower affinities. However, neither of the former are directly involved in the binding of various drugs and small molecules. No other organic molecule appears to be able to bind to the first high-affinity site except fatty acids and comparable compounds (14). It has been suggested that such binding involves a hydrophobic cleft in the albumin tertiary structure into which the aliphatic chain of the fatty acid is inserted (15). Despite the fact that drugs and fatty acids have different binding sites on the albumin molecule, the interaction of small molecules may be modulated by the presence of fatty acids. For example, the unbound L-tryptophan plasma concentration is finely regulated by the circulating fatty acid level. As a result, brain concentrations of the amino acid and its major metabolite, serotonin, are dependent on the nutritional state of the individual (16). The mechanism of this type of displacement, at least at physiological concentrations, appears to be allosteric rather than direct competition (14), although the latter probably occurs at higher levels.

B. α_1-Acid Glycoprotein

While the plasma binding of many small molecules and acidic drugs may in most instances be almost exclusively accounted for by albumin, the situation with basic compounds is less clear. It appears, however, that the acute-phase protein α_1-acid glycoprotein (orosomucoid) plays a major role in the binding of such compounds. This protein is a globulin with several unique properties, including a large number of sialyl residues and a very high carbohydrate content, accounting for about 10% of the total protein-bound carbohydrate of the plasma. Its molecular weight is about 44,000, and the carbohydrate and polypeptide moieties account for about 45% and 55%, respectively. Turnover studies using the ^{131}I-labeled globulin indicate a half-life of 5.5 days, although shorter values (1–2 days) have also been noted. In healthy normals, the plasma concentration of α_1-acid glycoprotein is quite variable, at about 50–100 mg/ml. However, up to four- to fivefold elevated levels are known to be associated with short- and long-term inflammation and various unrelated disease states. These include myocardial infarction, Crohn's disease, ulcerative colitis, rheumatoid arthritis, malignancy, burns, infections, and surgery (17). In contrast, pregnancy and oral contraceptives reduce the plasma concentration of α_1-acid glycoprotein, which is also low in the fetus and newborn (17).

Evidence for a significant binding role of α_1-acid glycoprotein is based primarily on the correlation of the extent of binding of basic drugs to the globulin's plasma concentration, but not that of albumin, in those disease states where the former is elevated to a varying extent. More recently, direct binding studies with the isolated purified protein have been performed. In this fashion, the binding of quinidine, lidocaine, dipyrimadole, local anesthetics, tricyclic antidepressants, chloropromazine, and β-adrenergic blocking agents have been demonstrated to be extensive to α_1-acid glycoprotein (17).

C. Lipoproteins

The plasma lipoproteins constitute an extremely heterogeneous group of proteins that are complexes, often in variable proportions, of lipid, protein, and carbohydrate. Operationally, they are classified on the basis of their ultracentrifugal properties into chylomicrons, very low density lipoproteins (VLDL), low-density lipoproteins (LDL), high-density lipoproteins (HDL), and very high density lipoproteins (VHDL). The protein content of lipoproteins ranges from as low as 2% in the chylomicrons to a high of about 50% in the HDL; the lipid content changes reciprocally from 95% to 40%. The major roles of the lipoproteins in various aspects of the transport and synthesis of fatty acids, triglycerides, phospholipids, and cholestrol are well established. Because of these functions, plasma levels of the lipoproteins rapidly and markedly change in response to nutritional status. In addition, a number of pathophysiological states can lead to elevated, and also reduced, plasma concentrations of the various types of lipoproteins.

There is increasing evidence that the lipoproteins play a role in drug binding, especially of very lipophilic and/or basic moieties, and lipoprotein binding may be comparable to that to albumin. Among those drugs reported to exhibit such binding are quinidine, chlorpromazine, imipramine, reserpine, propranolol, tetracycline, and insecticides (17). Simple solubilization of the drug is a probable mechanism for these interactions, and correlations exist between the extent of binding and lipiproteinemia (17,18). On the other hand, saturable binding of chlorpromazine and quinidine has been reported (17).

D. Other Binding Sites

A variety of very specific proteins are responsible for the plasma binding and transport of certain hormones and other physiologically/biochemically important compounds. For example, thyroxine binding and prealbumin globulins, transcortin, transferrin, hemopexin, ceruloplasmin, and retinol binding protein. Certain muscle relaxants, such as D-tubocurarine and pancuronium, have been demonstrated to bind to α_1-globulins, and a similar situation applies to certain opiates (17). In addition, the membrane of red and white blood cells as well as platelets can bind drugs, especially bases. In general, however, such binding is of only minor relevance to the overall interaction (19).

III. MEASUREMENT OF PLASMA BINDING

A variety of techniques have been used to characterize the plasma binding of small molecules. These may be broadly classified into two groups: methods, often spectroscopic, directed toward a qualitative understanding of the molecular aspects of the interaction (20), and those based on the physical separation of the bound and unbound moieties in order to quantify the extent of binding (21). None of the latter approaches are ideal, and each technique has both advantages and disadvantages. In the few instances where the various methods have been systematically compared, different binding values have often been observed (21−23).

A. Equilibrium Dialysis

Equilibrium dialysis is the most widely used method for determining the extent of binding because of its apparent ease and simplicity. In this method the plasma sample and a buffer solution containing neither protein nor ligand are placed on either side of a semipermeable membrane, such as cellulose. Unbound drug in the plasma passes through the membrane until, at equilibrium, the concentration of drug in the buffer solution and that of unbound drug in the plasma are equal. Measurement of the drug level on both sides of the membrane provides estimates of the total (plasma) and unbound (buffer) ligand concentrations from which the degree of binding can be determined. In its simplest form, dialysis may be performed with a tied length of dialysis tubing containing the plasma suspended in buffer solution. Increasing use is, however, being made of specially designed microcells which provide greater reproducibility and efficiency, and also permit the use of smaller volumes of plasma (< 1ml).

A critical factor in equilibrium dialysis is the time required to reach equilibrium. This is so highly dependent on the dialysis system and the ligand of interest that it is essential that the time course to equilibrium be characterized prior to any other studies. While overnight equilibrium is generally necessary when using the dialysis bag approach, with microcells as short a period as 2 hr may be satisfactory. An additional temporal aspect relates to the stability of the dialysis system. First, it must be recognized that the composition of the plasma may alter during storage and dialysis, especially at temperatures above 4°C. Levels of free fatty acids produced by lipolysis of triglycerides increase on storage (24), and this is particularly so if heparin has been administered in vivo prior to collection of the blood sample (25). In addition, lipoproteins may denature during the dialysis procedure.

As a consequence, the unbound fraction may increase with time, and the extent of binding may decrease subsequent to attainment of an apparent equilibrium. This appears to be especially problematic for basic compounds (22). Changes in plasma pH also occur with time, mainly due to the loss of HCO_3^-, and while these may be relatively small and of little importance with regard to the degree of ionization of the ligand, more significant consequences may arise due to changes in the binding macromolecule. This occurs because the conformational state of human albumin is pH-dependent in the neutral region due to the neutral-to-base (N-B) transition. Binding at both the warfarin (26) and benzo-diazepine (27) sites of albumin has been shown to be dependent on these conformational states of the protein. In many dialysis systems, it is quite difficult to ensure the maintenance of a constant physiological pH during the attainment of equilibrium. A further consideration is the stability of the ligand under study and the specificity of the analytical procedure used to determine the compound. When degradation occurs during dialysis and a nonspecific assay, such as radioanalysis, is used, considerable error may occur in the assessment of binding if the product(s) has different binding characteristics than the parent ligand (28).

There is increasing evidence that the nature of the buffer solution against which the plasma is dialyzed may be of more importance than generally considered. Frequently, a phosphate buffer is employed with emphasis on pH control. As a consequence, water may move from the buffer solution into the plasma as a result of the osmotic gradient. It is difficult to correct for such dilution of the binding macromolecule (29–31). Use of this type of buffer also leads to dilution of the various ions originally present in the plasma. The N-B transition of human albumin is sensitive to the presence of both Ca^{2+} and Cl^-, to the extent that there is an almost twofold change in the binding of diazepam dependent on whether or not the buffer solution contains these ions (27). A similar phenomen occurs with warfarin binding (26) and also quinidine, with respect to chloride ion (32).

A major problem with dialysis is that the equilibrium of the binding interaction is altered as unbound drug moves across the membrane. As a result, the final total concentration at which binding is assessed is lower than that in the original plasma sample. The magnitude of the difference between the initial and final concentration is dependent on the extent of binding and the design of the dialysis system (i.e., the volume of the buffer solution). Consideration of this situation is especially relevant when the experiment is performed in the concentration-sensitive portion of the binding isotherm. Direct measurement of the equilibrium concentration of total ligand in all forms (bound and unbound, labeled and unlabeled) in the plasma obviates interpretive complications of this nature (33). The same approach also overcomes the problems associated with adsorption of the ligand to the membrane and other parts of the dialyzing system. In many instances, the

amount of drug lost by these processes can be sufficiently significant
that an estimate of binding based on the initial plasma concentration
rather than the final equilibrium value can be grossly erroneous (21).
Finally, it must be recognized that if the ligand is ionized, and especially when either the unbound factor is large or the ionic strength of
the buffer solution is low, the Donnan effect must be taken into account since the unbound drug concentration will then overestimate that
in the plasma (34).

B. Ultrafiltration

Ultrafiltration through a semipermeable membrane has been successfully used to a considerable degree to determine the extent of plasma
binding. The major reasons for this appear to be its simplicity and
that it can be performed rapidly without storage or addition of potentially interactive buffer component and electrolytes. A significant
problem of this approach is adsorption of ligand onto the membrane.
This results in the unbound drug concentration in the ultrafiltrate
being artifactually low initially relative to that in the plasma. As filtration proceeds, the two concentrations become equal, and it is often
necessary to discard the first portion of the ultrafiltrate. In addition,
if adsorption is large, it may significantly reduce the plasma concentration of the total ligand. As the volume of ultrafiltrate increases, the
concentration of protein increases together with that of total and unbound ligand. To prevent the interpretive difficulties that such
changes cause, it is generally considered advisable to limit the volume
of the ultrafiltrate to no more than 15–20% of the plasma volume (21).
Leakage of protein through the membrane is also fairly common, even
within a single batch of membrane. This appears to be particularly
troublesome with a number of commercially available preformed membrane systems. Testing for the presence of protein in the solution
used to determine the unbound ligand concentration is, therefore, considerably more necessary on a routine basis than with other techniques. Again, the study of highly ionized ligands requires consideration of the Donnan effect.

C. Ultracentrifugation

From many aspects, ultracentrifugation is the most ideal method for
determining plasma binding. The separation of the small unbound moiety from the high-molecular-weight ligand-macromolecule complex by
high-speed centrifugation does not disturb the binding equilibrium and
the concentrations of ligand, protein, and other plasma constituents
are unaltered. Problems may, however, arise if adsorption occurs to
the tube and if the binding involves lipoproteins, since they will be
floated to the top of the tube. It is also possible for a concentration

gradient of unbound drug to develop due to sedimentation, even for ligands with low molecular weight (21). The availability of suitable equipment, the long period of centrifuging, and the large volume of plasma required has, however, limited application of this approach. The development of a simple, small bench ultracentrifuge with low-volume capacity (< 0.5 ml) and easy sampling (Airfuge, Beckman) may overcome these disadvantages.

Discrepancies in the extent of binding determined by two or more separate techniques are not uncommon (21–23). Occasionally, there may be a rational explanation, but in many instances this is not possible. Moreover, since there is no way to standardize any methodology, it is difficult to determine which is the more correct value with regard to the in vivo situation. In certain situations in vivo and in vitro binding may be correlated, and such relationships can be useful in assessing the validity of the technique used in the latter. For example, the translocation of drug into the cerebrospinal fluid (CSF) is generally considered to be limited to the unbound moiety and, therefore, in vivo binding may be determined by measuring the drug concentrations in CSF and the plasma. Such an approach indicated that ultrafiltration provided a more valid estimate of binding than dialysis for desmethylchlorimipramine (22). A similar conclusion was drawn using an analogous approach based on the transport of unbound phenytoin across the erythrocyte membrane (23). Passage of drugs into the saliva has also been used for this purpose, but with more limited success since factors other than binding affect the saliva/plasma concentration ratio (35).

IV. INTERPRETATION OF BINDING DATA

Ligand-macromolecule interactions in the plasma are generally considered to follow the law of mass action for a reversible process.

$$P + D_f \underset{k_2}{\overset{k_1}{\rightleftharpoons}} PD \tag{1}$$

where D_f, P, and PD are the concentrations of unbound ligand (drug) protein, and ligand (drug)-protein complex, respectively. Also, k_1 and k_2 are the first-order rate constants of the forward and reverse reactions, which generally have half-lives in the order of a few milliseconds. The ratio k_1/k_2 is termed the equilibrium association constant (K_a), and the larger this value, the greater the affinity of the ligand for the macromolecule. Frequently, the inverse of this ratio, the dissociation constant (K_d), is also used to characterize the interaction. In many instances, several identical and independent binding sites (n) are present on the macromolecule (i.e., K_a is the same and cooperativity is absent), in which case the fraction of the ligand that is bound (D_b/D_{tot}) is given by

$$\frac{D_b}{D_{tot}} = \frac{1}{1 + K_d/nP_t + D_f/nP_t} \qquad (2)$$

This indicates that the extent of binding, and therefore the concentration of unbound ligand, are dependent on the unbound (D_f) and total (D_{tot}) ligand concentrations, the number of binding sites (n), the total concentration of the binding macromolecule (P_t), and the dissociation constant (K_d). In many clinical situations simple knowledge of the extent of binding, and the unbound concentration, is an adequate description of the interaction. However, in most other cases, it is necessary to characterize the process more precisely in terms of the dissociation constant and the number of binding sites on either an absolute or molar basis. Because of the nonlinearity of the binding isotherm [equation (2)] most analyses in the past have been based on linearization techniques analogous to those used in interpreting Michaelis-Menten enzyme kinetics. By far the most commonly used approach is the Scatchard analysis, in which the bound/unbound concentration ratio (D_b/D_f) is plotted against the concentration of bound ligand.

$$\frac{D_b}{D_f} = K_a(nP_t - D_b) \qquad (3)$$

Accordingly, for a single class of binding sites, a straight line is obtained with an intercept on the abscissa of $K_a nP_t$ and a slope of $- K_a$. If the concentration of binding macromolecule (P_t) is known, the number of sites may be estimated; otherwise, only the total binding capacity (nP_t) can be characterized. Unfortunately, this approach is deceptively simple and may provide estimates that are considerably in error (36). Both the ratio D_b/D_f and the bound concentration determinations are subject to error and, therefore, neither one is truly an independent variable. Moreover, the errors in these two terms are highly correlated; an erroneously high value for D_b/D_f will be associated with and overestimate of D_b, and vice versa. Accordingly, the variance is nonuniform and unweighted linear regression is, from the statistical standpoint, invalid and yields erroneous estimates.

More significantly, the Scatchard plot frequently exhibits nonlinearity. This may be due to a number of factors, but it is probably indicative of heterogeneous binding (i.e., the presence of two or more classes of binding sites with different affinity and capacity characteristics), in which case binding is complex and follows the general relationship

$$D_b = \sum_{i=1}^{i=N} \frac{n_i P_t D_f}{K_{d_i} + D_f} \tag{4}$$

where the integer (i) indicates the number of different binding sites. Generally, experimental error and the limited amount of data makes it very difficult to characterize more than two classes of sites. In many cases, slight nonlinearity of the Scatchard plot is ignored and all the data are fitted to a single straight line! Alternatively, only the points in the high-affinity region are fitted. In either case, incorrect estimates of the binding parameters are obtained. Theoretically, the graphical curve-peeling method developed by Rosenthal provides an appropriate means of separating the different binding sites (37), and it has been used extensively for the analysis of steroid binding. However, in practice it is a tedious approach and provides only approximate estimates which are highly subjective. Many of these problems may be overcome by weighted least-squares curve fitting of the data to a defined model of binding. The availability of suitable programs (36) and computing facilities (often a desk-top calculator/computer is satisfactory) makes the latter approach the only acceptable one for precise characterization of ligand binding interactions.

V. FACTORS AFFECTING PLASMA BINDING

Equation (2) indicates a complex relationship between binding and the three variables determining the binding process; the total drug concentration, the binding capacity, and the dissociation constant. At any given total drug and binding macromolecule concentrations, the unbound fraction rises with decreasing affinity (i.e., increasing dissociation constant) (Figure 1). The large differences in the extent of binding between drugs and other ligands are primarily a reflection of the differences in binding affinity. This may also contribute in part to the variation in the degree of binding that occurs within any given population. In general, such intersubject variability and, also, binding perturbations are of importance only when the extent of binding is high, about 90% or greater. In this situation a small change in binding causes a relatively large alteration in the unbound fraction. For example, an approximately 5% reduction in binding from 95% to 90% causes a 100% increase in the unbound fraction (from 5% to 10%). Binding may be altered if the total ligand or binding macromolecule(s) concentrations are perturbed or other substances are present which can either affect binding by an allosteric effect or act as competitive displacers.

At low levels of total ligand a proportion is unbound, but with increasing concentration this increases in a sigmoid fashion (Figure 1). The precise shape of the binding isotherm depends on the affinity of the

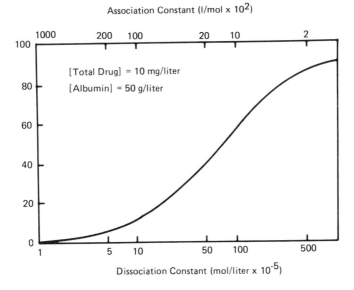

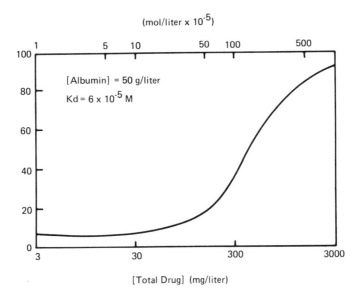

Figure 1 Effect on ligand binding to albumin of changes in dissociation constant (top panel) and total drug concentration (bottom panel). (Modified and reproduced and permission from *N. Engl. J. Med. 294*: 311-316,1976.)

interaction and the range of the concentration changes. The dissociation constant is equal to the unbound concentration at which 50% of the binding site is saturated. Hence at low levels relative to the dissociation constant the change in binding is modest but then as the binding sites become increasingly occupied a sharp increase in the unbound fraction occurs. No matter how high the affinity, the maximal possible binding capacity equals the molar concentration of the involved macromolecule(s) times the number of binding sites for the ligand. The concentration of albumin in healthy subjects is about 0.75×10^{-3} M. For a ligand with a molecular weight of about 300 this means that plasma concentrations of about 200 μg/ml or greater are required before saturation of binding is apparent. Moreover, significant concentration dependent binding is present at these levels only if the dissociation constant is less than about $10^{-4}–10^{-5}$ mol/liter. In general, such situations occur only with compounds that are administered or accumulate in large amounts and/or they are not widely distributed outside the vascular system (e.g., salicylate, sulfonamides). From a theoretical standpoint, saturation is more likely for ligands bound to α_1-acid glycoprotein since its plasma concentration is only about 1 to 3 $\times 10^{-5}$ M. However, in practice this does not appear to occur too frequently because the ligands that bind to this protein are administered in small doses and/or they have large volumes of distribution. In certain instances, a ligand may bind with different affinities to several types of plasma proteins. The relative contribution of each of these macromolecules to the overall binding may change as the ligand concentration increases. For example, thyroxine and certain corticosteroids are usually transported in the plasma bound with high affinity to specific globulins. However, the capacity of such sites is limited; hence when the ligands are present in high concentrations, the binding shifts to secondary low-affinity sites on albumin.

As indicated earlier, the plasma concentration of the binding molecule may show considerable intra- and intersubject variability. In the case of albumin, disease states such as cirrhosis (38), the nephrotic syndrome (39), malnutrition (40), and kwashiorkor (41) may lead to profound hypoalbuminemia and decreased binding. In contrast, inflammatory diseases and stress lead to elevated levels of α_1-acid glycoprotein, and ligands that are bound to this macromolecule exhibit a decrease in the unbound fraction in these situations (17). The fluctuations in lipoprotein composition and concentration would also be expected to affect the interaction of ligands bound to these macromolecules. However, this has not been extensively documented; in fact, the available information suggests that binding is hardly affected except when pronounced abnormalities are present (18,42). In the situation where more than one plasma lipoprotein is involved in the overall binding, changes in the relative amounts of any of these may also lead to redistribution of the ligand between the various binding sites (42).

It is generally assumed that the binding characteristics of the ligand-protein interaction are independent of the protein concentration, in which case, and provided that the unbound concentration is much less than the dissociation constant, it is theoretically possible to estimate the binding constant by using a fixed ligand concentration and varying that of the protein, rather than the more conventional reverse approach (30,43). However, in practice this technique has several statistical and interpretive shortcomings (30). More important is the possibility that binding results obained by varying the protein concentration may not be the same as those obtained by changing the ligand concentration. In several instances the binding constants are inversely dependent on the protein concentration (29,31). As a result, extrapolation of the parameters obtained in dilute protein solutions to the more physiological level may yield inappropriately high estimates of binding compared to that directly measured (29). The mechanism(s) involved in this phenomenon is not well understood. Impurities associated with both the ligand and the protein (albumin) preparation, together with some form of cooperative process or protein-protein interaction, have been suggested (31).

When a major fraction of the binding sites are occupied, this may reduce the binding of other concomitantly present ligands by direct displacement or allosteric mechanisms. Such competition may occur in vivo either because of endogenous displacers or by concurrent administration of another ligand (drug). The extent of the interaction depends on the relative binding affinities and concentrations of the competing ligands, and the kinetics and interpretation of the competition may be quite complex (44). Uremia frequently causes an impairment in the plasma binding of many drugs of an acidic nature which are bound to albumin (45). Treatment of the plasma with activated charcoal or dialysis, either in vitro or in vivo, frequently restores the binding toward a more normal value (46,47). It has therefore been concluded that renal failure leads to an accumulation of unidentified endogenous substances which act as competitive inhibitors of binding (46–48). Uremia may also increase the number of binding sites as well as altering the affinity, presumably as a result of displacement of ligand from primary to secondary sites (47). The separate binding sites on the albumin molecule appear to be differentially affected by the endogenous displacers (47, 48). This differential effect is even more accentuated in plasma from patients with liver cirrhosis; the diazepam binding site being more profoundly affected than the warfarin site (49). Such a competitive interaction further reduces the extent of binding caused by the frequently concomitant presence of hypoalbuminemia. It is also likely that endogenous displacers, including bilirubin, are responsible for the impaired plasma binding of many drugs in patients with acute viral hepatitis (38).

Endogenous binding inhibitors appear to be normally present in the plasma of healthy individuals, since binding to purified human albumin is often different from that in plasma (47,49). Intra- and interindividual variability in the binding of ligands may therefore be related to alterations in the plasma levels of such displacers. In this respect, the role of circulating nonesterified free fatty acids may be important; particularly fluctuations associated with prandial and nutritional status. For example, oleic acid decreases the in vitro binding of diazepam at all molar ratios of fatty acids: albumin (50). A similar effect is produced by high concentrations of palmitic acid, but when the molar ratio is less than unity, enhanced binding is present (50). In vivo, the net effect of displacement may therefore depend not only on the quantitative changes in the total level, but also in the ratio of the specific fatty acids to each other. Interestingly, the plasma concentration of diazepam exhibits pronounced diurnal fluctuations which are associated with changes in the unbound fraction secondary to food intake (51). Since free fatty acids are decreased following a meal, it is tempting to speculate that the observed plasma level fluctuations of diazepam, and possibly other drugs, is modulated by a competitive binding phenomenon (52).

Competitive binding inhibitors may also be important in certain artifacts of binding associated with the manner in which the blood sample is collected and handled. Small volumes of heparin solution are frequently injected to facilitate the collection of blood samples, and in clinical situations such as hemodialysis and cardiopulmonary bypass the patient is extensively heparinized. It is well established that the administration of heparin to both humans and animals causes a release of both lipoprotein lipase from the capillary endothelium and hepatic lipase into the blood. This leads to an increase in the circulating concentration of nonesterified fatty acids by hydrolysis of triglycerides. As little as 100 units of intravenous heparin has been reported to double the total free fatty acid plasma level within 5–10 min, and the dose-related effect is greater after a meal than in the fasting state (53). Several studies have demonstrated a significant relationship between these heparin-induced fatty acid changes and decreases in the in vitro binding of several drugs (53–56). With some ligands such as warfarin, heparin administration increases plasma binding (57). However, it is likely that such binding perturbations are, to a large extent, artifactual and related to the continued in vitro formation of free fatty acids by the in vivo liberated lipases subsequent to withdrawal of the blood sample. Thus when in vivo heparinized plasma is rapidly incubated at 0°C to reduce the lipase activity, or the enzymes are inactivated with an inhibitor, the increase in free fatty acids at subsequent times after collection is minimal (23). The lack of effect of heparin administration on the in vivo binding of phenytoin as assessed by the cerebrospinal fluid/serum concentration ratio (58) supports this hypothesis. Additionally, the presence in vitro of heparin per se, and possibly other anticoagulants, may affect ligand binding; the serum binding of warfarin, salicyclic acid, and phenytoin in the rat being smaller than that in plasma, while the reverse was found for bilirubin (59). These effects may, however, be species dependent since they are not present in humans (60).

Artifacts in the binding of basic drugs to α_1-acid glycoprotein can also occur as a consequence of the collection system used to obtain the blood sample. In particular, the tube into which the blood is placed after withdrawal is critical for these types of ligands. Many studies have documented that the stoppers of certain commercial collection tubes, Vacutainer in particular, contain a binding inhibitor(s) which may leak out when in contact with the blood (17). Not only is the extent of binding reduced, but also the drug redistributes in the formed elements of the blood, leading to a decrease in the plasma concentration. It is suspected that the plasticizer, trisbutoxyethylphosphate ester, is responsible in large part for this phenomenon (61). A similar binding displacement interaction may also occur if the blood sample is obtained through certain types of cannulae (62).

VI. EFFECTS OF PLASMA BINDING ON IN VIVO DRUG DISPOSITION

Intra- and interindividual differences in plasma binding are primarily studied in vitro, and they are frequently readily demonstrable. However, the significance of such differences on the manner in which the ligand is handled by the body, and in many instances the elicited pharmacological effects, vary considerably according to the pharmacokinetic characteristics of the ligand, in particular, the distribution of the ligand outside the vascular system and the determinants of the processes of eliminating the ligand from the body. Considerable binding differences may be demonstrated in vitro, but these may have little in vivo significance.

Drug distribution subsequent to tissue equilibration is usually assessed by the volume of distribution (Vd), which relates at any given time the amount of drug in the body to the plasma concentration. While this volume is a measure of the extent of extravascular distribution and determined by several physiological factors, it rarely corresponds to a real volume. Distribution is usually to a combination of tissues and fluids of the body, which vary from drug to drug. Moreover, binding to tissue components may be so great that the pharmacokinetic volume is very much larger than actual body size. Because only unbound ligand can penetrate biological membranes, the extent of distribution at equilibrium is dependent on binding in both the plasma and tissues. The simplest quantitative expression of the involved relationship is shown in equation (5):

$$Vd = V_P + V_T \frac{f_P}{f_T} \qquad (5)$$

where V_P is the plasma volume, V_T the volume of other body tissue water, and f_P and f_T the fractions of unbound drug in the plasma and tissue, respectively (63,64). It is therefore apparent that as long as tissue binding remains unchanged, the volume of distribution of a drug will increase as the unbound fraction in the plasma increases (Figure 2). Moreover, the change is almost directly proportional to the alteration in the free fraction except for extensively bound drugs distributed in a small volume (i.e., a large f_T). Drug distribution may also be expressed in terms of the unbound drug (Vd/f_P). While this term is essentially independent of the degree of binding for drugs which have

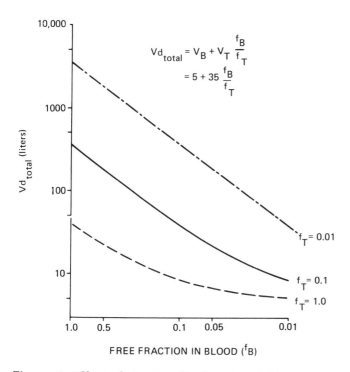

Figure 2 Effect of altering the fraction of binding in the blood on the volume of distribution of total drug. The three curves represent different degrees of tissue binding ($1 - f_T$). (From Ref. 64.)

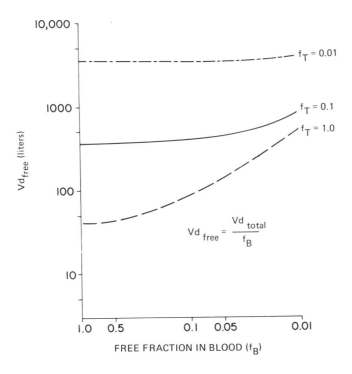

Figure 3 Effect of altering the fraction of binding in the blood on the volume of distribution of unbound (free) drug. The three curves represent different degrees of tissue binding $(1 - f_T)$ and correspond to those in Figure 2).

large volumes of distribution (i.e., small f_T), an increase in the unbound fraction in the plasma leads to a reduction in the value for drugs that are less extensively distributed (figure 3). This is especially so when the plasma binding is high. A large number of studies with a variety of drugs have confirmed the general validity of such predictions. Equation (5) is clearly an oversimplification since it does not take into account that plasma proteins may be distributed throughout the extracellular fluids. However, this consideration may be incorporated into the relationship (65) and such an approach probably provides a more physiologically appropriate way of examining the effects of altered plasma binding on distribution, especially if binding is extensive and the volume of distribution is small. Drug distribution may also be altered by a change in the unbound fraction in the tissues. It is possible that the causative factor of altered plasma binding may also affect tissue binding, in which case the resulting change in distribution is a balance of the two effects, including the possibility of offsetting alterations leading to no change in Vd. The problems of quantitatively determining tissue binding have limited investigation of this possibility, but certain binding interactions can be explained only if displacement occurs both in the plasma and the extravascular tissues (66,67).

In considering the effects of plasma binding on elimination processes such as metabolic and renal clearance, it is also necessary to recognize the other involved physiological determinants. For any organ these are the rate of drug delivery as controlled by the organ's blood flow (Q), the ability of the elimination process to irreversibly remove the drug from tissue water, termed free intrinsic clearance (Cl^u_{int}), and the fraction of drug unbound in the blood (f_B). The latter is related to the more conventionally determined unbound fraction in the plasma (f_p) by the blood/plasma concentration ratio, which may itself be dependent on plasma binding [$f_B = f_p/(1 - H + HK_pf_p)$], where H is the hematocrit and K_p is partition ratio of drug concentration in the formed elements of the blood to the unbound level in the plasma. The quantitative interrelationship of the three determinants is given by equation (6) (64, 68,69), where the term in parentheses is equivalent to the organ's extraction ratio (E).

$$Cl = QE = Q\left(\frac{f_B Cl^u_{int}}{Q + f_B Cl^u_{int}}\right) \qquad (6)$$

Accordingly, the effect of an alteration in drug binding on extraction and clearance depends on the relative magnitude of the free intrinsic clearance to the organ blood flow. When Cl^u_{int}/Q is small, binding is the limiting factor in clearance, and the two parameters are almost linearly related (Figure 4). Such "restrictive" elimination is well established for excretion via glomerular filtration and also for poorly extracted compounds metabolized by the liver [e.g., warfarin (70,71) and tolbutamide (72)]. In fact, in the latter case, acute viral hepatitis has a greater effect on plasma binding relative to the liver's ability to metabolize the drug (free intrinsic clearance) that the rate of elimination is faster in such patients than in normal healthy individuals. In contrast, when an organ is very efficient at elimination (i.e., $Q \ll Cl^u_{int}$), clearance is predominantly controlled by and dependent on organ blood flow, and elimination is less sensitive to alterations in binding (Figure 4). The relative independence from the degree of plasma binding of renal clearance by active secretion in the proximal tubule is typical of this situation, as is the hepatic clearance of drugs such as propranolol, where the free intrinsic clearance process is so efficient that it strips drugs from the vascular binding sites during passage through the liver (73,74).

In extending the consequences of drug binding to its effect on the frequently determined parameter of elimination, the half-life, it must

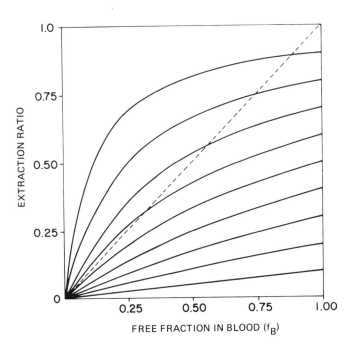

Figure 4 Effect of altering the unbound fraction of drug in the blood
(f_B) on an eliminating organ's extraction ratio. The individual curves
represent different values of Cl^u_{int}/Q corresponding to 10% stepwise
changes in extraction when $f_B = 1$; the dashed line indicates when $E = f_B$. (From Ref. 64.)

be recognized that this term is inversely related to clearance but directly proportional to the volume of distribution. Since both of the
latter change to varying extents with plasma binding, the net effect
is complex. It depends not only on the unbound fraction, but also the
free intrinsic clearance and the extent of tissue binding (64). When
the elimination process in "restrictive" (i.e., low Cl^u_{int} and f_p), an increase in the unbound fraction in the plasma increases both clearance
and the volume of distribution. The net effect is usually either no
change or a shortening of the elimination half-life (70—72). At the
other extreme, when the free intrinsic clearance is high relative to
eliminating organ blood flow, an increase in f_p has essentially no effect
on clearance but distribution is still affected. Accordingly, the half-
life is prolonged (73).
    A further way of considering the effects of plasma binding on drug
elimination is by examining the consequences on the total area under
the blood concentration/time curve (AUC). The AUC may be estimated

Table 1 Relationship Between AUC for Total and Free Drug and the Physiological Determinants of Hepatic Clearance and Route of Administration

Route of administration	AUC_{total}	AUC_{free}
Intravenous General	$\dfrac{D(Q + f_B Cl^u_{int})}{Q f_B Cl^u_{int}}$	$\dfrac{D(Q + f_B Cl^u_{int})}{Q Cl^u_{int}}$
$Q \ll Cl^u_{int}$	$\dfrac{D}{Q}$	$\dfrac{Df_B}{Q}$
$Q \gg Cl^u_{int}$	$\dfrac{D}{f_B Cl^u_{int}}$	$\dfrac{D}{Cl^u_{int}}$
Oral, all cases	$\dfrac{D}{f_B Cl^u_{int}}$	$\dfrac{D}{Cl^u_{int}}$

following acute drug administration or chronic dosing, since in the latter case the AUC is related proportionally to the average steady-state blood level by the dosage interval. Hence the effects of binding differences following acute and steady-state dosing can both be considered. Even if the drug is only metabolized by the liver following complete absorption of the administered dose (D), the situation is fairly complex (Table 1). After intravenous administration there are two extremes of behavior. If $Q \ll Cl^u_{int}$ and therefore extraction is high, the total drug level is relatively independent of the degree of binding in the blood, and unbound drug concentrations are simply related by f_B. On the other hand, if $Q \gg Cl^u_{int}$ and hepatic extraction is low, the total drug level is inversely proportional to the free fraction, whereas binding has little effect on free concentrations. It is important that after oral administration, regardless of the value of Cl^u_{int}, total drug levels depend on binding but free concentrations are controlled only by the free intrinsic clearance, although changes in the shape of the curve may be present due to alterations in systemic clearance.

Although the considerations above have proven extremely useful in pharmacokinetic prediction and data interpretation when plasma binding has been perturbed by a variety of mechanisms, they are dependent on the limitation that binding is independent of drug concentration over the range of interest. The effects of nonlinear binding in both the

plasma and tissues are beginning to be explored, especially as they relate to the time course of drug elimination. As would be expected, the
situation is extremely complex and dependent on the particular distribution and clearance characteristics of the drug; the log-concentration/
time course of both unbound and total drug having either linear, con-
vex, or concave profiles (75,76).

A somewhat special case of plasma binding and its effects on disposition and pharmacokinetics is when a displacing agent is introduced
into the body. Two aspects require consideration: the immediate and
the long-term consequences of displacement, which are dependent on
the rate of administration/accumulation of the displacer. The simplest
situation occurs when the displacing drug is administered in a fashion
that produces an immediate steady state, and plasma levels then remain
constant. The sudden addition of a second ligand at a concentration
producing displacement leads to a sudden elevation in the unbound
fraction of the drug, which in turn increases the plasma level of the
free drug and decreases that of the total drug (77–79). The change
in concentration is dependent not only on the magnitude of the binding
perturbation but also on the distribution characteristics of the drug,
since immediately upon the binding being disturbed, redistribution occurs. This has the effect of rapidly buffering the displacement interaction. As a result, the increase in the unbound drug level in the
plasma appears to last for only a few minutes after rapid administration
of the displacer (78,79). Furthermore, the magnitude of the increase
is generally only significant, especially in terms of any enhanced pharmacological response of the displaced drug, if the volume of distribution
of the unbound drug is small and the original level of binding is extensive (80,81).

Provided that the plasma level of the displacer then remains constant,
the subsequent changes in the unbound and total drug concentrations
are dependent on the clearance characteristics of the drug. If clearance is "restrictive" and dependent on the plasma binding (i.e.,
$Cl_{int}^u \ll Q$ and therefore Cp_{ss} = drug delivery rate/$fpCl_{int}^u$), the total
steady-state drug levels (Cp_{ss}) fall until a new steady state is
achieved at some time between three to five times the new elimination
half-life. However, the unbound plasma concentration will be the same
level as before the displacement occurred (81). Consequently, if the
biological effects of the drug are related to the unbound concentration,
displacement produces only a transient increase in this value. In contrast, , when the free intrinsic clearance of the drug is high, drug
elimination and the steady-state plasma level are essential independent
of plasma binding. Accordingly, the reverse situation occurs so that
displacement ultimately leads to no change in the concentration of total
drug but to an increase in the unbound level (81,82). In such cases the
drug's effects will be enhanced as long as the displacer is present.
Discontinuing administration slowly returns both of the drug's concentration levels back to their original values irrespective of the elimination

characteristics. The foregoing considerations are somewhat removed from many practical in vivo situations where the displacer may not be administered as a rapid and effective loading dose followed by maintenance of steady-state conditions. When a slower introduction into the body occurs which produces accumulation to a displacing concentration, the sharp increase in the unbound plasma level probably does not occur, although this has not been extensively investigated.

VII. PERSPECTIVES

The binding of small molecules, including drugs, hormones, endogenous substrates, and nutrients, to plasma constituents has been recognized for many years (1). Similarly, the consequences of such interactions have been well appreciated, but only in general terms. Progress over the past few years has, however, significantly enhanced the predictability of the interactions in both the qualitative and quantitative areas. The role of important proteins other than albumin in binding has become better defined, and factors affecting the interaction, such as disease states, have been elucidated. It is now possible to predict with reasonable accuracy the effects of altered plasma binding on the ligand's handling by the various disposition processes of the body.

The role of plasma binding has not been extensively investigated as a factor in the effects of nutrition on drug and hormone disposition and activity. Yet a number of types, and also stages, of malnutrition have well-known effects on the composition and concentration of the plasma proteins. Studies with a variety of drugs in several disease states, such as liver and renal disease, have clearly demonstrated the essential need to define the dispositional fate of both the unbound and total drug within the body. Without such considerations the experimental findings are often uninterpretable, and may lead to incorrect conclusions. This experimental approach would appear equally applicable to studies involving nutritional interactions, and it is to be hoped that future investigations in this particular area will be more cognizant of the potential effects of perturbed plasma binding.

REFERENCES

1. Goldstein, A. (1949). The interaction of drugs and plasma proteins. *Pharmacol. Rev.* 1:102-165.
2. Meyer, M. C., and Guttman, D. E. (1968). The binding of drugs by plasma proteins. *J. Pharm. Sci.* 57:895-918.
3. Jusko, W. J., and Gretch, M. (1976). Plasma and tissue protein binding of drugs in pharmacokinetics. *Drug Metab. Rev.* 5:43-140.

4. Vallner, J. J. (1977). Binding of drugs by albumin and plasma proteins. *J. Pharm. Sci.* *66*:447-465.
5. Sellers, E. M., Lang-Sellers, M. L., and Koch-Weser, J. (1977). Comparative warfarin binding to albumin from various species. *Biochem. Pharmacol.* *26*:2445-2447.
6. Sudlow, G., Birkett, D. J., and Wade, D. N. (1975). The characterization of two specific drug binding sites on human serum albumin. *Mol. Pharmacol.* *11*:824-832.
7. Sudlow, G., Birkett, D. J., and Wade, D. N. (1976). Further characterization of specific drug binding sites on human serum albumin. *Mol. Pharmacol.* *12*:1052-1061.
8. Sjöholm, I., Ekman, B., Kober, A., Ljungstedt-Påhlman, I., Seiving, B., and Sjödin, T. (1979). Binding of drugs to human serum albumin. XI. The specificity of three binding sites as studied with albumin immobilized in microparticles. *Mol. Pharmacol.* *16*:767-777.
9. Müller, W. E., and Wollert, U. (1979). Human serum albumin as a "silent receptor" for drugs and endogenous substances. *Pharmacology* *19*:59-67.
10. Fehske, K. J., Müller, W. E., and Wollert, U. (1979). The lone tryptophan residue of human serum albumin as part of the specific warfarin binding site: binding of dicoumarol to the warfarin, indole and benzodiazepine binding sites. *Mol. Pharmacol.* *16*:778-789.
11. Brodersen, R., Sjödin, T., and Sjöholm, I. (1977). Independent binding of ligands to human serum albumin. *J. Biol. Chem.* *252*:5067-5072.
12. Fehske, K. J., Müller, W. E., and Wollert, U. (1979). A highly reactive tyrosine residue as part of the indole and benzodiazepine binding site of human serum albumin. *Biochim. Biophys. Acta* *577*:346-359.
13. Sjöholm, I. (1980). The specificity of the drug binding sites of human serum albumin. *Acta Pharm. Suec.* *17*:76-77.
14. Spector, A. A., Santos, E. C., Ashbrook, J. D., and Fletcher, J. E. (1973). Influence of free fatty acid concentration on drug binding to plasma albumin. *Ann. N. Y. Acad. Sci.* *226*:247-258.
15. Spector, A. A. (1975). Fatty acid binding to plasma albumin. *J. Lipid. Res.* *16*:165-179.
16. Wurtman, R. J., and Fernstrom, J. D. (1976). Control of brain neurotransmitter systems by precursor availability and nutritional state. *Biochem. Pharmacol.* *25*:1691-1696.
17. Piafsky, K. M. (1980). Disease-induced changes in the plasma binding of basic drugs. *Clin. Pharmacokinet.* *5*:246-262.
18. Danon, A., and Chen, Z. (1979). Binding of imipramine to plasma proteins: effects of hyperlipoproteinemia. *Clin. Pharmacol. Ther.* *25*:316-321.

19. Bickel, M. H., (1975). Binding of chlorpromazine and imipramine to red cells, albumin, lipoproteins and other blood components. *J. Pharm. Pharmacol.* 27:733-738.

20. Chignell, C. F. (1971). Physical methods for studying drug-protein binding. In *Handbook of Experimental Pharmacology, Vol. 28/1, Concepts in Biochemical Pharmacology*, Part 1, B. B. Brodie, and J. R. Gillette, Eds., Springer-Verlag, New York, pp. 175-212.

21. Kurz, H., Trunk, H., and Weitz, B. (1977). Evaluation of methods to determine protein-binding of drugs. *Arzneim. Forsch.* 27:1373-1380.

22. Bertilsson, L., Braithwaite, R., Tybring, G., Garle, M., and Borgå, O. (1979). Techniques for plasma protein binding of demethylchlorimipramine. *Clin. Pharmacol. Ther.* 26:265-271.

23. Kurata, D., and Wilkinson, G. R. (1974). Erythrocyte uptake and plasma binding of diphenylhydantoin. *Clin. Pharmacol. Ther.* 16:355-362.

24. Sampson, D., and Hensley, W. J. (1975). A rapid gas chromatographic method for the quantitation of underivatized individual free fatty acids in plasma. *Clin. Chim. Acta* 61:1-8.

25. Giacomini, K. M., Swezey, S. E., Giacomini, J. C., and Blaschke, T. F. (1980). Administration of heparin causes in vitro release of non-esterified fatty acids in human plasma. *Life Sci.* 27:771-780.

26. Wilting, J., van der Giesen, W. F., Janssen, L. H. M., Weideman, M. M., and Otagiri, M. (1980). The effect of albumin conformation on the binding of warfarin to human serum albumin. *J. Biol. Chem.* 255:3032-3037.

27. Wilting, J., Hart, B. J. T., and deGier, J. J. (1980). The role of albumin conformation in the binding of diazepam to human serum albumin. *Biochim. Biophys. Acta* 626:291-298.

28. Yacobi, A., and Levy, G. (1975). Importance of assay specificity for plasma protein binding determinations. *J. Pharmacokinet. Biopharm.* 3:439-441.

29. Boobis, S. W., and Chignell, C. F. (1979). Effect of protein concentration on the binding of drugs to human serum albumin. I. Sulfadiazine, salicylate, and phenylbutazone. *Biochem. Pharmacol.* 28:751-756.

30. Aarons, L. J. (1979). A comment on estimating binding constants at variable protein concentrations. *J. Pharm. Pharmacol.* 31:655-656.

31. Bowmer, C. J., and Lindup, W. E. (1980). Inverse dependence of binding constants upon albumin concentration: results for L-tryptophan and three anionic dyes. *Biochim. Biophys. Acta* 624:260-270.

32. Nilsen, O. G., and Jacobsen, S. (1976). The influence of salts and differences in protein isolation procedure on the binding of quinidine to human serum albumin. *Biochem. Pharmacol.* 25:1261-1266.

33. Behm, H. L., and Wagner, J. G. (1979). Errors in the interpretation of data from equilibrium dialysis protein binding experiments. *Res. Commun. Chem. Pathol. Pharmacol.* 26:145-160.
34. Keen, P. M. (1966). The binding of penicillins to bovine serum albumin. *Biochem. Pharmacol.* 15:447-463.
35. Mucklow, J. C., Bending, M. R., Kahn, G. C., and Dollery, C. T. (1978). Drug concentration in saliva. *Clin. Pharmacol. Ther.* 24:563-570.
36. Rodbard, D., Munson, P. J., and Thakur, A. K. (1980). Quantitative characterization of hormone receptors. *Cancer* 46: 2907-2918.
37. Rosenthal, H. E. (1967). A graphic method for the determination and presentation of binding parameters in a complex system. *Anal. Biochem.* 20:525-532.
38. Blaschke, T. F. (1977). Protein binding and kinetics of drugs in liver disease. *Clin. Pharmacokinet.* 2:32-44.
39. Gugler, R., Shoeman, D. W., Huffman, D. H., Cohlmia, J. B., and Azarnoff, D. L. (1975). Pharmacokinetics of drugs in patients with the nephrotic syndrome. *J. Clin. Invest.* 55: 1182-1189.
40. Krishnaswamy, K., Ushasri, V., and Naidu, A. N. (1981). The effect of malnutrition on the pharmacokinetics of phenylbutazone. *Clin. Pharmacokinet.* 6:152-159.
41. Buchanan, N., Robinson, R., Koornhof, H. J., and Eyberg, C. (1979). Penicillin pharmacokinetics in kwashiorkor. *Am. J. Clin. Nutr.* 32:2233-2236.
42. Kates, R. E., Sokoloski, T. D., and Comstock, T. J. (1978). Binding of quinidine to plasma proteins in normal subjects and in patients with hyperlipoproteinemias. *Clin. Pharmacol. Ther.* 23:30-35.
43. Romer, J., and Bickel, M. H. (1979). A method to estimate binding constants at variable protein concentrations. *J. Pharm. Pharmacol.* 31:7-11.
44. Aarons, L. J., Schary, W. L., and Rowland, M. (1979). An in vitro study of drug displacement interactions: warfarin-salicylate and warfarin-phenylbutazone. *J. Pharm. Pharmacol.* 31:322-330.
45. Reidenberg, M. M. (1976). The binding of drugs to plasma proteins from patients with poor renal function. *Clin. Pharmacokinet.* 1:121-125.
46. Craig, W. A., Evenson, M. A., Sarver, K. P., and Wagnild, J. P. (1976). Correction of protein binding defect in uremic sera by charcoal treatment. *J. Lab. Clin. Med.* 87:637-647.
47. Sjöholm, I., Kober, A., Odar-Cederlöf, I., and Borgå, O. (1976). Protein binding of drugs in uremic and normal serum: the role of endogenous binding inhibitors. *Biochem. Pharmacol.* 25:1205-1213.

48. Kober, A., Sjöholm, I., Borgå, O., and Odar-Cederlöf, I. (1979). Protein binding of diazepam and digitoxin in uremic and normal serum. *Biochem. Pharmacol.* 28:1037-1042.
49. Kober, Å., Jenner, A., Sjöholm, I., Borgå, O., and Odar-Cederlöf, I. (1978). Differentiated effects of liver cirrhosis on the albumin binding sites for diazepam, salicylic acid and warfarin. *Biochem. Pharmacol.* 27:2729-2735.
50. Wong, G. B., and Sellers, E. M. (1979). Intravascular factors affecting diazepam binding to human serum albumin. *Biochem. Pharmacol.* 28:3265-3270.
51. Naranjo, C. A., Sellers, E. M., Giles, H. G., and Abel, J. G. (1980). Diurnal variations in plasma diazepam concentrations associated with reciprocal changes in free fraction. *Br. J. Clin. Pharmacol.* 9:265-272.
52. Naranjo, C. A., Sellers, E. M., and Khouw, V. (1981). Fatty acids modulation of meal-induced variations in diazepam free fraction. *Br. J. Clin. Pharmacol.* 10:308-310.
53. Desmond, P. V., Roberts, R. K., Wood, A. J. J., Dunn, G. D., Wilkinson, G. R., and Schenker, S. (1980). Effect of heparin administration on plasma binding of benzodiazepines. *Br. J. Clin. Pharmacol.* 9:171-175.
54. Wood, M., Shand, D. G., and Wood, A. J. J. (1979). Altered drug binding due to the use of indwelling heparinized cannulas (heparin lock) for sampling. *Clin. Pharmacol. Ther.* 25:103-107.
55. Kessler, K. M., Leech, R. C., and Spann, J. F. (1979). Blood collection techniques, heparin, and quinidine protein binding. *Clin. Pharmacol. Ther.* 25:204-210.
56. Wood, A. J. J., Robertson, D., Robertson, R. M., Wilkinson, G. R., and Wood, M. (1980). Elevated plasma free drug concentrations of propranolol and diazepam during cardiac catherterization. *Circulation* 62:1119-1122.
57. Routledge, P. A., Bjornsson, T. D., Kitchell, B. B., and Shand, D. G. (1979). Heparin administration increases plasma warfarin binding in man. *Br. J. Clin. Pharmacol.* 8:281-282.
58. Chou, R. C., and Levy, G. (1981). Effect of heparin or salicylate infusion on serum protein binding and on concentrations of phenytoin in serum, brain and cerebrospinal fluid of rats. *J. Pharmacol. Exp. Ther.* 219:42-48.
59. Wiegand, U. W., Slattery, J. T., Hintze, K. L., and Levy, G. (1979). Differences in the protein binding of several drugs and bilirubin in serum and heparinized plasma of rats. *Life Sci.* 25:471-478.
60. Weigand, U. W., Hintz, K. L., Slattery, J. T., and Levy, G. (1980). Protein binding of several drugs in serum and plasma of healthy subjects. *Clin. Pharmacol. Ther.* 27:297-300.

61. Borgå, O., Piafsky, K. M., and Nilsen, O. G. (1977). Plasma protein binding of basic drugs. I. Selective displacement from α_1-acid glycoprotein by tris(2-butoxyethyl)phosphate. *Clin. Pharmacol. Ther.* 22:539-544.

62. Cotham, R. H., and Shand, D. G. (1975). Spuriously low plasma propranolol concentrations resulting from blood collection methods. *Clin. Pharmacol. Ther.* 18:535-538.

63. Gillette, J. R. (1971). Factors affecting drug metabolism. *Ann. N. Y. Acad. Sci.* 179:43-66.

64. Wilkinson, G. R., and Shand, D. G. (1975). A physiological approach to hepatic drug clearance. *Clin. Pharmacol. Ther.* 18:377-390.

65. Øie, S., and Tozer, T. N. (1979). Effects of altered plasma protein binding on apparent volume of distribution. *J. Pharm. Sci.* 68:1203-1205.

66. Jähnchen, E., Wingard, L. B., and Levy, G. (1973). Effect of phenylbutazone on the distribution, elimination and anticoagulant action of dicumarol in rats. *J. Pharmacol. Exp. Ther.* 187: 176-184.

67. Thiessen, J. J., and Rowland, M. (1977). Kinetics of drug-drug interactions in sheep: tolbutamide and sulfadimethoxine. *J. Pharm. Sci.* 66:1063-1070.

68. Rowland, M., Benet, L. Z., and Graham, G. G. (1973). Clearance concepts in pharmacokinetics. *J. Pharmacokinet. Biopharm.* 1:123-136.

69. Pang, K. S., and Rowland, M. (1977). Hepatic clearance of drugs. I. Theoretical considerations of a "well-stirred" model and a "parallel tube" model. Influence of hepatic blood flow, plasma and blood cell binding, and the hepatocellular enzymatic activity on hepatic drug clearance. *J. Pharmacokinet. Biopharm.* 5:625-653.

70. Yacobi, A., and Levy, G. (1975). Comparative pharmacokinetics of coumarin anticoagulants. XIV. Relationship between protein binding, distribution and elimination kinetics of warfarin in rats. *J. Pharm. Sci.* 64:1660-1664.

71. Yacobi, A., Udall, J. A., and Levy, G. (1976). Serum protein binding as a determinant of warfarin body clearance and anticoagulant effect. *Clin. Pharmacol. Ther.* 19:552-558.

72. Williams, R. L., Blaschke, T. F., Meffin, P. J., Melmon, K. L., and Rowland, M. (1977). Influence of acute viral hepatitis on disposition and plasma binding of tolbutamide. *Clin. Pharmacol. Ther.* 21:301-309.

73. Evans, G. H., Nies, A. S., and Shand, D. G. (1973). The disposition of propranolol. III. Decreased half-life and volume of distribution as a result of plasma binding in man, monkey, dog, and rat. *J. Pharmacol. Exp. Ther.* 186:114-120.

74. Shand, D. G., Cotham, R. H., and Wilkinson, G. R. (1976). Perfusion-limited effects of plasma drug binding on hepatic drug extraction. *Life Sci.* *19*:125-130.

75. McNamara, P. J., Levy, G., and Gibaldi, M. (1979). Effect of plasma protein and tissue binding on the time course of drug concentration in plasma. *J. Pharmacokinet. Biopharm.* 7:195-206.

76. Øie, S., Guentert, T. W., and Tozer, T. N. (1980). Effect of saturable binding on the pharmacokinetics of drugs: a simulation. *J. Pharm. Pharmacol.* *32*:471-477.

77. McQueen, E. G., and Wardell, W. M. (1971). Drug displacement from protein binding: isolation of a redistribution drug interaction in vivo. *Brit. J. Pharmacol.* *43*:312-324.

78. Øie, S., and Levy, G. (1979). Effect of sulfisoxazole on pharmacokinetics of free and plasma-protein bound bilirubin in experimental unconjugated hyperbilirubinemia. *J. Pharm. Sci.* *68*:6-9.

79. Øie, S., and Levy, G. (1979). Effect of salicyclic acid on pharmacokinetics of free and plasma-protein bound bilirubin in experimental unconjugated hyperbilirubinemia. *J. Pharm. Sci.* *68*:1-5.

80. Gillette, J. R. (1973). Overview of drug-protein binding. *Ann. N. Y. Acad. Sci. 226*:6-17.

81. Shand, D. G., Mitchell, J. R., and Oates, J. A. (1975). Pharmacokinetic drug interactions. In *Concepts in Biochemical Pharmacology*, Part 3, J. R. Gillette, and J. R. Mitchell, Eds., *Handbook of Experimental Pharmacology*, Vol. 28/3, Springer-Verlag, New York, pp. 272-314.

82. Guentert, T. W. and Øie, S. (1980). Effect of plasma protein binding on quinidine kinetics in the rabbit. *J. Pharmacol. Exp. Ther. 215*:165-171.

3
Dietary Lipids and
Foreign Compound (Carcinogen) Metabolism

Bandaru S. Reddy and Peggy Smith-Barbaro*
*Naylor Dana Institute for Disease Prevention,
American Health Foundation, Valhalla, New York*

I. INTRODUCTION

The recognition that diet and nutrition play a significant role in the metabolism of exogenous (foreign) and endogenous compounds has received attention in recent years (1). Current data suggest that the nutritional state—nutrient excess and imbalances—has an influence on the metabolism of a variety of these substances. Indeed, progress has also been made in recent years in the understanding of the relationship between dietary fat and the metabolism of foreign compounds (environmental contaminants, xenobiotics, drugs and potential carcinogens, and cocarcinogens).

The production of cancer by foreign compounds or chemicals is a very special aspect of an adverse toxicological reaction (2). For example, chemical carcinogens in a given experimental setting show dose-response relationships and undergo biotransformation, as would any similarly structured pharmacologic agents. In addition, the response to chemical carcinogens varies with the species, strain, sex, and nutritional status of the experimental animal, as in the case with other pharmacologic agents or foreign compounds (2).

The importance of dietary factors in the development of experimental cancer induced by a foreign compound was realized in connection with the early studies involving carcinogenic azo dye, 4-dimethylaminoazobenzene (3,4). Low-protein low-riboflavin diets appeared essential to induce liver cancer by the carcinogenic azo dye in rats. Low dietary riboflavin resulted in reduced activity of the enzyme system, azo dye

---

*Present affiliation: Frito-Lay, Inc., Irving, Texas

reductase, involved in the reduction of the azo link. Subsequent studies have demonstrated that diet can affect chemical carcinogenesis at every critical step in the process: formation of activated carcinogens, interaction of the activated metabolite with cellular targets, enhanced sensitivity to carcinogens, and expression of initiated tumor cell. Wattenberg (5) has detailed the effect of a variety of laboratory diets and their active components on the aryl-hydrocarbon hydroxylase system in several organs.

Another way in which diet can affect chemical carcinogenesis is by interfering with the interaction of ultimate carcinogens with cellular macromolecules as proposed by the Millers (6). They also suggested that nucleophiles might be provided to act as competitive traps for the ultimate electrophilic reactants. In addition, diet also controls, in part, the level of other nucleophilic cell constituents, such as glutathione, which are good competitors with DNA. Another possibility is that diet can affect carcinogenesis by altering the tissue sensitivity to carcinogens. This hypothesis was studied in experiments aimed at examining the role of diet-induced liver cirrhosis in liver cancer development (7). Finally, the fact that diet can alter the process of tumor development has been most extensively studied in experiments designed to examine the role of dietary fat in mammary and colon tumorigenesis in animal models (8,9). In these situations, the high-fat diet appears to enhance carcinogenesis through its elevation of agents that act as promoters of tumor development. In many instances, the mechanisms by which the dietary lipids operate are incompletely understood. However, liver drug-metabolizing enzymes broadly known as mixed-function oxidases (MFO), which are responsible for the metabolism of a variety of substances, such as carcinogens, cocarcinogens, drugs, and many other foreign compounds, may be a mediating factor in the relationship between diet and carcinogenesis (10). Recent evidence suggest that many extrahepatic tissues, such as gastrointestinal mucosa, lung, kidney, and skin, exhibit MFO activities (11).

This review briefly covers studies on the metabolism and carcinogenic properties of a variety of foreign compounds, and on the effect of dietary lipids on the metabolism of these compounds.

II. CHEMICAL CARCINOGENS

Historically, several types of foreign compounds were discovered to have carcinogenic potential in experimental systems after having first been suspected of causing cancer in humans. On the basis of mode of action and other factors, cancer-causing agents can be classified into various broad classes (Table 1).

Table 1 Main Classes of Carcinogenic Chemicals

Class	Mode of action	Example
Direct-acting ultimate carcinogen	Electrophile, organic compound genotoxic, interacts with DNA	Ethylene imine, methylnitrosourea, N-methyl-N'-nitro-N-nitrosoguanidine, β-propiolactone, bis(chloromethyl)ether, diazomethane
Procarcinogen	Requires conversion through metabolic activation by host or in vitro to type 1	Vinyl chloride, dimethylaminoazobenzene, benzo(a)pyrene, aflatoxin B, safrole, 2-naphthylamine, 1,2-dimethylhydrazine, dimethylnitrosamine, 3,2'-dimethyl-4-aminobiphenyl
Solid-state carcinogen	Exact mechanism unknown; usually affects only mesenchymal cells and tissues; physical form vital	Polymer or metal foils, asbestos
Inorganic carcinogen	Not directly genotoxic; leads to changes in DNA by selective alteration in fidelity of DNA replication	Nickel, chromium
Hormone	Usually not genotoxic; mainly alters endocrine system balance and differentiation; often acts as promoter	Estradiol, diethylstilbestrol
Immunosuppressor	Usually not genotoxic; mainly stimulates "virally induced," transplanted, or metastatic neoplasms	Azathioprene, antilymphocytic
Cocarcinogen	Not genotoxic or carcinogenic, but enhances effects of type 1 or type 2 agent when given at the same time; may modify conversion of type 2 to type 1	Phorbol esters, catechol, pyrene n-do-decane
Promoter	Not genotoxic or carcinogenic, but enhances effect of type 1 or type 2 agent when given subsequently	Phorbol esters, phenol, bile acids, tryptophan metabolites, saccharine

Source: Adapted from Ref. 2.

A. Direct-Acting Carcinogens

A direct-acting carcinogenic compound which by itself is the ultimate carcinogen does not require metabolic activation to produce an active metabolite (12). Most direct-acting carcinogens are products of industry as chemical intermediates or developed as drugs for specific purposes (Table 1). Because these agents are generally highly reactive, they readily undergo detoxification or inactivation. In many cases, their reactivity is so great that their effect can be demonstrated only in vitro. On the other hand, if such a compound has a sufficient half-life in vivo to reach target organs, it may be a powerful carcinogen without regard for other environmental or dietary conditions.

Nitrosation of alkylureas, alkylamides, and esters produces some of the most potent direct-acting carcinogens. Some of these chemicals are fairly stable in the anhydrous state and do not require specific enzymic activation but spontaneously release an active carcinogen intermediate in the presence of water or buffer solution of an appropriate pH such as that of body fluids. This class of carcinogen, which includes alkylnitrosourethan and alkylnitrosoureas, yields cancer directly in the area of application.

Alkylnitrosoureas, alkylnitrosourethan, and the closely related N-methyl-N'-nitro-N-nitrosoguanidine, nitrosobiuret, and N-methyl-N'-acetyl-N-nitrosourea when administered orally produce tumors in the gastrointestinal tract, while intrarectal instillation induce colorectal tumors in animal models (13–15). The latter three compounds are chemicals of choice to induce cancer of the glandular stomach, a frequent lesion in humans in Japan, parts of Latin America, Iceland, Scandinavia, and certain parts of Europe. Treatment of food with nitrate, especially fish or beans, which are frequently consumed in areas where gastric cancer is high, yields mutagenic activity, which recently has been shown to induce cancer of the glandular stomach in rats (16).

Given intravenously, some of the alkylnitrosoureas (particularly the ethyl derivative) produce tumors of the brain (17). Some are also active transplacentally, producing a high incidence of cancer in the offspring after a single dose to a pregnant female (18).

B. Chemicals Requiring Metabolic Activation

Direct-acting ultimate carcinogens also result from the metabolic activation of precursor compounds, often known as pre- or procarcinogens (Table 1). Metabolic activation depends on the endogenous and exogenous factors, including species, sex, diet, and the effect of other agents. Most of the chemical carcinogens known fall into this category and hence are carcinogenic under more selective conditions than are the direct-acting carcinogens (6). The majority of procarcinogens are obviously in need of metabolic activation because they produce tumors only under certain conditions at specific sites and never at the point of

Table 2 Organotropic Effects of Carcinogenic Nitroso Compounds,
Dialkylhydrazines, and Aromatic Amines

Compounds	Organs affected
Examples of nitrosamines	
Dimethylnitrosamine	Liver, kidneys, lung
Diethylnitrosamine	Liver, lung, esophagus
Di-n-butylnitrosamine	Bladder, liver
Methylphenylnitrosamine	Esophagus
Pyrrolidine	Liver
Piperidine	Liver, esophagus, para-nasal sinuses
Morpholine	Liver, kidney, paranasal sinuses
Nornicotine	Esophagus, pharynx, para-nasal sinuses
Examples of dialkylhydrazines and analogs	
1,2-Dimethylhydrazine	Intestine, liver, kidney, ear duct
Azoxymethane	Intestine, liver, kidney, ear duct
Cycasin	Intestine, liver, kidney
Methylazoxymethanol	Intestine, liver, kidney
Examples of aromatic amines	
3,2'-Dimethyl-4-aminobiphenyl	Intestine, ear duct, salivary gland, mammary gland, prostate
N-2-Fluorenylacetamide	Liver
2-Naphthylamine	Bladder, liver

application (Table 2). Carcinogenesis in specific organs can be related in many instances to either specific enzymic activation processes
in some types of cells or the release of active intermediates from transport forms of the activated intermediate. Endogenous or genetic, as
well as exogenous or environmental, conditions that favor the activation
reaction increase carcinogenicity. In contrast, such conditions that
increase detoxification lower carcinogenicity. Thus whether a given
chemical is oncogenic under a specified condition depends on the relative ratio of metabolic activation versus detoxification pathways (6).

1. Polycyclic Aromatic Hydrocarbons and Their Derivatives

Polycyclic aromatic hydrocarbons (PAHs) contain some of the most extensively studied chemical carcinogens and occur in a wide variety of environmental products (e.g., soots, coal tar products, petroleum oils, and cigarette smoke). Many rodent species are highly sensitive to chemical carcinogens of this type (19,20). Many of the results obtained can be interpreted in terms of chemical structure and susceptibilty to biochemical activation and detoxification. Many of the PAHs that are carcinogenic are derived from benz[a]anthracene skeleton. Anthracene itself is not carcinogenic, but benz[a]anthracene appears to have a weak carcinogenicity. Addition of another benzene ring in select positions results in powerful carcinogenic agents such as dibenz[a,h]anthracene (DBA) or benzo[a]pyrene (B[a]P). Alkyl-substituted PAHs have specific structure-activity relationships which are somewhat different from those of the parent compounds. Thus the activity of the methylbenz[a]anthracene depends considerably on the point of substitution of the methyl group. 7,12-Dimethylbenzanthracene (DMBA) and 5-methylchrysene are powerful carcinogens, whereas benzo[a]anthracene and chrysene are weak carcinogens and 4-methylchrysene is noncarcinogenic (21). It appears that the 5-methyl substituent directs the metabolic activation into the A ring, and this unique biochemical reaction may account for the carcinogenicity of this particular compound (21).

Skin application of the more powerful agents, such as 3-methylcholanthrene, DMBA, and B[a]P, leads to carcinoma formation in mice, whereas subcutaneous injection in rats and mice produces sarcomas (20). Oral administration in sesame oil to 60-day-old female Sprague-Dawley rats results in the rapid induction of breast cancer (20). The fact that small amounts of PAH are highly oncogenic to mouse skin or the subcutaneous tissue of rats suggests that this activation reaction occurs efficiently and indicates that detoxification reactions are less pronounced in these tissues. A number of such PAHs are also active, inducing mammary tumors in rats and mice, suggesting that this tissue possesses the necessary enzymes for activation. On the other hand, except for some sensitive strains of hamsters, the intestines of most rodents are not target organs, suggesting either a lack of activation reaction or, more likely, an effective detoxification system. Although ring-hydroxylated metabolites of PAH are usually not carcinogenic, 2-hydroxybenzo[a]pyrene is as active as the hydrocarbon itself to mouse skin, presumably because this metabolite is not readily eliminated through detoxification reactions, and thus the activation reaction occurs on mouse skin as it does with the parent hydrocarbon (22).

2. Aromatic Amines

Among compounds of this class are large-volume industrial chemicals, intermediates, consumer products, and specialized laboratory chemicals

(23,21,2). Aromatic amines and derivatives yield neoplasms at sites remote from the point of entry. The site affected depends on the structure of the chemical; the species, strain, and sex of the animal tested; and the presence of other agents. Carcinogenicity in various sites, including mammary gland, urinary bladder, ear duct, and intestinal tract, is found with linear multiring amines such as 4-aminobiphenyl and benzidine and their analogs and substituted amines such as 3,3'-dichlorobenzidine, 4,4'-methylene-bis(2-chloraniline), o-tolidine, and 3-methyl-4-aminobiphenyl. Of interest is the fact that 4-biphenylamine, a human urinary bladder carcinogen, leads to mammary cancer in female rats and is relatively inactive in male rats, whereas 3-methyl-4-aminobiphenylamine and analogs with an o-methyl-arylamine structure induce mammary gland cancer in female rats and cancer of the large intestine in male and female rats (24–27).

The aromatic amines demonstrate even more stringent structure-related effects than PAH (23). 2-Fluorenamine and derivatives but not the 1-,3-, and 4-isomers are powerful carcinogens (28). 2-Naphthalimine is carcinogenic, whereas 1-isomer is not carcinogenic. The underlying explanation rests on the relative extent of the activation and detoxification reactions.

Carcinogenic aromatic and heterocyclic amines undergo many biochemical oxidation reactions (6,29–31). Ring carbon hydroxylation is often a detoxification reaction, mainly because the resulting phenols are readily conjugated and excreted as sulfate or glucuronic acid conjugates. Hydroxylation on the nitrogen of arylamines giving hydroxylamines is the first step of an activation process which is structure dependent. Amines such as 1-naphthalamine are much less susceptible, and thus not carcinogenic. Nitroaryl compounds are reduced by mammalian and bacterial enzymes to arylhydroxylamines. For liver, a second activation step is esterification by sulfate. For extrahepatic tissues, an acyl transferase or a peroxidase may be the second step. These reactions yield ultimately a nitrenium ion. However, arylamines, especially polynucleararylamines, can also be activated through epoxidation of the ring system, at positions activated by the nitrogen electron pair. The function of the amino group is to direct epoxidative attack at specific ring positions. Since aromatic amines are carcinogenic because of biochemical activation to a hydroxylamino intermediate, it is evident that the corresponding arylhydroxylamines are also carcinogenic. In fact, synthetic hydroxylamino derivatives based on certain of the inactive aromatic amines, such as 1-naphthylhydroxylamine, 1-fluorenylhydroxylamine, and N-hydroxy-N-2-fluorenylbenzamide, are powerfully carcinogenic (28).

Many alkyl- or alkylarylnitrosamines have been tested for carcinogenic action in a large number of animal species (32,33). In rodents, the symmetric dialkyl compounds under some conditions exhibit delicate and yet specific organotropism. For example, dimethyl- and diethylnitrosamine usually cause liver cancer in rats, while the dibutyl derivative and diamyl compound cause cancer of the urinary bladder and cancer of the lung, respectively, in rats. Asymmetric nitrosamines, especially those with at least one methyl group, result in cancer of the esophagus, as do some nitrosamines based on cyclic secondary amines. In hamsters, on the other hand, diethylnitrosamine also causes cancer in the respiratory tract, and diketopropylnitrosamine or 2,6-dimethylnitrosomorpholine in the ductal pancreas.

Several nitrosamines derived from alkaloids such as nicotine, in particular nitrosonornicotine and related compounds, are found in tobacco and in tobacco smoke (34,35). In rats, they mainly cause cancer of the esophagus and in hamsters cancer of the upper respiratory tract. The contribution of these chemicals to carcinogenesis in humans who smoke cigarettes or chew tobacco products is not yet known. Individuals who smoke and also drink alcoholic beverages have a high risk of cancer of the oral cavity and esophagus. The relevant mechanism may be an induction by alcohol of enzymes capable of metabolizing nitrosamines such as nitrosonornicotine, or polycyclic aromatic hydrocarbons found in smoke, in the target tissue (36).

Nitrosamines are converted to active electrophilic reactants through oxidation (23,37,38). With the prototype dimethylnitrosamine, an active intermediate has been thought to be the unstable hydroxymethyl compound, which is converted to a methyl carbonium ion: Cyclic nitrosamines can be metabolized by hydroxylation (alpha or beta) to the N-nitroso function. Recent developments demonstrate that the key activation reaction appears to be alpha hydroxylation (35). The structural requirement for carcinogenicity is that at least one alkyl group capable of metabolism be attached to the nitrosamine. If the alkyl group is bulky, for example, a tertiary butyl group, and is metabolically difficult to oxidize, the nitrosamine is unlikely to be carcinogenic.

Certain carcinogenic nitrosamines need not be consumed as such but can be formed endogenously from precursor nitrite or nitrate and the appropriate secondary amine (39,40). Identical types of cancer were observed at the same location after similar latent periods whether the preformed nitrosamine or sodium nitrite and the amine were given. More recently, the question was raised whether these hazardous compounds could be formed in the upper gastrointestinal tract by reaction of nitrate with naturally occurring or dietary amines, amides, and peptides. The required nitrite may stem from nitrite-preserved foods or bacterial reduction of ubiquitous nitrate (41).

Nitrosamines can be formed not only from the classic reaction of nitrite with secondary amines or amides, but also with tertiary amines as a substrate (39). Inasmuch as a number of drugs have a dialkylaminoaryl structure, it has been proposed that the simultaneous intake of nitrite and such drugs may yield potentially hazardous nitrosamines, and specifically dimethyl- or diethylnitrosamine, since many drugs bear diethyl- or diethylamine substituents (42).

3. Dialkylhydrazines

The carcinogenic properties of meal prepared from the nuts of the cycad plant, *Cycas circinalis*, were discovered by Laqueur (43) while studying the possible relationship between flour made from the cycad nut and a neurotoxic syndrome seen on some Pacific islands. Cycad meal fed at 200–400 ppm in the diet of rats for 6–9 months produced a variety of tumors, including colon, liver, and kidney. It was subsequently established that the active principle was cycasin, the β-glucoside of methylazoxymethanol (MAM) (43). Cycasin was carcinogenic in weanling or older conventional animals but not in germ-free rats when administered orally, but it was inactive parenterally. On the other hand, MAM itself or the chemically more stable MAM acetate yielded tumors irrespective of the route of administration in any animals at any age, germfree or conventional (43–45). These combined experiments on cycasin and MAM can be explained by the β-glucosidic linkage of cycasin being hydrolyzed by the intestinal bacteria but not in the tissues of conventional animals. Subcutaneous or intraperitoneal administration of cycasin transferred insufficient amounts of the glucoside to the large bowel, so that little hydrolysis by the bacteria to the active MAM took place. However, oral administration of this compound led to bacterial enzymic hydrolysis in the gut, which released the active intermediate, MAM, in the large intestine. Although this compound is not entirely stable at physiologic pH, its organospecificity suggested the need to search for enzymatically mediated activation mechanisms. Fiala et al. (46) have evidence that this enzyme may be related to alcohol dehydrogenase, which yields eventually, in several steps, methyl carbonium ion to be the active ultimate carcinogen formed in the cell from precursor material.

The discovery of the carcinogenicity of cycasin led Druckrey (47) to test its synthetic analogs, azoxymethane (AOM) and 1,2-dimethylhydrazine (DMH), which are the most effective carcinogens for the specific induction of tumors of the colon and rectum in rats and mice. The most suitable dose in rats was 15–20 mg/kg body weight weekly or 150 mg/kg body weight once, and in mice 30 mg/kg body weight weekly by subcutaneous injection. Recently, Reddy et al (48) produced colon tumors in rats by weekly intrarectal administration of DMH at a dose of 20 mg/kg body weight. In Fisher rats, given 10 weekly injections of AOM at 14.8 mg/kg body weight, Ward (49) obtained carcinomas exclusively in the duodenum and descending colon, but with 7.4 mg/kg body weight, the tumors were generally distributed in the colon. It was also possible to induce colonic tumors in rats by weekly intrarectal instillation of azoxymethane at a dose of 10 mg/kg body weight (50).

Studies on the pathogenesis of the colonic and rectal carcinomas induced by DMH and AOM revealed striking similarities to those seen in humans (47,49). This was true not only with respect to gross appear-

ance and histologic types of tumors, but also to the distribution of the
tumors in the various parts of the colon.

Metabolism of symmetric dialkylhydrazines by mammalian enzymes has
been studied by Fiala (51). A typical example is DMH, which is metabolized to a methyl carbonium ion in several stages. The first step
yields azomethane, which is oxidized to azoxymethane and finally to
MAM in the liver (51). The intestinal specificity of this material is
through a final activation step to the methyl carbonium ion, possibly
by alcohol dehydrogenase.

4. Microbial and Natural Products and Food Contaminants

A number of carcinogens are formed in nature by microorganisms or
plants. The mechanism of action of a number of these agents, particularly the antibiotics, is unknown. However, most of these naturally occurring carcinogens clearly require metabolic activation.

The dramatic discovery of the aflatoxins is well known. About 1960,
an epidemic destroyed half of the commercial turkey production in
Great Britain. Examination of the possible causes soon focused atten-
tiontion on a dietary factor and incriminated a peanut meal with an apparent mold contamination by certain species of *Aspergillus flavus* (52,
53). Cultures of the mold produced a toxin, small amounts of which
were fatal to ducklings. Several chemically closely related aflatoxins
were identified: aflatoxin B1, B2, G1. and G2 (54). There are major
differences in toxicity and carcinogenicity of these compounds. Aflatoxin B1 is the most toxic and carcinogenic in rats and several other
species, including monkeys. Affected organs are mainly the liver, and
less frequently the kidneys, stomach, and colon. In rats, even 1 μg/
kg diet was carcinogenic. Interestingly, mice (except when exposed
as newborns) do not show liver tumors, but some strains are sensitive to lung tumor induction (54). The reasons for this are not yet
clear.

Aflatoxin G1 is less carcinogenic, and aflatoxin B2 and G2 are only
slightly active. Aflatoxin B2 is converted to aflatoxin B1 by enzymic
dehydrogenation and it is thought that the activity of the B2 analog is
due to a small extent of conversion to the B1 isomer. A number of
other metabolites have been identified. Aflatoxin M1 was found in the
milk of cattle consuming aflatoxin-contaminated food. Aflatoxin P1,
stemming from the oxidation of the methoxy group, was thought to be
useful in evaluating possible human exposure, but has not been reliably
detectable. Other metabolites identified include aflatoxin Q1, stemming
from hydroxylation of the five-membered ring system in the coumarin
end of the molecule.

Among natural products, several antibiotics that enter the human
environment as drugs were found to induce tumors (55,56). These
include daunomycin, dactinomycin, griseofulvin, and streptozotocin.
Azaserine, originally thought to be an antimetabolite, was shown to

produce primarily pancreas, liver, and kidney tumors in rats. This organotropism correlates with localization of the agent (57).

In investigating the causes of hematuria and bladder cancer in cattle in Turkey and other regions, it was found that consumption of bracken fern was etiologically related to the development of lesions (58). In rats, administration of bracken fern has an effect not only on the urinary bladder, but also on the upper intestinal tract (59). There is possible human exposure to the carcinogen in bracken fern since it has been identified in the milk of cows consuming this plant (60). The components listed above have not yet been identified. In some countries, cooked or raw bracken fern is used for human consumption.

III. METABOLISM OF FOREIGN COMPOUNDS WITH EMPHASIS ON CHEMICAL CARCINOGENESIS

With few exception, endogenous as well as exogenous chemicals undergo metabolic reactions (6). In contrast to direct-acting carcinogens, which are chemically reactive and therefore do not persist in the environment, procarcinogens or chemicals that require activation are often chemically stable entities. The Millers have postulated that chemical carcinogens without reactivity must be enzymatically activated to a reactive electrophilic form, and that the electrophilic "ultimate carcinogens" covalently bind to tissue macromolecules to initiate the neoplastic lesion (31).

The relative effectiveness of a foreign compound, under given conditions, depends on the efficiency of the activation reactions over the competing detoxification reactions. Numerous factors, including genotypic and phenotypic influences such as species, strain, sex, and action of other endogenous or exogenous agents, ultimately express their major effect on the ratio of the activation over the detoxification metabolites. However, there are also secondary forces affecting this relationship, such as the availability of cellular and molecular receptors and other host factors. Therefore, biochemical activation and detoxification process are crucial to the entire carcinogenic process (2,6,31) (Table 3).

It is outside the scope of this chapter to elaborate on all the known metabolic activation/detoxification reactions for chemical carcinogens. Instead, the general principles of these activation/detoxification reactions, as well as inhibition of chemical carcinogenesis by inducers of MFO system, will be discussed briefly.

As discussed above, the enzyme system responsible for this activation of carcinogens, co-carcinogens, and other foreign compounds is thought to be "drug-metabolizing enzyme system or mixed-function oxidase (MFO) system." The MFO system exhibits high activity in the liver, but important activities are also found in a variety of other tissues; gastrointestinal mucosa, lung, kidney, and skin. Carcinogens

Table 3 Sequence of Events Leading to Cancer

Events in carcinogenesis[a]	Modifiers[b]
Detoxification, excretion	
Chemical carcinogen ⟶	Species, strain, age, sex, diet, mixture of agents, intestinal flora, change of activation/detoxification enzymes, cocarcinogens
↓ activation steps	
Ultimate carcinogen ⟶	Nucleophilic trapping agents? Availability of receptors? Modifiers of repair? Modifier of growth?
specific receptor / blocks repair — repair system	
Altered receptor ⟵	Repair systems, inhibit messenger biosynthesis
↓ expression	
Latent tumor cell	Promoters, growth stimulants or inhibitors, nutritional status, endocrine status, immunologic competence
↓ growth, development	
Differentiated tumor	Immunologic status? Fidelity in DNA synthesis
↓ progression	
Undifferentiated cancer	Surgery, radiation, chemotherapy, immunotherapy

[a]A chemical carcinogen is activated, reacts with specific receptors, neutralizes repair mechanisms. Expression of the information on the abnormal, transformed receptor, possibly DNA, and growth of the resultant tumor cell leads to a differentiated neoplasm, which can undergo further progression to anaplastic forms.
[b]Although certain modifiers could affect several of the steps, only the key ones are itemized.
Source: Ref. 2

are active at certain sites because of the presence of the necessary activating enzyme system. If the activity of the MFP system were totally absent, carcinogens requiring activation by this system would be inactive. It is the feature that accounts in great part for the organ-specific localization of the action of individual chemical carcinogens.

In a cell, the MFO enzyme is bound to membranes on the smooth particles of the endoplasmic reticulum. The system has been solubilized and partially purified. The overall reaction activates molecular oxygen and yields oxidized or hydroxylated substrates, and the equivalent of water. Studies with isotropic oxygen-18 proved that the oxygen in the metabolite comes from atmospheric oxygen and not from oxygen in the water. The system is composed of a number of coupled reactions utilizing NADPH, NADP, and magnesium, as well as other components, such as flavines and cofactors. The first enzyme system cycles between oxidized and reduced NADP-cytochrome P-450 reductase, which in turn is coupled to the cytochrome P-450 system. The substance is attached to the cytochrome P-450 during the oxidation or hydroxylation process (1).

Inhibition of chemical carcinogenesis by the modification of MFO activity has been discussed in detail by Wattenberg (5), who listed some potential mechanisms for inhibition. Thus far, a substantial number of instances have been found in which the inhibitors alter the metabolism of the carcinogen through the decreased activation, increased detoxification, or combination of both. The second mechanism of inhibition of carcinogenesis is by scavenging of active molecular species of carcinogens, thus preventing them from reaching critical target sites in the cell. However, no clear in vivo evidence of this mechanism is available at the present time. The third possible mechanism of chemical carcinogenesis inhibition is by prior administration of a competitive inhibitor. Studies have shown the presence of a binding protein in the cytoplasm and existence of competition among various PAHs as well as other compounds for this binding site (61).

A number of studies have demonstrated that it is possible to protect against chemical carcinogens by administration of inducers of increased microsomal MFO activity. The inducers used included compounds such as polycyclic hydrocarbons, which themselves are noxious agents, to chemicals such as flavones, which have low toxicity (62). In early studies it was shown that administration of polycyclic hydrocarbon inducers inhibited the occurrence of hepatic cancer resulting from feeding 3'-methyl-4-dimethylaminoazobenzene (63). Polycyclic hydrocarbon inducers reduce the incidence of tumors of the liver, mammary gland, ear duct, and small intestine in rats fed N-2-fluorenylacetamide (63).

More recently, studies have been carried out in which protection against the carcinogenic effects of a number of other compounds has been observed (5). Employing the pulmonary adenoma test system in the mouse, it has been shown that flavone inducers will inhibit the formation of pulmonary neoplasms resulting from oral administration of DMBA or B[a]P. An experimental model that has been widely used to study the effects of inducers of increased MFO activity is that of mammary tumor formation in rats given DMBA. Several different types of inducers, such as PHAs, phenothiazines, and flavones, administered prior to DMBA will inhibit tumor formation.

One of the factors that may be of importance in explaining carcinogen inhibition by induction of increased MFO activity is that in many instances chemical carcinogens are subjected to detoxification, whereas hydroxylation of the nitrogen is an activation reaction (6). Thus administration of inducers of MFO activity in these instances may result in a relatively greater proportion of the carcinogen being detoxified rather than activated to a carcinogenic metabolite. Changes in proportion of detoxified metabolites to carcinogenic metabolites simply could be the results of relative responses of the two pathways to the inducer. An alternative possibility suggested by the studies with butylated hydroxyanisole (BHA) is that a basic alteration in metabolism may occur, resulting in a changed metabolite pattern. In this instance, alteration of metabolite pattern could be independent of magnitude of induction and, in fact, as in the case of BHA, might occur without any overall increase in MFO activity (5).

If the activity of the microsomal MFO system were totally absent, carcinogens requiring activation by this system would be inactive. Efforts have been made to achieve inhibition of chemical carcinogenesis by this mechanism. Studies of suppression of polycyclic hydrocarbon-induced epidermal neoplasia have been carried out employing 7,8-benzoflavone, a potent inhibitor of microsomal MFO activity. In experiments in which DMBA was the carcinogen, inhibition of epidermal neoplasia has been obtained (64). A problem with exploitation of inhibition of MFO activity as a means of suppressing chemical carcinogenesis might occur if the enzyme inhibition was only partial. Under these conditions, almost any result would be possible if the assumption is correct that slow activation of carcinogens can be effective in carcinogen activation (5). An additional negative aspect of inhibiting the microsomal MFO system is that it would render the organism more susceptible to the noxious effects of xenobiotic compounds detoxified by this system (5).

IV. EFFECT OF DIETARY LIPIDS ON MIXED-FUNCTION OXIDASE SYSTEM

Several recent reviews discuss both general and specific aspects of the effect of dietary lipids on drug-metabolizing enzymes or the MFO system (65). The drug-metabolizing MFO system is composed of a group of enzymes located on the lipoprotein membrane of the endoplasmic reticulum (65). Basically, the MFO system consists of several oxidative enzymes which are responsible for metabolizing numerous foreign compounds such as carcinogens, drugs, and other exogenous substances, and endogenous substrates such as steroids and bile acids.

A. Dietary Lipids and Hepatic Cytochrome P-450 Levels

Cytochrome P-450 and NADPH-cytochrome P-450 reductase are part of the flavoprotein reductase system which contains specific electron donors and acceptors (1). The most commonly utilized methodological approach to examining the role of dietary fat on hepatic cytochrome (Cyt) P-450 levels is the short-term feeding experiment. Rats are generally fed diets containing various levels and types of fats for 4–5 weeks, at which time rats are killed and tissues to be studied are removed, and microsomal pellets for specific MFO analysis are prepared by centrifugation. No change in hepatic Cyt P-450 levels was reported in 8-week-old female Wistar rats fed diets containing either 17.5% sunflower seed oil (P/S = 6.9) or 17.5% tallow diets (P/S = 1.0) for 4 weeks (66). However, the addition of pentobarbital, a MFO inducer, to the drinking water of these rats caused an increase in hepatic Cyt P-450 levels, regardless of the type of diet fed, with rats receiving beef tallow saturated fat diet having significantly elevated hepatic Cyt P-450 levels compared to rats fed the sunflower seed oil polyunsaturated fat diet. Hopkins and West (66) also reported an inverse relationship between diet-induced changes in hepatic Cyt P-450 levels and pentobarbitone-induced sleeping times. Pentabarbitone-induced sleeping times are one of the few in vivo methods available to evaluate rates of drug metabolism (66).

The results reported above are contradictory to those previously reported by Marshall and McLean (67). Marshall and McLean (67) demonstrated induction of hepatic Cyt P-450 in rats fed a high polyunsaturated fatty acid diet (15% herring oil) but not in saturated fat (15% coconut oil) fed rats. These differences may be attributed to several factors. Hopkins and West (66) used female rats in their experiment, while Marshall and McLean (67) used male rats. We have reported that the level of hepatic Cyt P-450 in rats fed high-fat diets appears to be sex dependent, with male rats fed high-beef-fat diets exhibiting lower hepatic levels of Cyt P-450 relative to microsomal protein then male rats fed high-vegetable-oil (corn oil) diets (Table 4). Female rats fed high-beef-fat diets had slightly higher Cyt P-450 levels than female rats fed a high-vegetable-oil diet (68). These results are supported by the data of McLeod et al. (69). Another difference between experiments of Hopkins and West (66) and Marshall and McLean (67) was the age of the animals studied. Although we know of no reported work that was aimed directly at evaluating developmental changes in hepatic Cyt P-450 levels, studies have been reported that show the activity of specific MFO enzymes varies with the age of the test animal (68,70).

Several investigators have examined the effect of altering the level of fat in the diet on hepatic Cyt P-450 levels (71,72). Hepatic Cyt P-450 levels are not significantly altered by feeding a high-unsaturated fat diet (20% corn oil versus 5% corn oil) (71). These results were

Table 4 Effect of Diet on Hepatic Mixed-Function Oxidase Enzymes in Male and Female Rats[a]

	Cytochrome P-450 (nmol mg^{-1} protein)	Benzpyrene hydroxylase (nmol mg protein^{-1} min^{-1})	Aminopyrene demethylase (nmol HCHO mg protein^{-1} min^{-1})
Females			
Corn oil (5%)	0.55 ± 0.07	0.28 ± 0.02	4.6 ± 0.35
Beef fat (6%)	0.62 ± 0.05	0.21 ± 0.03	3.3 ± 0.34[b]
High corn oil (25%)	0.71 ± 0.07	0.27 ± 0.03	4.5 ± 0.34
High beef fat (25%)	0.72 ± 0.03	0.27 ± 0.06	3.4 ± 0.46
Males			
Corn oil (5%)	0.85 ± 0.02	0.23 ± 0.04	3.6 ± 0.33
Beef fat (6%)	0.89 ± 0.04	0.59 ± 0.10[c]	5.6 ± 0.21[c]
High corn oil (25%)	1.0 ± 0.83	0.31 ± 0.05	4.0 ± 0.28
High beef fat (25%)	0.94 ± 0.03	0.69 ± 0.07[c]	5.9 ± 0.18[c]

[a]Mean ± SEM for eight animals per group.
[b]Significantly different from opposite diet, $P < 0.05$.
[c]Significantly different from opposite diet, $P < 0.01$.

substatiated by those of Gaillard et al. (72), who fed diets containing either 1% or 25% peanut oil, as well as those of Martin et al. (68), who fed high-beef-fat or high-corn-oil diets (Table 4). In addition, when rats from the Gaillard et al. (72) experiment were exposed to the pesticide Morestan, hepatic Cyt P-450 levels were significantly reduced in both the 1% and 25% lipid groups.

Hietanen et al. (73) suggested that fatty acids may act to alter drug-induced changes in the activity of MFO enzymes by changing the microenvironment of these membrane-bound constituents. They reported that the phospholipid content of the microsomal membrane was lowered by giving elevated (200 mg/kg body weight) intraperitoneal doses of linoleic acid or elaidic acids (73). Phenobarbital caused the proportion of linoleic acid in phosphatidylcholine and phosphatidylethanolamine to increase 120–140% of the control animal fed a commercially available laboratory diet, while the proportion of oleic, arachidonic, and decosahexaneoic acid decreased (21). The phenobarbital-induced increase in linoleic acid content of the hepatic phospholipid membrane occurred simultaneously with an increased Cyt P-450 concentration and increased activity of the drug hydroxylating enzymes. Results from experiments of Davidson and Wills (74) suggested that phosphatidyl choline containing linoleic acid in the β position was necessary for drug-induced oxidative demethylation reactions carried out by the MFO system in the endoplasmic reticulum.

B. Dietary Fat and Specific Hepatic MFO Enzymes

Examination of hepatic Cyt P-450 levels yields general information on the "broad" substrate specificity of the drug metabolizing enzymes for numerous foreign compounds (75–79). However, examination of Cyt P-450 levels alone may not elucidate clearly its contributory role as a metabolic activation system for certain other drugs (80,81). Perhaps one of the most striking examples of this is that aminopyrine metabolism appears to be mediated by the endogenous Cyt P-450-dependent monooxygenase system of hepatic microsomes inducible by barbiturates, whereas benzpyrene hydroxylase involves the transient methylcholanthrene-inducible Cyt P-448-dependent mixed-function oxidase system (82,83). With these differences in mind, it is of considerable interest to examine the role of dietary fat in altering specific drug-metabolizing enzymes. Martin et al. (68) reported that feeding a high-fat diet did not change the activity of benzpyrene hydroxylase or aminopyrene-N-demethylase, regardless of whether the fat was unsaturated and from a vegetable source (corn oil) or saturated and from a beef source (Table 4). However, it was observed that in male rats benzpyrene hydroxylase and aminopyrene-N-demethylase were related to the quan-

tity and not the quality of fat in the diet (68,72). Male rats fed high-
meat diets had significantly higher enzyme activity than those fed high-
vegetable-fat diet at both low and high levels of dietary fat (Table 4).
Stimulation of benzpyrene hydroxylase and aminopyrene-N-demethylase
in the liver of female rats was seen after feeding a high-vegetable-oil
diet rather than a high-beef-fat diet (68). Although the mechanism
for this sex-related difference is unclear, it is possible that the greater amount of unsaturated fat (i.e., corn oil) associated with the vegetarian diet may have altered the substrate binding (K_m) and the subsequent metabolic rates (V_{max}) in female rats (84).

Lambert and Wills (85,86) demonstrated that the activity of aminopyrine demethylase and benzpyrene hydroxylase was enhanced by feeding
a 10% corn oil diet (P/S = 5.4) or a 10% herring oil diet (P/S = 4.2)
when compared to values from a 10% lard (P/S = 1.25) group. These
results appear to directly contradict those of Martin et al. (68). However, after a comprehensive examination aimed at determining the exact
dietary constituent responsible for altering enzyme activity, Lambert
and Wills (85) concluded that the unsaponifiable fraction of the fat,
rather than the polyunsaturated fatty acid content, was of major importance in producing the increased rate (V_{max}) of hepatic oxidative
demethylation by aminopyrine, while cholesterol itself was less effective in increasing the rate of oxidative demethylation. In addition, adding cholesterol to a 10% lard diet caused an 8.6% increase in benzpyrene hydroxylase activity (86). Therefore, the higher cholesterol content of the beef diet when compared to the vegetable diet, in Martin
et al.'s (68) experiments, might in part be responsible for the elevated
hepatic aminopyrine demethylase and benzpyrene hydroxylase activity
exhibited in male rats.

The addition of cholesterol to olive oil or cocoa butter diets caused
significant elevation in hepatic UDP glucuronosyl transferase activity
when compared to values from rats fed diets containing olive oil or
cacao butter without cholesterol (87). In addition, ρ-nitrosoanisole-
O-demethylase activity was doubled in hepatic microsomes of rats fed
high-fat diets irrespective of the composition of the fat fed. It was the
contention of these authors that the activities of drug-metabolizing enzymes was dependent on the structure of the membrane, which, in
turn, was altered by the cholesterol content of the lipid content of the
diet (87). This concept is supported by studies in which elaidic and
linoleic acid was administered intraperitoneally to male rats (73). Simultaneous decreases in UDP-glucuronosyltransferase, ρ-nitroanisole-O-
demethylase, and the phospholipid structure of the microsomal membrane were observed (73). These results suggested that the fatty
acid-induced changes in the activities of the particular drug-metabolizing enzymes may be due to changes in the microenvironment of the enzymes bound to the membrane.

C. Cholesterol and Hepatic Mixed-Function Oxidase Systems

Cholesterol derived from the diet (85,86,88) as well as that synthesized in the body tissue (17,89) has been shown to have a profound effect on hepatic Cyt P-450 levels. Lambert and Wills (85) fed rats diets containing either 10% lard (P/S = 1.25; 90 mg of cholesterol/kg diet), 10% corn oil (P/S = 5.05; no cholesterol in diet), or 10% herring oil (P/S = 4.2; 745 mg of cholesterol/kg diet). In addition, the authors included a 10% lard + 0.2% cholesterol group (P/S = 1.25; 2180 mg of cholesterol/kg diet). A 300% increase in phenobarbital-induced Cyt P-450 levels was observed when 0.2% cholesterol was added to the 10% lard diet. The authors used these results as partial evidence to suggest that cholesterol directly induced elevation of hepatic Cyt P-450 levels. However, the percent increase in phenobarbital-induced Cyt P-450 levels was relatively similar in all three high-fat groups with a 59% increase in the 10% corn oil group and a 49% increase in the herring oil group. If dietary cholesterol alone was responsible for increased hepatic Cyt P-450 levels, the herring oil group should have had higher hepatic Cyt P-450 levels than the 10% corn oil and 10% lard group, since the cholesterol content in the herring oil diet is higher than that found in either the corn oil or lard groups (758 times and 9.3 times, respectively). Lambert and Wills (85) do suggest that a relationship between cholesterol content of the diet and the particular type of fatty acids present in the diet (i.e., saturated versus unsaturated) may also play a role in determining the level of Cyt P-450 in the liver. This explanation is plausible; however, it cannot be tested by the experimental design of Lambert and Wills (85), since they neglected to include a 10% corn oil–0.2% cholesterol and a 10% herring oil–0.2% cholesterol group.

A second possible explanation for Lambert and Wills (85) findings is the possibility that endogenous cholesterol levels (i.e., those found in the liver itself) may, in fact, regulate the level of Cyt P-450. Numerous studies have indicated that the rate of cholesterol synthesized in the liver as well as the amount of cholesterol stored in hepatic tissues can be altered by diet (90–94). We have demonstrated that by feeding various types and amounts of fiber, the level of cholesterol stored in the liver and hepatic Cyt P-450 levels can be simultaneously altered. Rats fed a 15% citrus pulp diet had the lowest level of hepatic cholesterol, Cyt P-450, and Cyt b_5. As the concentration of hepatic cholesterol increases (i.e., in the 15% wheat bran group), Cyt P-450 and Cyt b_5 levels increased. Rats consuming the control diets (5% alphacel) demonstrated the greatest hepatic cholesterol, Cyt P-450, and Cyt b_5 levels.

One puzzling observation in the study above was that the level of cholesterol present in the liver was not directly related to the changes

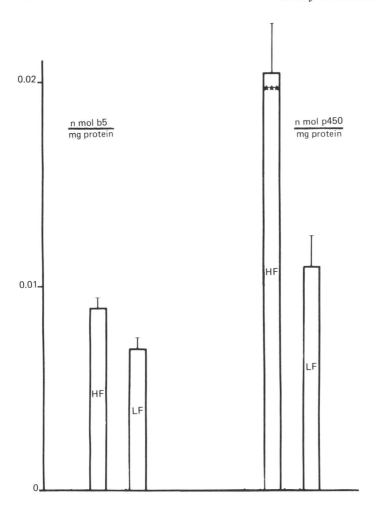

Figure 1 Effect of high- and low-fat diet on colonic cytochrome P-450 and cytochrome b_5 levels in F344 rats. Each bar denotes the mean ± SEM of pooled mucosa of 12 rats. A triple star represents significance at $P < 0.05$.

in activity of HMG-CoA reductase (E.C. 1.1.1.34), the key rate-limiting enzyme in cholesterol biosynthesis (93). This might be explained by the suggestion that the conversion of cholesterol to bile acids via 7α-hydroxylase may be different in the various fiber groups. 7α-Hydroxylase activity may be dependent on a Cyt P-450 which is similar, but not electrophoretically identical to Cyt P-450, essential for drug hydroxylation (89).

Table 5 Effect of Diet on Small Intestine Mucosal Mixed-Function Oxidase Enzymes in Male and Female Rats[a]

	Cytochrome P-450 (nmol mg protein^{-1})	Benzpyrene hydroxylase (nmol mg protein^{-1} min^{-1})	Aminopyrene demethylase (nmol HCHO mg protein^{-1} min^{-1})
Females			
Corn oil (5%)	0.04 ± 0.006	12.1 ± 2.0	1.5 ± 0.1
Beef fat (6%)	0.05 ± 0.001	5.51 ± 1.3[b]	0.5 ± 0.09[c]
High corn oil (25%)	0.09 ± 0.004	0.6 ± 2.0	1.7 ± 0.3
High beef fat (25%)	0.97 ± 0.007	10.2 ± 1.3	0.4 ± 0.08[c]
Males			
Corn oil (5%)	0.03 ± 0.004	2.8 ± 0.4	0.6 ± 0.1
Beef fat (6%)	0.06 ± 0.006[c]	3.8 ± 0.7	0.7 ± 0.1
High corn oil (25%)	0.04 ± 0.006	2.9 ± 0.4	0.9 ± 0.1
High beef fat (25%)	0.05 ± 0.004[b]	2.9 ± 0.5	0.6 ± 0.1

[a]Mean ± SEM for eight animals per group.
[b]Significantly different from opposite diet, $P < 0.01$.
[c]Significantly different from opposite diet, $P < 0.05$.

D. Dietary Fat and Extrahepatic Mixed-Function Oxidase Systems

Although the liver appears to be the major site of drug metabolism,
extrahepatic tissues such as the small intestine and colon contain MFO
systems capable of metabolizing drugs (68,71,87,88,95,96). A 14%
increase in small intestine mucosal and a 50% increase in colonic mucosal Cyt P-450 levels was observed in male rats fed a 20% corn oil
diet when compared to values observed in male rats fed a 5% corn oil
diet (71) (Figure 1). These results substantiated those previously
reported by Martin et al. (68), who found that increasing the amount
of vegetable fat fed to male and female rats caused an increase in
the level of Cyt P-450 present in the small intestine (Table 5).
However, increasing the amount of saturated fat caused no change in
small intestine mucosal Cyt P-450 levels in male rats (66,88), while a
30% increase in the small intestine of female rats fed a high-satu-
rated-fat diet has been reported (68) (Table 5). These results present a complex interaction between the level of fat, the type of fat,
the sex of the experimental animal, and extrahepatic Cyt P-450 levels.

A sex-related stimulation of benzpyrene hydroxylase activity in the
small intestine of male rats fed a high-vegetable-fat diet was reported
by Martin et al. (68) (Table 5). These results contradict those of
Chhabra and Fouts (97), who reported that there were no sex-related
differences in the extrahepatic metabolism of benzpyrene by small intestine microsomes, whereas Hietanen (87) showed that female Wistar
rats had a lower capacity to hydroxylate benzpyrene than male rats
and that castration of male rats did not alter enzyme activities significantly. Although the mechanism for these differences is not clear, it
is possible that the differences in the source of dietary fat or the sex
of the rat may have altered substrate binding (K_m) and the subsequent
metabolic rate (V_{max}) in female rats (84,98).

V. LIPIDS AND EXPERIMENTAL CARCINOGENESIS

During the past two decades, epidemiologic studies have elaborated on
the influence of the environment in general and particularly the role
of dietary factors on the development of certain forms of cancer (99).
These studies suggest that as we identify the ways in which environmental factors increase the risk of cancer we may be in a position to
manipulate the environment and reduce to a minimum the risk of cancer
in future generations.

Following up on leads advanced by epidemiologists (100,101), exper-
mentalists have found that nutrition is related to the development of
cancer in three ways: (1) food additives or contaminants may act
as carcinogens, cocarcinogens, or both; (2) nutrient deficiencies may
lead to biochemical alterations that produce neoplastic processes; and
(3) changes in the intake of selected macronutrients such as fat, pro-

tein, or carbohydrate may produce metabolic and biochemical abnormalities, either directly or indirectly, which increase the risk of cancer. This part of the review presents an evaluation of the current status of the relationship between dietary fat and chemical carcinogenesis in the animal model and will question the inconsistencies and make recommendations for additional research.

A. Early Studies

An early study in which tumors were produced by skin painting with B[a]P, 3-MC, or dibenz[a,h]anthracene showed that in the case of five different fats, three different basal diets, and two strains of mice, the tumor incidence increased when the dietary fat level exceeded 15% (102). Tannenbaum (103) and Silverstone and Tannenbaum (104) showed that a regimen that contained enhanced levels of fat led to an increased incidence of B[a]P-induced skin tumors in Swiss, C57 Black, and DBA mice. With mammary tumors in DBA mice, either the latency period was reduced or the number of tumors increased. Lavik and Baumann (105), showed that enhancement of skin tumorigenesis in mice was related to the triglyceride component of dietary fat, rather than the nonsaponifiable fraction. Dietary fat appears to affect primarily the developmental stage of tumorigenesis (106). It is difficult to rule out completely the possibility that dietary fat exerts some effect on the carcinogenic agent, but it seems more probable that fat acts by providing a more favorable environment for the development of latent tumor cells.

The importance of the type of fat in the diet is well documented by the DAB-induced hepatomas. Substitution of hydrogenated coconut oil for corn oil reduced the number of hepatomas (107), although the more potent carcinogenic 3'-methyl derivative did not show a similar effect (108). The fatty acids obtained from hydrogenated coconut oil and corn oil produced similar DAB-induced tumor yield (109).

B. Experimental Studies in Colon Carcinogenesis

Research on the mechanisms of cancer causation in the large bowel (Table 6) has been assisted by the discovery over the last 20 years of several animal models that mirror the type of lesions seen in humans. These models are (1) induction of large bowel cancer in rats through chemicals such as 3-methyl-4-aminobiphenyl or 3-methyl-2-naphthylamine; (2) derivatives and analogs of cycasin and methylazoxymethanol (MAM) such as azoxymethane (AOM) and 1,2-dimethylhydrazine (DMH), which work well in rats and mice of selected strains; (3) intrarectal administration of direct-acting carcinogens of the type of alkylnitrosoureas, such as methylnitrosourea (MNU) or N-methyl-N'-

Table 6 Modifying Factors in Colon Cancer

Dietary fat[a]	Dietary fibers[a,b]	Micronutrients[c]
1. Increases bile acid secretion into gut	1. Certain fibers increase fecal bulk and dilute carcinogens and promoters	1. Modify carcinogenesis at activation and detoxification level
2. Increases metabolic activity of gut bacteria	2. Modify metabolic activity of gut bacteria	2. Act also at promotional phase of carcinogenesis
3. Increases secondary bile acids in colon	3. Modify the metabolism of carcinogens and/or promoters	
4. Alters immune system		
5. Stimulation of mixed-function oxidase system		

[a]Dietary factors, particularly high total dietary fat and a relative lack of certain dietary fibers and vegetables, have a role.
[b]High dietary fiber or fibrous foods may be a protective factor even in the high dietary fat intake.
[c]Include vitamins, minerals, antioxidants, etc.

nitro-N-nitrosoguanidine (MNNG), which lead to cancer of the descending large bowel in every species tested so far; and (4) the oral administration of large doses of 3-methylcholanthrene, which leads to large-bowel cancer in selected strains of hamsters (24).

1. Effect of Dietary Fat on Chemically Induced Colon Carcinogenesis

Investigations were carried out to study the possible role of dietary fat in large-bowel carcinogenesis using the animal models and direct-acting carcinogens, as well as those requiring activation. However, the data generated from certain studies could not be compared validly with other studies because of variations in experimental parameters, including composition of experimental diets, selective differences in the food intake by the animals, differences in the nature of the carcinogen used, and alterations in the susceptibility of a particular animal strain to carcinogen treatment.

The stage of carcinogenesis at which the effect of dietary fat is exerted appears to be during the promotional phase of carcinogenesis rather than during initiation phase (9). Enhancement of carcinogenesis by high-fat diet can be blocked by some, but not all, antioxidants and may be related to the ability of antioxidants to induce MFO or other enzymes. In addition, absorption, distribution, metabolic activation, and inactivation, as well as excretion of carcinogens and other chemicals, may be influenced by the actions of dietary fat on gastrointestinal motility, metabolism of absorptive cells, transport mechanisms, MFO and other enzymes, bacterial metabolism in the gut, and possibly excretory pathways. However, definitive pharmacokinetic and metabolic data are not available to give a complete view of the influence of dietary fat on the metabolism of any one carcinogen.

Nigro et al. (110) induced intestinal tumors in male Sprague-Dawley rats by subcutaneous administration of AOM at a weekly dose rate of 8 mg/kg body weight for about 24 weeks and compared animals fed Purina chow with 35% beef fat to those fed Purina chow containing about 5% fat. Animals fed the high-fat diet developed more intestinal tumors and more metastases into abdominal cavity, lungs, and liver than the rats fed the low-fat diet. In this study, however, the two experimental diets were not adjusted isocalorically and rats consumed less food when given the high-fat diet than when on a low-fat diet. In addition, the simple addition of fat to a complete diet dilutes all nutrients in the diet and reduces dietary intake because of increased caloric density of the diet.

In another study, W/Fu rats fed a 30% lard diet had an increased number of DMH-induced large-bowel tumors compared to the animals fed the standard diet (111). Rogers and Newberne (112) found that a diet marginally deficient in lipoproteins but high in fat enhanced DMH-induced colon carcinogenesis in Sprague-Dawley rats. These results suggest that total dietary fat may have a function in the pathogenesis of colon cancer.

Table 7 Colon Tumor Incidence in Rats Fed Diets High in Fat and Treated with Carcinogenesis

Source of dietary fat	Percentage in diet	Source of dietary protein	Percentage in diet	Carcinogen	Percentage of rats with colon tumors
Lard	5	Casein	25	DMH[a]	17
Lard	20	Casein	25	DMH[a]	67
Corn oil	5	Casein	25	DMH[a]	36
Corn oil	20	Casein	25	DMH[a]	64
Beef fat	24	Beef	40	DMH[a]	57
Beef fat	6	Beef	19	DMH[a]	35
Corn oil	24	Soybean	40	DMH[a]	54
Corn oil	6	Soybean	19	DMH[a]	35
Beef fat	20	Casein	22	DMH[b]	60
Beef fat	5	Casein	22	DMH[b]	27
Beef fat	20	Casein	22	MNU[c]	73
Beef fat	5	Casein	22	MNU[c]	33
Beef fat	20	Casein	22	MAM acetate[d]	80
Beef fat	5	Casein	22	MAM acetate[d]	45
Beef fat	20	Casein	20	DMAB[e]	74
Beef fat	5	Casein	20	DMAB[e]	26

[a]Female F344 rats, at 7 weeks of age, were given weekly s. c. DMH at a dose rate of 10 mg/kg body weight for 20 weeks and autopsied 10 weeks later.

[b]Male F344 rats, at 7 weeks of age, were given a single dose of s. c. DMH, 150 mg/kg body weight, and autopsied 30 weeks later.

[c]Male F344 rats, at 7 weeks of age, were given i. r. MNU, 2.5 mg/rat twice in one week, and autopsied 30 weeks later.

[d]Male F344 rats, at 7 weeks of age, were given i. p. MAM acetate, 35 mg/kg body weight once, and autopsied 30 weeks later.

[e]Male F344 rats, at 7 weeks of age, were given weekly s. c. DMAB, 50 mg/kg body weight for 20 weeks, and autopsied 20 weeks later.

Inasmuch as humans in various populations usually follow comparable dietary regimens over generations, Reddy et al. (113) designed experiments to study the effect of a particular type and amount of dietary fat for two generations before animals were exposed to treatment with a carcinogen. Virgin female rats fed diets containing 5% corn oil, 20% corn oil, 5% lard, or 20% lard were bred and the litters were weaned to the same diet consumed by the mothers. At 7 weeks of age, all second-generation animals, except controls, received 20 weekly subcutaneous doses of DMH (10 mg/kg body weight) and were continued on their respective diets. Animals fed 20% lard or 20% corn oil were more susceptible to colon tumor induction by DMH than those in other groups (Table 7). The type of fat appears to be immaterial at the 20% level, although at the 5% fat level there is a suggestion that unsaturated fat (corn oil) predisposes to more DMH-induced colon tumors than saturated fat (lard). In a similar experimental design, combinations of high beef protein (40%) and high beef fat (20%) or high soybean protein (40%) and high corn oil (20%) led to more DMH-induced colon tumors in F344 rats than did control diets of beef protein (20%) and low beef fat (6%) or soybean protein (20%) and low-corn-oil diet (6%) (114) (Table 7). Broitman et al. (115) showed that rats fed a 20% safflower oil diet had more DMH-induced large-bowel tumors than did those animals fed either the 5% or 20% coconut oil diets. These studies provide no evidence that dietary polyunsaturated fat per se is more effective than saturated fat in augmenting tumorigenesis by DMH. However, these data indicate that at low density fat levels, diets rich in polyunsaturated fats are more effective tumor promoters than diets rich in saturated fats. With regard to the relationship between dietary fat and colon cancer, one fundamental point that remains to be solved is the question of the specific roles played by essential polyunsaturated fatty acids vis-à-vis saturated fatty acids.

Investigations were also carried out to test the effect of high dietary fat on colon tumor induction by a variety of carcinogens, DMH, MAM acetate, DMAB, or MNU, which not only differ in metabolic activation but also represent a broad spectrum of exogenous carcinogens (27,116) (Table 7). Male F344 weanling rats were fed semipurified diets containing 20 or 5% beef fat. At 7 weeks of age, animals were given DMH (subcutaneous, 150 mg/kg body weight, one dose), MAM acetate (intraperitoneal, 35 mg/kg body weight, one dose), DMAB (subcutaneous, 50 mg/kg body weight, weekly for 20 weeks), or MNU (intrarectal, 2.5 mg per rat weekly for 2 weeks) and autopsied 30–35 weeks later. Irrespective of the colon carcinogen, animals fed a diet containing 20% beef fat had a greater incidence of colon tumors than did rats fed a diet containing 5% beef fat (Table 7).

The suggestion that promotion may be involved in intestinal cancer has been supported by the observation that the carcinogenic response to a variety of intestinal carcinogens is enhanced by the dietary fat, which in itself is not carcinogenic (9). Recent studies indicate that

the enhanced tumorigenesis in the animals fed the high-fat diet is due
to promotional effects (117). Ingestion of high-fat diet increased the
intestinal tumor incidence when fed after carcinogen (AOM) administration, but not during or before AOM treatment. Therefore, the high-
fat diet in this model exhibited most of the properties of promoters
developed from mouse-skin cancer (118). The carcinogenic process in
the human may have similar characteristics since there is a good correlation between the findings in a variety of animal studies and those
done in humans (9). Due to the wide variety of initiating agents and
the possible difficulties in removing them from the environment, the
promotional phase of carcinogenesis may be a more promising area of
development of preventive measures.

In order to understand specifics of the mechanisms whereby dietary
fat influences colon cancer, the effect of high dietary fat on biliary
and fecal bile acid pattern was investigated. Many secondary bile acids
have been shown to act as colon tumor promoters. Biliary excretion
of total bile acids, as well as cholic acid, β-muricholic acid, ursodeoxy-
cholic acid, and deoxycholic acid, was higher in rats fed a diet containing 20% corn oil or 20% lard than in rats fed diets containing 5% corn
oil or 5% lard. High fat (corn oil or lard at 20% level) intake was associated with an increased excretion of fecal neutral sterols and bile
acids. The excretion of deoxycholic acid, lithocholic acid, and 12-
ketolithocholic acid was increased in rats fed high-fat diets (119).

2. Bile Acids and Cholesterol in Colon Carcinogenesis

The role of bile acids in colon carcinogenesis has received some support
from studies in animal models. In one study, the carcinogenic effect of
AOM in rats was increased by surgically diverting bile to the middle
of the small intestine, which also raised the fecal excretion of bile salts
(120). The evidence of the importance of bile acids as colon tumor
promoters came from studies by Narisawa et al. (121) and Reddy et al.
(122,123) (Table 8). The development of adenomas significantly increased among those conventional rats initiated with limited amounts of
intrarectal MNNG to give a definite low yield of colon cancer and administered with intrarectal lithocholic acid or taurodeoxycholic acid as
promoters compared to the groups that was given only the carcinogen.
Deoxycholic acid applied topically to the colon increased MNNG-induced
colon adenocarcinomas in germ-free rats. The bile acids themselves
did not produce any tumors.

A recent study also indicates that the primary bile acids, cholic acid
and chenodeoxycholic acid, also produced a MNNG-induced colon-tumor-
promoting activity in rats (123). Cholic acid and chenodeoxycholic acid
given intrarectally to conventional rats are subjected to bacterial 7α-
dehydroxylation to deoxycholic acid and lithocholic acid, respectively.

Table 8 Colon Tumor Incidence in Germ-Free and Conventional Rats Treated with Intrarectal MNNG and(or) Bile Acids[a]

	Germ-free		Conventional	
	Rats with tumors (%)	Tumors/rat	Rats with tumors (%)	Tumors/rat
Cholic acid (10–12)[b]	0	0	0	0
Chenodeoxycholic acid (10–12)	0	0	0	0
Lithocholic acid (10–12)	0	0	0	0
MNNG (22–30)	27	0.27	37	0.55
MNNG + cholic acid (24–30)	50	0.63	67[c]	0.87
MNNG + chenodeoxycholic acid (24–30)	54	1.08	70[c]	1.23
MNNG + lithocholic acid (24)	71[c]	1.04	83[c]	1.83

[a]Cholic acid, chenodeoxycholic acid, or lithocholic acid group received intrarectally 20 mg of sodium salt of respective bile acid three times weekly for 48 weeks; MNNG group received intrarectally 2 mg of MNNG twice a week for 2 weeks followed by vehicle for 46 weeks; MNNG + lithocholic acid, or MNNG + chenodeoxycholic acid group received intrarectally MNNG for 2 weeks and bile acid thereafter for 16 weeks.

[b]Number of rats are shown in parentheses.

[c]Significantly different from rats given MNNG alone by chi-square test, P < 0.05.

Cohen et al. (124) reported that cholic acid in the diet increases MNU-induced colon carcinogenesis in rats. Total fecal bile acids, particularly deoxycholic acid output, was elevated in animals fed cholic acid compared to controls. This increase in fecal deoxycholic acid was due to bacterial 7α-dehydroxylation for cholic acid in the colonic contents. These studies demonstrate that these secondary bile acids have a promoting effect in colon carcinogenesis.

The colon-tumor-promoting effect of cholesterol, cholesterol-5α,6α-epoxide (epoxide), and cholestane-3β,5α,6β-triol (triol) was studied in F344 rats (125). Our results indicate that cholesterol epoxide and triol do not exhibit any colon-tumor-promoting activity in both germ-free and conventional rats.

The mechanisms of action of bile acids in colon carcinogenesis has not been elucidated. Bile acids have been shown to affect cell kinetics in the intestinal epithelium, although the structural specificity of this effect has not been examined extensively (126,127). In the intestine, the data do not permit a critical distinction between a direct effect of bile acids on cell division and an indirect or physiological stimulus secondary to increased cell loss from sloughing or damage (126). The cell renewal system is dynamic and may be influenced by changes in a number of factors, including the composition of gut microflora (128) and bile acids in the intestine (129). Recently, Cohen et al. (124) reported an enhanced colonic cell proliferation in rats fed cholic acid, as well as in animals treated with intrarectal MNU. This increased cell proliferation involved in DNA synthesis induced by cholic acid feeding would favor the expression of damage at a far higher level than with the carcinogen MNU alone, bringing about not only a greater overall incidence of MNU-induced colon tumors, but also an enhanced number of tumors in rats fed cholic acid. Lipkin (130) demonstrated that during neoplastic transformation of colonic cells, a similar sequence of changes leading to uncontrolled proliferative activity develops in colon cancer in humans and in rodents given a chemical carcinogen that induces colon cancer.

Although the molecular mechanisms of tumor-promoting action of bile acids are not completely understood, recent studies of Takano et al. (131) suggest that the induction of colonic epithelial ornithine decarboxylase (ODC) and S-adenosyl-L-methionine decarboxylase (SAMD) activities by the bile acids may play a role in these mechanisms. The studies reported by Takano et al. (131) indicate that the colonic epithelial responses of the polyamine-biosynthetic enzymes ODC and SAMD to applications of bile acids are among the earliest changes to occur in this tissue in response to promoting agents.

Irrespective of the mechanism by which bile acids enhance cell proliferations, decrease the generation time of proliferating cells, and/or increase the colonic ODC and SAMD biosynthesis, the phenomenon may have important implications for colon carcinogenesis.

C. Experimental Studies in Breast Cancer

Within the past few years, animal models have been developed to induce mammary tumors by the administration of 2-AAF, DMBA, and MNU (8,132,133). After a single oral dose of 5–10 mg of DMBA in corn oil, female Sprague-Dawley rats develop mammary tumors within 4 months. Gullino et al. (132) first reported experiments in which high yields of mammary tumors were found in three strains of rats following multiple injections of MNU. Metastasis to bone marrow and spleen and hypercalcemia were reported, suggesting that MNU model may more closely mimic human breast cancer than the more commonly used DMBA tumor model, which does not metastasize or induce hypercalcemia. Chan et al. (133) have developed a protocol in which a single intravenous dose of MNU (25 mg or 50 mg/kg body weight) was used. An essential aspect of this tumor model is its sensitivity to changes in the experimental variables under study such as diet. With regard to low-fat diets, mammary tumor incidence in animals receiving 50 mg of MNU/kg body weight is approximately 40%. Using these models, the effects of qualitative and quantitative aspects of fats were studied.

1. Dietary Fat as a Tumor-Promoting Agent

Carroll and Khor (106) showed that, in the DMBA model, the high fat effect could be demonstrated only when the diet was administered after initiation with DMBA. When a high-fat diet was given before initiation and then replaced by a low-fat diet, no enhancement was seen. Hence it appears that the dietary effect is exerted at the promotion, but not the initiation phase of breast carcinogenesis. Available evidence suggests that as the carcinogen dose increases, the promoting effect of dietary fat becomes less and less pronounced, a finding of considerable importance with regard to the human disease. The fact that ubiquitous environmental carcinogens are present at very low concentrations suggests that promoting factors may have a preponderant influence on the eventual outcome of the neoplastic process in humans.

2. Quantity and Quality of Dietary Fat

Using the MNU model, Chan et al. (133) studied the effect of high- or low-fat diet on breast cancer incidence in female F344 rats (Figure 2). MNU was administered intravenously at 55 days of age and the animals were then fed a high-fat diet (20% lard) or a low-fat diet (5% lard). The median latent period was 83 days in the high-fat group and 103 days in the low-fat group. The tumor incidence differed significantly from the 18-days-after-MNU administration; high intake of dietary fat increased the incidence of MNU-induced mammary tumors.

Using the DMBA model, Carroll and Khor (8,106) also studied the effect of a variety of fats and oils on breast cancer development. When tumor incidence was the end point measured, high-fat diets promoted

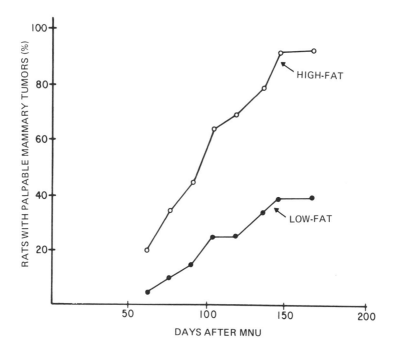

Figure 2 Effect of high- or low-fat diet on methylnitrosourea-induced breast cancer incidence in female F344 rats.

tumor development in most but not all cases. However, when total tumor yield was the end point measured (i.e., the total number of tumors per animal), consistent differences emerged. Animals fed fats that were deficient in or contained low levels of the essential fatty acid linoleate, such as coconut oil and tallow, exhibited significantly lower total tumor yields than did animals fed fats rich in linoleate, such as corn or sunflower seed oil. These results were confirmed under somewhat different experimental conditions by Nishizuka (134) and Hopkins et al. (135).

The reason for the discrepancy between results obtained from tumor incidence measurements and tumor multiplicity measurements is unclear at present. Part of the problem may lie in the fact that the conditions under which these experiments were conducted differed particularly with regard to key intervening variables, such as carcinogen dose, animal strain, and diet composition.

Another aspect of the high-fat effect on breast carcinogenesis is the finding in the DMBA model that the tumorigenic response to fat intake is not linear in nature. When corn oil was the source of dietary fat, a

threshold was reached beyond which increases in fat intake had no
further influence on tumor incidence. When the corn oil content of the
diet was increased from 5 to 20%, a significant difference in tumor incidence occurred. However, increasing dietary fat above 20% or decreasing it below 5% had no discernible effect on tumor incidence. Apparently, in the DMBA model, physiological responses were triggered
only when fat comprises 8—12% of the diet.

The relationship between dietary linoleic acid intake and tumor yield
is not linear. Animals fed high-fat diets containing lard or olive oil,
which contain 11% and 7% linoleate, respectively, develop almost as
many tumors as those fed high-fat diets rich in linoleate, such as corn
oil and sunflower seed oil (56% and 75% linoleate, respectively). In a
recent study by Hopkins and Carroll (136), mixtures of linoleic acid-
rich and linoleic acid-poor fats were added at 20% to the diet. It was
found that DMBA-treated animals exhibited comparable tumor yields,
provided that greater than 2% linoleate was present in the diet. In addition, when carcinogen-treated animals were fed low-fat diets (20%),
total tumor yields were significantly decreased in the low-fat groups.
These results suggest that a certain amount of linoleic acid as well as
a high-fat diet are required for optimal tumor growth enhancement.

Major themes that emerged from this survey of experimental studies
on dietary fat and breast carcinogenesis are as follows: (1) dietary
fat exerts its effects on the promotional phase of breast carcinogenesis; (2) promoting agents, such as excess dietary fat, play a more significant role in determining the eventual outcome of the neoplastic process when the initiating carcinogen dose is low than when it is high;
(3) the total quantity of dietary fat, irrespective of qualitative factors,
is a central factor in the high-fat effect; and (4) a certain threshold
quantity of essential fatty acids is a necessary requirement for full expression of the high-fat effect.

3. Mechanism(s) of Action of Dietary Fat

Detailed reviews of the possible mechanism(s) by which dietary fat
may exert its effect on breast cancer have been published by Hopkins
and West (137), Hankin and Rawlings (138), and Miller (139). Two
mechanistic hypotheses have emerged from these reviews: (1) direct
effects at the level of the mammary gland, and (2) indirect effects mediated by host systems remote from the mammary gland.

Direct effects are based on the physical and chemical properties of
fat, the formation of lipid peroxides, alterations in membrane structures and/or function, and enhanced prostaglandin synthesis.

The role of adipose tissue in breast carcinogenesis (either acting as
a reservoir or depot for carcinogens) has been studied, since adipose
tissue rapidly takes up and slowly releases lipid-soluble agents. It has
been proposed that the adipose tissue surrounding ductal cells may
contribute to the susceptibility of tissue cells to cancer by prolonged

exposure to lipid-soluble carcinogens of endogenous or exogenous origins (140,141). Dao et al. (142) suggested that mammary adipose tissue functioned as a storage depot for hydrocarbons. However, this model appears unlikely since tumor incidence is not affected by a high-fat or a low-fat diet given prior to DMBA treatment, with subsequent placement of the experiental animal on a high-fat diet (8).

Since polyunsaturated fatty acids are converted by free radical reactions to lipid peroxides, a model involving breast cancer and lipid peroxidation has been advanced. Lipid peroxidation has been associated with carcinogenesis (143). It is possible that increased peroxidation of membrane lipids results in alterations in the function of transformed mammary cell membranes, which, in turn, permit increased rates of growth (137). However, available evidence suggests that lipid peroxidation and free radical processes accompanying it are associated primarily with the activation of procarcinogens (144) and not with the promotion of tumor development. Little evidence is available to suggest a role for peroxidation processes in the past transformation events, where dietary fat exerts its stimulatory effect.

Direct changes in the lipid composition of cell membranes induced by diet could have far-reaching structural and functional effects on membrane permeability and the activity of membrane-bound enzyme systems. The relevance of these membrane changes to the stimulatory effect of a high-fat diet remains to be established, however.

Indirect mechanisms are those in which dietary fat secondarily stimulates mammary tumor growth by modifying the physiology of the host. Some evidence exists that dietary fat intake alters the function of at least two major systems that regulate the internal environment: (1) mixed-function oxidases (MFO), and (2) endocrine control systems. These mechanisms are not necessarily mutually exclusive and may interact with each other. Evidence suggests that nutritional factors can markedly influence activity of microsomal MFO enzymes (1). It is well established that mixed-function exidase systems are the key in the biotransformation of chemical carcinogens (145) and steroids (146). Steroids such as androgens and estrogens have been implicated in breast carcinogenesis, and alterations in steroid-metabolizing enzyme systems such as MFO by diet could, in turn, influence breast cancer development. Although the biotransformation of carcinogens to their active metabolites is a major role of MFO, it is unlikely that this aspect of MFO function is involved in the fat effect, since the influence of fat is exerted days or weeks after carcinogen administration.

The work of Furth (147), Pearson (148), and Meites (149) demonstrated that although a variety of hormones are involved in mammary tumor growth, prolactin is the predominant factor in rodent breast cancer development. Meites (149) showed in the DMBA model that experimental procedures that elevate serum prolactin increased tumor yield. It should be noted that tumor yield is enhanced only if the prolactin-elevating procedure is introduced after DMBA administration, a response strikingly reminiscent of the fat effect on breast carcinogenesis.

Based on the foregoing considerations, Chan and Cohen (150) designed a series of experiments to assess the relationhips between high-fat intake, prolactin secretion, and mammary carcinogenesis. Drugs that antagonize estrogen action and block prolactin secretion retarded tumor development as expected. Only the antiprolactin drug abolished the differential in tumor incidence characteristic of animals fed high- and low-fat diets. Although indirect, the results suggested that the fat effect was mediated by prolactin. It was also found that rats fed a high-fat diet exhibited significantly higher serum prolactin levels than did rats fed a low-fat diet (151).

Direct proof that dietary fat alters circulating prolactin levels, but not estrogen levels, was obtained by simultaneous measurement of prolactin and estrogen levels in the serum of MNU-treated animals 20 weeks after carcinogen treatment. The high-fat groups exhibited (1) elevated prolactin levels, (2) unchanged total estrogens; and (3) elevated prolactin to estrogen ratios at both proestrus-estrous and metestrous-diestrous.

Boyns et al. (152) and Hawkins et al. (153) found that in three strains of rats with different genetically determined susceptibilities to the carcinogenic action of DMBA, tumor yield was directly proportional to plasma prolactin levels, whereas estrogen levels were unchanged, again suggesting that rat mammary tumor development is a function of the relative proportions of circulatory prolactin and estrogen.

VI. CONCLUSION

During the last decade, as this review indicates, impressive progress has been made in the understanding of numerous steps involved in the metabolism of foreign or carcinogenic compounds, as well as the role played by the dietary constituents in general and specifically the role of lipids in the metabolism of carcinogenic compounds. Although there is much need for further research to understand the modification of carcinogenic process, the successes thus achieved have expanded into some understanding of the numerous steps involved in the action and detoxification of various chemical carcinogens and promoters by a variety of means.

The population with high incidences of cancer of the breast and large bowel are characterized by consumption of a high level of dietary fat. Thus alteration of dietary habits leading to a lower intake of fat would be indicated to decrease the risk of these important cancers. Beginning this dietary pattern early in life may prove most beneficial.

The demonstration of two stages in experimentally induced cancer in animal models suggests that there are two stages in environmentally induced cancer in humans (118). Most human cancers probably result from a complex interaction of carcinogens, cocarcinogens, and tumor promoters. Most of nutritional or dietary factors act at the promotional phase of carcinogenesis. Because promotion is a reversible process, in contrast to the rapid, irreversible process of initiation by carcinogens, manipulation of promotion would seem to be the best method of cancer prevention (9,118). Such studies have not been conducted to any great extent in animal systems and should be considered for future research programs.

In addition to pinpointing harmful environmental agents and their elimination, which is also one of the practical methods of preventing cancer, there seems to be on the horizon the promise of select methods of prevention. Application of a number of such basic tools, elimination of harmful agents from the environment, reduction of biochemical activation processes, and a concomitant increase in detoxification reactions, as well as trapping of active intermediates by harmless nucleophilic reagents point to a promising future for preventive efforts. Thus there is hope that these important types of cancer can be controlled by modifying not only environment with respect to genotoxic carcinogens, but also that of epigenetic carcinogens and thus human cancer risk feasibly can be reduced.

ACKNOWLEDGMENTS

The authors' research is supported by Grants CA-16382 through the National Large Bowel Cancer Project, CA-12376, and CA-17613 (Cancer Center Support Grant), and Contracts CP-85659 and CP-05721 from the National Cancer Institute. The authors thank Ms. Arlene Banow for preparation of the manuscript.

REFERENCES

1. Campbell, T. C. (1978). *Adv. Nutr. Res.* 2:29.
2. Weisburger, J. W., and Williams, G. (1980). In *Casarette and Doull's Toxicology*, 2nd ed., J. Doull, C. D. Klaassen, and M. O. Amdur, Eds., Macmillan, New York, p. 84.
3. Searle, C. E. (1976). *Chemical Carcinogens*, ACS Monograph 173, American Chemical Society, Washington, D. C.
4. Miller, E. C., and Miller, J. A. (1947).
5. Wattenberg, L. W. (1978). *Adv. Cancer Res.* 26:197.
6. Miller, E. C. (1978). *Cancer Res.* 38:1479.
7. Warwick, G. P. (1971). *Fed. Proc.* 30:1760.
8. Carroll, K. K. (1975). *Cancer Res.* 35:3374.

9. Reddy, B. S., Cohen, L. C., McCoy, G. D., Hill, P., Weisburger, J. H., and Wynder, E. L. (1980). *Adv. Cancer Res.* 32:237.
10. Lu, A. Y. H. (1976). *Fed. Proc.* 35:2460.
11. Chhabra, R. S., and Fouts, J. R. (1976). *Drug Metab. Dispos.* 4:208.
12. Lawley, P. D. (1976). In *Chemical Carcinogens,* C. E. Searle, Ed., ACS Monograph 173, American Chemical Society, Washington, D. C., p. 83.
13. Sugimura, T., and Kawachi, T. (1973). *Methods Cancer Res.* 7:245.
14. Narisawa, T., and Weisburger, J. H. (1975). *Proc. Soc. Exp. Biol. Med.* 148:166.
15. Druckrey, H. (1973). In *Topics in Chemical Carcinogenesis,* W. Nakahara, S. Takayama, T. Sugimura, and S. Odashima, Eds., University Park Press, Baltimore, Md., p. 73.
16. Weisburger, J. H., Marquardt, H., Hiroto, N., Mori, H., and Williams, G. M. (1980). *J. Natl. Cancer Inst.* 64:163.
17. Druckery, H. (1975). *Gann Monogr.* 17:107.
18. Rajewsky, M. F., Augenlicht, L. H., Biessmann, H., Goth, R., Hulser, D. F., Laerum, O. D., and Lomakina, L. Y. (1977). In *Origins of Human Cancer,* H. H. Hiatt, J. D. Watson, and J. A. Winstein, Eds., Cold Spring Harbor Laboratory, Cold Spring Harbor, N. Y., p. 709.
19. Arcos, J. C. (1978). *J. Environ. Pathol. Toxicol.* 1:433.
20. Jones, P. W., and Freudenthal, R. I. (1978). *Polynuclear Aromatic Hydrocarbons. Carcinogenesis—A Comprehensive Survey,* Vol. 3, Raven Press, New York.
21. Hecht, S., Loy, M., Mazzarese, R., and Hoffmann, D. (1978). *J. Med. Chem.* 21:38.
22. Jerina, D., Yagi, H., Lehr, R. E., Thakker, D. R., Schaefer-Ridder, M., Karle, J. M., Levin, W., Wood, A. W., Chang, R. L., and Conney, A. H. (1978). In *Polycyclic Hydrocarbons and Cancer: Environment, Chemistry, Molecular and Cell Biology,* H. V. Gelboin and P. O. P. Ts'o, Eds., Academic Press, New York.
23. Magee, P. N., Montesano, R., and Preussmann, R. (1976). In *Chemical Carcinogens,* C. E. Searle, Ed., ACS Monograph 173, American Chemical Society, Washington, D. C., p. 491.
24. Bralow, S. P., and Weisburger, J. H. (1976). *Clin. Gastroenterol.* 5:527.
25. Walpole, A. L., Williams, M. H., and Roberts, D. C. (1952). *Br. J. Ind. Med.* 9:255.
26. Reddy, B. S., and Watanabe, K. (1978). *J. Natl. Cancer. Inst.* 61:1269.

27. Reddy, B. S., and Ohmori, T. (1981). *Cancer Res.* *41*:1363.
28. Gutmann, H. R., Leaf, D. S., Yost, Y., Rydell, R. E., and Chen, C. C. (1970). *Cancer Res.* *30*:1485.
29. Jollow, D. J. (1977). *Biological Reactive Intermediates: Formation, Toxicity and Inactivation,* Plenum Press, New York.
30. Magee, P. N. (1977). In *Origins of Human Cancer,* H. H. Hiatt, J. D. Watson, and J. A. Winstein, Eds., Cold Spring Harbor Laboratory, Cold Spring Harbor, N. Y., p. 629.
31. Miller, J. A., and Miller, E. C. (1977). In *Origins of Human Cancer,* H. H. Hiatt, J. D. Watson, and J. A. Winstein, Eds., Cold Spring Harbor Laboratory, Cold Spring Harbor, N. Y., p. 605.
32. Schmähl, D., and Habs, M. (1980). *Oncology* *37*:237.
33. Druckrey, H., Preussmann, R., Ivankovic, S., and Schmähl, D. (1967). *Z. Krebsforsch.* *69*:103.
34. Schmeltz, I., and Hoffmann, D. (1977). *Chem. Res.* *77*:295.
35. Hecht, S. S., Chen, C. B., and Hoffmann, D. (1979). *Accounts Chem. Res.* *12*:92.
36. McCoy, G. D., Hecht, S. S., and Wynder, E. L., (1980). *Prev. Med.* *9*:622.
37. Preussmann, R. (1973). In *Handbuch der allgemeinen Pathologie,* Vol. VI/6, Part 2, Springer-Verlag, Berlin, p. 421.
38. Walker, E. A., Castegnaro, M., Griciute, L., and Lyle, R. E., Eds. (1978). *IARC Scientific Publications No. 19,* International Agency for Research on Cancer, Lyon, France.
39. Lijinsky, W., (1980). *Oncology* *37*:223.
40. Mirvish, S. S. (1975). *Toxicol. Appl. Pharmacol.* *31*:325.
41. Tannenbaum, S. R., Moran, D., Rand, W., Cuello, C., and Correa, P. (1979). *J. Natl. Cancer. Inst.* *62*:9.
42. Odashima, S. (1980). *Oncology* *37*:282.
43. Laqueur, G. C. (1970). In *Carcinoma of the Colon and Antecedent Epithelium,* W. J. Burdette, Ed., Charles C Thomas, Springfield, Ill., p. 305.
44. Zedeck, M. S., and Sternberg, S. S. (1974). *J. Natl. Cancer Inst.* *53*:1419.
45. Reddy, B. S., Watanabe, K., and Weisburger, J. H. (1977). *Cancer Res.* *37*:4156.
46. Fiala, E. S., Kulakis, C., Christiansen, G., and Weisburger, J. H. (1978). *Cancer Res.* *38*:4515.
47. Druckrey, H. (1970). In *Carcinoma of the Colon and Antecedent Epithelium,* W. J. Burdette, Ed., Charles C Thomas, Springfield, Ill., p. 267.
48. Reddy, B. S., Weisburger, J. H., Narisawa, T., and Wynder, E. L. (1974). *Cancer Res.* *34*:2368.
49. Ward, J. M. (1975). *Vet. Pathol.* *12*:165.

50. Reddy, B. S., Narisawa, T., Wright, P., Vukusich, D., Weisburger, J. H., and Wynder, E. L. (1975). *Cancer Res.* 35:287.
51. Fiala, E. S. (1977). *Cancer* 40:2435.
52. Newberne, P. M. (1976). *Cancer Detect.* 1:129.
53. Wogan, G. N. (1975). *Cancer Res.* 35:3499.
54. Schoental, R. (1976). In *Chemical Carcinogens*, C. E. Searle, Ed., ACS Monograph 173, American Chemical Society, Washington, D. C., p. 626.
55. Schmahl, D., Thomas, C., and Auer, R. (1977). *Carcinogenesis*, Springer-Verlag, Berlin.
56. Uraguchi, K., and Yamazaki, M., Eds. (1978). *Toxicology, Biochemistry, and Pathology of Micotoxins*, Halsted Press, New York.
57. Longnecker, D. S., and Curphey, T. J. (1975). *Cancer Res.* 35:2249.
58. Jarrett, W. F., NcNeil, P. E., Grimshaw, W. T. R., Selman, T. E., and McIntyre, W. I. M. (1978). *Nature* 274:215.
59. Hirano, I., Ushimaru, Y., Kato, K., Mori, H., and Sasaoka, I. (1978). *Gann* 69:383.
60. Pamukcu, A. M., Erturk, E., Yalciner, S., Milli, U., and Bryan, G. T. (1978). *Cancer Res.* 38:1556.
61. Poland, A., Glover, E., and Kinde, A. S. (1976). *J. Biol. Chem.* 251:4936.
62. Wattenberg, L. W., Loub, W. D., Lam, L. K. T., and Speier, J. L. (1976). *Fed. Proc.* 35:1327.
63. Miller, E. C., Miller, J. A., Brown, R. R., and MacDonald, J. (1958). *Cancer Res.* 18:469.
64. Slaga, T., and Bracken, W. M. (1977). *Cancer Res.* 37:1631.
65. Wade, A. E., and Norred, W. P. (1976). *Fed. Proc.* 35:2475.
66. Hopkins, G. J., and West, C. E. (1976). *Lipids* 11:736-740.
67. Marshall, W. J., and McLean, A. E. M. (1971). *Biochem J.* 122:569.
68. Martin, C. W., Fjermestad, J., Smith-Barbaro, P., and Reddy, B. S. (1980). *Nutr. Rep. Int.* 22:395.
69. McLeod, S. M., Renton, K. W., and Eade, N. R. (1972). *J. Pharmacol. Exp. Ther.* 183:289.
70. Hietanen, E. (1977). *Biol. Neonate* 31:135.
71. Smith-Barbaro, P., Hanson, D., and Reddy, B. S. (1981). *Lipids, in press.*
72. Gaillard, D., Chamoiseau, G., and Derache, L. (1977). *Toxicology* 8:23.
73. Hietanen, E., Hanninen, O., Laitanen, M., and Lang, M. (1978). *Enzyme* 23:127.
74. Davison, S. C., and Wills, E. D. (1974). *Biochem. J.* 140:461.

75. Chhabra, R. S., Pohl, R. J., and Fouts, J. R. (1974). *Drug Metab. Dispos.* 2:443.
76. Conney, A. H., Pantuck, E. L., Hsiao, K. C., Garland, W. A., Anderson, K. E., Alvares, A. P., and Kappas, A. (1976). *Clin. Pharmacol. Index Ther.* 21:158.
77. Hoensch, H., Woo, C. H., Raffin, S. B., and Schmidt, R. (1976). *Gastroenterology* 70:1063.
78. Chhabra, R. S., and Fouts, J. R. (1976). *Drug Metab. Dispos.* 4:208.
79. Stohs, S., Grafstrom, R. C., Burke, M. D., and Orrenius, S. (1970). *Drug Metab. Dispos.* 4:517.
80. Hendelberger, C. (1975). *Annu. Rev. Biochem.* 44:79.
81. Czygan, P., Greim, H., Garro, A., Schattner, F., and Popper, H. (1974). *Cancer Res.* 34:119.
82. Abbot, V., Deloria, L., Guenthuen, T., Jeffrey, E., Kotake, A., Nerland, D., and Mannering, G. (1976). *Drug Metab. Dispos.* 4:215.
83. Lu, H. Y. H., Kuntzman, I., West, S., Jacobson, M., and Conney, A. H. (1972). *J. Biol. Chem.* 247:1727.
84. Norred, W. P., and Wade, A. E. (1972). *Biochem. Pharmacol.* 21:2887.
85. Lambert, L., and Wills, E. D. (1977). *Biochem. Pharmacol.* 26:1417.
86. Lambert, L., and Wills, E. D. (1977). *Biochem. Pharmacol,* 26:1423.
87. Hietanen, E., Laitinen, M., Vainio, H., and Hanninen, O. (1975). *Lipids* 10:467.
88. Hietanen, E., and Laitinen, M. (1977). *Biochem. Pharmacol.* 27:1095.
89. Atkin, S. D., Palmer, G. D., English, P. D., Morgan, B., Cawthorne, M. A., and Green, J. (1972). *Biochem. J.* 128:237.
90. Avigan, J., and Steinberg, D. (1958). *Proc. Soc. Exp. Biol. Med.* 97:814.
91. Frantz, I. D., Jr., and Carey, J. B. (1965). *Proc. Soc. Exp. Biol. Med.* 106:800.
92. Dietschy, J. M., and Siperstein, M. D. (1967). *J. Lipid Res.* 8:97.
93. Goldfarb, S., and Pitot, H. C. (1972). *J. Lipid Res.* 13:797.
94. Lakshmanan, M. R., Dugan, E., Nepokeroeff, C. M., Ness, G. C., and Porter, J. A. (1975). *Arch. Biochem. Biophys.* 168:89.
95. Strobel, H. W., Fang, W. F., and Oshinsky, R. J. (1980). *Cancer* 45:1060.
96. Craven, P. A., and DeRubertis, F. R. (1980). *Biochem. Biophys. Res. Commun.* 94:1044.

97. Chhabra, R. S., and Fouts, J. R. (1974). *Drug Metab. Dispos.* 2:375.
98. Defrawy, E. L., Masry, S., Cohen, G. M., and Mannering, G. J. (1974). *Drug Metab. Dispos.* 2:257.
99. Wynder, E. L., and Gori, G. B. (1977). *J. Natl. Cancer Inst.* 58:825.
100. Doll, R., Muir, C., and Waterhouse, J., Eds. (1970). *Cancer Incidence in Five Continents,* Vol. II, International Union Against Cancer, New York.
101. Wynder, E. L., Kajitani, T., Ishakawa, S., Dodo, H., and Takano, A. (1969). *Cancer* 23:1219.
102. Jacobi, H. P., and Baumann, C. A. (1946). *Am. J. Cancer* 39:338.
103. Tannenbaum, A. (1945). *Cancer Res.* 5:616.
104. Silverstone, H., and Tannenbaum, A., (1951). *Cancer Res.* 11:200.
105. Lavik, P. S., and Baumann, C. A. (1941). *Cancer Res.* 1:181.
106. Carroll, K. K., and Khor, H. T. (1975). *Prog. Biochem. Pharmacol.* 10:308.
107. Miller, J. A., Kline, B. E., Rusch, H. P., and Baumann, C. A. (1944). *Cancer Res.* 4:756.
108. Giese, J. E., Clayton, C. C., Miller, E. C., and Baumann, C. A. (1946). *Cancer Res.* 6:679.
109. Kline, B. E., Miller, J. A., Rusch, H. P., and Baumann, C. A. (1946). *Cancer Res.* 6:5.
110. Nigro, N. D., Singh, D. V., Campbell, R. L., and Pak, M. S. (1975). *J. Natl. Cancer. Inst.* 54:429.
111. Bansal, B. R., Rhoads, J. E., Jr., and Bansal, S. C. (1978). *Cancer Res.* 38:3293.
112. Rogers, A. E., and Newberne, P. M. (1975). *Cancer Res.* 35:3427.
113. Reddy, B. S., Narisawa, T., Vukusich, D., Weisburger, J. H., and Wynder, E. L. (1976). *Proc. Soc. Exp. Biol. Med.* 151:237.
114. Reddy, B. S., Narisawa, T., and Weisburger, J. H. (1976). *J. Natl. Cancer Inst.* 57:567.
115. Broitman, S. A., Vitale, J. J., Vavrousek-Jakuba, E., and Gottlieb, L. S. (1977). *Cancer* 40:2455.
116. Reddy, B. S., Mangat, S., Weisburger, J. H., and Wynder, E. L. (1977). *Cancer Res.* 37:3533.
117. Bull, A. W., Soullier, B. K., Wilson, P. S., Hayden, M. T., and Nigro, N. D. (1979). *Cancer Res.* 39:4956.
118. Diamond, L., O'Brien, T. G., and Baird, W. M. (1980). *Adv. Cancer. Res.* 32:1.

119. Reddy, B. S., Mangat, S., Sheinfil, A., Weisburger, J. H., and Wynder, E. L., (1977). *Cancer Res.* 37:2132.
120. Chomchai, C., Bhadrachari, N., and Nigro, N. D. (1974). *Dis. Colon Rectum* 17:310.
121. Narisawa, T., Magadia, N. E., Weisburger, J. H., and Wynder, E. L., (1974). *J. Natl. Cancer Inst.* 36:1379.
122. Reddy, B. S., Narisawa, T., Weisburger, J. H., and Wynder, E. L. (1976). *J. Natl. Cancer. Inst.* 56:441.
123. Reddy, B. S., Watanabe, K., Weisburger, J. H., and Wynder, E. L., (1977). *Cancer Res.* 37:3238.
124. Cohen, B. I., Raicht, R. F., Deschner, E. E., Takahashi, M., Sarwal, A. N., and Fazzini, E. (1980). *J. Natl. Cancer Inst.* 64:573.
125. Reddy, B. S., and Watanabe, K. (1979). *Cancer Res.* 39:1521.
126. Bagheri, S. A., Bolt, M. G., Boyer, J. L., and Palmer, R. H. (1978). *Gastroenterology* 7:188.
127. Roy, C. C., Laurendeau, G., Doyon, G., Chartrand, L., and Rivest, M. R. (1975). *Proc. Soc. Exp. Biol. Med.* 149:1000.
128. Matsuzawa, T., and Wilson, R. (1965). *Radiat. Res.* 25:15.
129. Meslin, J. C., Sacquet, E., and Raiband, P. (1974). *Ann. Biol. Anim. Biochem. Biophys.* 14:709.
130. Lipkin, M. (1975). *Cancer* 36:2319.
131. Takano, S., Matsushima, M., Erturk, E., and Bryan, G. (1981). *Cancer Res.* 41:624.
132. Gullino, P. M., Pettigrew, H. M., and Grantham, F. H. (1975). *J. Natl. Cancer Inst.* 54:401.
133. Chan, P. C., Head, J. F., Cohen, L. A., and Wynder, E. L. (1977). *J. Natl. Cancer Inst.* 59:1279.
134. Nishizuka, Y. (1978). *Prev. Med.* 7:218.
135. Hopkins, G. J., West, C. E., and Hard, G. C. (1976). *Lipids* 2:328.
136. Hopkins, G. J., and Carroll, K. K. (1979). *J. Natl. Cancer Inst.* 62:1009.
137. Hopkins, G. J., and West, C. E. (1976). *Life Sci.* 19:1103.
138. Hankin, J. H., and Rawlings, V. (1978). *Am. J. Clin. Nutr.* 31:2005.
139. Miller, A. B. (1977). *Cancer* 39:2704.
140. Beer, A. E., and Billingham, R. E. (1978). *Lancet* 2:296.
141. Tannenbaum, A., and Silverstone, H. (1957). In *Cancer*, Vol. 1, R. W. Raven, Ed., Butterworth, London, p. 306.
142. Dao, T. L., Bock, F. G., and Crouch, S. (1959). *Proc. Soc. Exp. Biol. Med.* 102:635.
143. Shamberger, R. J., Andreone, T. L., and Willis, C. E. (1974). *J. Natl. Cancer Inst.* 53:1771.

144. Floyd, R. A., Soong, L. M., Stuart, M. A., and Reigh, D. L. (1978). *Arch. Biochem. Biophys. 185*:450.
145. Weisburger, J. H., and Williams, G. M. (1981). In *Etiology of Cancer*, 2nd ed., J. F. Holland and E. Frei, III, Eds., Lea & Febiger, Philadelphia, p. 42.
146. Gustafsson, B. F., Einarsson, K., and Gustafsson, J. E. (1975). *J. Biol. Chem. 250*:8496.
147. Furth, J. (1973). In *Human Prolactin*, J. L. Pasteels and C. Robyn, Eds., American Elsevier, New York, p. 233.
148. Pearson, O. H., (1972). In *Current Research in Oncology*, C. B. Anfinson, M. Potter, and A. N. Schechter, Eds., Academic Press, New York, p. 125.
149. Meites, J. (1977). In *Comparative Endocrinology of Prolactin*, H. D. Dellman, J. A. Johnson, and D. M. Klachko, Eds., Plenum Press, New York, p. 135.
150. Chan, P. C., and Cohen, L. A. (1974). *J. Natl. Cancer. Inst. 52*:25.
151. Chan, P. C., Didato, F., and Cohen, L. A. (1975). *Proc. Soc. Exp. Biol. Med. 149*:133.
152. Boyns, A. E., Buchan, R., Cole, E. N., Forest, A. P. M., and Griffiths, K., (1973). *Eur. J. Cancer. 9*:169.
153. Hawkins, R. A., Drewitt, D., Greedman, B., Killen, E., Jenner, D. A., and Cameron, E. H. D. (1976). *Br. J. Cancer 34*:546.

4

Retinoids and Drug-Metabolizing Enzymes

Rajendra S. Chhabra
National Institute of Environmental Health Sciences, Research Triangle Park, North Carolina

I. INTRODUCTION

Vitamin A, an essential lipid-soluble nutrient, was first discovered in eggs, milk, butter, and fish liver oils. Plants contain vitamin A in the form of its provitamin, β-carotene. In recent years the term "retinoids" has been designated as a general term that includes both natural forms of vitamin A and its synthetic analogs. Vitamin A is necessary for the support of growth, health, and life of all vertebrates and for the prevention of night blindness. Vitamin A is necessary for the maintenance of differentiated epithelia, for reproduction, and for glycoprotein production. The trans-vitamin A alcohol or trans-retinol is the parent substance and its naturally occurring oxidation products are trans-retinal (vitamin A aldehyde) and trans-retinoic acid (vitamin A acid). The retinoid molecule can be chemically modified in many ways into unlimited numbers of compounds. The nutritional role of vitamin A has been extensively reviewed.

The association of vitamin A deficiency and a high incidence of cancer has been known for a long time (Bollag, 1970). For the past decade a number of investigations have shown that the susceptibility of many epithelial tissues to a number of carcinogens is enhanced by vitamin A deficiency. Vitamin A and its synthetic analogs have also been found to possess anticarcinogenic activity. For example, Nettesheim and Williams (1976) have shown that susceptibility of rats to pulmonary carcinogenesis induced by 3-methylcholanthrene is increased in the absence of dietary vitamin A. Chu and Malmgren (1965) have shown that large doses of vitamin A could influence the induction of stomach, in-

testine, vaginal, and cervical cancer by 7,12-dimethylbenzanthracene
(DMBA)- or benzpyrene-induced appearance of dyskeratosis, papillomas, and carcinomas in the esophagus, stomach, and intestine of
hamsters was delayed or prevented by the addition of 0.5% vitamin A
palmitate to the animal diet. The vitamin palmitate-treated animals
showed lower incidences of both squamous metaplasia of the bronchial
mucosa and of squamous cell carcinomas produced by intratracheal instillation of benzpyrene (Saffiotti et al., 1967). The number of skin
papillomas in animals treated with a single application of 7,12-dimethyl-
benzanthracene was far smaller in the animals fed with vitamin A-supplemented diets when compared to the animals on control diets (Davies,
1967). Newberne and Suphakaran (1977) have reported that dietary
deficiency of vitamin A can increase susceptibility to N-nitrosodimethylamine (DMH)-induced colon tumors in rats as well as liver tumors in rats
exposed to aflatoxin B_1. Recently, Siddik et al. (1980) have reported
that vitamin A deficiency in rats may play a protective role against
chemical toxicity. Significantly increased hepatic glutathione S-aryltransferase activities measured in vitro against 1,2-dichloro-4-nitro-
benzene and sulfobromophthalein were noticed in rats on vitamin A-
deficient diet.

There are also some contradictory reports which show little or no
antineoplastic effect of vitamin A. For example, the effect of retinyl
acetate on the incidence of mammary carcinomas was totally negative in
a study conducted by Maiorana and Gullino (1980), which is at variance
with the results of other studies (Moon et al., 1976,1977; McCormick
et al., 1979). Narisawa et al. (1976) have studied the effect of vitamin
A deficiency on rat colon carcinogenesis induced by N-methyl-N'-nitro-
N-nitrosoguanidine (MNNG). Vitamin A-deficient rats showed significantly suppressed large-bowel tumor induction in MNNG-treated animals compared to rats fed adequate vitamin A; however, a high incidence of squamous cell papillomatosis of the urinary bladder was noticed in rats fed vitamin A-free diet, and suggesting that the large
intestine has a susceptibility that is different from that of the respiratory and urinary tract to tumorigenic stimulation in vitamin A-deficient
studies. However, despite confusing and contradictory reports the
majority of reports indicate antineoplastic effects; therefore, a number
of synthetic vitamin A analogs are being tested for their potential antineoplastic effect (Sporn et al., 1976; Sporn and Newton, 1979). Effects of vitamin A and its analogs on normal and neoplastic cells have
been recently reviewed by Lotan (1980) and by Nettesheim (1980).

Various hypotheses have been offered to explain the protective action
of vitamin A toward toxicity and carcinogenicity of the chemicals. For
example, Sporn et al. (1976) have proposed that the antineoplastic
action of retinoids is associated with the control of DNA synthesis and
mitotic activity in target epithelia. Felix et al. (1976) have shown that
retinoids could enhance the cellular immune responses since they observed the ability of vitamin A to destroy injected melanoma nodules in

the murine system and in three patients with multiple dermal metastasis. Earlier, Bollag (1970) had suggested that the hormonelike
action of vitamin A on cell differentiation may be a possible mechanism
for the anticarcinogenic effect of vitamin A. One of the mechanisms
for antineoplastic effect of retinoids could be alteration in metabolism
of potential carcinogens (Hill and Shih, 1974). Most of the foreign
chemicals including carcinogens are metabolized by the microsomal
drug-metabolizing enzyme system. In the following section some characteristics of drug-metabolizing enzymes and influence of changes in
dietary components on these enzymes are discussed.

II. SOME CHARACTERISTICS OF DRUG-
METABOLIZING ENZYMES

The hepatic endoplasmic reticulum contains a group of nonspecific
enzymes termed "microsomal drug-metabolizing enzymes" which metabolize a wide variety of chemicals, including drugs, pesticides, carcinogens, herbicides, food additives, and industrial organic solvents, as
well as endogenous substrates such as fatty acids and steroids. These
enzymes catalyze diverse reactions such as the oxidation of alkanes and
aromatic compounds; the epoxidation of alkanes, polycyclic hydrocarbons, and halogenated benzenes; the dealkylation of the secondary and
tertiary amines; the conversion of amines to N-oxides, hydroxylamines,
and nitroso derivatives; the oxidative cleavage of ethers and organic
thiophosphate ethers; and conversion of phosphothionates to their
phosphate derivatives. These enzymes also catalyze the reduction of
azo compounds and nitro compounds to primary aromatic amines (Gillette et al., 1972). These enzyme systems have in common several
properties, including their location in the endoplasmic reticulum and
the requirement for NADPH, molecular oxygen, and an electron transport system which consists of NADPH-cytochrome c reductase, lipid,
and a carbon monoxide binding pigment generally known as cytochrome
P-450. Frequently, these enzyme systems are referred to as "mixed-
function oxidases" since they require both NADPH (or NADH) and oxygen (Mason, 1957). Compounds metabolized by this system are usually
quite lipid soluble prior to metabolism. The reaction products are less
lipid soluble and are excreted as such or after conjugation. The details of hepatic drug metabolism have been reviewed extensively (Gillette et al., 1972; Gillette, 1966; Conney, 1967; Remmer, 1972; Lu and
Levin, 1974; Neims et al., 1976).

Although the liver is the major site where metabolism of foreign chemicals occurs, in the past few years it has become increasingly evident
that extrahepatic tissues such as the lung, skin, and intestine can
transform foreign chemicals to inactive or active metabolites (Bickers
et al., 1974; Pohl et al., 1976; Hook and Bend, 1976; Bend et al.,
1972; Gram, 1973; Litterest et al., 1977; Hartiala, 1973; Chhabra and

Tredger, 1978). Generally, the rates of metabolism of foreign chemicals by extrahepatic tissues are much lower than in the liver, but the
ability of these tissues to transform chemicals to active toxic metabolites
may affect general or target organ toxicity of the chemicals.

It is well known that physiological factors (sex, age, species, strain)
and environmental factors (diet, foreign chemicals) and disease state
of animals can influence the activities of hepatic drug-metabolizing enzymes (Conney and Burns, 1962). The influence of changes in composition of macronutrients of diet on hepatic drug-metabolizing enzymes
has been extensively studied (Campbell and Hayes, 1974; Erikson et
al., 1975; Rowe and Willis, 1976; Dickerson et al., 1976; Sato and Zannoni, 1976; Hafeman and Hoekstra, 1977; Truex et al., 1977). These
studies show that macronutrient composition of diet as well as the presence of chemical contaminants and food additives can modify the activities of these enzymes. The most extensively studied macronutrient
is protein. Protein deficiency causes depression of hepatic drug-metabolizing enzymes. A variety of in vitro microsomal reaction rates
have been shown to be depressed for a number of drug substrates,
such as phenobarbital, strychnine, aminopyrine, benzpyrene, zoxazo-
lamine, pyramidon, ethylmorphine, and aniline. The toxicities of chemicals in animals on protein-deficient diets depend on whether the principal reaction rate affected is toxication or detoxication (Campbell and
Hayes, 1974). The role of carbohydrates on drug-metabolizing enzymes has been limited to a few studies. High amounts of sugars in
the diet increase the duration of sleep induced by barbiturates in mice,
which correlates with decreases in the metabolism of barbiturates
(Strother et al., 1971). Norred and Wade (1972) have studied the role
of lipids on hepatic drug-metabolizing enzymes by comparing rats fed
either fat-free or 3% corn oil diets for 3 weeks. Cytochrome P-450 levels were decreased and were accompanied by decreases in V_{max} and K_m
estimations for ethylmorphine demethylation and hexobarbital oxidation.
The effects of vitamins and mineral deficiencies on hepatic drug-metabolizing enzymes have been studied but the results are not as striking as those observed for protein deficiency. When studied individually, dietary minerals such as copper, iron, and zinc do alter drug metabolism in rodents, but no data exist to indicate the effect of such
minerals on drug metabolism in domestic animals or in humans. Interrelationship of these minerals and their relationship to drug metabolism
need to be further investigated (Becking, 1978). Among vitamins affecting drug metabolism, vitamin C has been extensively studied by
Zannoni and his associates. Vitamin C deficiency in guinea pig lowers
the hepatic drug-metabolizing enzyme activities. The activities are
augmented when diets are supplemented with vitamin C (Sato and Zannoni, 1976). Kuenzig et al. (1977), in their study on the effect of
ascorbic acid deficiency on extrahepatic microsomal metabolism in the
guinea pig, have shown that the effect of ascorbate deficiency on the
microsomal metabolism of drugs and carcinogens varies with different

tissues and substrates. A recent study (Dashman and Kamm, 1979) has shown that large doses of vitamin E administered intramuscularly could decrease the rate of drug-metabolizing enzymes and then decrease the hepatotoxicity of DMN by inhibiting its metabolism to a presumed active metabolite. Chronic riboflavin deficiency in male and female rats resulted in a decrease in the rate of hepatic drug metabolism and cytochrome P-450 contents (Patel and Pawar, 1974). Administration of riboflavin to deficient animals reversed the effects of vitamin deficiency.

The role of vitamin A in regulation of drug-metabolizing enzymes has been studied in a number of laboratories, including ours. The following sections deal with data primarily from our laboratories and its discussion in relation to results from other laboratories.

III. VITAMIN A DEFICIENCY AND DRUG-METABOLIZING ENZYMES

In our laboratory the effect of vitamin A deficiency on hepatic and extrahepatic in vitro metabolism of prototype drug substrates in male guinea pigs and male New Zealand rabbits was studied. Animals were divided into three groups and fed a complete semipurified diet (Tekland Test Diets, Madison, Wisconsin) with or without retinyl palmitate. The control diet contained retinyl palmitate concentration of 35 IU/g of guinea pig diet and 15 IU/g of rabbit diet. The control diet was given in restricted amounts (pair-fed controls) to equal the food intake of animals fed vitamin A and to another control group the food was given ad libitum. The guinea pigs were fed for 9 weeks and rabbits for 12 weeks. The activities of various enzymes were studied in liver, intestine and lungs of the animals. Table 1 shows the effects of vitamin A-deficient diet on body weight and hepatic vitamin A contents. Guinea pigs or rabbits fed vitamin A-deficient diet for 12 weeks had body weight similar to those of the corresponding pair-fed controls. The levels of vitamin A in both guinea pigs and rabbits fed deficient diet were significantly lower than the pair-fed controls.

The effect of vitamin A-deficient diet on various drug-metabolizing enzymes in the guinea pig is shown in Table 2. Specific drug-metabolizing enzyme activities and cytochrome P-450 content in liver remained unchanged after feeding the deficient diet for 3 weeks (data not shown). However, by 9 weeks, aminopyrine demethylase, aniline hydroxylase, 7-ethoxycoumarin deethylase, and aryl hydrocarbon hydroxylase (AHH) activities, and cytochrome P-450 contents were significantly reduced in the vitamin A-deficient animals as compared to controls. Epoxide hydrase and glutathione S-transferase activities were not altered by vitamin A deficiency. No significant differences in the drug-metabolizing enzyme activities were observed between pair-fed and ad libitum control animals. None of the drug-metabolizing

Table 1 Effects of Vitamin A-Deficient Diet on Growth and Liver Vitamin A Content of Guinea Pig and Rabbit[a]

Dietary group	Weeks on test	Final body weight (g)	Liver vitamin A (μg/g)
Guinea pig			
Deficient	9	531 ± 18 (14)[b]	0.468 ± 0.09 (4)[b,c]
Pair-fed control	9	522 ± 13 (13)[b]	145 ± 19 (4)
Ad libitum control	9	616 ± 14 (15)	158 ± 19 (4)
Rabbit			
Deficient	12	2853 ± 93 (8)	1.32 ± 0.23 (4)[b,c]
Pair-fed control	12	2694 ± 101 (7)	71 ± 4.3 (4)
Ad libitum control	12	2961 ± 170 (7)	95 ± 6 (4)

[a]Values are mean ± SE. The number of animals is given in parentheses.
[b]Significantly different from ad libitum control, $P < 0.05$.
[c]Significantly different from pair-fed control, $P < 0.05$.
Source: Data similar to Miranda et al. (1979).

Table 2 Effects of Vitamin A-Deficient Diet on Hepatic Drug Metabolism in Guinea Pig Liver, Lung, and Small Intestine[a]

Tissue	Cytochrome P-450	Aminopyrine demethylase	Aniline hydroxylase	Aryl hydrocarbon hydroxylase (AHH)	7-Ethoxy-coumarin deethylase	Epoxide hydrase	Glutathione S-transferase (GST)
Liver							
Deficient	0.552 ± 0.11[b]	3.18 ± 0.71[b,c]	0.39 ± 0.08[b,c]	830 ± 99[b,c]	0.32 ± 0.13[b]	13.1 ± 0.66	266 ± 14
Pair-fed control	0.896 ± 0.17	5.84 ± 0.33	0.75 ± 0.03	1722 ± 303	0.69 ± 0.06	13.8 ± 0.83	256 ± 17
Ad libitum control	0.943 ± 0.11	5.72 ± 0.19	0.68 ± 0.01	1803 ± 77	0.87 ± 0.10	14.0 ± 0.63	261 ± 21
Lung							
Deficient	0.17 ± 0.04	0.70 ± 0.07	0.19 ± 0.001	75 ± 13	0.15 ± 0.02	0.53 ± 0.04	19 ± 1.3
Pair-fed control	0.10 ± 0.02	0.88 ± 0.18	0.25 ± 0.04	97 ± 19	0.28 ± 0.05	0.49 ± 0.03	19 ± 2.6
Ad libitum control	0.11 ± 0.02	0.86 ± 0.18	0.25 ± 0.05	72 ± 9	0.29 ± 0.05	0.50 ± 0.04	17 ± 1.7
Small intestine							
Deficient	0.23 ± 0.03	0.98 ± 0.11[b,c]	0.07 ± 0.003[b,c]	185 ± 24[b,c]	0.07 ± 0.005[b,c]	5.4 ± 0.27	24 ± 2.8
Pair-fed control	0.16 ± 0.02	0.59 ± 0.04	0.04 ± 0.003	118 ± 19	0.05 ± 0.01	5.3 ± 0.44	24 ± 3.9
Ad libitum control	0.19 ± 0.01	0.70 ± 0.03	0.06 ± 0.004	115 ± 15	0.05 ± 0.004	5.2 ± 0.33	23 ± 3.8

[a]Values are expressed as the mean ± SE. Tissues were pooled from four animals (N = 4 individual pooled samples). Enzyme activities are expressed as nmol/mg of microsomal protein/min except for AHH and GST. AHH is expressed as relative fluorescence units/mg of microsomal protein/min. GST is expressed as nmoles if conjugate formed with benzo[a]pyrene 4,5-oxide/min/mg of supernatant protein.
[b]Significantly different from ad libitum controls, P < 0.05.
[c]Significantly different from pair-fed controls, P < 0.05
Source: Data similar to Miranda et al. (1979).

Table 3 Effects of Vitamin A-Deficient Diet on Drug Metabolism in Rabbit Liver, Lung, and Small Intestine[a]

Tissue	Cytochrome P-450	Aminopyrine demethylase	Aniline hydroxylase	Aryl hydrocarbon hydroxylase	7-Ethoxy-coumarin deethylase	Epoxide hydrase	Glutathione S-transferase
Liver							
Deficient	0.55 ± 0.12	4.24 ± 0.87	0.20 ± 0.02[b,c]	319 ± 70[b,c]	0.27 ± 0.02[b,c]	7.82 ± 0.54	6.61 ± 1.7
Pair-fed control	0.64 ± 0.03	5.62 ± 0.60	0.40 ± 0.05	691 ± 102	0.46 ± 0.06	9.16 ± 0.69	5.45 ± 0.45
Ad libitum control	0.64 ± 0.02	6.17 ± 0.74	0.40 ± 0.03	682 ± 93	0.70 ± 0.14	9.71 ± 0.99	4.53 ± 0.46
Lung							
Deficient	0.28 ± 0.03	1.94 ± 0.13	0.26 ± 0.04	77 ± 2.2	0.46 ± 0.10	0.45 ± 0.03	0.67 ± 0.05
Pair-fed control	0.29 ± 0.03	2.44 ± 0.19	0.32 ± 0.06	85 ± 3.3	0.66 ± 0.06	0.45 ± 0.02	0.67 ± 0.05
Ad libitum control	0.31 ± 0.01	2.41 ± 0.21	0.30 ± 0.04	62 ± 9.4	0.54 ± 0.05	0.45 ± 0.02	0.69 ± 0.08
Small intestine							
Deficient	0.33 ± 0.02	0.44 ± 0.03[b,c]	0.14 ± 0.01	65 ± 2.0[c]	0.06 ± 0.01	6.79 ± 0.30	2.32 ± 0.16
Pair-fed control	0.35 ± 0.02	0.31 ± 0.04	0.16 ± 0.04	69 ± 16	0.06 ± 0.003	7.01 ± 0.39	1.97 ± 0.27
Ad libitum control	0.30 ± 0.03	0.27 ± 0.06	0.10 ± 0.02	35 ± 9	0.05 ± 0.005	6.41 ± 0.40	1.73 ± 0.15

[a]Enzymic activities are expressed as in Table 2.
[b]Significantly different from pair-fed control, $P < 0.05$.
[c]Significantly different from ad libitum control, $P < 0.05$.
Source: Data similar to Miranda et al. (1979).

Table 4 Effects of Vitamin A-Deficient Diets on Hepatic Drug-Metabolizing Enzymes and Cytochrome P-450 Contents in Rats

Drug substrate	Percent change from control	Days on test diet	Reference
Aminopyrine	−38[a]	20	Becking (1973)
Aniline	−29[a]	25	
	−37[a]	20	
p-Nitrobenzoic acid	−37[a]	25	
	+7	20	
	−6	25	
Ethylmorphine	−49[a]	42–56	Colby et al. (1975)
Aniline	−37[a]	42–56	
Cytochrome P-450	−39[a]		
Ethylmorphine	−7	35	Hauswirth and
Aminopyrine	−13[a]	35	Brizuela (1976)
Aniline	+2	35	
Cytochrome P-450	−30[a]	35	
Aminopyrine	−46	70	Kalamegham and
Benzo[a]pyrene	−52	70	Krishnaswamy (1980)

[a]Significantly different from controls.

enzyme activities in the lung were significantly altered by vitamin A deficiency. In the small intestine, aminopyrine demethylase, aniline hydroxylase, 7-ethoxycoumarin deethylase, and AHH activities were significantly higher in guniea pigs fed the vitamin A-deficient diet.

Rabbits on vitamin A-deficient diet for 12 weeks had significantly lower hepatic aniline hydroxylase, AHH, and 7-ethoxycoumarin deethylase activities than the pair-fed controls (Table 3). However, intestinal aminopyrine demethylase activity was significantly increased in the vitamin A-deficient rabbits. The lung enzymic activities were not altered by vitamin A-deficient diet in rabbit. The epoxide hydrase or glutathione S-transferase activities were not altered in any of the tissues examined.

The studies from other laboratories have also shown effects of vitamin A-deficient diet on drug-metabolizing enzyme activities. For example, Becking (1973) reported reduction in cytochrome P-450 levels in rats fed vitamin A-deficient diet for 20 to 25 days. Colby et al. (1975) looked at effects of retinol deficiency on hepatic oxidative metabolism in rat and reported a decrease in cytochrome P-450 contents and a decrease in ethylmorphine demethylase and aniline hydroxylase activities in the rats on retinol-deficient diet for 8 weeks (Table 4). Retinol administration for 6 weeks completely reversed the effects of retinol deficiency. Hauswirth and Brizuela (1976) maintained Sprague-Dawley rats on a vitamin A-deficient diet for 5 weeks and did not find any changes in ethylmorphine N-demethylase or aniline hydroxylase activities, while cytochrome P-450 and aminopyrine N-demethylase activities were reduced slightly but significantly. Vitamin A is known to have a protective influence against the incidence of aflatoxin-induced tumors or toxicity. Bassir et al. (1978) investigated the relationship between dietary vitamin A levels and metabolism of aflatoxins. In vitamin A-deficient rabbits the activities of aflatoxin B_1 (AFB_1) demethylase were significantly reduced, but AFB_1 hydroxylase activities were found to increase in deficient animals, suggesting that the affect of vitamin A on AFB_1 demethylation and hydroxylation is perhaps exerted through different mechanisms (Table 5).

The in vitro addition of drug substrates to liver microsomes results in typical type I and type II binding spectra produced by apparent affinity of drug substrates to microsomal cytochrome P-450 (Schenkman et al., 1967). Colby et al. (1975) studied the apparent spectral affinity of cytochrome P-450 from vitamin A-deficient rat liver for several type I oxidative drug substrates. The binding affinities for ethylmorphine and hexobarbital were reduced but for ethylbenzene and naphthlene were increased in retinol-deficient rats.

For the last several years it has been known that a number of aromatic compounds are not carcinogenic or toxic per se until they are converted to intermediary metabolites by the microsomal drug-metabolizing enzymes. These enzymes catalyze the formation of epoxides which are highly reactive to a variety of nucleophiles, including such

Table 5 Metabolism of Aflatoxin B_1 During Vitamin A Depletion and Supplementation

	Metabolic reaction	
	Demethylation (nmol H·CHO/mg protein/hr ± SEM)	Hydroxylation (mol toxin metabolized or product/mg protein ± SEM)
Deficient	0.0092 ± 0.0015[a]	0.122 ± 0.024
Control	0.0133 ± 0.0017	0.104 ± 0.013
Excess	0.0130 ± 0.0017	0.081 ± 0.014

[a]Significantly lower than control values.
Source: Data compiled from Bassir et al. (1978).

cellular micromolecules as DNA, RNA, and protein. These epoxides, which are also referred to as arene oxides, bind to the macromolecules within the cell. In general, this binding is correlated with the toxic effects elicited by the aromatic compounds. The epoxides may be converted to phenols, to dihydrodiols by microsomal enzyme epoxide hydrase, and could be conjugated with glutathione. The rates of inactivation of epoxides determines the toxicity of these aromatic compounds (Daly et al., 1972; Jerina and Daly, 1974). It is possible that in vitamin A-deficient animals the alterations in the rate of inactivation of arene oxides or epoxides may be the reason for the increased susceptibility of vitamin A-deficient animals to toxic and carcinogenic effects of specific aromatic compounds. Adekunle et al. (1979) have studied the kinetic parameters of styrene oxide as a prototype epoxide in rats on vitamin A-deficient and supplemented diets. The K_m and V_{max} values for epoxide hydrase where styrene oxide was used as substrate showed that both colon mucosal and liver K_m values of the reaction are lower. Based on these observations the authors have postulated that vitamin A-deficient animals have abundant free epoxides for binding to the macromolecules in the cell which is correlated with the expression of toxicity by a specific chemical. In the animals on vitamin A-supplemented diet where K_m values were higher, only very small amounts of free epoxides are available for binding to macromolecules; thus less severe or no toxic effects are postulated in that situation.

One of the hypotheses—that retinoids may exert anticarcinogenic effects by inhibiting the activation of procarcinogens to ultimate carcinogen—is further supported by the studies of Baird and Birnbaum (1979). The mutagenicity of 2-fluorenamine (2-FA), which requires activation, was inhibited in *Salmonella typhimurium TA98* microsome assay system in the presence of retinol, but mutagenesis induced by adriamycin, which does not require activation for its mutagenic activity, was not affected by the presence of retinol. Busk and Ahlborg (1980) have shown that retinol inhibited the mutagenic activity of aflatoxin B_1 (AFB_1) when added to the *Salmonella*/mammalian microsome assay. The mutagenicity of diepoxybutane, a mutagen that does not require metabolic activation, was not affected by the presence of retinol. In a study where human fibroblasts in culture were used, vitamin A palmitate or all-trans-retinoic acid were found to prevent the 2,3,7, 8-tetrachlorodibenzo-p-dioxin-induced increase of benzo[a]pyrene metabolism (Kohl and Rüdiger, 1980). The decreased metabolism of benzopyrene in vitamin A-deficient rats could lead to delayed clearance of the reactive metabolite, thus making the animals more susceptible to carcinogenesis in vitamin A deficiency (Kalamegham and Krishnaswamy, 1980). On the other hand, a report from Bornstein et al. (1978) showed that vitamin A deficiency did not alter benzo[a]pyrene metabolism in Syrian hamsters. In our studies (Tables 2 and 3) the epoxide hydrase or glutathione S-transferase activities were not changed in vitamin A-deficient or vitamin A-supplemented animals. This may be due to species differences since our studies were confined to rabbits and guinea pigs. Further studies are needed in this direction to understand better the mechanism(s) of protective effects of vitamin A in chemical toxicity, including carcinogenicity.

IV. HYPERVITAMINOSIS A AND DRUG-METABOLIZING ENZYMES

The studies on effects of hypervitaminosis in microsomal drug-metabolizing enzymes are few. A report from Tuchweber et al. (1976) revealed that rats given 30,000 IU of vitamin A orally, once daily for 20 days, produced a moderate accumulation of smooth endoplasmic reticulum with no alteration in the duration of zoxazolamine-induced paralysis. Rogers et al. (1973) reported that hepatic p-nitroanisole demethylase activity of rats fed diets with excess vitamin A for 3, 5, or 7 weeks remained at the control level. A study was undertaken in our laboratory to determine whether the activities of the enzymes involved in hepatic and extrahepatic metabolism of prototype drug substrates is altered by the high vitamin A contents in the diet. The guinea pigs and rabbits were used for this study. The control and test diets for guinea pigs contained 34 and 500 IU of vitamin A plamitate per gram of diet, respectively. The control rabbit diet contained 15 IU of vitamin A palmitate per gram, while the test diet contained 250 IU/g. The guinea pigs and rabbits were fed ad libitum for 6 and 7 weeks, respectively. A number of drug-metabolizing enzymes were measured after the completion of control and test fed regimen in guinea pig liver and in intestine, lungs, and liver from rabbits.

Table 6 Effects of Excess Dietary Vitamin A on Weight Gain, Food Intake, Liver Weight, and Liver Vitamin A of Guinea Pig and Rabbit[a]

Group	Days on diet	Total weight gain (g)	Daily food intake (g)	Liver weight (g)	Liver vitamin A (µg/g)
Guinea pig					
Control	42	110 ± 33	26 ± 1.7	19 ± 3.7	152 ± 13
Excess A	42	96 ± 15	25 ± 1.5	17 ± 2.4	911 ± 171[b]
Rabbit					
Control	48	527 ± 59	77 ± 4.2	73 ± 12	79 ± 15
Excess A	48	584 ± 181	85 ± 4.7	97 ± 8	1083 ± 276[b]

[a]Values are the mean ± SE from four animals.
[b]$p < 0.05$.
Source: Data from Miranda and Chhabra (1981).

Table 7 Effects of Excess Dietary Vitamin A on Microsomal Protein and Cytochrome P-450 Content of Guinea Pig and Rabbit Tissues[a]

Tissue	Microsomal protein (mg/g)		Cytochrome P-450 (nmol/mg)	
	Control	Excess A	Control	Excess A
Guinea pig liver	17 ± 0.4	17 ± 1.0	1.57 ± 0.12	1.39 ± 0.04
Rabbit				
Liver	12 ± 2.2	15 ± 1.1	0.68 ± 0.05	0.55 ± 0.10
Lung	5 ± 0.4	7 ± 0.8[b]	0.27 ± 0.01	0.17 ± 0.01[b]
Small intestine	10 ± 0.6	9 ± 2.5	0.27 ± 0.02	0.13 ± 0.04[b]

[a]Values are mean ± SE from four animals.
[b]$p < 0.05$.
Source: Data from Miranda and Chhabra (1981).

Feeding of vitamin A in high concentration had no effect on body weight, food intake, and liver weight of guinea pigs and rabbits (Table 6). However, the hepatic levels of vitamin A of both guinea pigs and rabbits and microsomal protein of lung (Table 7) were significantly increased by the high vitamin A in diet. On the other hand, the levels of microsomal cytochrome P-450 in lung and small intestine of rabbit were significantly decreased by the high-vitamin A diet (Table 7). Despite the presence of large amounts of vitamin A in liver, and clinical signs or gross lesions indicative of hypervitaminosis A observed in the treated animals, excess dietary vitamin A had no effect on hepatic microsomal protein and cytochrome P-450 of guinea pig.

The activities of various drug-metabolizing enzymes in the liver of guinea pigs and rabbits are shown in Table 8. Feeding excess vitamin A increased the activities of aminopyrine demethylase and aniline hydroxylase in guinea pig liver but not in rabbit liver. In contrast, the activities of 7-ethoxycoumarin deethylase and glutathione S-transferase were increased in rabbit liver but not in guinea pig liver by a high vitamin A containing diet.

The activities of drug-metabolizing enzymes in lung and small intestine of rabbit are given in Table 9. Unlike in rabbit liver, the activities of aminopyrine demethylase and aniline hydroxylase in rabbit lung and small intestine were significantly reduced by high-vitamin A diet. Aryl hydrocarbon hydroxylase activity in rabbit lung was similarly lowered by excess vitamin A.

Direct additions of vitamin A (as retinyl acetate dissolved in acetone) to incubation mixtures containing normal rabbit liver or intestinal microsomes produced an inhibition of AHH activity when 120 μM concentration of the vitamin was reached in the incubation mixture (Table 10). A much greater inhibition of AHH activity was observed when higher concentrations of vitamin A were added to the incubation mixtures.

In general, these studies show that some drug-metabolizing enzymes were altered in animals on high-vitamin A diet but the effect was species dependent. For example, the activities of aminopyrene demethylase and aniline hydroxylase were elevated in guinea pig liver but not in rabbit liver by excess vitamin A. Substrate-specific differences were also noted, as shown by the increase in the activities of 7-ethoxycoumarin deethylase and glutathione S-transferase in rabbit liver by feeding excess vitamin A. Drug-metabolizing enzymes in the liver, lung, and small intestine did not respond uniformly in the animals on diet containing high vitamin A content. Liver enzyme activities were increased but the lung and intestinal enzyme activities were reduced. The reduction of enzyme activity in lung and small intestine may be explained in part by the decrease in cytochrome P-450 content of these tissues. The presence of high levels of vitamin A in the tissues may not explain tissue differences in drug-metabolizing enzyme activities. If high levels of vitamin A in lung and small intestine are inhibitory to drug-metabolizing enzymes, it may be expected that the liver enzymes

Table 8 Effects of Excess Dietary Vitamin A on Hepatic Drug-Metabolizing Enzyme Activities in Guinea Pig and Rabbit

| Group | Enzyme activities[a] | | | | |
	Aminopyrine demethylase	Aniline hydroxylase	Aryl hydrocarbon hydroxylase	7-Ethoxycoumarin deethylase	Glutathione S-transferase
Guinea Pig:					
Control	11.0 ± 1.0	1.28 ± 0.24	2590 ± 155	1.15 ± 0.15	186 ± 13
Excess A	14.0 ± 0.9^b	2.52 ± 0.09^b	2661 ± 93	1.16 ± 0.11	170 ± 4
Rabbit:					
Control	9.4 ± 1.13	0.61 ± 0.07	2585 ± 323	0.52 ± 0.06	111 ± 3
Excess A	8.5 ± 1.0	0.84 ± 0.14	2218 ± 294	1.00 ± 0.07^b	154 ± 10^b

[a]Values are mean $\pm$ SE from four animals. Enzymic activities are expressed as in Table 2.
[b]$P < 0.05$.
Source: Data from Miranda and Chhabra (1981).

Table 9 Effects of Excess Dietary Vitamin A on Drug-Metabolizing Enzyme Activities in Lung and Small Intestine of Rabbit

Tissue and group	Enzyme activities[a]				
	Aminopyrine demethylase	Aniline hydroxylase	Aryl hydrocarbon hydroxylase	7-Ethoxy- coumarin deethylase	Glutathione S-transferase
Lung					
Control	2.17 ± 0.18	0.37 ± 0.01	264 ± 17	0.42 ± 0.07	25 ± 4.8
Excess A	1.67 ± 0.11^b	1.29 ± 0.02^b	174 ± 5^b	0.34 ± 0.01	19 ± 2.3
Small intestine					
Control	0.81 ± 0.25	0.25 ± 0.05	112 ± 16	0.10 ± 0.02	2.4 ± 0.06
Excess A	0.47 ± 0.11^b	0.05 ± 0.01^b	73 ± 13	Not detected	2.0 ± 0.39

[a]Enzymic activities are expressed as in Table 2.
[b]$p < 0.05$.
Source: Data from Miranda and Chhabra (1981).

Table 10 Effect of In Vitro Addition of Vitamin A (Retinyl Acetate) to Incubation Mixtures on Rabbit Hepatic and Intestinal Microsomal Aryl Hydrocarbon Hydroxylase Activity[a]

	Aryl hydrocarbon hydroxylase activity	
	Liver	Small intestine
Microsomes and acetone	679 ± 38	161 ± 8
Microsomes and vitamin A (μM)		
12	775 ± 31^{b}	165 ± 9
30	635 ± 65	160 ± 15
60	601 ± 48	140 ± 15
120	546 ± 32^{b}	113 ± 14^{b}
360	378 ± 11^{b}	90 ± 10^{b}
600	172 ± 39^{b}	62 ± 8^{b}

[a]Acetone or retinyl acetate in acetone, 0.1 ml, was added to incubation mixtures containing 2.5 mg (liver) or 5 mg of microsomal protein (small intestine). Final volume was 2.5 ml. Values are mean $\pm$ SE of four determinations in duplicate.
[b]$p < 0.05$, compared to corresponding control.
Source: Data from Miranda and Chhabra (1981).

should also be inhibited. Vitamin A concentrates high in the liver relative to other tissues in animals fed diet containing high vitamin A content. The lack of effect of excess dietary vitamin A on AHH activity is surprising since the inhibition of the enzyme was observed when vitamin A was added in vitro to incubation mixtures containing liver microsomes from untreated rabbits. However, the concentration of vitamin A added in vitro to cause enzyme inhibition is much greater than that found in liver microsomes from the vitamin A-fed rabbits. Moreover, vitamin A may affect drug metabolism in a different manner in the in vivo system.

V. CONCLUSIONS

The role of retinoids in protection of toxicologic and carcinogenic effects of chemicals has been the subject of investigation by several laboratories in recent years. One of the several possible mechanisms of protective effect of retinoids could be the alteration in metabolism of potential toxic chemicals. Our laboratory has investigated the effect of vitamin A-deficient and vitamin A-supplemented diets on microsomal drug-metabolizing enzyme activities in guinea pig and rabbit hepatic and extrahepatic tissues. The results of these studies suggest that the effects of dietary levels of retinoids on drug-metabolizing enzymes are species and organ specific. The interaction between dietary contents of retinoids and foreign chemicals warrants further experimental investigation since it is known that levels of hepatic vitamin A in experimental animals are reduced by the administration of a number of toxic chemicals, such as 2-aminoanthraquinone (Reddy and Weisburger, 1980), methoxychlor (Davison and Cox, 1976), and polychlorinated biphenyls (Innami et al., 1976).

REFERENCES

Adekunle, A. A., Campbell, T. C., and Campbell, S. C. (1979). Effect of vitamin A deficiency on rat hepatic and colon epoxide hydrase. *Experientia* 35:241-242.

Baird, M. B., and Birnbaum, L. S. (1979). Inhibition of 2-fluorenamine-induced mutagenesis in *Salmonella typhimurium* by vitamin A. *J. Natl. Cancer Inst.* 63:1093-1096.

Bassir, O., Adekunle, A. A., and Okoye, Z. S. C. (1978). Effects of vitamin A deficiency and excess on aflatoxin metabolism in the rabbit. *Biochem. Pharmacol.* 27:833-838.

Becking, G. C. (1973). Vitamin A status and hepatic drug metabolism in the rat. *Can. J. Physiol. Pharmacol.* 51:6-11.

Becking, G. C. (1978). Dietary minerals and drug metabolism. In *Nutrition and Drug Interactions*, J. N. Hathcock and J. Coon, Eds., Academic Press, New York, pp. 371-398.

Bend, J. R., Hook, G. E. R., Esterling, R. E., Gram, T. E., and Fouts, J. R. (1972). A comparative study of the hepatic and pulmonary microsomal mixed-function oxidase system in the rabbit. *J. Pharmacol. Exp. Ther.* 183:206-217.

Bickers, D. R., Kappas, A., and Alvares, A. P. (1974). Differences in inducibility of cutaneous and hepatic drug metabolizing enzymes and cytochrome P-450 by polychlorinated biphenyls and DDT. *J. Pharmacol. Exp. Ther.* 188:300-309.

Bollag, W. (1970). Vitamin A and vitamin A acid in prophylaxis and therapy of epithelial tumors. *Int. J. Vet. Res.* 40:299-314.

Bornstein, W. A., Lamden, M. P., Chuang, A. H. L., Gross, R. L., Newberne, P. M., and Bresnick, E. (1978). Inability of vitamin A deficienty to alter benzo[a]pyrene metabolism in Syrian hamsters. *Cancer Res.* 38:1497-1501.

Busk, L., and Ahlborg, U. G. (1980). Retinol (vitamin A) as an inhibitor of the mutagenicity of aflatoxin B_1. *Toxicol. Lett.* 6:243-249.

Campbell, T. C., and Hayes, J. R. (1974). Role of nutrition in the drug-metabolizing enzyme system. *Pharmacol. Rev.* 26:171-197.

Chhabra, R. S., and Tredger, J. M. (1978). Interactions of drugs and intestinal mucosal endoplasmic reticulum. In *Nutrition and*

Drug Interrelations, J. N. Hathcock and J. Coon, Eds., Academic Press, New York, pp. 253-277.

Chu, E. W., and Malmgren, R. A. (1965). An inhibitory effect of vitamin A on the induction of tumors of forestomach and cervix in the Syrian hamster by carcinogenic polycyclic hydrocarbons. *Cancer Res.* 25:884-895.

Colby, H. D., Kramer, R. E., Greiner, J. W., Robinson, D. A., Krause, R. F., and Canady, W. J. (1975). Hepatic drug metabolism in retinol-deficient rats. *Biochem. Pharmacol.* 24:1644-1646.

Conney, A. H., and Burns, J. J. (1962). Factors influencing drug metabolism. *Adv. Pharmacol.* 1:31-58.

Conney, A. H., (1967). Pharmacological implications of microsomal enzyme induction. *Pharmacol. Rev.* 19:317-366.

Daly, J. W., Jerina, D. M., and Witkop, B. (1972). Arene oxides and the NIH shift: the metabolism, toxicity and carcinogenicity of aromatic compounds. *Experientia* 28:1129-1264.

Dashman, T., and Kamm, J. J. (1979). Effects of high doses of vitamin E on dimethyl nitrosamine hepatotoxicity and drug metabolism in the rat. *Biochem. Pharmacol.* 28:1485-1490.

Davies, R. E. (1967). Effect of vitamin A on 7,12-dimethylbenz(α)-anthracene-induced papillomas in Rhino mouse skin. *Cancer Res.* 27:237-241.

Davison, K. L., and Cox, J. H. (1976). Methoxychlor effects on hepatic storage of vitamin A in rats. *Bull. Environ. Contam. Toxicol.* 16:145-148.

Dickerson, J. W., Basu, T. K., and Parke, D. V. (1976). Effect of protein-energy nutrition on the activity of hepatic microsomal drug-metabolizing enzymes in growing rats. *J. Nutr.* 106:258-264.

Erikson, M., Catz, C., and Yaffe, S. J. (1975). Effect of weanling malnutrition upon hepatic drug metabolism. *Biol. Neonate* 27:339-351.

Felix, E. L., Cohen, M. H., and Loyd, B. C. (1976). Immune and toxic antitumor effects of systemic and intralesional vitamin A. *J. Surg. Res.* 21:307-312.

Gillette, J. R. (1966). Biochemistry of drug oxidation and reduction by enzymes in hepatic endoplasmic reticulum. *Adv. Pharmacol.* 4:219-261.

Gillette, J. R., Davis, D. C., and Sasame, H. A. (1972). Cytochrome P-450 and its role in drug metabolism. *Annu. Rev. Pharmacol.* 12:57-84.

Gram, T. E. (1973). Comparative aspects of mixed function oxidation by lung and liver of rabbits. *Drug. Metab. Rev.* 2:1-32.

Hafeman, D. G., and Hoekstra, W. G. (1977). Protection against carbon tetrachloride-induced lipid peroxidation in the rat by dietary vitamin E, selenium and methionine as measured by ethane evolution. *J. Nutr. 107*:656-665.

Hartiala, K. (1973). Metabolism of hormones, drugs, and other substances by the gut. *Physiol. Rev. 53*:496-534.

Hauswirth, J. W., and Brizuela, B. S. (1976). The differential effects of chemical carcinogens on vitamin A status on microsomal drug metabolism in normal and vitamin A-deficient rats. *Cancer Res. 36*:1941-1946.

Hill, D. L., and Shih, T.-W. (1974). Vitamin A compounds and analogs as inhibitors of mixed-function oxidases that metabolizes carcinogenic polycyclic hydrocarbons and other compounds. *Cancer Res. 34*:564-570.

Hook, G. E. R., and Bend, J. R. (1976). Pulmonary metabolism of xenobiotics. *Life Sci. 18*:279-290.

Innami, S., Nakamura, A., Miyazaki, M., Nagayama, S., and Nishide, E. (1976). Further studies on the reduction of vitamin A content in the livers of rats given polychlorinated biphenyls. *J. Nutr. Sci. Vitaminol. 22*:409-418.

Jerina, D. M., and Daly, J. W. (1974). Arene oxides: a new aspect of drug metabolism. *Science 185*:573-582.

Kalamegham, R., and Krishnaswamy, K. (1980). Benzo[a]pyrene metabolism in vitamin A dependent rats. *Life Sci. 27*:33-38.

Kohl, F.-V., and Rüdiger, H. W. (1980). Retinoids inhibit 2,3, 7,8-tetrachlorodibenzo-p-dioxin induced activity of benzo[a]-pyrene metabolizing enzymes in human diploid fibroblasts. *Carcinogenesis 1*:733-737.

Kuenzig, W., Tjaczevski, V., Kamm, J. J., Conney, A. H., and Burns, J. J. (1977). The effect of ascorbic acid deficiency on extrahepatic microsomal metabolism of drugs and carcinogens in the guinea pig. *J. Pharmacol. Exp. Ther. 201*:527-533.

Litterest, C. L., Minnhaugh, E. G., and Gram, T. E. (1977). Comparative alterations in extrahepatic drug metabolism by factors known to affect hepatic activity. *Biochem. Pharmacol. 26*:749-756.

Lotan, R. (1980). Effects of vitamin A and its analogs (retinoids) on normal and neoplastic cells. *Biochim. Biophys. Acta 605*:33-91.

Lu, A. Y. H., and Levin, W. (1974). The resolution and reconstitution of the liver microsomal hydroxylation system. *Biochim. Biophys. Acta 344*:205-240.

Maiorana, A., and Gullino, P. M. (1980). Effect of retinyl acetal on the incidence of mammary carcinomas and hepatomas in mice. *J. Natl. Cancer Inst. 64*:655-663.

Mason, H. S. (1957). Mechanisms of oxygen metabolism. *Science 125*:1185-1188.

McCormick, D. L., Burns, F. J., and Albert, R. E. (1979). The inhibition of rat mammary tubors by dietary retinyl acetate at various times during and after treatment with a carcinogen. *Proc. Am. Assoc. Cancer Res. 20:*99.

Miranda, C. L., and Chhabra, R. S. (1981). Effects of high dietary vitamin A on drug metabolizing enzyme activities in guinea pigs and rabbits. *Drug-Nutr. Interact. 1:*55-61.

Miranda, C. L., Mukhtar, H., Bend, J. R., and Chhabra, R. S. (1979). Effects of vitamin A deficiency on hepatic and extra-hepatic mixed function oxidase and epoxide-metabolizing enzymes in guinea pigs and rabbits. *Biochem. Pharmacol. 28:*2713-2716.

Moon, R. C., Grubbs, C. J., Sporn, M. B., and Goodman, D. G. (1977). Retinyl acetate inhibits mammary carcinogenesis induced by N-methyl-N-nitrosourea. *Nature 267:*620-621.

Moon, R. C., Grubbs, C. J., and Sporn, M. B. (1976). Inhibition of 7,12-dimethylbenz[a]anthracene-induced mammary carcinogenesis by retinyl acetate. *Cancer Res. 36:*2626-2630.

Narisawa, T., Reddy, B. S., Wong, C.-Q., and Weisburger, J. H. (1976). Effect of vitamin A deficiency on rat colon carcinogenesis by N-methyl-N-nitrosoguanidine. *Cancer Res. 36:*1379-1383.

Neims, A. H., Warner, M., Loughman, P. M., and Avanda, J. V. (1976). Developmental aspects of the hepatic cytochrome P-450 monooxygenase system. *Annu. Rev. Pharmacol. Toxicol. 16:* 427-445.

Nettesheim, P., and Williams, M. L. (1976). The influence of vitamin A on the susceptibility of the rat lung to 3-methylcholanthrene. *Int. J. Cancer 17:*351-357.

Nettesheim, P. (1980). Inhibition of carcinogenesis by retinoids. *Can. Med. Assoc. J. 122:*757-765.

Newberne, P. M., and Suphakaran, V. (1977). Preventive role of vitamin A in colon carcinogenesis in rats. *Cancer 40:*2553-2556.

Norred, W. P., and Wade, A. E. (1972). Dietary fatty acid-induced alterations of hepatic microsomal drug metabolism. *Biochem. Pharmacol. 21:*2887-2897.

Patel, J. M., and Pawar, S. S. (1974). Riboflavin and drug metabolism in adult male and female rats. *Biochem. Pharmacol. 23:*1467-1477.

Pohl, R. J., Philpot, R. M., and Fouts, J. R. (1976). Cytochrome P-450 content and mixed function oxidase activity in microsomes isolated from mouse skin. *Drug. Metab. Dispos. 4:*442-450.

Reddy, T. V., and Weisburger, E. K. (1980). Hepatic vitamin A status of rats during feeding of the hepatocarcinogen 2-aminoanthraquinone. *Cancer Lett. 10:*39-44.

Remmer, H. (1972). Induction of drug metabolizing enzyme system in the liver. *Eur. J. Clin. 5:*116-136.

Rogers, A. E., Herndon, B. J., and Newberne, P. M. (1973). Induction by dimethylhydrazine of intestinal carcinoma in normal rats and rats fed high or low levels of vitamin A. *Cancer Res. 33:*1003-1009.

Rowe, L., and Willis, E. D. (1976). The effect of dietary lipids and vitamin E on lipid peroxide formation, cytochrome P-450 and oxidative demethylation in the endoplasmic reticulum. *Biochem. Pharmacol.* 25:175-179.

Saffiotti, U., Montesano, R., Sellakumar, R. R., and Borg, S. A. (1967). Experimental cancer of the lung. Inhibition by vitamin A of the induction of tracheobronchial squamous metaplasia and squamous cell tumors. *Cancer* 20:857-864.

Sato, P., and Zannoni, V. G. (1976). Ascorbic acid and hepatic drug metabolism. *J. Pharmacol. Exp. Ther.* 198:295-307.

Schenkman, J. B., Remmer, H., and Estabrook, R. W. (1967). Spectral studies of drug interaction with hepatic microsomal cytochrome. *Mol. Pharmacol.* 3:113-123.

Siddik, Z. H., Drew, R., and Gram, T. E. (1980). Metabolism and biliary excretion of sulfobromophthalein in vitamin A deficiency. *Biochem. Pharmacol.* 29:2583-2588.

Sporn, M. B., Dunlop, N. M., Newton, D. L., and Smith, J. M. (1976). Preventions of chemical carcinogenesis by vitamin A and its synthetic analogs. *Fed. Proc.* 35:1332-1338.

Sporn, M. B., and Newton, D. L. (1979). Chemoprevention of cancer with retinoids. *Fed. Proc.* 38:2528-2534.

Strother, A., Throckmorton, J. K., and Herzer, C. (1971). The influence of high sugar consumption by mice on the duration of action of barbiturates of in vitro metabolism of barbiturates, aniline and p-nitroanisole. *J. Pharmacol. Exp. Ther.* 179:490-498.

Truex, C. R., Brattsten, L., and Visek, W. J. (1977). Changes in the mixed function oxidase enzymes as a result of individual amino acid deficiencies. *Biochem. Pharmacol.* 26:667-670.

Tuchweber, B., Garg, B. D., and Salas, M. (1976). Microsomal enzyme inducers and hypervitaminosis A in rat. *Arch. Pathol. Lab. Med.* 100:100-105.

5

Availability of Cosubstrates
as a Rate-Limiting Factor

Gerard J. Mulder and Klaas R. Krijgsheld
State University of Groningen, Groningen, The Netherlands

I. RATE-LIMITING FACTORS IN CONJUGATION: GENERAL ASPECTS

When a drug is administered to an animal a complex interplay between many factors results in the metabolites that finally are excreted. One of these factors, the availability of cosubstrates for conjugation, is the main subject of this chapter. The various conjugation reactions and their special requirements for cosubstrates are given in Table 1.

However, several factors other than cosubstrate availability may influence conjugation rates in vivo, and some of these are discussed briefly in this introductory section. They include route and mode of administration, dose of the drug, pharmacokinetics and enzyme kinetics of conjugation, and mutual competition between the transferases for conjugation of the same drugs. These factors may limit the rate and extent of conjugation of a drug by the various competing pathways. A number of potentially rate-limiting steps in conjugation are indicated in Figure 1 and discussed further throughout this chapter.

A. Route of Administration

The route of administration determines the rate of drug entry into the systemic circulation, and whether first-pass effects may occur in certain organs (Table 2). Obviously, oral administration of a drug leads to a relatively slow uptake and relatively low blood concentrations of the drug. In contrast, the intravenous bolus injection yields a high peak in the blood concentration and results in an immediate, complete

Table 1   Main Conjugation Reactions and Their Requirements of Special Precursors

Conjugation reaction	Special requirements in the food	Cosubstrate precursor(s)	Cosubstrate	Required per mol conjugated substrate[a]	Activating enzyme(s)
Glucuronidation		UDP-glucose	UDP-glucuronate	1 UTP; 2 NAD;[a] 1 glucose-6-P	UDPG-dehydrogenase
Methylation	Methionine or homocysteine	Methionine	S-adenosylmethionine	1 ATP	Methionine adenosyl-transferase
Sulfation	Inorganic sulfate, cysteine, or methionine	Sulfate	Adenosine 3'-phosphate, 5'-sulfato-phosphate	2 ATP	ATP sulfurylase; APS kinase
Glutathione conjugation	Cysteine or methionine	Glycine, cysteine, glutamate	Glutathione	2 ATP	γ-Glutamylcysteine-synthetase, gluta-thione synthetase
Taurine conjugation	Taurine, cysteine, or methionine	b	Taurine[c]	1 ATP[c]	Acyl-CoA synthetase
Amino acid conjugation	-	b	Glycine,[c] gluta-mate[c]	1 ATP[c]	Acyl-CoA synthetase
Acetylation	Coenzyme A	b	Acetyl-CoA	1 ATP	b

[a] ATP or UTP consumed in the activation reactions is converted to ADP, AMP, or adenosine, depending on the reaction; for details see the respective sections in the chapter.
[b] Various precursors may be utilized to synthesize the cosubstrate; different enzymes are involved.
[c] The acceptor substrate (a carboxylic acid) is activated by transfer to the -SH group of coenzyme A to form an activated acyl~S-CoA derivative.

TABLE 2 Potential First-Pass Organs After Various Routes of Administration of Drugs

Route of administration	First organ passed	Percentage of the dose that is first exposed to this organ in unconjugated form	Second organ passed
Oral	Gut mucosa	100% of absorbed fraction	Liver (lymph)
Rectal	Gut mucosa	100% of absorbed fraction	Lung (a small percentage may go to the liver)
Sublingual	Buccal mucosa; a high percentage will be swallowed (then as oral)	Variable[a] Buccal mucosa (Oral: gut mucosa)	Lung (Liver)
Inhalation spray	Lung; a high percentage will be swallowed	Variable[b] Lung (Oral: gut mucosa)	General circulation (Liver)
Intravenous	Lung	100%	General circulation
Intraarterial	Via general circulation to various organs (such as liver[c])		
In hepatic vein	Liver	100%	Lung
Subcutaneous } Transdermal }	Skin	100% of absorbed fraction	Lung
Intramuscular	Muscle	100%	Lung

[a]The distribution between sublingual absorption and swallowing will depend to a very high extent on the rate of absorption of the drug and the skills and attitude of the patient; therefore, wide variation will be found.
[b]Most of the drug will be swallowed. Only approximately 2% of the inhalation dose of cromoglycate is absorbed in the lung, while 98% is swallowed (1).
[c]The blood flow through the liver for various species is given in Refs. 2 and 3.

bioavailability of the drug. The consequences of this difference in pharmacokinetics of drug absorption for drug metabolism are discussed in Section I.B. Food components or the use of other drugs may affect the rate of absorption of an orally administered drug since these may slow down (or accelerate) the rate of drug absorption by various mechanisms (4,5).

Although the liver is considered to be quantitatively the main site of metabolism for most drugs, extrahepatic metabolism may be very important for some drugs (see Ref. 6 for a review) and may have been underestimated so far. Recent findings on the conjugation of phenol in the rat in vivo have drawn attention to the prominent role of the lungs in the metabolism of this compound (7). The authors have compared pharmacokinetics and conjugation of phenol administered by four different routes: oral (first-pass metabolism in the gut, and, subsequently, the liver), intravenous (first pass in the lungs), arterial (first distributed throughout the body), and intravenous in the portal vein (first pass in the liver). Their results indicate that the liver contributes only to a minor extent to the conjugation of phenol, but that the major part of the conjugation takes place in the lungs. Even when phenol was injected into the portal vein, relatively little conjugation occurred in the liver. It should be realized that after intravenous injection (except for administration in the portal vein, or course) the complete dose will be delivered "first pass" to the lungs. The liver, on the other hand, gets only approximately 25% of the cardiac output (2,3). This puts the lungs in an advantageous position as far as availability of the drug for uptake and metabolism is concerned. When phenol was given orally, the gut mucosa was the major site of conjugation, and little unconjugated phenol reached the circulation. This is in agreement with previous findings that pointed at the important role of the gut mucosa for metabolism of orally administered drugs (6,8–10).

One important advantage that the liver may have over various other drug-metabolizing organs is that it takes up many substances at an extremely high efficiency (10–12): extraction percentages over 90% are often found in the perfused rat liver. In combination with high activities of the conjugating enzymes in the liver and the size of the organ, the liver will play a major role in conjugation. Possibly, the uptake mechanisms of the liver determine to a certain degree whether a compound is conjugated to a high extent in the liver or extrahepatically. The lung, on the other hand, has the advantage of being most extensively exposed to the drug in blood, because it receives the total cardiac output when the blood is returned to the heart.

As yet, few data are available on the first-pass metabolism in the skin of drugs that are percutaneously absorbed (13); such metabolism is probably very low since the skin has rather low levels of the conjugating enzymes (14). Subcutaneous and intramuscular injections may be given in such a pharmaceutical form that the release of the drug from its site of injection is enhanced or retarded (15). Such effects on the rate of drug absorption will affect the resulting blood levels of the drug and, thereby, may change its pattern of metabolism.

The discussion above shows that first-pass effects may occur, depending on the route of administration (see Ref. 10 for a review). Another factor that has to be considered in this respect is the dose, because it is to be expected that the extent of first-pass metabolism is dose dependent. For instance, at increasing dose of an orally administered drug the first-pass conjugation in the gut mucosa may become saturated; as more unconjugated drug escapes the gut mucosa cells, hepatic metabolism will become more important. Such a situation may give rise to very complex dose-dependent shifts in the pattern of conjugation of orally administered drugs when the ratio between the activities of two competing enzymes is different in the gut mucosa and in the liver. Unless a detailed and complete pharmacokinetic analysis of the conjugates and the parent compound is performed, however, such phenomena will probably be overlooked.

An interesting species difference in the conjugation of benzoic acid illustrates that the enzyme activities in the first-pass organ determine the nature of the conjugates formed. In the dog and the ferret, benzoic acid, after oral administration, is conjugated to an appreciable extent with glucuronic acid, while in herbivorous and omnivorous mammals it is conjugated almost exclusively with glycine. The explanation seems to be that the liver of the ferret and the dog is relatively deficient in hippuric acid synthesis; therefore, in these species first-pass conjugation in the liver will lead to appreciable glucuronidation, the competing conjugation reaction (16).

B. Pharmacokinetics and Enzyme Kinetics of Conjugation

A drug can be administered in a single dose, for instance orally, or as an intravenous bolus injection. Alternatively, a continuous, constant supply of the drug can be provided by, for instance, an osmotic minipump or an intravenous infusion. When a single dose is given, the supply of the drug to the conjugating enzymes decreases in time. Depending on the degree of saturation of (one of) the enzyme(s) involved, the decrease of the substrate concentration in vivo will be linear or exponential in time. In the study of the kinetics of conjugation in vivo under such conditions, therefore, the rate of the reaction may change with time. Usually, it is impossible to measure the substrate concentration at the active site of the conjugating enzyme. In general, therefore, it seems advisable to give a constant infusion of the drug, leading to a steady state, in order to study properly the rate of conjugation in vivo. However, this may result in accumulation of the conjugation products in vivo that may interact with the conjugation of the parent compound, for instance by product inhibition, or that may affect the condition of the experimental animal otherwise. This is one

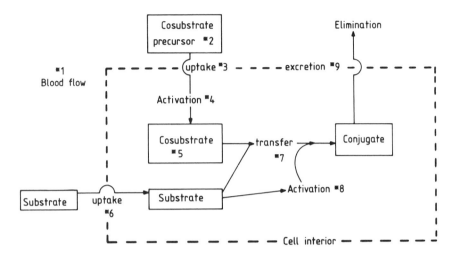

Figure 1 Potentially rate-limiting steps in the conjugation of a substrate and the elimination of its conjugate. 1, Blood flow through the organ (supply of substrate and cosubstrates or their precursors); 2, availability of precursors of cosubstrates for activation; 3, uptake of precursors of cosubstrates, or the cosubstrates; 4, activation of precursor to group-donating cosubstrates; 5, availability of cosubstrate; 6, uptake of substrate; 7, transfer reaction; 8, activation of the substrate; 9, elimination of the conjugate to blood, urine, or bile.

of the reasons why the use of a single-pass perfused organ is preferred above the recirculating perfusion for kinetic studies on conjugation (17,18), even though certain cellular metabolic intermediates may be depleted in the perfused organ by continuous washing out with fresh medium in the single-pass perfusion.

A complete pharmacokinetic profile of the conjugation of a drug should be obtained before a rate-limiting step can be pinpointed at any level of its metabolism (see Figure 1). A detailed analysis of the rate of disappearance of the substrate and the rates of appearance and disappearance of the conjugates in blood, urine, and bile may reveal whether the rate of conjugation was limited by, for instance, the capacity of (one of) the conjugation(s), the rate of supply of the substrate to the sites of conjugation, or by the blood flow through the organ where the conjugation takes place. Usually, in vivo experiments are not sufficient but, in addition, experiments with isolated perfused organs, isolated cell preparations, and purified enzymes will be required.

At increasing dose of a drug (i.e., at increasing substrate concentration) the conjugating enzymes in vivo will become saturated at a certain dose level. The in vivo operative K_m value will determine at which blood level of the substrate saturation occurs, and the maximum velocity will depend on the V_{max} value; obviously, the concentration of the substrate at the site of conjugation may be very different from that in blood or plasma. The rate at which the substrate is supplied to the site of conjugation inside the cell may be limiting, for instance when a rather poorly lipid-soluble substrate has to cross a membrane before it reaches the enzyme; in that case the V_{max} of a transport carrier across the membrane may be the actual V_{max} for such a conjugation in vivo.

The rate at which a cosubstrate for conjugation is supplied can under certain circumstances be a further rate-limiting factor in vivo or in intact cell preparations. Then it is often possible to enhance the rate of conjugation by increasing the rate of synthesis of the cosubstrate. Thus sulfate conjugation may be limited by the rate at which adenosine 3'-phosphate 5'-sulfatophosphate (PAPS), the cosubstrate of sulfation, is synthesized because this process most likely has a rather high K_m for inorganic sulfate (19). Consequently, the synthesis of PAPS can probably be enhanced by increasing the concentration of inorganic sulfate in the blood, and the sulfation rate of all those compounds should be increased, whose rate of conjugation was limited by availability of PAPS. Substrates that had saturated their sulfate conjugation at the level of the sulfotransferase at a low PAPS requirement (i.e., at a low V_{max} of sulfation, limited by transferase activity) may be expected to demonstrate little further increase in sulfation rate upon administration of inorganic sulfate.

When the maximum velocity of conjugation is determined by the cosubstrate supply, a high dose of the substrate that depletes the cosubstrate will thereby decrease the rate of conjugation. Administration of a precursor of the cosubstrate can compensate for the depletion, provided that the rate of synthesis of the cosubstrate is high enough. This depletion and replenishment occurs with sulfation, methylation, taurine conjugation, and glutathione conjugation (see the various sections on these conjugations). When high doses of a substrate for a certain conjugation are administered for a prolonged time, the rate-limiting step may change from, for instance, the transfer reaction initially to the availability of the cosubstrate lateron, when depletion of the cosubstrate progresses slowly.

For all these reasons, the in vitro determined K_m and V_{max} values for a transferase may not be relevant for the in vivo situation, although they are required for a complete characterization of the conjugating system. The interpretation of the in vitro-determined kinetic constants of the transferases is further complicated by the fact that some of these enzymes are located in subcellular organelles. Thus UDP-glucuronosyltransferase is firmly bound to the membrane of the endoplasmic reticulum, and glycine conjugation of carboxylic acids takes place inside the mitochondrion. The purified enzymes clearly represent artifacts, yet these have to be accepted because meaningful in vitro kinetic constants can only be determined with purified enzymes, in the absence of any interfering substances. At the same time, however, such substances may be involved in the physiological regulation of the enzyme activity.

If two or more enzymes compete for the same substrate, for instance phenol sulfotransferase and UDP-glucuronosyltransferase for a phenolic drug, their affinities for the substrate will usually be different. Therefore, at increasing blood levels of the substrate changing ratios between the rates of formation of both conjugates will be found as one of the conjugations becomes saturated. This will lead to dose-dependent shifts in the pattern of conjugation. These have been observed for several drugs. Thus, usually glucuronidation increases relative to sulfation at increasing dose under conditions in which no depletion of sulfate occurred (19-22). Similar data were found for other conjugation reactions (23-25). Changes in the rate of absorption of an orally administered drug may be reflected in changing ratios between various conjugates of the drug if more than one conjugating enzyme converts it. When conjugation takes place in two or more organs (compartments) (e.g., gut mucosa and liver after oral dosage) it depends on the pharmacokinetics of drug entry into these compartments whether saturation of a particular enzyme in both compartments occurs at the same blood concentration of the drug or at different levels. If in one compartment the substrate is taken up at a higher rate than in the other, this will lead to saturation of the enzyme in the former compartment at a lower *blood* concentration than in the other compartment. Several reviews on the pharmacokinetics of biotransformation have been published (26-28).

C. Competing Pathways of Conjugation In Vivo

When two or more different conjugations can occur with a substrate, the transferases involved will compete for the same substrate; the affinities and maximum velocities of the enzyme systems then play an important role, as discussed in the preceding section. Further, the group-donating cosubstrate of one of the conjugations may be depleted, thus favoring the competing conjugation(s). This happens, for instance, at very high doses of substrates for sulfation, in which case the competing glucuronidation takes over (29). Interestingly, the rate of elimination of the substrate need not be seriously affected by the loss of sulfation, because the glucuronidation process has a very high capacity and a rate that is almost as fast as that of sulfation at the same substrate concentration (30).

A further complicating factor may be the tissue distribution of competing enzymes. If part of the substrate is taken up by one tissue, and part by another, the respective ratios of conjugate A to B formed in the two tissues will depend on the ratios of transferase activities in those tissues; these may be widely different.

In vivo, the result of conjugation can be followed in the metabolite pattern found in urine and bile. It is important to realize that the rate of excretion of different conjugates from the same compound may be different, so that the time course of their elimination does not necessarily reflect their rate of synthesis. Further, some conjugates can be hydrolyzed again in vivo (31).

From a pharmacological point of view it is often rather unimportant which of two competing transferases converts a substrate, because the conjugates usually are pharmacologically inactive. However, in some cases conjugation leads to extremely toxic metabolites; thus the N-O-sulfate conjugate of N-hydroxy-2-acetylaminofluorene is very chemically reactive, whereas its N-O-glucuronide counterpart is relatively stable. The N-O-sulfate has been implicated in the carcinogenic action of the parent compound, while the N-O-glucuronide seems to be "safe" (32). In this and similar cases, therefore, it remains not without consequences whether one or the other conjugation prevails.

D. Elimination of the Conjugates

Once the conjugates have been formed, they usually will be eliminated by urinary and biliary excretion. Although in the rat excretion in bile, especially of conjugates with higher molecular weight (above 300) is very important, this is less so in many other species (33). Yet in a study on the total metabolism of a drug it is hazardous to collect only urine after dosing an animal with the drug, because in most species a part of the dose is excreted in bile. This fraction may increase as the dose increases because the metabolism may change to metabolites that are more readily excreted in bile. Indeed, the pattern of the metabolites excreted in bile is usually different from that excreted in urine. For instance, glucuronide conjugates are more readily excreted in bile, whereas sulfate conjugates will be excreted predominantly in urine in the rat (31). Therefore, both eliminatory routes should be investigated.

When the drug conjugates are excreted in bile, the possibility of enterohepatic recirculation exists, when the conjugate can be hydrolyzed to the parent compound by enzymes in the gut such as β-glucuronidase. If only urine is collected in such a situation, these "primary" conjugates in bile will be missed, and only those that ultimately "escape" in urine after enterohepatic recirculation and bacterial modification ("secondary" metabolites) will be found in urine. The interruption of enterohepatic recirculation by an inhibitor of such bacterial hydrolysis, administered orally, may lead to a shortening of the pharmacological action of substances subject to such recirculation (34).

E. Species Differences and Genetic Defects

In different species, even in different strains of the same species, the rate-limiting step in conjugation may be different. As yet, few species differences have been analyzed as to the mechanisms involved. Thus the cat and most Felidae are relatively deficient in glucuronidation; yet they do conjugate several substrates with glucuronate (35). Therefor, they possess the machinery for glucuronidation, but may lack a glucuronidation "isoenzyme." Phenols that are almost exclusively sulfated in the cat are almost completely glucuronidated in the pig; again, the latter species does sulfate various other phenols.

    Genetically determined deficiencies within a species or a strain usually will be easier to pinpoint, since they involve often one single step, most pronounced in the homozygous animal. Thus the homozygous Gunn rat is unable to conjugate bilirubin with glucuronic acid because it is absolutely deficient in the functional form of UDP-glucuronosyltransferase that converts bilirubin (36). A less absolute deficiency in the formation of the cosubstrate for sulfation, PAPS, has been observed in brachymorphic mice (37). The genetically determined difference between slow and fast acetylators (38) is well known, and recently similar differences have been detected for catechol-O-methyltransferase (39). So far, few absolute deficiencies have been observed in conjugation, presumably because they are incompatible with life.

II. GLUCURONIDATION: UDP-GLUCURONATE

A. Biosynthesis and Functions of UDPGA

UDP-glucuronic acid (UDPGA) (Figure 2) is synthesized in a two-step reaction from glucose-1-phosphate and UTP, catalyzed by, subsequently, UDP glucose pyrophosphorylase (UTP: α-D-glucose-1-phosphate uridylyl transferase, E. C. 2.7.7.9) and UDP glucose dehydrogenase (UDPglucose:NAD$^+$ 6-oxidoreductase, E. C. 1.1.1.22). Its biosynthesis and the following glucuronide conjugation have recently been extensively reviewed by Dutton (36).

$$\text{UTP + glucose-1-P} \rightleftharpoons \text{UDP-glucose + PP}_i \tag{1}$$

$$\text{UDP-glucose + 2NAD}^+ + \text{H}_2\text{O} \rightleftharpoons \text{UDPGA + 2NADH + 2H}^+ \tag{2}$$

$$\text{UDPGA + substrate} \rightleftharpoons \text{UDP + } \beta\text{-D-glucuronide conjugate} \tag{3}$$

    In most animal tissues both UDPGA-synthesizing enzymes are present and, therefore, UDPGA synthesis may occur in probably every tissue. It cannot be decided at present whether the rate of formation of UDPGA or the transfer of the glucuronic acid moiety to the acceptor substrate is rate limiting in glucuronidation in vivo in the various tissues. It

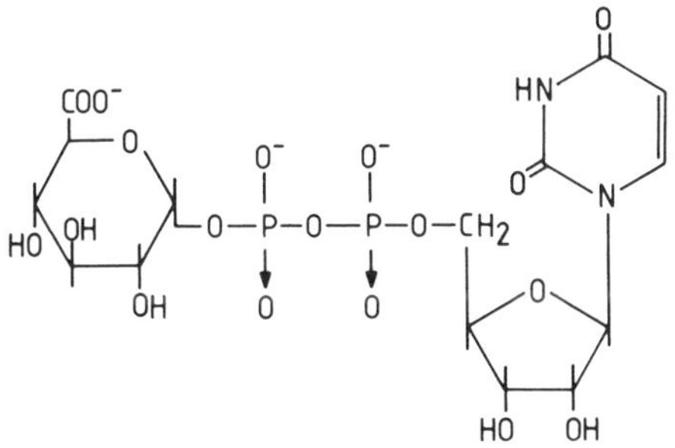

Figure 2 Chemical structure of UDP-glucuronic acid (UDPGA).

seems that at least in the liver the rate of synthesis of UDPGA can cope with even very high demands for this substance. Assuming that the liver is the main site for glucuronidation of xenobiotics, especially at high dose, the fact that no saturation of glucuronidation is found at increasing doses of these substrates in vivo shows that UDPGA can be resynthesized very rapidly under normal conditions. In the rat liver 0.15−0.25 μmol of UDPGA is present per gram of tissue (see Section II.B). Glucuronidation of harmol in the single-pass perfused rat liver reached a rate of 0.1 μmol/min per gram of liver, and this rate was sustained for more than 60 min, indicating that UDPGA synthesis has a very high capacity (40). Few xenobiotics will be so little toxic that such high amounts can be administered in vivo, requiring these high rates of UDPGA supply for their conjugation; therefore, depletion of UDPGA in vivo, even by very high doses of xenobiotics, seems very unlikely (unless, of course, the drug interferes with UDPGA synthesis).

UDPGA is not only used for the glucuronide conjugation of various exogenous and endogenous low-molecular-weight substances, but is also required for several other metabolic processes. It is an intermediate in the D-glucuronic acid pathway (41,42) that leads to the synthesis of glucaric acid and L-ascorbic acid. This pathway is induced by many foreign compounds that, as a result, stimulate the urinary excretion of ascorbic acid, glucaric acid, and xylulose (43). Further, UDPGA is required for the synthesis of various glucuronic acid-containing macromolecules (36,44).

At present it is unknown whether UDPGA in the cell is restricted to the cytosol, or whether it also occurs inside subcellular particles. It does not occur in the blood, and probably is not taken up by the cells from the extracellular medium. UDPGA is rather chemically stable, but several enzymes may break it down in homogenous and in vivo, as reviewed by Dutton (36).

Table 3 Concentrations of UDP-Glucuronate and UDPGglucose in
Various Tissues of the Rat and Some Other Species[a]

Tissue	Species	UDP-glucuronate (μmol/g tissue)	UDPglucose (μmol/g tissue)
Liver	Rat	0.12 ± 0.01	0.28 ± 0.02
	Rabbit	0.18 ± 0.02	0.29 ± 0.02
	Guinea pig	0.41 ± 0.03	0.21 ± 0.01
	Pig	0.29 ± 0.02	0.11 ± 0.01
Small intestine	Rat	0.06 ± 0.01	0.10 ± 0.01
Kidney	Rat	0.04 ± 0.00	0.15 ± 0.02
Lung	Rat	Trace	0.09
Testis	Rat	0.00	0.11 ± 0.01

[a]The results are given as means ± SEM.
Source: Data from Ref. 52.

B. Assay and Tissue Concentrations

UDPGA can be purified from the tissues and quantitated by its absorbance (45,46). However, this purification is a time-consuming procedure, and in most methods the amount of UDPGA present in an aqueous extract of a tissue is determined without further purification by
the amount of a glucuronide conjugate that can be formed from it.
Several substrates have been used in this assay, such as tyramine
(47), 2-aminophenol (36,48), 4-nitrophenol (49), and harmol (50). Recently, 3-hydroxybenzo[a]pyrene has been introduced as substrate,
which offers a very sensitive assay (51). Obviously, the reverse reaction should be negligible, so that at equilibrium the reaction yields almost completely the glucuronide product. Table 3 shows the UDPGA
and UDPglucose contents of several tissues; more data can be found in
Ref. 52.

C. Methods to Decrease the Availability of UDPGA In Vivo

So far, no highly selective methods to reduce the intracellular concentration of UDPGA in the tissues in vivo have been found. However, in
a nonspecific way UDPGA may be decreased by either administration of
galactosamine (in vivo and in hepatocyte incubations) or ethanol (in
hepatocyte incubations only).

D-Galactosamine is metabolized by the liver to UDP-galactosamine; at
high doses of galactosamine the uridine pool may become depleted, so
that all uridine-dependent reactions are profoundly affected (53).
Hence the effect of galactosamine is not limited to UDPGA availability,
and severe liver damage results at higher doses. At moderate dose,

however, galactosamine will reversibly decrease hepatic UDPGA without causing too many untoward side effects (46,49). As a result, glucuronidation in vivo of various compounds such as bilirubin, 1-naphthol, and harmol was decreased (19,54). This is only a short-lasting effect because of the low dose used to ensure reversibility; such doses did not decrease the glucuronidation of paracetamol (55). In isolated rat hepatocytes the effect is more pronounced, and galactosamine (2—5 mM) may almost completely inhibit the glucuronidation of harmol, paracetamol, and 1-naphthol (56—58).

Ethanol (10 mM) inhibits glucuronidation if it is included in the incubation medium of isolated hepatocytes. Presumably, this is due to the shift of the $NAD^+/NADH$ ratio to a more reduced state by ethanol oxidation (41), because the effect of ethanol on glucuronidation was completely prevented by the inclusion of pyrazole, an inhibitor of alcohol dehydrogenase (59). The chronic administration of ethanol in vivo, however, did not have such an effect on glucuronidation in isolated hepatocytes prepared from the liver of these pretreated rats; in contrast, an increase of glucuronidation was observed (60). Presumably, the $NAD^+/NADH$ ratio is not so easily disturbed in vivo. Ethanol pretreatment indeed had no major effects on UDPGA in the rat liver in vivo (42). Diethyl ether narcosis was reported to decrease rapidly the UDPGA concentration in the liver (60a).

D. Hormonal, Nutritional, and Drug Effects on UDPGA in the Liver

Insulin, corticosteroids, and testosterone affect the biosynthesis of UDPGA by as yet poorly defined mechanisms (61—66). When rats were made diabetic, the glucuronidation of bilirubin and 2-aminophenol was impaired due to a decreased content of UDPGA in the liver; administration of insulin and tolbutamide prevented this. Functionally intact adrenals were required for the tolbutamide effect (63). A sex difference in the hepatic concentration of UDPGA was observed in the rat, males having a higher concentration and, therefore, glucuronidation activity (in slices in vitro) than females (62). The activity of UDPG-dehydrogenase was higher in male than in female rat liver, which might explain this sex difference in UDPGA content. However, UDPG-dehydrogenase probably is not rate limiting in the formation of UDPGA, and therefore its activity cannot be used as an index of UDPGA availability in general (36,37). These findings are rather complex and indicate that effects at many levels of overall glucuronidation are involved. Later it was suggested that UDP-glucuronosyltransferase can be induced by administration of glucagon in the rat (67).

In mouse and pig liver the UDPGA content gradually increases from very low levels in the fetus, via higher levels after birth, to the still higher adult level (48,52). Few further data are available on developmental aspects of UDPGA availability (36,68).

Table 4 Effects of Various Drugs on UDP-Glucuronate and UDPGlucose Content in Rat Liver In Vivo[a]

Drug	Dose [mg/kg (route)]	UDP-glucuronate (μmol/g liver)	UDPglucose (μmol/g liver)
Control	—	0.26 ± 0.02	0.23 ± 0.02
Barbital	150 (i.p.)	0.50 ± 0.04[b]	0.29 ± 0.02
Phenobar-bital	130 (i.p.)	0.69 ± 0.02[b]	0.37 ± 0.03[b]
Nikethamide	130 (i.p.)	0.70 ± 0.03[b]	0.44 ± 0.03[b]
D-Galacto-samine	600 (i.p.)	0.16 ± 0.01[b]	0.11 ± 0.01[b]
Chlorbutol	150 (p.o.)	0.36 ± 0.04[b]	0.37 ± 0.03[b]
DDT	60 (p.o.)	0.69 ± 0.04[b]	0.33 ± 0.03[b]

[a]Male rats were given two doses, at zero time and at 4 hr; the livers were taken out for analysis 8 hr after the first dose. Values are means ± SEM. i.p., intraperitoneally; p.o., per os.
[b]Significantly different from control, $P < 0.05$.
Source: Data from Ref. 42.

Fasting decreases hepatic UDPGA levels in the rat (69), in parallel with a fall in UDPG-dehydrogenase activity. These effects of a 72-hr fast were reversible in 24 hr upon refeeding. Interestingly, the UDPglucose level was not affected by the fast. Phenobarbital pretreatment prevented these effects on UDPGA levels, and increased the UDPGA content of the liver considerably in normally fed rats (69). Fasting also changed UDP-glucuronosyltransferase activity in the liver; both an increase and a decrease have been reported (34,70,71). These conflicting findings may be the result of the use of different assay procedures in these studies; this needs further clarification.

A carbohydrate-rich diet may increase glucuronidation, although the evidence that increased UDPGA supply may be the explanation is still rather limited (72). In isolated rat liver cells, however, an increase in glucuronidation was indeed observed when glucose was added to the incubation medium; cells from 48-hr -starved rats were used in this study (58). Several drugs, notably barbiturates (42,49), nikethamide, and DDT (42), increase the levels of UDPGA in rat liver (Table 4).

III. METHYLATION: S-ADENOSYLMETHIONINE

A. Biosynthesis and Functions of SAM

S-Adenosyl-L-methionine (SAM) (Figure 3) is synthesized in vivo by the enzyme methionine adenosyltransferase (ATP: L-methionine S-

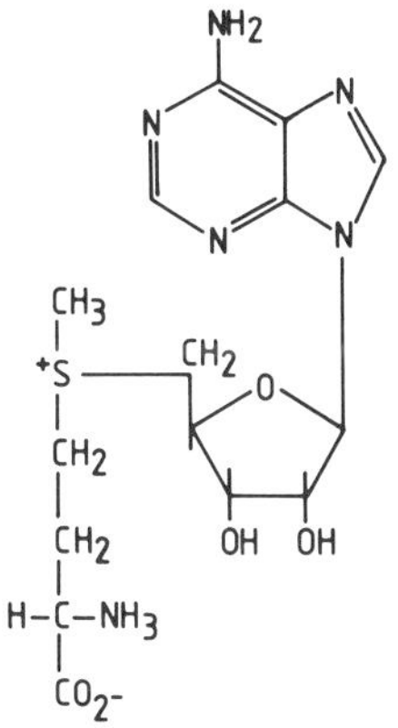

Figure 3   Chemical structure of S-adenosylmethionine (SAM).

adenosyltransferase, E. C. 2.5.1.6) from ATP and L-methionine. Its biosynthesis and many biological roles have been discussed extensively in several recent reviews (73–75). The specificity of methionine adenosyltransferase is rather broad, so that S-adenosyl-D-methionine can be synthesized from D-methionine (76), and ethionine is activated to S-adenosylethionine (see Section III.C).

$$\text{L-Methionine} + \text{ATP} \rightleftharpoons \text{S-adenosyl-L-methione} + \text{PP}_i + \text{P}_i \qquad (4)$$

$$\text{SAM} + \text{substrate} \rightleftharpoons \text{S-adenosylhomocysteine} + \text{substrate-CH}_3 \quad (5)$$

The biologically active diastereomer of SAM has the S configuration at the sulfonium center (77); its R isomer is not active in methylation reactions. The active S isomer is formed in vivo in probably all tissues in animals, plants, and microorganisms. SAM provides activated methyl groups for methylation of xenobiotic and endogenous low-molecular-weight substances, especially those containing catecholic hydroxyl groups. In addition, it is required for the methylation of endogenous macromolecules such as RNA and protein (73–75,78). It further serves as precursor for the synthesis of polyamines such as spermidine (73–75,79,80). The mechanism of methylation is a direct transfer of the S-methyl group by an S_N2 reaction, without a methylated enzyme intermediate (81).

The availability of methionine is critical for the supply of SAM in the cells. Methionine is rapidly incorporated into SAM in the liver, as observed after intravenous injection of radiolabeled methionine. This process is somewhat slower in brain, probably because the activity of methionine adenosyltransferase in brain is much lower than in the liver

(82–84). Therefore, a rapid adaptation of SAM levels in the liver to increased methionine supply is to be expected, especially since the concentrations of methionine in various tissues (85) are usually well below the K_m of methionine adenosyltransferase for L-methionine: 0.3–1.0 mM (84,86–90). In rat liver two forms of methionine adenosyltransferase are found, a minor form with K_m of 21 μM, and a major form with a K_m of 1 mM for methionine (91). Thus administration of additional methionine, either orally or intraperitoneally, leads to increased serum methionine levels and to increases of SAM in various tissues (82,86,92–95). Uptake of methionine by the cells does not seem to be rate limiting, at least not in liver and heart (96).

Since methylation is one of the main conjugation reactions for several neurotransmitters in brain, its presence in that tissue has drawn much attention. Although the rate of synthesis of SAM is slower than in liver (82–84), in brain the SAM concentration increases when serum methionine is enhanced, even though L-methionine in brain does not in all cases follow such a rise in blood (97,98).

By transfer of the methyl group to an acceptor, SAM is converted into S-adenosylhomocysteine, which is a very potent inhibitor of transmethylation reactions. This product is either reloaded with a methyl group through 5-methyltetrahydrofolate, or further metabolized by transsulfurylation (see Section VIII). Under conditions of methionine deprivation the methionine metabolism is adapted by a strong reduction of transsulfurylation such that this amino acid and also homocysteine are conserved as much as possible for their transmethylating function. Serine is used as a methyl donor for the conversion of homocysteine to methionine, mediated by tetrahydrofolate (99).

A low concentration of SAM is found in serum, approximately 1 μM (92). Isolated rat hepatocytes take up SAM from the medium, probably in unchanged form (100). The uptake of SAM by the isolated perfused rat liver from the perfusion medium was rather slow (101,102). It seems unlikely, therefore, that in vivo uptake of SAM from blood plays a major role (82). Surprisingly, some SAM seems to be taken up as such after oral administration in the rat; only little reaches the general circulation, presumably because of first-pass uptake and metabolism in the gut and the liver (103).

B. Assay and Tissue Concentrations

SAM is often determined enzymatically according to the method of Baldessarini and Kopin (82,92). In this method hydroxyindole-O-methyltransferase (S-adenosyl-L-methionine:N-acetylserotonine-O-methyltransferase, E. C. 2.1.1.4) is employed to methylate ^{3}H-labeled N-acetylserotonine with ^{14}C-labeled SAM. When a sample of unlabeled SAM of unknown concentration is added, the ^{3}H/^{14}C ratio in the methylated product is increased, and this increase is correlated with the

Table 5 Methionine Adenosyltransferase Activity and Concentrations of SAM and S-Adenosylhomocysteine in Various Rat Tissues[a]

Organ	Methionine adenosyl-transferase activity (pmol/min/mg protein)	SAM (nmol/g tissue)	S-adenosyl-homocysteine (nmol/g tissue)
Liver	7700	68	44
Pancreas	558	40	11
Kidneys	192	47	23
Adrenals	86	52	16
Testis	70	21	6
Brain	43	25	3
Heart	42	39	4

[a]Male rats aged 3 weeks and fed ad libitum were used for the analysis.
Source: Data from Ref. 94.

amount of unlabeled SAM in the sample, which can then be calculated from a calibration curve.

Isotope dilution methods have been devised by several authors; radiolabeled SAM is added to the sample in which SAM has to be determined; before further workup. SAM is subsequently purified by column chromatography or thin-layer chromatography, and the amount of SAM present is determined by ultraviolet (UV) absorbance, while the recovery of radioactivity indicates the percentage of recovery for the whole extraction procedure (92,104–108). SAM and its analogs can also be separated and determined by high-performance liquid chromatography (109), eventually in the form of a fluorescent derivative (110). The tissue concentrations of SAM and S-adenosylhomocysteine in various tissues and different species are given in Tables 5 and 6.

C. Decreased Availability of SAM In Vivo

A decrease of SAM in the tissues by a high requirement for methylation reactions in vivo tends to be rapidly adjusted by resynthesis from methionine. However, short-lasting depletion of SAM by administration of high doses of drugs that are methylated indeed does occur. Particularly strong is the effect of pyrogallol, which is methylated by catechol-O-methyltransferase; this drug thereby inhibits methylation reactions very effectively (111). L-Dopa similarly depletes SAM, especially in brain and less so in the liver (86,89,111), which may be related to the lower rate of synthesis of SAM in the brain (92). Various polyphenols also deplete SAM in various tissues to some extent

Table 6 Species Differences in the Concentrations of SAM and S-
Adenosylhomocysteine in the Liver

Species	SAM (nmol/g tissue)	S-adenosylhomocysteine (nmol/g tissue)
Rabbit	70	70
Calf	55	55
Rat	53	63
Chicken	58	47
Eel	37	39

Source: Data from Ref. 104.

(86,89,92,95,111,112); since these compounds do not seem to affect
methionine adenosyltransferase activity, the mechanism of action
probably is depletion of SAM by a high requirement of this substrate
in the methylation of these phenols. This decreased availability of
SAM may reduce methylation of physiological substrates in brain (86,
111,113), which may be prevented by the concomitant administration
of methionine or even SAM itself (95,114).

The decrease of SAM after administration of pyrogallol and similar
drugs is not very long lasting, and further doses have to be administered to keep the concentration of SAM low (111). This has very toxic
consequences and, therefore, results obtained by this treatment have
to be interpreted with caution.

When the methionine analog ethionine is given in large doses, accumulation of S-adenosylethionine occurs, leading to the depletion of the
adenine pool and of SAM; various methylation reactions are severely
affected (115–117). Another type of methionine analog, represented
by methionine sulfoximine and related oximines, also inhibits the methylation reaction, probably due to a decreased level of SAM (93,118).
However, these sulfoximines also inhibit glutathione synthesis and thus
are not specific for methylation in their inhibitory effect (118,119).

Various nucleoside-modified analogs of SAM, and the methionine analog
L-2-amino-4-methoxy-trans-3-butenoic acid, inhibit methylation via a
mechanism that probably involves (analogs of) S-adenosylhomocysteine
(120–122); modified nucleosides also effectively inhibited spermine and
spermidine synthesis (79,80).

A number of cyclic amino acids are very strong inhibitors of methionine adenosyltransferase (123). Guanidinoacetic acid lowers SAM in the
liver by 45% for prolonged periods of time when it is fed regularly
(124).

D. Nutritional and Hormonal Effects on SAM in the Tissues

As indicated above, the dietary supply of methionine determines to a large extent the availability of SAM in the tissues (82,86,90,92–95, 104). Reviews about the regulation of methionine metabolism in mammals are available (99,125); the further metabolism of methionine is discussed in Section VIII.

Fasting decreases the SAM concentration of the liver, presumably due to a deficiency of methionine. A sudden great loss of blood has the same effect: within 30 min after cardiac puncture the SAM content in the liver reached its lowest level, approximately 30% below control (126).

A decrease of the SAM content of brain with age has been reported in several species (82,94,112). For the liver the data are controversial: a decrease (82), an increase (94), and no change (112) have all been reported. The product of transmethylation, S-adenosylhomocysteine, was found to increase with age in rat liver (94).

A circadian rhythm of the SAM concentration in brain has been observed in the rat, with a peak at 4 a.m. (97,127), which has a complex relationship with a diurnal variation of methionine in serum and brain (97).

Although pyridoxine deficiency in the food does not decrease SAM in the rat, it leads to a decreased rate of breakdown of S-adenosylhomocysteine. The result is an accumulation of this product and, thereby, inhibition of methylation. The mechanism of this slower catabolism is the pyridoxine requirement of enzymes that metabolize homocysteine, such as cystathionine synthase and cystathionase (106).

So far, no drugs have been found that increase SAM in the tissues. Only an "overshoot" phenomenon has been observed after doses of L-dopa that first depleted SAM in the brain, but several hours later resulted in a concentration 30–40% higher than normal (86,128).

A sex difference in methionine adenosyltransferase in liver has been noted, female rats having twice the activity found in males. After castration the male level increased to the female level. Yet no sex difference was found in the SAM content in liver in the rat (94).

IV. SULFATION: ADENOSINE 3'-PHOSPHATE 5'-SULFATOPHOSPHATE

A. Biosynthesis and Functions of PAPS

Adenosine 3'-phosphate 5'-sulfatophosphate (PAPS) (Figure 4) is synthesized in a two-step reaction from inorganic sulfate and ATP. The first step, catalyzed by ATP sulfurylase (ATP: sulfate adenylyltransferase; E. C. 2.7.7.4), yields adenosine 5'-sulfatophosphate (APS); the product of the second step, catalyzed by APS kinase (ATP: adenylylsulfate 3'-phosphotransferase; E. C. 2.7.1.25), is PAPS. By

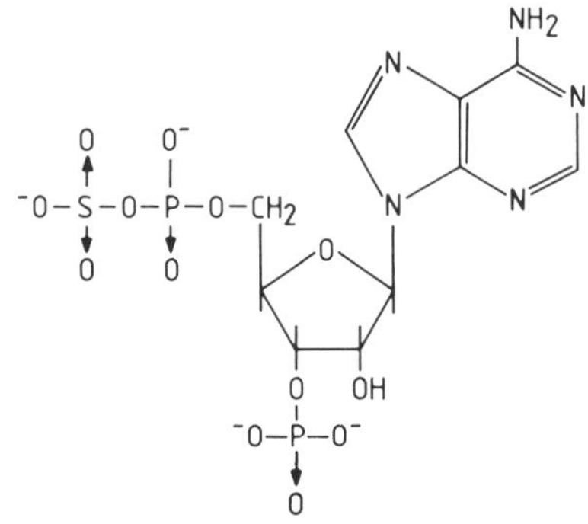

Figure 4 Chemical structure of adenosine 3'-phosphate 5'-sulfatophos-
phate (PAPS).

the sulfate transfer reaction adenosine 3',5'-bisphosphate (PAP) is
formed; this is strongly inhibitory toward sulfation and probably is
rapidly further metabolized in vivo. Biosynthesis of PAPS and sulfate
conjugation have been extensively reviewed recently (129,129a); the
activating enzymes can be found probably in all mammalian tissues.

$$ATP + SO_4^{2-} \rightleftharpoons APS + PP_i \tag{6}$$

$$APS + ATP \rightleftharpoons PAPS + ADP \tag{7}$$

$$PAPS + substrate \rightleftharpoons PAP + sulfate\ conjugate \tag{8}$$

When [35S]-labeled sulfate is administered intravenously, it is rapidly
incorporated into sulfate conjugates of low-molecular-weight substrates
such as phenol (130) and harmol (131), indicating a rapid mixing of inorganic sulfate in blood with the tissue sulfate pool (probably mainly
the liver and the lung for the sulfation of these two substrates), and a
rapid subsequent activation to PAP[35S]. In agreement with this a rapid
uptake of inorganic sulfate was observed in isolated hepatocyte incubations; at low sulfate concentration in the medium the hepatocytes accumulated sulfate at a higher level than in the medium, but at physiological sulfate levels no such accumulation occurred (132). Since in
vivo the equilibrium between the radioactivity of intravenously injected
[35S] sulfate in blood and that in the harmol sulfate conjugate is established within a few minutes (131), the pools of PAPS in the conjugating
organs probably are very small. This seems an advantage, because
PAPS is rather biochemically labile: several hydrolytic enzymes in the
liver and other tissues may break it down. Further, the thermodynam-
ics of the first step in the biosynthesis of PAPS are very unfavorable

for the formation of APS, so that the reaction probably occurs at an appreciable rate only when APS is rapidly utilized for the formation of PAPS required for a sulfation reaction (129,133). Yet PAPS can be synthesized at a high rate by the rat liver when it is continuously required for conjugation: In the single-pass perfused rat liver, sulfation of harmol in the perfusion medium occurred at a rate of approximately 0.1 μmol/min per gram of liver for at least 60 min (40). Since only about 0.3 μmol of PAPS seems to be available per gram of liver (134), this high rate of sulfate conjugation indicates that the rate of PAPS synthesis is determined in vivo by the rate of utilization of this cosubstrate rather than by the activities of the two activating enzymes (as long as inorganic sulfate is supplied at a constant level). The K_m for sulfate of sulfate activation to PAPS is rather high: values from 0.1 to 3.5 mM have been reported (129). In the rat in vivo (134a), the perfused rat liver, and isolated rat hepatocytes similar high values were found (56,135), although a K_m of only 75 μM for sulfate was found in the sulfation of 1-naphthol in hepatocytes (58). In hepatocyte incubations 4-nitrophenyl sulfate was an even better sulfate donor than inorganic sulfate or cysteine in the sulfation of harmol (58).

The serum concentration of inorganic sulfate in various species lies between 0.3 mM (humans) and 2.5 mM (chicken), with rat and mouse somewhere in between at 1.0 and 1.4 mM, respectively (136). Therefore, inorganic sulfate may not be saturating for overall sulfation in vivo; in that case, a depletion of serum sulfate will lead to a decreased rate of sulfate activation to PAPS (see Section IV.C). Probably for that reason also, administration of large amounts of sulfate or a sulfate precursor such as cysteine leads usually to an increased rate of sulfation of xenobiotics (137–139; see Ref. 19 for a review).

PAPS serves as the sulfate-donating cosubstrate for many sulfation reactions in vivo. Not only endogenous and exogenous low-molecular-weight substrates, but also many macromolecules such as glycosaminoglycans and proteins are sulfated (140,141). Also, the synthesis of sulfolipids requires PAPS (142). In several microorganisms APS and PAPS are utilized as final electron acceptors (143).

B. Assay and Tissue Concentrations of PAPS

The assay of PAPS in tissue extracts is usually performed by measuring the amount of a sulfate ester that can be formed from a sample of PAPS-containing material by purified phenol sulfotransferase. Various substrates have been used, such as harmol, 2-naphthol, and 4-methylumbelliferone (134,144,145). 4-Nitrophenol should not be used, because its reaction with PAPS is freely reversible (88,144,146). An alternative method uses the luciferin-luciferase system of the sea pansy *Renilla reniformis*, which is sensitive to adenosine 3',5'-bisphosphate (PAP). Before determination PAPS has to be converted to PAP, which

Table 7 Concentrations of PAPS in Various Organs

	Species	PAPS concentration (nmol/g tissue)
Liver	Guinea pig	33
	Rat	29
	Rabbit	8
	Mouse	5
	Dog	0
	Monkey	0
Brain, gut, and several other organs	Rat	0

Source: Data from Ref. 134.

can then be assayed by the bioluminescence of the luciferin-luciferase system (147).

Purification of PAPS by ion-pair chromatography, and its quantitation by UV absorbance using a high-performance liquid chromatographic method, is possible (148) but has not yet been applied to tissue extracts. Electrophoresis is another, rather time-consuming alternative (149).

Table 7 gives some data on the concentration of PAPS in mammalian tissues (134,149a); as yet it is uncertain whether the concentration of PAPS is affected by the length of time it takes to prepare the tissue extract. It seems advisable to freeze-clamp the tissue, since PAPS is metabolically very labile. Therefore, it is not clear whether the failure to detect PAPS in monkey and dog liver, or in several other tissues of the rat, such as the kidney, small and large intestine, heart, and brain, is due to its low concentration in those tissues or to a rapid breakdown during preparation and workup of the tissue extract.

C. Decreased Availability of PAPS In Vivo

The only method presently available to decrease the availability of PAPS in vivo is to decrease the availability of inorganic sulfate. No selective inhibitors of the activating enzymes have yet been discovered. Sulfate can relatively easily be depleted in vivo. This depletion, of course, will affect all physiological processes that are dependent on PAPS. Yet for short periods this presumably will not be too harmful to the organism, and the effects are probably fully reversible.

Inorganic sulfate is depleted in vivo by the administration of a high dose of a substrate for sulfation, as observed originally by Bray et al.

(29) and later confirmed by other authors (21,137,150; see Ref. 19 for a review). A drawback of this method is that these substrates are usually toxic, and that the sulfate level rapidly returns to normal after administration of the drug is discontinued. Thus considerable unconjugated acetaminophen was still present when the serum sulfate level in the rat started to return to the control level (151).

Surprisingly, oral administration of sodium chloride under diethyl ether anesthesia also reduces serum sulfate in the rat (151). This is a mild, rather variable decrease in serum sulfate for 2 hr, after which the sulfate level starts to return to the control level. The advantage of this method is that very little disturbance is caused in the physiology of the rat; on the other hand, the effect is short lasting.

Finally, the feeding of a diet deficient in protein and sulfate results in a prolonged decrease of serum sulfate to $0.1-0.4$ mM in the rat, presumably because the supply of cysteine becomes rate limiting in the generation of inorganic sulfate (151). This diet can be given for extended periods of time; however, other adaptive changes may occur, such as changes in the levels of the conjugating enzymes (70), which make the interpretation of the findings under these diet conditions more complicated.

The depletion of sulfate in vivo by a substrate of sulfation requires rather high doses because sulfate is continuously generated from cysteine and, probably, from the catabolism of sulfate-containing macromolecules (152). Therefore, it is advisable to measure serum sulfate levels to determine whether a decreased rate of sulfation is indeed due to a decreased serum sulfate level. An increase of sulfation by administration of (a) sulfate (precursor) does not necessarily mean that sulfate had been depleted, because of the rather high K_m of overall sulfation for inorganic sulfate; the additional sulfate may increase the sulfate levels and, thereby, the sulfation rate above normal (19).

D. Nutritional, Hormonal, and Drug Effects on PAPS In Vivo

Starvation decreases the activity of the first enzyme in sulfate activation, ATP sulfurylase, in the liver (153,154). However, it is questionable whether this would result in a decreased rate of sulfation in vivo, since the activity of this enzyme probably is not rate limiting (see Section IV.A). Fasting did not decrease the serum sulfate level during the first 72 hr (Table 8), probably because of the resulting catabolic state and sulfate retention by the kidneys (151). No data on in vivo sulfation of drugs during fasting are available.

As mentioned in Section IV.A, the feeding of inorganic sulfate or sulfate precursors increases serum sulfate and thereby sulfation. Inorganic sulfate is rapidly and completely absorbed from the gut (129, 154).

Table 8 Effect of Fasting on Serum Sulfate Concentration and the
Urinary Excretion of Inorganic Sulfate in the Rat[a]

Days fasted	Serum sulfate (mM)		Urinary sulfate (μmol/day)	
	Fasted	Control	Fasted	Control
1	1.00 ± 0.06[b]	0.85 ± 0.02	165 ± 12[b]	334 ± 21
3	0.94 ± 0.00	0.83 ± 0.06	224 ± 33	319 ± 58

[a]Control rats (200 g body weight) were fed ad libitum, while fasted
rats received only water for 24 or 72 hr, respectively. The mean ±
SEM are given.
[b]Means significantly different from control, $P < 0.05$.
Source: Data from Ref. 151.

Little is known about developmental aspects of sulfate activation. In
most cases overall sulfation has been measured; it appears that sulfation is functioning at birth at an almost adult level of activity, while
even in fetal liver high activities are found (129,155–159). In the
chick cornea it seems that during development the availability of PAPS,
rather than the sulfotransferase activity, is rate limiting in sulfation
of macromolecules in that tissue (149,160).

The effect of various drugs on PAPS levels in the liver of guinea pigs
and rats has been determined. The thyroid hormones, thiouracil, sucrose, pyridoxine, and an atherogenic diet with and without ascorbic
acid had relatively minor effects, which were not further analyzed in
terms of mechanism (161–166).

Vitamin A deficiency led to defective sulfation. Although it has been
suggested that ATP sulfurylase was involved in this effect because it
was thought to require some form of vitamin A as a cofactor for its
catalytic activity, the data so far have been too conflicting and confusing to permit a definite conclusion. During vitamin A deficiency, food
consumption is decreased, which in itself causes a decrease in ATP sulfurylase activity. These results have been reviewed extensively recently (129). Somatomedin, a growth hormone, stimulates the incorporation of sulfate into macromolecules; the mechanism of action has
not yet been clarified (167,168).

A genetic defect in the activation of sulfate in a special strain of
mice, brachymorphic mice, has been pinpointed to an extremely low
level of APS kinase in extracts from cartilage in these mice (37). No
studies on sulfation of drugs in this strain have yet been reported.

V. GLUTATHIONE CONJUGATION: GLUTATHIONE

A. Biosynthesis and Functions of Glutathione; the γ-Glutamyl Cycle

Glutathione (L-γ-glutamyl-L-cysteinylglycine) occurs in probably all living cells, often in appreciable concentrations. Several recent reviews on the metabolism and the various roles of glutathione are available (169,170). Reed and Beatty have published an excellent review of the biosynthesis and regulation of glutathione in 1980 (171). Synthesis and degradation of glutathione are linked by the γ-glutamyl cycle (172) (Figure 5). The synthesis consists of two consecutive steps, catalyzed by γ-glutamylcysteine synthetase (E. C. 6.3.2.2) and glutathione synthetase (E. C. 6.3.2.3).

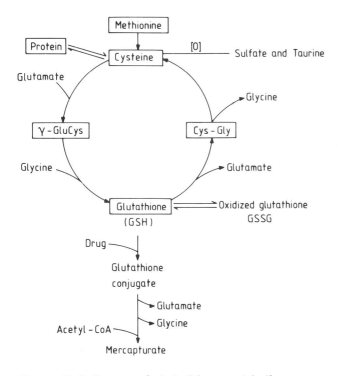

Figure 5 Pathways of glutathione metabolism.

$$L\text{-}Glu + L\text{-}Cys + ATP \rightleftharpoons L\text{-}\gamma\text{-}Glu\text{-}L\text{-}Cys + ADP + P_i \qquad (9)$$

$$L\text{-}\gamma\text{-}Glu\text{-}L\text{-}Cys + Gly + ATP \rightleftharpoons glutathione + ADP + P_i \qquad (10)$$

Glutathione is a feedback inhibitor of γ-glutamylcysteine synthetase and thereby is involved in the regulation of its own synthesis (173). Depending on the structure of a low-molecular-weight substrate, glutathione conjugation is either an addition reaction or a nucleophilic displacement.

Several inborn errors of glutathione metabolism are known (see Refs. 172 and 241 for reviews). Thus deficiency of glutathione synthetase causes 5-oxoprolinuria (see below), with a reduced glutathione level in the tissues. Patients with this enzyme deficiency exhibit an overproduction of γ-glutamylcysteine, in agreement with the reduced feedback inhibition by glutathione of γ-glutamylcysteine synthetase. The excess of γ-glutamylcysteine gives rise to greatly increased amounts of 5-oxoproline, which is excreted in urine.

The availability of L-cysteine is limiting in the synthesis of glutathione; indeed, the K_m of γ-glutamylcysteine synthetase for cysteine is of the same order as the tissue concentrations of this amino acid (171,174). When starved rats that have a reduced hepatic glutathione content were fed a protein-free diet, the increase in liver glutathione was dependent on the amount of cyst(e)ine added to the diet (174). The increase occurred within a few hours, indicating that biosynthesis of glutathione responds rapidly to an increased supply of cysteine. Comparison of turnover of glutathione in various organs of mice and rats revealed that the highest turnover rate occurs in the kidney, followed by the liver, pancreas, and skeletal muscle (175). Dietary experiments led to the hypothesis that there are two pools of glutathione in rat liver: a "labile" pool with a $t_{1/2}$ value of 1.7 hr, comprising about 50—60% of total hepatic glutathione that may be functioning as a reservoir for cysteine, and a "stable" pool with a $t_{1/2}$ value of 28.5 hr which cannot easily be depleted (174,176). The pool with the short half-life has also been demonstrated in the mouse and the rabbit (177).

Glutathione is the most abundant nonprotein sulfhydryl compound in the cell. It is present in the cell mainly in the reduced form (GSH), while very low concentrations of oxidized glutathione (GSSG) occur (169,170,178,179). Reduction of oxidizing agents by glutathione in the cell is catalyzed by glutathione peroxidase. The resulting GSSG can be reduced again by glutathione reductase at the expense of NADPH (169—171). Perturbation of the GSSG/GSH ratio results in the deregulation of many physiological processes (180). The perfused rat liver releases predominantly reduced glutathione in the perfusion medium (181), but during cytochrome P-450-catalyzed drug oxidation or hydroperoxide reduction the GSSG efflux was significantly increased, while the GSH efflux remain unchanged (171,182). Salicylate depleted rat liver glutathione, possibly by an increased glutathione leakage from the liver (183).

Glutathione is broken down by γ-glutamyltranspeptidase (E. C. 2.3.2.2) as shown in reaction (11). Cysteinylglycine is

$$\text{Glutathione + L-amino acid} \rightleftharpoons \text{L-}\gamma\text{-Glu-amino acid + L-CysGly} \quad (11)$$

further degradated by a peptidase to the constituent amino acids. γ-Glutamyltranspeptidase is bound to the membranes of epithelial cells at sites known to be involved extensively in the transport of amino acids, in which the γ-glutamyl group covalently binds the amino acid to be transported by a transpeptidation reaction (172). The γ-glutamyl-amino acid depeptide is cleaved within the cell by γ-glutamylcyclotrans-ferase, yielding the amino acid and 5-oxoproline; the latter is converted to glutamate by 5-oxoprolinase.

Glutathione in plasma is almost completely present in the oxidized form. It is rapidly removed from the circulation, the $t_{1/2}$ value of total glutathione in human plasma being only 1.6 min (184). The kidneys play an important role in the catabolism of extracellular glutathione (185,186). The extraction percentage of glutathione by the kidneys is about 90%; even at very high plasma glutathione concentrations in the renal blood supply (up to 200-fold above control), 60—70% extraction in the kidneys is found. However, extrarenal catabolism of glutathione also occurs (171,186), in which the intestinal mucosa may play an important role (187).

Many functions are ascribed to glutathione. It is though to protect the -SH groups of proteins and it is required in disulfide exchange reactions. It protects the cell by scavenging peroxides and free radicals, and also traps electrophilic reactive intermediates in drug metabolism. As indicated above, it is involved in the transport of amino acids across cell membranes and it serves as a cosubstrate for several metabolic reactions (169,170).

B. Assay and Tissue Concentrations of Glutathione

Many assay methods for glutathione have been described (see the review in Refs. 188 and 189). Most are based on a chemical reaction with the thiol group of reduced glutathione after deproteinization of a tissue extract. Although these methods are not specific for glutathione, they can be used satisfactorily because glutathione is usually the major nonprotein thiol-group-containing substance present. Thus Ellmann's reagent [5,5'-dithio-bis(2-nitrobenzoic acid), or DTNB] has been employed in a number of assays (178,190). This assay is applicable to glutathione determination in whole blood and tissues. It gives the total glutathione concentration (GSH + GSSG) if a glutathione reductace plus NADPH has been used in a preincubation to convert any GSSG into GSH. Pretreatment of tissue extracts with N-ethylmaleimide or 2-vinyl-pyridine to block the -SH group of reduced glutathione present allows the determination of the (low levels of) oxidized glutathione present in a tissue extract; after reduction of the free -SH groups GSSG is sub-sequently converted to free reduced glutathione by the reductase under conditions in which the -SH reagent is no longer active (178, 191). Specific for glutathione is the fluorimetric assay based on the reaction of glutathione with o-phthaldialdehyde at alkaline pH, yielding a product of which the fluorescence at 420 nm is proportional to the concentration of reduced glutathione (192). More recently, highly specific high-performance liquid chromatographic methods have been reported for the determination of reduced and oxidized glutathione in whole blood (193) and tissue extracts (194—197).

The glyoxalase reaction has often been used for the specific enzyma-tic determination of glutathione (198); glutathione reacts with methyl-glyoxal to S-lactoylglutathione (catalyzed by glyoxylase I), which can be determined spectrophotometrically. It is important to take precau-tions during the assay procedures to prevent oxidation of reduced glutathione.

Histochemical methods have been developed for reduced glutathione; they show, for instance, a different concentration of glutathione in dif-ferent regions of the rat liver lobule (199,200). The concentration of reduced glutathione is subject to diurnal variation; the highest concen-tration is found early in the morning, and the lowest (approximately half the maximum concentration) early in the evening, as observed in mouse and rat liver (201,202). This diurnal decrease in free gluta-thione parallels an increase in mixed disulfides between glutathione and the SH groups of proteins; these mixed disulfides can be determined separately (203). As much as 25% of total glutathione may be in the form of mixed disulfides with other thiol-containing substances, es-pecially proteins (204,205). In addition, glutathione is bound to glu-tathione S-transferases, probably in a noncovalent fashion. Induction of this transferase and other proteins that bind reduced glutathione may explain the increase in total hepatic glutathione by phenobarbital pretreatment: bound glutathione was increased while free glutathione was unaffected (183).

Although the reported values differ widely, in general the highest glutathione levels are found in the liver and erythrocytes, followed by the kidney and the spleen (Table 9). In various organs such as the liver (200), kidney (190), and brain (194) the distribution of gluta-thione may be nonhomogeneous over the different cell types and areas of the organ.

Table 9 Tissue Glutathione Levels
In Mice[a]

Tissue	Glutathione (μmol/g)
Brain	2.08 ± 0.15
Heart	1.35 ± 0.10
Lung	1.52 ± 0.13
Liver	7.68 ± 1.22
Pancreas	1.78 ± 0.31
Kidney	4.13 ± 0.15
Small intestine mucosa	2.94 ± 0.16
Colon mucosa	2.11 ± 0.19
Skeletal muscle	0.78 ± 0.05

[a]Mice were fed ad libitum.
Source: Data from Ref. 175.

C. Decrease of Glutathione Availability and Drug Toxicity

A standard procedure to decrease glutathione in the liver is the treatment of animals with diethylmaleate (206,207). This drug is conjugated
with glutathione and at higher doses utilizes all available glutathione
in the liver. It has few toxic effects if it is not dosed too high, and
results in a rapid, reversible depletion of glutathione that is rather
short lasting, because glutathione is rapidly resynthesized. Glutathione in other organs is also depleted, although less so than in the
liver (Figure 6).

Since glutathione conjugation has an important function in detoxification (208), especially of electrophilic reactive intermediates of drug
metabolism (209), this depletion of glutathione may have profound toxicological consequences. Every substrate for glutathione conjugation,
either after catalysis by glutathione S-transferase or after nonenzymatic reaction because of its high chemical reactivity, will be expected to
deplete glutathione at increasing dose, primarily in the liver but possibly also in other organs (207). The glutathione conjugates that are
formed are degraded to mercapturic acids by removal of the glutamate
and glycine moieties, and subsequent N-acetylation of the remaining
cysteine residue. The resulting decrease in the availability of glutathione in the various tissues will reduce the capacity of this detoxifying
pathway and will increase the risk of tissue lesions (22,208). Paracetamol (acetaminophen) is metabolized for a minor part (at low dose) to an
electrophilic intermediate which is detoxified by formation of a glutathione conjugate; this conjugation prevents the covalent binding of the

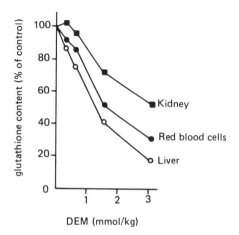

Figure 6 Depletion of glutathione in various organs in the rat by administration of diethylmaleate (DEM). Glutathione was determined $2\frac{1}{2}$ hr after the injection of DEM. (Data from Ref. 207).

reactive intermediate to cell constituents. This drug has been used in many studies on the relationship between glutathione depletion and toxicity (22,209,209a). For instance, in the hamster liver a complete depletion of glutathione can be achieved as the dose of paracetamol is increased; as soon as that occur, the covalent binding of the reactive intermediate to cellular macromolecules increases very rapidly. No depletion of glutathione was observed in rat erythrocytes, even at high doses of paracetamol, probably indicating a lack of metabolism of paracetamol to the reactive intermediate in these cells (210). Similarly, in mouse ocular lens no glutathione depletion occurred, yet ocular toxicity was observed after paracetamol (211).

If the substrate for glutathione conjugation is first generated by, for instance, oxidative metabolism, obviously the degree of glutathione depletion will be affected by treatments that change the rate of generation of the intermediate (209). Several drugs have been identified that deplete glutathione, such as paracetamol, and whose effect in this respect is influenced by pretreatment with inducers of cytochrome P-450, such as bromobenzene, furan derivatives, and N-hydroxyphenacetin (171,209,212).

Low-protein diets and starvation decrease the glutathione concentration in the liver (171,213−215), presumably by a shortage of cysteine. A chronic exposure of rats to ethanol also decreases the hepatic glutathione levels. In isolated hepatocytes it was shown that this effect was due to acetaldehyde formation; the effect of both ethanol and acetaldehyde on the glutathione availability could be prevented by inclusion of methionine in the incubation medium (216).

Methionine sulfoximine and related drugs strongly inhibit glutathione synthesis in vivo by inhibition of γ-glutamylcysteine synthetase. The most effective drug of this series so far is buthionine sulfoximine (S-n-butyl homocysteine sulfoximine) (117,118,175,216a). This may be a very useful tool to decrease glutathione availability; S-adenosyl-methionine is also affected, however.

Glycylglycine enhances the utilization of glutathione by γ-glutamyl-transpeptidase during transport of glycine, which leads to a consider-able decrease of glutathione (217,218).

D. Nutritional, Hormonal, and Drug Effects on Glutathione Availability

As discussed in Section V.A, the availability of cysteine is an import-ant factor in the biosynthesis of glutathione, and an increased supply of sulfur-containing amino acids may increase the glutathione levels above normal (171,219), as found in the liver. After starvation of rats for 1 or 2 days the liver glutathione content is between two-thirds and one-half of the normal level (174,213–215); upon reflecting it rapidly returns to normal (220). When starved rats are fed a protein-free diet, the increase in liver glutathione is dependent on the amount of cysteine added to the diet (174). A low-protein diet resulted in a liver glutathione content even lower than starvation, about one-third of control (213). The same was found for mouse erythrocytes: a diet free of methionine and cysteine caused a reduction of glutathione of about 30% in 3 weeks, which was larger than the reduction during fasting (221).

L-Methionine is incorporated into glutathione after transsulfurylation via cystathionine to cysteine; propargylglycine, an inhibitor of the cy-stathionine pathway, therefore prevents the incorporation of methionine and homocysteine into glutathione (219). Large doses of methionine, however, decreased glutathione in the kidneys to about 50% of normal in acute experiments; concomitantly, there was an increase in 5-oxopro-line in the kidney. Inhibition of γ-glutamyltranspeptidase prevented these effects (217). This suggests that under those conditions gluta-thione in the kidneys is consumed (for transport of methionine into the cell) at a much faster rate than it is resynthesized. In rat liver a re-duction of glutathione was observed after intraperitoneal injection of N-acetylcysteine or cysteine, but not after a large dose of methionine (222). Mixed disulfides between administered -SH-group-containing compounds and glutathione may have been formed.

In isolated hepatocytes the glutathione content decreases steadily during incubation. This decrease can be prevented by methionine, N-acetylcysteine, and homocysteine (223,224). In hepatocytes from starved rats, which contained about 50% of the normal level of gluta-thione, not only was this decrease during incubation prevented by the inclusion of methionine in the incubation medium, but the glutathione concentration in the cells even increased during the incubation (224). Cysteine was effective only if present in the reduced form, probably because cysteine is poorly taken up by the cells (223). At high concentrations of cysteine a loss of glutathione was observed, possibly by the same mechanism as the in vivo effect of high cysteine dose: the formation of mixed disulfides (222,224). Isolated hepatocytes from diethylmaleate-pretreated rats synthesized glutathione at approximately an in vivo rate; added cysteine as well as methionine stimulated the formation (225).

Glutathione levels increase steadily during development, from very low in fetal liver and lung to higher neonatal levels, and still higher adult levels (171,226—228). The overall activities of the glutathione-synthesizing enzymes increase in parallel in the liver (226,228). Later, during aging, the glutathione levels decrease again (171,179,229—231). The concentration of oxidized glutathione remains constant, however. In rapidly growing hepatomas the glutathione concentration was lower than normal (232,233).

Various hormonal treatments influence the glutathione levels in the tissues directly or indirectly. Thus daily treatment with estradiol-17β increased the concentration of reduced glutathione in the uterus, while GSSG remained constant (234). Propylthiouracil, which increased hypothyroidism, increased glutathione in the liver by 30% (235), which agrees with the finding that the level of reduced glutathione is inversely correlated with thyroid function (236).

The breakdown of glutathione by isolated kidney cells was strongly inhibited by the drug AT-125, a potent inhibitor of γ-glutamyltranspeptidase (237). As yet, no data on the in vivo effect of this compound have been published.

Various metal salts induce the formation of glutathione, probably after first binding to this compound. Thus treatment with cobalt chloride and arsenic chloride results in enhanced glutathione levels (238, 239). Finally, the continuous administration of some carcinogens, such as 2-acetylaminofluorene, may lead to increased glutathione levels in the liver (232). Various deficiencies in glutathione metabolism have been reviewed by Finkelstein (240).

VI. AMINO ACID CONJUGATION: TAURINE

A. Amino Acids as Acceptors: Activation of the Substrate

Many aromatic carboxylic acids, especially arylacetic acids, are conjugated with amino acids after activation of the carboxylic group through thioester formation with coenzyme A [reactions (12) and (13)]. The amino acids glycine and taurine most often are the acceptors in mammals; glutamate is less common. In birds ornithine is an important acceptor substrate for conjugation. Reviews on amino acid conjugation have appeared recently (241,242). Important physiological substrates for amino acid conjugation are the bile salts that are conjugated with taurine or glycine (243).

The first step in this conjugation is the activation of the carboxylic acid substrate by the formation of a coenzyme A derivative. Reactions (12) and (13) are catalyzed by Acyl-CoA synthetase,

$$R\text{-}COOH + ATP \rightleftharpoons R\text{-}CO\text{-}AMP + PP_i \quad (12)$$

$$R\text{-}CO\text{-}AMP + CoA\text{-}SH \rightleftharpoons R\text{-}CO\text{-}SCoA + AMP \quad (13)$$

$$R\text{-}CO\text{-}SCoA + H_2N\text{-}R'\text{-}COOH \rightleftharpoons R\text{-}CO\text{-}NH\text{-}R'\text{-}COOH + CoA\text{-}SH \quad (14)$$

(acid:CoA ligase (AMP forming), E. C. 6.2.1.3) and the final conjugation reaction by acyl-CoA: amino acid N-acyltransferase (E. C. 23.1.13). The substrate specificity in vivo for aromatic carboxylic acid xenobiotics had been investigated thoroughly in recent years (241,242). Glucuronidation of these substrates often competes with their activation to acyl-CoA derivatives.

It seems that in some species the final transfer reaction accepts both taurine and glycine as acceptor for the conjugation of bile salts, while in others only one of these can function as acceptor. In the guinea pig and the rat the affinity for taurine is much higher than that for glycine, while in the rabbit the reverse is found (244,245). The cat does not conjugate cholate with glycine but only with taurine (246). In humans the addition of taurine to the food increases the percentage of bile salts that is conjugated with taurine; additional glycine did not increase the corresponding glycine conjugates (247). In newborns bile salts are mainly conjugated with taurine, but in the first week conjugation with glycine rapidly increases. Adult levels are reached after 7−12 months (248).

Activation of the bile salts to their CoA derivatives takes place in the endoplasmic reticulum, and their transfer to glycine or taurine in the cytosol (249,250). In the case of the arylacetic acids the mitochondria are involved, and the final acyl transfer reaction takes place in the matrix (251,252). Activation of these substrates also occurs in the mitochondria. Relatively little work has been done on hippurate synthesis and other amino acid conjugations in vitro, so that many biochemical details of these conjugation reactions are unknown (252-254). For instance, it is not known whether specificity for uptake by the mitochondria may be one of the factors that determine substrate specificity or conjugation rate for the various substrates.

The activation step of the aromatic carboxylic acids may be rate limiting, since the N-acyl transfer has a higher activity than the activation reaction in mitochondria, at least for the substrates benzoate and sali-

cylate (251,253). Another factor that may be rate limiting is the availability of the amino acid used as acceptor. Under normal conditions,
glycine and glutamate will usually always be available from the intermediary metabolism. However, taurine is synthesized in many mammalian species from cysteine and because of the limited supply of cysteine,
taurine may be depleted at high doses of the substrates for taurine
conjugation (see Section VI.D). In the following sections only the
availability of taurine is reviewed.

B. Biosynthesis and Functions of Taurine

Taurine is ubiquitously present in animal tissues (for a review, see
Refs. 253 and 255); therefore, in carnivores the supply of this amino
acid in the food is sufficient, and the need for synthesis is low. However, plants do not contain taurine and herbivores must therefore make
their own taurine. Various biosynthesis routes are possible, and the
main pathway of biosynthesis has not yet been determined (in fact,

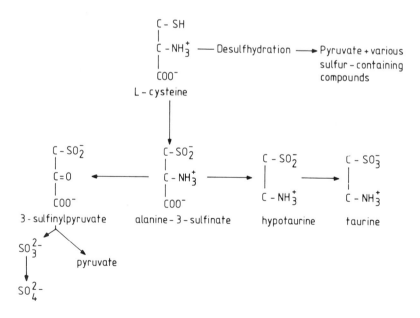

Figure 7 Pathways of cysteine metabolism.

Table 10 Taurine Pools in Humans and Rat

Species	Rapidly miscible pool		Slowly exchanging pool	
	nmol/kg	$t_{1/2}$	nmol/kg	$t_{1/2}$
Rat	6.5	3 days[a]	9.5	24 days
Humans	0.04	0.1 hr	14	3 days

[a]In the case of the rat a faster miscible pool may be present, but cannot be detected due to the experimental design used in Ref. 262.
Source: Data from Refs. 262 and 263.

this may be different in various species). So far, most attention has been given to the route from cysteine, through alanine 3-sulfinate ("cysteine sulfinate") and hypotaurine, to taurine (Figure 7). An alternative route leads first to cysteic acid, which is then converted to taurine by decarboxylation. Finally, cysteamine generated from cysteine may be oxidized further to hypotaurine and taurine. These routes have been discussed recently by Huxtable (256). In mammals, contrary to avians, taurine is not synthesized from inorganic sulfate to any extent under normal conditions (256,257), although the enzymes required for this are present (258). Several collections of papers on taurine are available (259–261) in which the roles that taurine may play in the heart and nervous system have been emphasized.

In the body two pools of taurine have been identified (Table 10): a relatively small pool with a short half-life, and a larger pool with a long half-life (262,263). Supplemental taurine in the food did not extensively equilibrate with the slowly exchangable pool (262). Yet it increased plasma taurine levels and the taurine content of most tissues, especially the liver (246,257,263). Hepatocytes rapidly take up taurine by a Na^+-dependent, carrier-mediated transport process (264). Intravenously injected ^{35}S-labeled taurine is rapidly eliminated from the liver and the kidney, whereas it has a rather slow turnover in the heart, muscle, and brain (265). A vitamin B_6-deficient diet affects the behavior of these pools in various ways (262).

In the rat taurine can be synthesized from cysteine as shown, for instance, in the isolated perfused rat liver. In the same preparation from the cat, however, the synthesis of taurine from cysteine is much slower (266,267). For this reason in the cat taurine has to be provided with the food and is an essential amino acid (246).

In some species the pool of taurine available for conjugation is rather large; when in the ferret the dose of phenylacetic acid was increased from 1.25 to 2.5 nmol/kg, the percentage that became conjugated with taurine remained approximately 23%, indicating that within a 24-hr period at least 0.5 mmol of taurine per kilogram is available (268). However, in other species the pool size may be smaller because it has been observed that in those species the addition of taurine to the diet increased the amount of bile salts that was excreted as taurine conjugate (246,269). This implies that in these species the availability of taurine determines the extent of conjugation with taurine. These data could be confirmed in the isolated rat liver (267). When cholate was infused it was initially conjugated mainly with taurine, but later glycine conjugation increased at the expense of the taurine conjugate. However, when taurine was continuously infused, no such decrease of taurine conjugation with time took place.

Much taurine is excreted in urine, since in mammals it is hardly further metabolized, except by the gut flora (263). The amount found in urine is very dependent on the composition of the diet (263,270–272); in particular, the consumption of meat, a high-taurine food, leads to high levels of taurine in the urine (270,273,274).

C. Assay and Tissue Concentrations of Taurine

Taurine can be determined in tissue extracts after homogenization and deproteinization. It is usually further purified by chromatography across Dowex W50-8X (265,271,275–277). Then taurine may be determined spectrophotometrically; as color reagents, ninhydrin or 2,4-dinitrofluorobenzene can be employed (267,275,278,279).

A double isotope assay has been developed with [^{35}S]taurine and [^{3}H]cholate. This assay utilizes the formation of [^{35}S]tauro-[^{3}H]cholate by rat liver microsomes, and is dependent on the dilution of the specific radioactivity of taurine by the unlabeled taurine present in perchloric acid extracts of homogenized tissues (278). It is more sensitive than the spectrophotometric procedures and requires less time. However, it is not superior to an amino acid analyzer procedure (278). Concentrations of taurine in various tissues are given in Tables 11 and 12.

D. Decreased Availability of Taurine In Vivo

An increase in the rate of synthesis of bile salt conjugates may lead to a decreased conjugation with taurine when this compound becomes depleted (280). This can also be observed when the elimination of specifically taurine-conjugated cholate in the feces is enhanced by the oral administration of cholestyramine; this compound binds the taurine conjugates much more strongly than the glycine conjugates. As a result, the enterohepatic recirculation of taurocholate is interrupted and taurine is depleted. The proportion of bile salts that is conjugated with glycine increases subsequently. When additional taurine is fed, this decrease of conjugation with taurine is prevented, confirming the rate-

Table 11   Species Differences in Taurine Content in Several Tissues[a]

Species	Taurine (mmol/g tissue)		
	Liver	Kidney	Heart
Rat	1.6 ± 0.2	7.4 ± 0.6	28.4 ± 10.5
Guinea pig	0	1.8	9.3
Rabbit	0	1.9	14.6
Pig	1.1	7.4	33.7
Beef	5.3	Not determined	3.5
Sheep	3.7	4.1	7.2

[a]Means ± SEM are given.
Source: Data from Ref. 272.

limiting character of taurine availability (281).   Thus oral administration of cholestyramine may lead to depletion of taurine.

An alternative method to decrease the availability of taurine in the
rat and mouse is to feed guanidoethyl sulfonate (Table 12); the mechanism of this effect is inhibition of uptake of taurine by the cells (282).
In the guinea pig this compound is not effective (283).   Several other
compounds also reduced taurine, such as β-alanine; treatment with
these agents leads to their accumulation in the cell.

Cardiotoxic doses of isoprenaline and methoxamine lead to decreases
in taurine in the heart, but an increase in the liver.   The underlying
mechanisms have not yet been elucidated (284).

The availability of taurine in vivo determines the extent of conjugation with this compound; so far no experiments have been reported
with xenobiotic agents such as the aromatic carboxylic acids, but it
seems likely that at higher doses they will deplete taurine.   However,
in that case the activated CoA form of the substrate will be conjugated
with glycine, or glucuronidation will take over, so that the elimination
of these carboxylic acids may be unaffected by such a depletion.

E.   Nutritional, Hormonal, and Drug Effects on Taurine Availability

As has been indicated above, the quality of the food determines to a
large extent the supply of taurine available for conjugation.   A diet
rich in meat will contain much taurine, whereas a vegetarian diet might
be very deficient in this component.

Fasting causes an increase in taurine in the tissues, especially in the
liver of male rats; in females no such effect was observed (172) (Table
13).   When food intake was only 50% of normal, a similar effect was
found (257); therefore, pair feeding is important in studies on the ef-

Table 12   Taurine Content of Various Organs and the Effect of Guanidinoethyl Sulfonate in the Rat[a]

	Taurine[b] (μmol/g tissue)	
Organ	Control	Guanidinoethyl sulfonate-treated
Heart	23.4 ± 1.1	4.6 ± 0.5
Lung	6.7 ± 0.5	2.0 ± 0.4
Kidney	4.6 ± 1.0	2.5 ± 0.3
Liver	4.5 ± 1.5	1.1 ± 0.3
Spleen	4.2 ± 1.1	1.2 ± 0.1
Intestine	5.6 ± 1.2	2.0 ± 0.4

[a]Male Sprague-Dawley rats were treated during 4 weeks with 1% guanidinoethyl sulfonate in the water before sacrifice.
[b]Data are given as means ± SEM.
Source: Data from Ref. 282.

fect on taurine availability in vivo of compounds added in the food. When the food is supplemented with inorganic sulfate, this results initially in a reduced rate of oxidation of cysteine to taurine; later, no differences were observed when the diet was given for more than a week (271). Nutritional aspects of taurine metabolism have recently been reviewed (261).

Table 13   Sex Differences in Taurine Content in the Rat, and the Effect of Fasting

	Taurine[a] (μmol/g tissue)	
Organ	Fed	Fasted 7 days
Male rats		
Liver	1.0 ± 0.2	6.1 ± 0.3
Kidney	7.4 ± 0.6	10.1 ± 0.7
Heart	28.4 ± 10.5	30.3 ± 1.7
Female rats		
Liver	5.3 ± 0.3	2.3 ± 0.3
Kidney	8.1 ± 0.8	9.3 ± 0.4
Heart	26.7 ± 0.6	26.2 ± 1.1

[a]Means ± SEM are given.
Source: Data from Ref. 272.

Data on developmental aspects of taurine levels are available in several species. Thus in the rabbit, monkey, humans, and the rat the taurine concentration in the liver decreases after birth to reach adult levels after a few days or weeks. However, in the guinea pig the concentration seems to remain constant (285,286). In female rats the liver concentration of taurine is about twice that in males (255).

VII. ACETYLATION: ACETYL-CoA

A. Biosynthesis and Function

Acetyl-CoA is the cosubstrate for the acetylation reaction; the acceptor group for this conjugation in most cases is the aromatic amino group, but hydroxyl groups in certain structures may also become acetylated.

Acetyl-CoA is synthesized from various precursors. One of the main sources in vivo is pyruvate metabolism by pyruvate dehydrogenase, which yields acetyl-CoA (287). Further, it is synthesized during the breakdown of fatty acids; the various pathways have been reviewed (287–289). Since it is one of the key substances in the intermediary metabolism, and required in pathways involved in the biosynthesis of numerous endogenous compounds (fatty acid synthesis, Krebs cycle, etc.), an overwhelming amount of literature is available on acetyl-CoA. Because of this it is outside the scope of this chapter to review these data, and the reader is referred to some recent reviews for more details (287–289). Unfortunately, little has been published, it seems, on the in vivo availability of acetyl-CoA and its regulation; probably several separate pools of acetyl-CoA are present inside the cell. In most cases the enzymes generating or consuming acetyl-CoA have been reviewed.

For the acetylation reaction coenzyme A is a necessary cofactor; it is regenerated by the acetyl transfer. Dietary sodium sulfate may increase the availability of coenzyme A in the liver (290).

VIII. THE CENTRAL ROLE OF METHIONINE AND CYSTEINE IN THE CONJUGATION WITH SULFUR-CONTAINING COSUBSTRATES

Four of the conjugation reactions use sulfur-containing cosubstrates for conjugation: conjugation with taurine and glutathione, sulfation, and methylation. In the latter reaction the sulfur-containing group itself is not transferred, but is either reloaded with a methyl group or is converted to cysteine. In the following discussion methionine and cysteine will mean L-methionine and L-cysteine, respectively, unless otherwise specified. The nutritional aspects of sulfur-containing substances were reviewed in 1970 (291).

In mammals methionine cannot be synthesized from cysteine since the cystathionine synthesis from methionine is virtually irreversible.

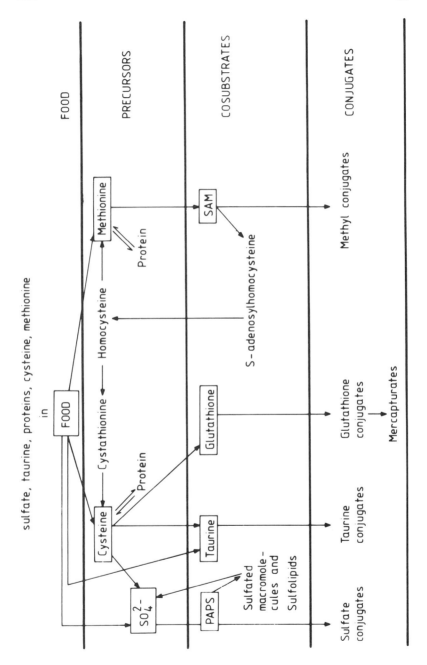

Figure 8 Interrelationship between various sulfur-containing compounds and conjugation reactions.

Methionine (or its potential precursor homocysteine), therefore, has to be provided with the food. Because cysteine can be synthesized from methionine, it is a dispensible amino acid; methionine can probably completely replace cysteine. This explains why cysteine in the food has a sparing effect on methionine: as much as two-thirds of the daily requirement of methionine can be replaced by cysteine. For the role of methionine as, for example, methyl donor and for the synthesis of proteins or polyamines, however, a sufficient supply of methionine should be available in the food (292–294). Surprisingly, if both methionine and cysteine are completely left out of a synthetic diet of human volunteers, the plasma levels of methionine and cysteine showed little decrease over an 8-day period, although urinary methionine and inorganic sulfate levels dropped markedly during this period (295). These findings can be explained by the catabolic state that results from such a diet.

As yet it is unknown to what extent inorganic sulfate present in the food contributes to the total sulfate requirement. Contrary to what is reported in many pharmacological handbooks, inorganic sulfate is well and almost completely absorbed from the gut when the dose is not so high that diarrhea results (155,296,297). Hence addition of inorganic sulfate salts to the food increases nitrogen retention or growth rate of several species, including humans (291,297,298). The explanation probably is that a sufficient supply of inorganic sulfate, required for sulfation of several endogenous macromolecules and of xenobiotics, reduces the need to oxidize cysteine, so that more of this amino acid becomes available for protein synthesis. This has been investigated especially in commercially grown animals such as sheep, where wool production requires much cysteine. Figure 8 summarizes the interrelationships between the various sulfur-containing compounds in relation to conjugation.

A. Methionine

Protein is usually the only source of methionine in the food. When an increased supply of this amino acid is required it can be added to the food as such or in the form of N-acetyl-L-methionine. The advantage of the latter compound is that it is chemically more stable and therefore does not give rise to objectionable odors as a result of chemical modification during processing. The N-acetyl derivative is absorbed and utilized to the same extent as methionine itself; the N-acetyl group is cleaved off by deacetylating enzymes after absorption (299,300).

A rapid rise in methionine in blood is observed after oral administration of methionine (82,86,90,92–95,104,300), even though the liver may take up a high percentage of the dose. Surprisingly, in human volunteers neither cysteine nor taurine in plasma increased, although

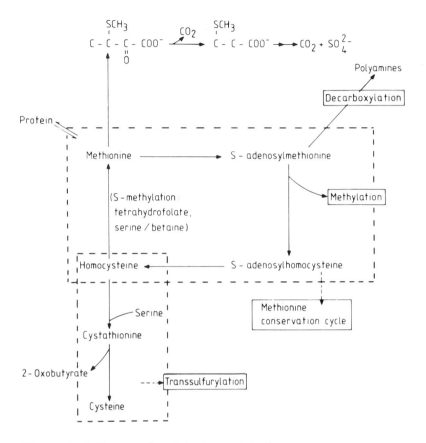

Figure 9 Pathways of methionine metabolism.

plasma methionine went up from 0.01 to 0.55 mM after an oral dose of 5 g of methionine (301). In monkeys the taurine concentration in serum was higher after methionine dosing, but cysteine was not (302). In rats fed additional methionine, however, the cysteine in serum did increase (303,303a,304).

Feeding high amounts of methionine leads to adaptive changes of the activities of several enzymes involved in the catabolism of methionine and cysteine (171,292,304,305). In general, their activity is enhanced. Further, in combination with low-protein diet, it causes a fatty liver as the result of high triglyceride synthesis (306).

Methionine is one of the most toxic amino acids when fed at high doses (307–310). This toxicity may, in part, be due to the formation of S-methyl-3-thiopropionate by transamination and subsequent de-

carboxylation (310) (Figure 9). Glycine and serine provide partial
protection against the toxic effects of methionine (308), but not of S-
methyl-3-thiopropionate (310), presumably because they enhance the
capacity of the cystathionine pathway of methionine detoxification.
Retinol similarly alleviates the toxicity of methionine, but not that of
cysteine or S-methylcysteine (309).

When the supply of methionine exceeds the requirement, it is broken
down along the pathways shown in Figure 9. The major pathway
probably is the conversion to SAM and, subsequently, to homocysteine
and cystathionine (99). The methyl group is used, in part, for the
formation of choline, sarcosine, and related methylated compounds
(311,312). At high concentration methionine inhibits the remethylation
of homocysteine by methyltetrahydrofolate and thereby ensures that
homocysteine is further metabolized by the cystathionine pathway. The
regulation of this pathway has been discussed by Krebs et al. (313).

An alternative route has been postulated to start with transamination
of methionine (314–316). This leads to a series of abnormal sulfur-
containing intermediates; the enzyme activities required in this pathway are present in rat liver (317).

Under conditions of a limited supply of methionine, homocysteine is
conserved and remethylated very efficiently (99). Using methionine
labeled with ^{3}H and ^{35}S only in the S-methyl group, Finkelstein (99)
has shown that the rate of turnover of this methyl group ($t_{1/2}$) is 5.5
min; approximately 50% is transsulfurylated in the isolated perfused rat
liver obtained from rats fed a normal diet. When the rats were fed a
protein-restricted diet, these values became 9.3 min and 10%, respectively, and in rats fed a high protein diet, 4.8 min and 70%. Similar
experiments demonstrated remethylation both in brain and liver, with
a higher rate in the liver (318). These data illustrate that under conditions that are rate limiting in methionine, transsulfurylation is prevented. Interestingly, after partial hepatectomy in the rat the transsulfurylation enzymes were increased, while remethylation of homocysteine and methionine conservation were reduced (319). Both remethylation of homocysteine and transsulfurylation can be reduced in
vivo by periodate-oxidized adenosine, which inhibits the hydrolysis
of S-adenosylhomocysteine (320).

The serum concentration of methionine shows a diurnal variation; in
the rat the nadir occurs around 6 p.m. and the peak at 6 a.m. (321).
In fasting human volunteers the peak was observed ay 7 a.m., while
consumption of protein led to a peak at night (322). The concentration
of methionine in brain does not follow this normal diurnal variation in
blood; yet SAM in brain changes in parallel with methionine in blood
(97,127). In patients with cirrhosis of the liver, plasma methionine
is higher than in normal subjects (323).

Many of the enzymes involved in the transsulfurylation pathway require pyridoxal phosphate as cofactor; therefore, a vitamin B$_6$ defi-

ciency in the food causes deregulation of methionine metabolism (324, 325), reflected, for instance, in an increased urinary excretion of cystathionine. A deficiency of vitamin B_{12} also results in various defects, leading for instance to homocysteinuria (240).

D-Methionine is relatively little metabolized in humans and monkeys, and excreted mainly unchanged (298), while rats excrete only small amounts of unchanged D-methionine in urine (326). It has been suggested that D-methionine can be converted to the L isomer by D-amino acid oxidase and a transaminase; in some species (but not in humans) D-methionine can partially replace L-methionine (298). Studies with labeled D-methionine will be required to study its metabolism in detail.

B. Cysteine

For mammals the main source of cysteine is protein in the food; digestion yields either cysteine directly or cysteine generated from methionine as discussed in Section VIII.A. Increasing the supply of cysteine results in higher serum levels of cystine, and in an increased breakdown when the requirement is exceeded. Oral administration of high doses of cysteine in the rat (where the normal serum level of cystine is below detection) leads to measurable cystine levels for several hours. Serum taurine and inorganic sulfate levels are increased for a much longer time, up to 24 hr after administration (327). This is the result of the fact that cysteine is largely broken down oxidatively, as shown in Figure 7 (304). The first, major product is alanine 3-sulfinate (less correctly but more commonly called cysteine sulfinate). The cysteine dioxygenase involved in this oxidation responds very rapidly and strongly to changes in dietary levels of cysteine or methionine, and is also very sensitive to hormonal influences (171). Alanine-3-sulfinate may then be decarboxylated to hypotaurine, or be transaminated to 3-sulfinylpyruvate. The first compound is subsequently oxidized to taurine, and the latter to sulfate (and pyruvate) through the intermediary sulfite. In humans a genetically determined deficiency in sulfite oxidase has been found. Patients deficient in this enzyme accumulate sulfate and probably lack a sufficient supply of sulfate. They are mentally retarded and acquire several neurological anomalies (328,329).

As discussed in Section VIII.A, methionine can provide the cysteine requirements by transsulfurylation; therefore, an adequate cysteine supply has a sparing effect on methionine (291,330). A correct balance between cysteine and methionine in the food ensures optimum growth conditions (291,294,331).

When cysteine is administered in high doses, part of it may be sequestered in the liver in the form of a labile glutathione pool (see Section V). The relationship between cysteine availability and glutathione synthesis in the perinatal period has been investigated by Takeishi et al. (228). Incorporation of cysteine in the glutathione pool can be demonstrated when fasted rats are fed a protein-deficient diet and cysteine is added at various doses. The effect occurs only when there is an excess of cysteine compared to the availability of other amino acids (174,226,332). Both methionine and cysteine increase the hepatic content of glutathione (see Section V).

Studies with the isolated perfused rat liver showed that a small percentage of cysteine is converted to glucose by a pathway other than alanine-3-sulfinate. Probably, desulfhydration takes place, yielding pyruvate by some as yet unidentified pathway (333), although a number of routes can be envisioned (304). However, presumably less than 5% of the dose of cysteine was thus metabolized. Adaptive changes in the enzymes involved may take place both in desulfhydrase activity and in alanine-3-sulfinate decarboxylase (L-systeine sulfinate carboxylase, E. C. 4.1.1.29), one of the enzymes in the oxidative metabolism of cysteine (334).

The discussion above implies that many responses may be found when a high dose of cysteine is given either with the food or in a single dose. The most prominent effect, however, is usually a rise in taurine and inorganic sulfate, both in plasma and in urine (304,335, 327). The same occurs when one of the other essential amino acids is deficient in the diet. The then existing relative excess of cysteine is oxidized to inorganic sulfate, and an increased urinary output of sulfate indicates an imbalanced diet (336).

The D isomer of cysteine is not oxidized to taurine in the rat (327, 337), indicating that one or more of the enzymes involved in the synthesis of taurine from L-cysteine is sterospecific. The concentration of cysteine in the liver is 0.3−0.5 mM (338); it is taken up in liver cells by a carrier-mediated transport (339).

REFERENCES

1. Walker, S. R., Evans, M. E., Richards, A. J., and Paterson, J. W. (1972). *J. Pharm. Pharmacol.* 24:525.

2. Pang, K. S., and Gillette, J. R. (1978). *Drug Metab. Dispos.* 6:567.

3. Boxenbaum, H. (1980). *J. Pharmacokinet. Biopharm.* 8:165.

4. Houston, J. B., and Wood, S. G. (1980). In *Progress in Drug Metabolism*, Vol. 4, J. W. Bridges and L. F. Chasseaud, Eds., Wiley, Chichester, England, p. 57.

5. Toothaker, R. D., and Welling, P. G. (1980). *Annu. Rev. Pharmacol.* 20:173.

6. Gram, T. E., (1980). *Extrahepatic Drug Metabolism.* Spectrum Publications, Jamaica, N. Y.

7. Cassidy, M. K., and Houston, J. B. (1980). *J. Pharm. Pharmacol.* 32:57.

8. Conolly, M. E., Davies, D. S., Dollery, C. T., Morgan, J. W., Paterson, J. W., and Sandler, R. (1972). *Brit. J. Pharmacol.* 46:458.

9. Powell, G. M., Miller, J. J., Olavesen, A. H., and Curtis, C. G. (1974). *Nature* 252:234.

10. Routledge, P. A., and Shand, D. G. (1979). *Annu. Rev. Pharmacol.* 19:447.

11. Wilkinson, G. R. (1975). *Annu. Rev. Pharmacol.* 15:11.

12. Bass, L. (1980). *J. Theor. Biol.* 86:365.

13. Chien, Y. W. (1982). *Novel Drug Delivery Systems*, Marcel Dekker, New York, Chap. 5.

14. Bickers, D. R. (1980). In *Current Concepts on Cutaneous Toxicity*, V. A. Drill and P. Lagar, Eds., Academic Press, New York, p. 95.

15. Wagner, J. G. (1971). *Biopharmaceutics and Relevant Pharmacokinetics*, Drug Intellegence Publications, Hamilton, Ill.

16. Kao, J., Jones, C. A., Fry, J. R., and Bridges, J. W. (1978). *Life Sci.* 23:1221.

17. Pang, K. S., and Gillette, J. R. (1979). *J. Pharmacokinet. Biopharm.* 7:275.

18. Keiding, S., Johansen, S., Midtbøll, I., Rabøl, A., and Christiansen, L. (1979). *Am. J. Physiol.* 237:E316.

19. Mulder, G. J. (1981). In *Sulfation of Drugs and Related Compounds*, G. J. Mulder, Ed., CRC Press, Boca Raton, Fla., Chap. 6.

20. Eyer, P., and Kampffmeyer, H. G. (1978). *Biochem. Pharmacol.* 27:2223.

21. Weitering, J. G., Krijgsheld, K. R., and Mulder, G. J. (1979). *Biochem. Pharmacol.* 27:757.

22. Jollow, D. J., Thorgeirsson, S. S., Potter, W. Z., Hashimoto, M., and Mitchell, J. R. (1974). *Pharmacology* 12:251.

23. Bridges, J. W., French, M. R., Smith, R. L., and Williams, R. T. (1970). *Biochem. J.* 118:47.

24. Mathieu, P., Charvet, J. G., Greffe, J. (1975). *Biochem. Pharmacol.* 28:43.

25. Grafstrom, R., Ormstad, K., Moldeus, P., and Orrenius, S. (1979). *Biochem. Pharmacol.* 28:3573.

26. Shand, D. G., Kornhauser, D. M., Wilkinson, G. R. (1975). *J. Pharmacol. Exp. Ther.* 195:424.

27. van Rossum, J. M., van Ginneken, C. A. M., Henderson, P. Th., Ketelaars, H. C. J., and Vree, T. B. (1977). In *Kinetics of Drug Action*, J. M. van Rossum, Ed., *Handbook of Pharmacology*, Vol. 47, Springer-Verlag, Berlin, p. 125.

28. Pang, K. S., Rowland, M., and Tozer, N. (1978). *Drug Metab. Dispos.* 6:197.

29. Bray, H. G., Humphris, B. G., Thorpe, W. V., White, K., and Wood, P. B. (1952). *Biochem. J.* 52:419.

30. Mulder, G. J., and Scholtens, E. (1977). *Biochem. J.* 165:553.
31. Powell, G. M., and Olavesen, A. H. (1981). In *Sulfation of Drugs and Related Compounds*, G. J. Mulder, Ed., CRC Press, Boca Raton, Fla., Chap. 7.
32. Irving, C. C. (1971). *Xenobiotica* 1:387.
33. Smith, R. L., (1973). *The Excretory Function of Bile: The Elimination of Drugs and Toxic Substances in Bile*, Chapman & Hall, London.
34. Marselos, M., Dutton, G. J., and Hänninen, O. (1975). *Biochem. Pharmacol.* 24:1855.
35. Capel, C. D., Millburn, P., and Williams, R. T. (1974). *Xenobiotica* 4:601.
36. Dutton, G. J. (1980). *Glucuronidation of Drugs and Other Compounds*, CRC Press, Boca Raton, Fla.
37. Sugahara, K., and Schwartz, N. B. (1982). *Arch. Biochem. Biophys.* 214:589.
38. Weber, W. W. (1971). In *Concepts in Biochemical Pharmacology*, B. B. Brodie and J. R. Gillette, Eds., *Handbook of Experimental Pharmacology*, Vol. 28, Part. 2, Springer-Verlag, Berlin, p. 564.
39. Weinshilboum, R. M. (1980). *Trends Pharmacol. Sci.* 1:378.
40. Pang, K. S., Koster, H., Halsema, I. C. M., Scholtens, E., and Mulder, G. J. (1981). *J. Pharmacol. Exp. Ther.* 219:134.
41. Miettinen, T. A., and Leskinen, E. (1970). In *Metabolic Conjugation and Metabolic Hydrolysis*, Vol. 1, W. H. Fishman, Ed., Academic Press, New York, p. 158.
42. Notten, W. R. F., and Henderson, P. Th. (1975). *Int. J. Biochem.* 6:111.
43. Lake, B. G., Longland, R. C., Harris, R. A., Severn, B. J., and Gangolli, S. D. (1978). *Biochem. Pharmacol.* 27:2357.
44. Gainey, P. A., and Phelps, C. F. (1972). *Biochem. J.* 128:215.
45. Zhivkov, V. (1970). *Biochem. J.* 120:505.
46. Zhivkov, V., and Chelibonova-Lorer, H. (1975). *Int. J. Biochem.* 6:429.
47. Wong, K. P., (1977). *Anal. Biochem.* 82:559.
48. Fyffe, J., and Dutton, G. J. (1975). *Biochim. Biophys. Acta* 411:41.
49. Bock, K. W., and White, I. N. H. (1974). *Eur. J. Biochem.* 46:451.
50. Wong, K. P., and Sourkes, T. L., (1967). *Anal. Biochem.* 21:444.
51. Singh, J., Schwarz, L. R., and Wiebel, F. J. (1980). *Biochem. J.* 189:369.
52. Zhivkov, V., Tosheva, R., and Zhivkova, Y. (1975). *Comp. Biochem. Physiol.* 51B:421.

53. Decker, K., and Keppler. D. (1972). In *Progress in Liver Disease*, Vol. 4, H. Popper and F. Schaffner, Eds., Grune & Stratton, New York, p. 183.

54. Otani, G., Abou el Makarem, M. M., and Bock, K. W. (1976). *Biochem. Pharmacol.* 25:1293.

55. Bolanowska, W., and Gessner, T. (1980). *Biochem. Pharmacol.* 29:1167.

56. Moldeus, P., Andersson, B., and Gergely, V. (1979). *Drug Metab. Dispos.* 7:416.

57. Singh, J., and Schwarz, L. R. (1981). *Biochem. Pharmacol.* 30:3252.

58. Schwarz, L. R. (1980). *Arch. Toxicol.* 44:137.

59. Moldeus, P., Andersson, B., and Norling, A. (1978). *Biochem. Pharmacol.* 27:2583.

60. Moldeus, P., Andersson, B., Norling, A., Ormstad, K. (1980). *Biochem. Pharmacol.* 29:1741.

60a. Eriksson, G., and Strath, D. (1981). *FEBS Lett.* 124:39.

61. Müller-Oerlinghausen, B., Hasselblatt, A., and Jahns, R. (1968). *Naunyn-Schmiedeberg's Arch. Pharmakol.* 260:254.

62. Müller-Oerlinghausen, B., and Künzel, B. (1968). *Life Sci.* 7(II):1129.

63. Müller-Oerlinghausen, B., Jahns, R., Künzel, B., and Hasselblatt, A. (1969). *Naunyn-Schmiedeberg's Arch. Pharmakol.* 262:17.

64. Künzel, B., and Müller-Oerlinghausen, B. (1969). *Naunyn-Schmiedelberg's Arch. Pharmakol.* 262:112.

65. Müller-Oerlinghausen, B. (1970). *Naunyn-Schmiedeberg's Arch. Pharmakol.* 265:372.

66. Müller-Oerlinghausen, B., and Schinke, G. (1970). *Naunyn-Schmiedeberg's Arch. Pharmakol.* 266:3.

67. Costantopoulos, A., and Matsaniotis, N. (1978). *Gastroenterology* 75:486.

68. Dutton, G. J. (1978). *Annu. Rev. Pharmacol.* 18:17.

69. Felsher, B. F., Carpio, N. M., and van Couvering, K. (1979). *J. Lab. Clin. Med.* 93:414.

70. Magdalou, J., Steinmetz, D., Batt, A. M., Poullain, B., Siest, G., and Debry, G. (1979). *J. Nutr.* 109:964.

71. Hietanen, E. (1980). *Gen. Pharmacol.* 11:443.

72. Reinke, L. A., Kauffman, F. C., Evans, R. K., Belinsky, S. A., and Thurman, R. G. (1979). *Res. Commun. Chem. Pathol. Pharmacol.* 23:185.

73. Salvatore, E., Borek, E., Zappia, V., Williams-Ashman, H. G., and Schlenk, F., Eds. (1977). *The Biochemistry of Adenosylmethionine*, Columbia University Press, New York.

74. Usdin, E., Borchardt, R., and Creveling, C. R., Eds. (1979). *Transmethylation*, Elsevier/North-Holland, Amsterdam.

75. Cavallini, D., Gaull, G. E., and Zappia, V., Eds. (1980). *Natural Sulfur Compounds: Novel Biochemical and Structural Aspects,* Plenum Press, New York.
76. Schlenk, F., Hannum, C. H., and Ferro, A. J. (1978). *Arch. Biochem. Biophys. 187*:191.
77. Cornforth, J. W., Reichard, S. A., Talalay, P., Carrell, H. L., and Glusker, J. P. (1977). *J. Am. Chem. Soc. 99*: 7292.
78. Oliva, A., Galletti, P., Zappia, V., Paik, W. K., and Kim, S. (1980). *Eur. J. Biochem. 104*:595.
79. Jänne, J., Pösö, H., and Raina, A. (1978). *Biochim. Biophys. Acta 473*:241.
80. Hibasami, H., Borchardt, R. T., Chen, S. Y., Coward, J. K., and Pegg. A. E. (1980). *Biochem. J. 187*:419.
81. Woodward, G. W., Tsai, M. D., Floss, H. G., Crooks, P. A., and Coward, J. K. (1980). *J. Biol. Chem. 255*:9124.
82. Baldessarini, R. J., and Kopin, I. J. (1966). *J. Neurochem. 13*:769.
83. Matthysse, S., Baldessarini, R. J., and Vogt, M. (1972). *Anal. Biochem. 48*:410.
84. Carl, G. F., Benesh, F. C., and Hudson, J. H., (1978). *Biol. Psychiatry 13*:661.
85. Lombardini, J. B., Burch, M. K., and Talalay, P. (1971). *J. Biol. Chem. 246*:4465.
86. Baldessarini, R. J. (1975). *Int. Rev. Neurobiol. 18*:41.
87. Pan, F., and Tarver, H. (1967). *Arch. Biochem. Biophys. 119*:429.
88. Chou, T. C., and Talalay, P. (1972). *Biochemistry 11*:1065.
89. Ordonez, L., and Wurtman, R. J. (1973). *Biochem. Pharmacol. 22*:134.
90. Liau, M. C., Chang, C. F., and Giovanella, B. C. (1980). *J. Natl. Cancer Inst, 64*:1071.
91. Liau, M. C., Lin, G. W., and Hurlbert, R. B. (1977). *Cancer Res. 37*:427.
92. Baldessarini, R. J. (1966). *Biochem. Pharmacol. 15*:741.
93. Schatz, R. A., and Sellinger, O. Z. (1975). *J. Neurochem. 24*:63.
94. Eloranta, T. O. (1977). *Biochem. J. 166*:521.
95. Taufek, H. R., and Bone, A. H. (1980). *Biochem. Soc. Trans. 8*:62.
96. Watkins, C. A., and Morgan, H. E. (1979). *J. Biol. Chem. 254*:693.
97. Rubin, R. A., Ordonez, L. A., and Wurtman, R. J. (1974). *J. Neurochem. 23*:227.
98. Burnet, F. R. (1979). *J. Neurochem. 33*:603.

99. Finkelstein, J. D. (1979). In *Transmethylation*, E. Ustin, G. E. Gaull, and V. Zappia, Eds., Elsevier/North-Holland, Amsterdam, p. 49.

100. Pezzoli, C., Stramentinoli, G., Galli Kienle, M., and Pfaff, E. (1978). *Biochem Biophys. Res. Commun.* 85:1031.

101. Zappia, V., Galletti, P., Porcelli, M., Ruggiero, G., and Andreana, A. (1978). *FEBS Lett.* 90:331.

102. Guaitani, A., Gualano, M., Villa, P., Stramentinoli, G., and Bartosek, I. (1979). *Eur. J. Drug Metabol. Pharmacokinet.* 4:187.

103. Stramentinoli, G., Gualano, M., and Galli-Kienle, M. (1979). *J. Pharmacol. Exp. Ther.* 209:323.

104. Salvatore, F., Utili, R., Zappia, V., and Shapiro, S. K. (1971). *Anal. Biochem.* 41:16.

105. Hoffman, J. (1975). *Anal. Biochem.* 68:522.

106. Eloranta, T. O., Kajander, E. O., and Raina, A. M. (1976). *Biochem. J.* 160:287.

107. Glazer, R. I., and Peale, A. L. (1978). *Anal. Biochem.* 91: 516.

108. Hyde, C. L., Rusten, R., and Poirier, L. A. (1980). *Anal. Biochem.* 106:35.

109. Floridi, A., Frisi, C., Palmerini, C. A., Mozzi, R., and Porcellati, G. (1979). *J. Liq. Chromatogr.* 2:1003.

110. Shugart, L. (1979). *J. Chromatogr.* 174:250.

111. Guldberg, H. C., and Marsden, C. A. (1975). *Pharmacol. Rev.* 27:135.

112. Hoffmann, D. R., Cornatzer, W. E., and Duerre, J. A. (1979). *Can. J. Biochem.* 57:56.

113 Bone, A. H., and Taufek, H. R. (1980). *Biochem. J.* 192: 703.

114. Stramentinoli, G., Catto, E., and Algeri, S. (1980). *J. Pharm. Pharmacol.* 32:430.

115. Villa-Trevino, S., Shull, K. H., and Farber, E. (1966). *J. Biol. Chem.* 241:4670.

116. Shull, K. H., McConomy, J., Vogt, M., Costillo, A., and Farber, E. (1966). *J. Biol. Chem.* 241:5060.

117. Tsukuda, K., Yamano, H., Abe, T., and Okada, G. (1980). *Biochem. Biophys. Res. Commun.* 95:1160.

118. Griffith, O. W., Anderson, M. E., and Meister, A. (1979). *J. Biol. Chem.* 254:1205.

119. Griffith, O. W., and Meister, A. (1979). *J. Biol. Chem.* 254:7558.

120. Zimmerman, T. P., Wolberg, G., Duncan, G. S., and Elion, G. B. (1980). *Biochemistry* 19:2252.

121. Kredich, N. M. (1980). *J. Biol. Chem.* 255:7380.

122. Tisdale, M. J. (1980). *Biochem. Pharmacol.* 29:501.

123. Sufrin, J. R., Coulter, A. W., and Talalay, P. (1979). *Mol. Pharmacol. 16*:661.
124. Matthysse, S. (1978). *Monogr. Gesamtgeb. Psychiatr. 18*: 119.
125. Zeisel, S. H., and Wurtman, R. J. (1979). In *Transmethylation*, E. Ustin, G. E. Gaull, and V. Zappia, Eds., Elsevier/North-Holland, Amsterdam, p. 59.
126. Bartosek, I., Guaitani, A., Villa, P., Stramentinoli, G., Gualano, M., and Pezzoli, C. (1978). *Biochem. Pharmacol. 27*: 2649.
127. Wurtman, R. J., Rose, C. M., Matthysse, S., Stephenson, J., and Baldessarini, R. (1970). *Science 169*:395.
128. Chalmers, J. P., Baldessarini, R. J., and Wurtman, R. J. (1971). *Proc. Natl. Acad. Sci. USA 68*:662.
129. Mulder, G. J. (1981). *Sulfation of Drugs and Related Compounds*, CRC Press, Boca Raton, Fla.
129a.Mulder, G. J., Caldwell, J., Van Kempen, G. M. J. and Vonk, R. J. (1982). *Sulfate Metabolism and Sulfate Conjugation*, Taylor & Francis, London.
130. Herbai, G. (1970). *Acta Physiol. Scand. 80*:470.
131. Mulder, G. J., and Scholtens, E. (1978). *Biochem. J. 172*: 247.
132. VonDippe, P., and Levy, D. (1982). *J. Biol. Chem. 257*:4381.
133. Robbins, P. W., and Lipmann, F. (1958). *J. Biol. Chem. 233*:681.
134 Wong, K. P., and Yeo, T. (1979). *Biochem. J. 181*:107.
134a.Krijgsheld, K. R., Scholtens, E., and Mulder, G. J. (1982). *Biochem. Pharmacol. 31*:3997.
135. Mulder, G. J., and Keulemans, K. (1978). *Biochem. J. 176*: 959.
136. Krijgsheld, K. R., Scholtens, E., and Mulder, G. J. (1980). *Comp. Biochem. Physiol. 67A*:683.
137. Büch, H., Rummel, W., Pfleger, K., Eschrich, C., and Texter, N. (1968). *Naunyn-Schmiedeberg's Arch. Pharmakol. 259*:276.
138. Bennett, P. N., Blackwell, E., and Davies, D. S. (1975). *Nature 258*:247.
139. Galinsky, R. E., Slattery, J. T., and Levy, G. (1979). *J. Pharm. Sci. 68*:803.
140. Katona, E. (1976). *Eur. J. Biochem. 63*:583.
141. Brunngraber, E. G. (1979). *Neurochemistry of Aminosugars*, Charles C. Thomas, Springfield, Ill.
142. Farooqui, A. A. (1978). *Int. J. Biochem. 9*:709.
143. Postgate, J. R. (1979). *The Sulfate-Reducing Bacteria*, Cambridge University Press, Cambridge.
144. Roy, A. B., and Trudinger, P. A. (1970). *The Biochemistry of Inorganic Compounds of Sulphur*, Cambridge University Press, Cambridge.

145. Van Kempen, G. M. J. and Jansen, G. S. I. M. (1973). *Anal. Biochem. 51*:324.
146. Robbins, R. W., and Lipmann, F. (1957). *J. Biol. Chem. 229*:837.
147. Stanley, P. E., Kelley, B. C., Tuovinen, O. H., and Nicholas, D. J. D. (1975). *Anal. Biochem. 67*:540.
148. Pennings, E. J. M., and van Kempen, G. M. J. (1979). *J. Chromatogr. 176*:478.
149. Conrad, G. W., and Woo, M. L. (1980). *J. Biol. Chem. 255*: 3086.
149a. Wong, K. P. (1982). In *Sulfate Metabolism and Sulfate Conjugation*, G. J. Mulder, J. Caldwell, G. M. J. van Kempen, and R. J. Vonk, Eds., Taylor & Francis, London, p. 85.
150. Greiling, H., and Schulder, B. (1963). *Z. Rheumaforsch. 22*: 47.
151. Krijgsheld, K. R., Scholtens, E., and Mulder, G. J. (1981). *Biochem. Pharmacol. 30*:1973.
152. Perry, M. A., Powell, G. M., Wusteman, F. S., and Curtis, C. G. (1977). *Biochem. J. 166*:373.
153. Geison, R. L., Rodgers, W. E., and Johnson, B. C. (1968). *Biochim. Biophys. Acta 165*:448.
154. Levi, A. S., Geller, S., Roor, D. M., and Wolf, G. (1968). *Biochem. J. 109*:69.
155. Krijgsheld, K. R., Frankena, H., Scholtens, E., Zweens, J., and Mulder, G. J. (1979). *Biochim. Biophys. Acta 586*:492.
156. Jansen, G. S. I. M., Van Elk, R., and Van Kempen, G. M. J. (1973). *J. Neurochem. 20*:9.
157. Miller, R. P., Roberts, R. J., and Fisher, L. J. (1976). *Clin. Pharmacol. Ther. 19*:284.
158. Rollins, D. E., Von Bahr, C., Glaumann, H., Moldeus, P., and Rane, A. (1979). *Science 205*:1414.
159. Gerlach, U. (1963). *Klin. Wochenschr. 41*:873.
160. Hart, G. W. (1978). *J. Biol. Chem. 253*:347.
161. Srinavas, L., and Rama, P. B. R. (1975). *Nutr. Metabol. 19*: 299.
162. Vijayakumar, S. T., and Kurup, P. A. (1975). *Atherosclerosis 21*:245.
163. Nambison, B., and Kurup, P. A. (1975). *Atherosclerosis 22*: 447.
164. Sushama, D. C. S., and Kurup, P. A. (1975). *Indian J. Biochem. Biophys. 12*:43.
165. Menon, P. V. C. and Kurup, P. A. (1976). *J. Nutr, 106*:555.
166. Vijayammal, P. L., and Kurup, P. A. (1978). *Aust. J. Biol. Sci. 31*:7.
167. Nevo, Z., and Laron, Z. (1979). *Am. J. Dis. Child. 133*:419.
168. Mohan, P. S., and Rao, K. S. J. (1980). *J. Nutr. 110*:868.

169. Arias, I. M., and Jakoby, W. B. Eds. (1976). *Glutathione, Metabolism and Function*, Raven Press, New York.
170. Sies, H., and Wendel, A., Eds. (1978). *Functions of Glutathione in Liver and Kidney*, Springer-Verlag, Berlin.
171. Reed, D. J., and Beatty, P. W. (1980). In *Reviews in Biochemical Toxicology*, Vol. 2, E. Hodgson, J. R. Bend, and R. M. Philpot, Eds., Elsevier, Amsterdam, p. 213.
172. Meister, A. (1978). In *Functions of Glutathione in Liver and Kidney*, H. Sies and A. Wendel, Eds., Springer-Verlag, Berlin, p. 43.
173. Richman, P., and Meister, A. (1975). *J. Biol. Chem. 250:* 1422.
174. Tateishi, N., Higashi, T., Naruse, A., Nakashima, K., Shiozaki, H., and Sakamoto, Y. (1977). *J. Nutr. 107:* 51.
175. Griffith, O. W., and Meister, A. (1979). *Proc. Natl. Acad. Sci. USA 76:* 5606.
176. Higashi, T., Tateishi, N., Naruse, A., and Sakamoto, Y. (1977). *J. Biochem. (Tokyo) 82:* 117.
177. Sekura, R., and Meister, A. (1974). *Proc. Natl. Acad. Sci. USA 71:* 2969.
178. Tietze, F. (1969). *Anal. Biochem. 27:* 502.
179. Hazelton, G. A., and Lang, C. A. (1980). *Biochem. J. 188:* 25.
180. Kosower, E. M., and Kosower, N. S. (1976). In *Glutathione, Metabolism and Function*, I. M. Arias and B. Jakoby, Eds., Raven Press, New York, p. 139.
181. Bartoli, G. M., and Sies, H. (1978). *FEBS Lett. 86:* 89.
182. Sies, H., Bartoli, G. M., Burk, R. F., and Waydhas, C. (1978). *Eur. J. Biochem. 89:* 113.
183. Kaplowitz, N., Kuhlenkamp, J., Goldstein, L., and Reeve, J. (1980). *J. Pharmacol. Exp. Ther. 212:* 240.
184. Wendel, A., and Cikryt, P. (1980). *FEBS Lett. 120:* 209.
185. Hahn, R., Wendel, A., and Flohe, L. (1978). *Biochim. Biophys. Acta 539:* 324.
186. Häberle, D., Wahlländer, A., Sies, H., Linke, I., and Lachenmaier, C. (1979). *FEBS Lett. 108:* 335.
187. Grafstrom, R., Stead, A. H., and Orrenius, S. (1980). *Eur. J. Biochem. 106:* 571.
188. Jocelyn, P. C. (1972). In *Biochemistry of the SH Group*, Academic Press, London. p. 137.
189. Meister, A. (1975). In *Metabolism of Sulfur Compounds*, D. M. Greenberg, Ed., Academic Press, New York, p. 101.
190. Brehe, J. E., and Burch, H. B. (1976). *Anal. Biochem. 74:* 189.
191. Griffith, O. W. (1980). *Anal. Biochem. 106:* 207.
192. Hissin, P. J., and Hilf, R. (1976). *Anal. Biochem. 74:* 214.

193. Rabenstein, D. L., and Saetre, R. (1978). *Clin. Chem. 24:* 1140.
194. Mefford, I., and Adams, R. N. (1978). *Life Sci. 23:*1167.
195. Reed, D. J., Babson, J. R., Beatty, P. W., Brodie, A. E., Ellis, W. W., and Potter, D. W. (1980). *Anal. Biochem. 106:* 55.
196. Jones, D. P., Moldeus, P., Stead, A. H., Ormstad, K., Jörnvall, H., and Orrenius, S. (1979). *J. Biol. Chem. 254:* 2787.
197. Reeve, J., Kuhlenkamp, J., Kaplowitz, N. (1980). *J. Chromatogr. 194:*424.
198. Berndt, E. (1974). In *Methods of Enzymatic Analysis,* 2nd Ed., Vol. 4, Chemie Verlag, Weinheim, p. 1643.
199. Asghar, K., Reddy, B. G., and Krishna, G. (1975). *J. Histochem. Cytochem. 23:*774.
200. Smith, M. T., Loveridge, N., Wills, E. D., and Chayen, J. (1979). *Biochem. J. 182:*103.
201. Isaacs, J., and Binkley, F. (1977). *Biochim. Biophys. Acta 497:*192.
202. Jaeger, R. J., Connolly, R. B., and Murphy, S. D. (1973). *Res. Commun. Chem. Pathol. Pharmacol. 6:*465.
203. Habeel, A. F. (1973). *Anal. Biochem. 56:*60.
204. Harisch, G., Eikemeyer, J., and Schole, J. (1979). *Experientia 35:*719.
205. Kosower, N. S., and Kosower, E. M. (1976). In *Glutathione, Metabolism and Function,* I. M. Arias and W. B. Jakoby, Eds., Raven Press, New York, p. 159.
206. Boyland, E., and Chasseaud, L. F. (1970). *Biochem. Pharmacol. 19:*1526.
207. Richardson, R. J., and Murphy, S. D. (1975). *Toxicol. Appl. Pharmacol. 31:*505.
208. Boyland, E., and Chasseaud, L. F. (1969). *Adv. Enzymol. 32:*173.
209. Mitchell, J. R., Hinson, J. A., and Nelson, S. D. (1976). In *Glutathione, Metabolism and Function,* I. M. Arias and W. B. Jakoby, Eds., Raven Press, New York, p. 357.
209a.Lauterburg, B. H., and Mitchell, J. R. (1982). *Hepatology 2:*8.
210. Miller, D. J., Pichanick, G. G., Fiskerstrand, C., and Saunders, S. J. (1977). *Am. J. Dig. Dis. 22:*1055.
211. Schichi, H., Tanaka, M., Jensen, N. M., and Nebert, D. W. (1980). *Pharmacology 20:*229.
212. Boyd, M. R. (1980). *CRC Rev. Toxicol. 7:*103.
213. McLean, A. E., and Day, P. A. (1975). *Biochem. Pharmacol. 24:*37.

214. Pessayre, D., Dolder, A., Artigou, J. Y., Wandscheer, J. C., Descatoire, V., and Degott, C. (1979). *Gastroenterology* 77: 264.
215. Wendel, A., Feuerstein, S., and Konz, K. H. (1979). *Biochem. Pharmacol.* 28:2051.
216. Vina, J., Estrela, J. M., Guerri, C., and Romero, F. J. (1980). *Biochem. J.* 188:549.
216a. Griffith, O. W. (1982). *J. Biol. Chem.* 257:13704.
217. Griffith, O. W., Bridges, R. J., and Meister, A. (1978). *Proc. Natl. Acad. Sci. USA* 75:5405.
218. Palekar, A. G., Tate, S. S., and Meister, A. (1975). *Biochem. Biophys. Res. Commun.* 62:651.
219. Beatty, P. W., and Reed, D. J. (1980). *Arch. Biochem. Biophys.* 204:80.
220. Tateishi, N., Higashi, T., Shinya, S., Naruse, A., and Sakamoto, Y. (1974). *J. Biochem. (Tokyo)* 75:93.
221. Batalden, P., Swain, W. R., and Lowman, J. T. (1968). *J. Lab. Clin. Med.* 71:312.
222. Vina, J., Romero, F. J., Estrela, J. M., and Vina, J. R. (1980). *Biochem. Pharmacol.* 29:2968.
223. Thor, H., Moldeus, P., and Orrenius, S. (1979). *Arch. Biochem. Biophys.* 192:405.
224. Vina, J., Hems, R., and Krebs, H. A. (1978). *Biochem. J.* 170:627.
225. Reed, D. J., and Orrenius, S. (1977). *Biochem. Biophys. Res. Commun.* 77:1257.
226. Higashi, T., and Tateishi, N. (1978). In *Functions of Glutathione in Liver and Kidney*, H. Sies and A. Wendel, Eds., Springer-Verlag, Berlin, p. 22.
227. Yam, J., Frank, C., and Roberts, R. J. (1978). *Proc. Soc. Exp. Biol. Med.* 157:293.
228. Tateishi, N., Higashi, T., Nakashima, K., and Sakamoto, Y. (1980). *J. Nutr.* 110:409.
229. Bartoc, R., Bruhis, S., Klein, R., Moldoveanu, E., Oeriu, I., and Oeriu, S. (1975). *Exp. Gerontol.* 10:161.
230. Abraham, E. C., Taylor, J. F., and Lang, C. A. (1978). *Biochem. J.* 174:819.
231. Lauterburg, B. H., Vaishnav, Y., Stillwell, W. G., and Mitchell, J. R. (1980). *J. Pharmacol. Exp. Ther.* 213:54.
232. Fiala, S., Mohindru, A., Kettering, W. G., Fiala, A. E., and Morris, H. P. (1976). *J. Natl. Cancer Inst.* 57:591.
233. With, P. J., and Thorgeirsson, S. S. (1978). *Cancer Res.* 38:2861.
234. Suojanen, J. N., Gay, R. J., and Hilf, J. R. (1980). *Biochim. Biophys. Acta* 630:485.

235. Linscheer, W. G., Raheja, K. L., Cho, C., and Smith, N. J. (1980). *Gastroenterology* 78:100.
236. Vuopio, P., Viherkoski, M., Nikkila, E., and Lamberg, B. A. (1970). *Ann. Clin. Res.* 2:184.
237. Reed, D. J., Ellis, W. W., and Meck, R. A. (1980). *Biochem. Biophys. Res. Commun.* 94:1273.
238. Sasame, H. A., and Boyd, M. R. (1978). *J. Pharmacol. Exp. Ther.* 205:718.
239. Pisciotto, P. T., and Graziano, J. H. (1980). *Biochim. Biophys. Acta* 628:241.
240. Finkelstein, J. D. (1975). In *Metabolic Pathways*, Vol. 7: 3rd ed., D. M. Greenberg, Ed., Academic Press, New York, p. 547.
241. Caldwell, J. (1982). In *Metabolic Basis of Detoxication*, W. B. Jakoby, J. Bend, and J. Caldwell, Eds., Academic Press, New York, p. 271.
242. Caldwell, J. (1978). In *Conjugation Reactions in Drug Biotransformation*, A. Aitio, Ed., Elsevier/North-Holland, Amsterdam, p. 111.
243. Schersten, T. (1970). In *Metabolic Conjugation and Metabolic Hydrolysis*, Vol. 2, W. H. Fishman, Ed., Academic Press, New York, p. 75.
244. Brueton, M. J., Berger, H. M., Brown, G. A., Ablitt, L., Iyngkaran, N., and Wharton, B. A. (1978). *Gut* 19:95.
245. Vessey, D. A. (1978). *Biochem. J.* 174:621.
246. Knopf, K., Sturman, J. A., Armstrong, M., and Hayes, K. C. (1978). *J. Nutr.* 108:773.
247. Sjövall, J. J. (1959). *Proc. Soc. Exp. Biol. Med.* 100:676.
248. Encrantz, J. C., and Sjövall, J. (1959). *Clin. Chim. Acta* 4:793.
249. Vessey, D. A., and Zakim, D. (1977). *Biochem. J.* 163:357.
250. Vessey, D. A., Crissey, M. H., and Zakim, D. (1977). *Biochem. J.* 163:181.
251. Gatley, S. J., and Sherratt, H. S. A. (1977). *Biochem. J.* 166:39.
252. James, M. O., and Bend, J. R. (1978). *Biochem. J.* 172:285.
253. Forman, W. B., Davidson, E. D., and Webster, L. T. (1971). *Mol. Pharmacol.* 7:247.
254. Killenberg, P. G., Davidson, E. D., and Webster, L. T. (1971). *Mol. Pharmacol.* 7:260.
255. Jacobsen, J. G., and Smith, L. H. (1968). *Physiol. Rev.* 48:424.
256. Huxtable, R. J. (1978). In *Taurine and Neurological Diseases*, A. Barbeau and R. J. Huxtable, Eds., Raven Press, New York, p. 5.
257. Lombardini, J. B., and Medina, E. V. (1978). *J. Nutr.* 108:428.

258. Groby, W. G., and Martin, W. G. (1975). *Proc. Soc. Exp. Biol. Med. 148*:544.
259. Barbeau, A., and Huxtable, R. J. (1978). *Taurine and Neurological Diseases*, Raven Press, New York.
260. *Fed. Proc. 39*:2678-2707. (1980).
261. Sturman, J. A., and Hayes, K. C. (1980). *Adv. Nutr. Res. 3*:322.
262. Sturman, J. A. (1973). *J. Nutr. 103*:1566.
263. Sturman, J. A., Hepner, G. W., Hofmann, A. F., and Thomas, P. J. (1975). *J. Nutr. 105*:1206.
264. Hardison, W. G. M., and Weiner, R. (1980). *Biochim. Biophys. Acta 598*:145.
265. Spaeth, D. G., and Schneider, D. L. (1974). *J. Nutr. 104*: 179.
266. Hardison, W. G. M., Wood, C. A., and Proffitt, J. H. (1977). *Proc. Soc. Exp. Biol. Med. 155*:55.
267. Hardison, W. G. M., and Proffitt, J. H. (1977). *Am. J. Physiol. 232*:E75.
268. Hirom, P. C., Idle, J. R., Millburn, P., and Williams, R. T. (1977). *Biochem. Soc. Trans. 5*:1033.
269. Hardison, W. G. M. (1978). *Gastroenterology 75*:71.
270. Thompson, D. E., and Vivian, V. M. (1977). *J. Nutr. 107*: 673.
271. Whittle, B., and Smith, J. T. (1974). *J. Nutr. 104*:666.
272. Awapara, J. (1956). *J. Biol. Chem. 218*:571.
273. Evered, D. F., Harvey, M. S., Luch, L. J., and Solari, M. E. (1969). *Life Sci. 8(II)*:601.
274. Roe, D. A., and Weston, W. O. (1965). *Nature 204*:287.
275. Sorbö, B. (1961). *Clin. Chim. Acta 6*:87.
276. Huxtable, R., and Bressler, R. (1976). In *Taurine*, R. Huxtable and A. Barbeau, Eds., Raven Press, New York, p. 45.
277. Guidotto, A., Badiani, G., and Papeu, G. (1972). *J. Neurochem. 19*:431.
278. Lombardini, J. B. (1974). *J. Pharmacol. Exp. Ther. 193*: 301.
279. Wilbraham, A. C., Owen, T. C., Johnson, B. G., and Roach, J. A. G. (1971). *Talanta 18*:997.
280. Garbutt, J. T., Lack, L., and Tyor, M. P. (1971). *Am. J. Clin. Nutr. 24*:218.
281. Cook, D. A., Hagerman, L. M., and Schneider, D. L. (1971). *Proc. Soc. Exp. Biol. Med. 138*:830.
282. Huxtable, R. J., Laird, H. E., and Lippincott, S. E. (1979). *J. Pharmacol. Exp. Ther. 211*:465.
283. Huxtable, R. J., Chubb, J., and Acari, J. (1980). *Fed. Proc. 39*:2685.
284. Lombardini, J. B. (1980). *J. Pharmacol. Exp. Ther. 213*:399.

285. Sturman, J. A., and Gaull, G. E. (1976). In *Taurine*, R. Huxtable and A. Barbeau, Eds., Raven Press, New York, p. 73.

286. Sturman, J. A., Rassin, D. K., and Gaull, G. E. (1977). *Life Sci. 21*:1.

287. Randle, P. J., Hutson, N. J., and Kerbey, A. L. (1977). In *Regulatory Mechanisms of Carbohydrate Metabolism*, FEBS Meeting Symposia, p. 3.

288. Lane, M. D., Moss, J., and Polakis, S. E. (1974). In *Current Topics in Cellular Regulation*, Vol. 8, B. L. Horecker and E. R. Stadtman, Eds., Academic Press, New York, p. 139.

289. McGarry, J. D., and Foster, D. W. (1980). *Annu. Rev. Biochem. 49*:395.

290. Verma, R. S., and Motzok, I. (1975). *Nutr. Rep. Int. 20*: 735.

291. Muth, O. H., and Oldfield, J. E. (1970). *Sulfur in Nutrition*, AVI, Westport, Conn.

292. Finkelstein, J. D., and Mudd, S. H. (1976). *J. Biol. Chem. 242*:873.

293. Clark, M. E., Howe, J. M., Shannon, B. M., Carlson, K., and Kolski, S. M. (1970). *Am. J. Clin. Nutr. 23*:731.

294. Stipanuk, M. H., and Benevenga, N. J. (1977). *J. Nutr. 107*:1455.

295. Lakshmanan, F. L., Perera, W. D. A., Scrimshaw, N. S., and Young, V. R. (1976). *Am. J. Clin. Nutr. 29*:1367.

296. Dziewiatkowski, D. D. (1949). *J. Biol. Chem. 178*:389.

297. Mulder, G. J. (1981). In *Sulfation of Drugs and Related Compounds*, G. J. Mulder, Ed., CRC Press, Boca Raton, Fla., Chap. 3.

298. Zezulke, A. Y., and Calloway, D. H. (1976). *J. Nutr. 106*: 1286.

299. Puigserver, A. J., Sen, L. C., Clifford, A. J., Feeney, R. E., and Whitaker, J. R. (1979). *J. Agric. Food. Chem. 27*:1286.

300. Steglink, L. D., Filer, L. J., and Baker, G. L. (1980). *J. Nutr. 110*:42.

301. Block, W. D., Markovs, M. E., and Steele, B. F. (1969). *Am. J. Clin. Nutr. 22*:33.

302. Steglink, L. D., Moss, J., Printen, K. J., and Cho, E. S. (1980). *J. Nutr. 110*:1240.

303. Sanchez, A., Swenseid, M. E., Clark, A. J., and Umezawa, C. (1972). *Am. J. Clin. Nutr. 25*:550.

303a. Shemer, M., and Perkins, E. G. (1976). *J. Nutr. 104*:1389.

304. Stipanuk, M. H. (1979). *J. Nutr. 109*:2126.

305. Fau, D., Bois-Joyeux, B., Delhomme, B., Chanez, M., and Peret, J. (1980). *Nutr. Rep. Int. 21*:577.

306. Noda, K., and Okita, T. (1980). *J. Nutr. 110*:550.
307. Benevenga, N. J. (1974). *J. Agric. Food Chem. 22*:2.
308. Benevenga, N. J. Yeh, M. H., and Lalich, J. J. (1976). *J. Nutr. 106*:1714.
309. Peng, Y. S., and Evenson, J. K. (1979). *J. Nutr. 109*:281.
310. Steele, R. D., Barber, T. A., Lalich, J., and Benevenga, N. J. (1979). *J. Nutr. 109*:1739.
311. Mitchell, A. D., and Benevenga, N. J. (1976). *J. Nutr. 106*:1702.
312. Case, G. L., and Benevenga, N. J. (1977). *J. Nutr. 107*:1665.
313. Krebs, H. A., Hems, R., and Tyler, B. (1976). *Biochem. J. 158*:341.
314. Case, G. L., and Benevenga, N. J. (1976). *J. Nutr. 106*:1721.
315. Mitchell, A. D., and Benevenga, N. J. (1978). *J. Nutr. 108*:67.
316. Everett, G. B., Mitchell, A. D., and Benevenga, N. J. (1979). *J. Nutr. 109*:597.
317. Livesey, G., and Lund, P. (1980). *Biochem. Soc. Trans. 8*:540.
318. Spector, R., Coakley, G., and Blakely, R. (1980). *J. Neurochem. 34*:132.
319. Finkelstein, J. D., Martin, J. J., Kyle, W. E., and Harris, B. J. (1980). *Proc. Soc. Exp. Biol. Med. 164*:510.
320. Hoffmann, J. L. (1980). *Arch. Biochem. Biophys. 205*:132.
321. Fernstrom, J., Larin, F., and Wurtman, R. J. (1971). *Life Sci. 10(I)*:813.
322. Fernstrom, J., Wurtman, R., Wiklund, B., Rand, W., Munro, H., Davidson, C. (1979). *Am. J. Clin. Nutr. 32*:1912.
323. Fernstrom, J. D., Wurtman, R. J., Hammerstrom-Wiklund, B., Rand, W. M., Munro, H. N., and Davidson, C. S. (1979). *Am. J. Clin. Nutr. 32*:1923.
324. Shin, H. K., and Linkswiler, H. M. (1974). *J. Nutr. 104*:1348.
325. Shannon, B. M., Smiciklas-Wright, H., Itzcovics, J., and Schearer, H. L. (1975). *J. Nutr. 105*:1334.
326. Cho, E. S., and Stegink, L. D. (1979). *J. Nutr. 109*:1086.
327. Krijgsheld, K. R., Glazenburg, E., Scholtens, E., and Mulder, G. J. (1982). *Biochim. Biophys. Acta 677*:7.
328. Irreverre, F., Mudd, S. H., Heizer, W. D., and Laster, L. (1967). *Biochem. Med. 1*:187.
329. Johnson, J. L., and Rajagopalan, K. V. (1980). In *Sulphur In Biology*, Ciba Foundation Symp. 72 (new series), Excerpta Medica, Amsterdam, p. 119.
330. Teeter, R. G., Baker, D. H., and Corbin, J. E. (1978). *J Nutr. 108*:291.

331. Featherston, W. R., and Rogler, J. C. (1978). *J. Nutr. 108*: 1954.
332. Reed, D. J., and Beatty, P. W. (1978). In *Functions of Gluta-thione in the Liver and Kidney*, H. Sies and A. Wendel, Eds., Springer-Verlag, Berlin, p. 18.
333. Simpson, R. C., and Freedland, R. A. (1976). *J. Nutr. 106*: 1272.
334. Whittle, B. A., and Lee, C. H. (1976). *J. Nutr. 106*:537.
335. Sabry, Z. I., Shadarevian, S. B., Cowan, J. W., and Camp-bell, J. A. (1965). *Nature 206*:931.
336. Lakshmanan, F. L., Vaughan, D. A., and Barnes, R. E. (1978). *Fed. Proc. 37*:783.
337. Cavallini, D., De Marco, C., and Mondovi, B. (1958). *J. Biol. Chem. 230*:25.
338. Anderson, G. H., Ashley, D. V. M., and Jones, D. J. (1976). *J. Nutr. 106*:1108.
339. Kilberg, M. S., Christensen, H. N., and Handlogten, M. E. (1979). *Biochem. Biophys. Res. Commun. 88*:744.

6

Glutathione Conjugation Systems and Drug Disposition

Donald J. Reed and Michael J. Meredith*
Oregon State University, Corvallis, Oregon

I. INTRODUCTION

Glutathione (L-γ-glutamyl-L-cysteinylglycine, GSH) is found in virtually all cells (except for certain mutant bacteria) as the most abundant low-molecular-weight thiol. This ubiquitous tripeptide has an important role in the detoxification of electrophilic and free radical metabolites of drugs and literally hundreds of thousands of other xenobiotics. Trapping of reactive intermediates by GSH leads to their rapid elimination and prevents their covalent binding to tissue macromolecules, thereby providing protection from loss of cellular viability and function.

This chapter focuses on recent findings concerning the intra- and extracellular status of glutathione and glutathione conjugates. New analytical methodologies, freshly isolated organ cell systems, and a greater understanding of the interorgan relationships of GSH and GSH conjugates as well as the enzymology of the metabolism of GSH and GSH conjugates have added enormously to our understanding of the relationship between nutrition and drug disposition.

II. RECENT DEVELOPMENTS IN METHODOLOGY

A. Quantitation of GSH, Glutathione Disulfide, and Mixed Disulfides

Estimation of GSH with an enzymic assay procedure developed by Tietze (1969) and based on glutathione reductase cleavage of the mixed disul-

Present affiliation: Vanderbilt University, Nashville, Tennessee

fide between 2-nitro-5-thiobenzoic acid and GSH is sensitive, specific, and reliable, with little interference from other thiols. However, efforts to utilize this method for glutathione disulfide (GSSG) measurement are still less than satisfactory, due to N-ethylmaleimide (NEM) inactivation of glutathione reductase after GSH elimination with NEM, as discussed by Akerboom and Sies (1981).

A recent modification (Griffith, 1980) is the replacement of NEM with 2-vinylpyridine to adduct formation with GSH prior to GSSG analysis. 2-Vinylpyridine does not inhibit glutathione reductase activity and it reacts with GSH at slightly acidic pH values where spontaneous formation of GSSG is minimal.

The method of Saville (1958) has been considered well suited for the measurement of nonprotein (or acid-soluble) thiols in biological extracts. This is based on the reaction of thiol group at low pH with nitrous acid to give S-nitroso derivations, which in turn can be selectively degraded and regenerated nitrous acid reacted with N-1-naphthylethylenediamine to yield absorbance at 550 nm. Caution should be exercised in evaluating the quantitative significance of data derived from this assay procedure since acid-soluble protein sulfhydryls are measured (Todd and Gronow, 1969; Gronow and Todd, 1969).

Hissin and Hilf (1976) extended the observation of Cohn and Lyle (1966) on the use of o-phthalaldehyde for sensitive fluorometric assays of glutathione (GSH) and glutathione disulfide (GSSG). Whereas the method is quite specific for GSH, the procedure is known to give unreliable values for GSSG in tissue samples (Beutler and West, 1977) and particularly in sera samples. In fact, caution should be exercised whenever this assay method is utilized with biological samples.

A rapid and sensitive high-performance liquid chromatography (HPLC) method for nanomole levels of GSH, GSSG, and related thiols and disulfides has been developed by Reed et al. (1980 a, b). The procedure is based on the initial formation of S-carboxymethyl derivatives with iodoacetic acid and then conversion of free amino groups to 2,4-dinitrophenyl derivatives by reaction with 1-fluoro-2,4-dinitrobenzene. Chromatography of the reaction mixture without sample isolation is on a 3-aminopropylsilane-derivatized silica column and elution with an acetate gradient. More than 20 thiols and disulfides have been characterized by this method (Reed et al., 1980a,b). This method appears to be the most sensitive and satisfactory method for analysis of mixed disulfides, including cysteinyl glutathione mixed disulfide. In contrast, lack of sensitivity and failure to separate certain mixed disulfides (i.e., cysteinylglycine) from phenylalanine with amino acid analyzer systems have been described (Perry and Hansen, 1981).

New and more sensitive methods for quantitative analysis of thiols in biological samples have been reported. Recently, picomole quantitation has been described with a new fluorescent reagent, monobromotrimethyl ammoniobimane (3,7-dimethyl-4-bromoethyl-6-trimethylammoniomethyl-1,

5-diazabicyclo[3.3.0]octa-3,6-diene-2,8-dione) (Fahey et al., 1980, 1981). In this procedure, thiols are converted to fluorescent derivatives by reaction with monobromobimane and the derivatives are separated by ion exchange HPLC and detected by fluorescence in a flow fluorometer. These workers utilized N-ethylmaleimide (NEM) to block thiols to determine nonthiol fluorescence background and dithiothreitol (DTT) to maintain thiols in a reduced state. Thiols present as disulfides must be chemically reduced prior to analysis. Since DTT cleaves disulfides, DTT was utilized to measure the combined free and disulfide thiol content of biological samples (Fahey et al., 1981). Reverse-phase HPLC on a C_{18} column with methanol, acetic acid, and water mixtures at pH 3.9 allowed separation of about 20 thiols, including some without an amino group. This method does not permit characterization of low-molecular-weight mixed disulfides, only the corresponding thiol. Yet this method may become the method of choice for low-molecular-weight thiols due to the degree of sensitivity and resolution obtained by the use of HPLC procedures.

Thus methodology has continued to be a limiting factor in understanding the status of intra- and extracellular glutathione and glutathione conjugates. As an example, Anderson et al. (1980) reported that GSSG represented about 70% of the total glutathione (GSH and GSSG) present in arterial plasma after L-(αS,5S)-α-amino-3-chloro-4,5-dihydro-5-isoxazoleacetic acid (AT-125) treatment of rats. In contrast, Reed and Ellis (1982) have observed that, after administration of AT-125 to rats, 48% of the total glutathione equivalents was not GSH or GSSG but the mixed disulfide of cysteine and GSH (CYSSG). The remaining glutathione equivalents were 7% GSH and 45% GSSG or 87% as GSSG based only on GSH and GSSG for total glutathione equivalents.

B. Detection and Quantitation of GSH Conjugates and Metabolites

One of the earliest general methods for the detection of premercapturic and mercapturic acids on paper chromatograms was developed by Knight and Young (1958). Quantities of the order of 5 μg could be detected by spraying the dried chromatogram with 0.1 M $K_2Cr_2O_7$ acetic acid (1:1) and then with 0.1 M $AgNO_3$. They observed that more than 30 premercapturic acids and mercapturic acids tested appeared as orange spots against a red-brown background.

Quantitation of glutathione conjugate products and resulting cysteine conjugates has been a major challenge. Solvent participation and various chromatographic procedures have been utilized for conjugate isolation and detection (for reviews, see Boyland and Chasseaud, 1969; Chasseaud, 1973a,1979; Reed and Beatty, 1980).

Recently, HPLC analysis procedures have been described for greater resolution and more sensitive quantitation than those provided by conventional chromatography systems. Reverse-phase columns have been utilized with solvents that permit ionic suppression with acetic acid as a modifier (Howie et al., 1977) or ion-pair systems with either alkylammonium or sulfonate counterions (Knox and Jurand, 1978). Efficient separation of the isomeric thioether metabolites of styrene oxide allows resolution of diastereoisomeric pairs (Hernandez et al., 1982). Isocratic elution with 15% methanol in buffered solutions of phosphoric acid-trihydroxymethyl aminomethane allowed the separation of positional and stereoisomers of styrene oxide conjugates of glutathione, cysteinylglycine, cysteine, and N-acetylcystein (Hernandez et al., 1982). Regiospecificity and stereospecificity in the enzymic conjugation of GSH with benzo[a]pyrene 4,5-oxide have been established by HPLC techniques (Hernandez et al., 1980a).

Glutathione conjugate metabolism has recently been shown to create metabolite patterns that require a continuation of highly developed chromatographic techniques and mass spectral analysis. Analysis techniques have shown that the metabolic activity of the intestinal microflora as well as tissue enzymes can result in glutathione conjugates being converted by C-S lyase systems to thiol derivatives which are subsequently metabolized by different pathways. Thiols produced in tissues are conjugated with glucuronic acid, whereas the thiols formed by the flora are methylated and oxidized to a series of methylsulfonyl-containing metabolite. Careful and systematic analysis of the glutathione conjugate and metabolites of the herbicide propachlor (2-chlora-N-isopropylacetanilide) (Bakke et al., 1976) and 2-acetamido-4-(chloromethyl)thiazole (Bakke et al., 1981d) have demonstrated convincingly that the intestinal microflora are involved in the metabolism of mercapturic acid pathway metabolites. Only with highly developed analytical tools will we begin to understand what such metabolism means to the biological events of polycyclic hydrocarbons such as benzo[a]pyrene.

C. Isolated Organ Cells

An increasing portion of the studies of glutathione conjugation reactions are being conducted in isolated cell and organ systems. The change in research methods to utilize isolated cells, as opposed to whole animals, has been stimulated by several generalized advantages. Among these are the ability to work with a defined cell population in a defined medium, with the option of making accurately measurable changes in the chemical environment of the cell. In addition, it is possible to isolate the effects and products of metabolic events within an organ by having excluded further metabolism which normally occurs by other organ systems or cell types.

The ability to attribute certain discrete steps in the process of glutathione conjugate formation and metabolism to specific cell and organ location has been essential in understanding the process as a whole.

1. Hepatocytes

The isolated hepatocyte has been used extensively to resolve complex multistep metabolic pathways to a series of measurable events free of the ultrastructural complication and heterogeneity found even in the perfused organ methods (Jungerman and Sasse, 1978). Although most toxicological studies have been done with primary suspension cultures, establishment of monolayer cultures has been noted (Chapman et al., 1973) to provide more uniform cell population. The ease of sampling and manipulation of extracellular environment of the isolated hepatocyte has made possible studies examining metabolite levels on an ever-decreasing time scale.

The early procedures for preparation of hepatocytes employed mechanical force, then chelators of Ca^{2+} and K^+ (Jacob and Bhavova, 1962; Rappaport and Howze, 1966). However, methods using mechanical force, even combined with digestive enzymes (Howard et al., 1967), did not produce acceptable viable hepatocytes. The introduction of the recirculating perfusion method by Berry and Friend (1969), in conjugation with the collagenase/hyaluronidase digestion procedure, leads to reproducible high yields of viable hepatocytes. Elimination of hyaluronidase (Wagle and Ingebretsen, 1975) and introduction of precollagenase perfusion to remove calcium as well as calcium-free medium (Seglen, 1973), and closer attention to the gas phase of the perfusion vessel and solutions (Moldeus et al., 1978a), have further improved the liver perfusion method to its current station of high reliability and utility. Discussions, in considerable detail, of methods of cell preparation and early applications of isolated liver cells have appeared elsewhere (Tager et al., 1976; Moldeus et al., 1978a).

The GSH complement of hepatocytes has been shown to be depleted by numerous agents reacting enzymatically either with glutathione S-transferase or with glutathione reductase. Those agents inhibiting glutathione reductase, such as some nitrosourea compounds, lead to accumulation of GSSG (Babson and Reed, 1978; Babson et al., 1981), whereas the transferase substrates eliminate GSH through conjugation reactions. The latter class of compounds has been used extensively experimentally to probe the functions of glutathione in the detoxification process. Because of the ubiquitous nature of glutathione S-transferases, a commonly used reagent is the α,β-unsaturated carbonyl compound diethylmaleate (DEM) (Chasseaud, 1973b; Plummer et al., 1981). DEM reacts nonenzymically with GSH, but at a slower rate (Boyland and Chasseaud, 1970). Possible undesirable effects of DEM treatment include increased hepatic microsomal heme oxygenase activity (Burk and Correia, 1979) and inhibition of monooxygenase activity (Anders, 1978; Burk and Correia, 1979; Chaung et al., 1978).

The turnover of GSH in the isolated rat hepatocyte was measured after depletion with DEM (Högberg and Kristoferson, 1978). After the rapid initial loss, GSH was found to be resynthesized in the presence of cysteine, at a rate of about 10 nmol/hr per 10^6 cells. However, later studies demonstrated an enhancement in the rate of GSH synthesis during periods of depletion (Lauterburg et al., 1980).

The enhancement of hepatotoxicity by GSH depletion has been noted during the metabolism of several compounds. Thor et al. (1978a-c), in a series of experiments examining the metabolism and hepatotoxicity of bromobenzene in hepatocytes from phenobarbital-treated rats, found GSH to be rapidly depleted by inclusion of bromobenzene in the incubation medium. However, no evidence of membrane damage (increased NADH leakage) was seen. When hepatocytes were pretreated with DEM, reducing intracellular GSH to about 30% of untreated samples, bromobenzene addition resulted in loss of glutathione to 5% of initial levels, and significant cell death (75% by 5 hr) was noted. Addition of cysteine, methionine, or N-acethylcysteine (Thor et al., 1979) prevented bromobenzene toxicity but did not prevent GSH depletion. Bromobenzene in the presence of a cysteine source reduced initial levels to about 40% of control (Thor et al., 1978b). In all cases, the presence of metyrapone, an inhibitor of cytochrome P-450-dependent monooxygenase reactions, eliminated bromobenzene toxicity. These data are consistent with a requirement for bromobenzene activation prior to GSH conjugation.

The correlation between the formation of GSH conjugates and the resultant reduction of intracellular GSH concentration in the isolated hepatocyte has been examined under general conditions of external stress. The observation that malondialdehyde production, indicative of lipid peroxidation, could be stimulated by DEM addition (Högberg et al., 1975) suggested that GSH was closely related to membrane integrity In addition, they found that ADP-Fe^{3+} as well as pyrophosphate-complexed ferric ion stimulated malondialdehyde production. However, common aspects of mechanism were not demonstrated, although a small reduction of cellular GSH (less than 40%) was observed during iron-induced peroxidation. Later studied (Högberg and Kristoferson, 1977), focusing on the role of GSH in the prevention of hepatocyte death, demonstrated that paracetamol (acetaminophen) could deplete hepatocyte GSH, even in the presence of complete medium. Furthermore, the GSH lost did not appear as GSSG, indicating consumption of GSH in a manner other than a simple redox cycle through glutathione peroxidase and reductase.

The depletion of hepatocyte glutathione by DEM has, in all cases, never been found to exceed 90--95% of total cell glutathione. Hepatocytes thus depleted have been found to remain viable for several hours, eventually resynthesizing the original complement of GSH. Without additional stress, such as acetaminophen (Högberg and Kristoferson, 1977) or ADP-Fe^{3+} (Högberg et al., 1975), lipid peroxidation and cell death were not observed. Recent studies in this laboratory (Babson et al., 1981) have shown that in hepatocytes depleted of GSH by 1,3-bis(2-chloroethyl)-1-nitrosourea (BCNU), no malondialdehyde was noted above control levels through 5 hr of incubation. If adriamycin is included, GSH levels are reduced to less than 5% by 3 hr, coincident with a dramatic increase in malondialdehyde production and lactate dehydrogenase leakage. Additional studies have shown that the pool of GSH which is uneffected by mild DEM and/or BCNU treatment is sequestered within the mitochondria (Meredith and Reed, 1981). The accessibility of BCNU to the mitochondrial matrix was shown by the rapid and complete inhibition of the mitochondrial glutathione reductase. Depletion of the mitochondrial pool of GSH, in a GSH S-transferase-dependent reaction with ethacrynic acid, was accompanied by a rapid leakage of lactate dehydrogenase (Meredith and Reed, 1981).

Liver cell culture has been very useful for the study of chemical activation, metabolism, and toxicity (Sirica and Pitot, 1980). From such studies come some interesting relationships between the intracellular content of GSH, the concentration of cytochrome P-450, and the nutritional status of the media for rat cell culture. The concentration of cytochrome P-450 decreases 60–70% during the first 24 hr of culture if cysteine is present in the culture medium (Paine and Legg, 1978). Elimination of cystine from the medium permits maintenance of P-450 but not GSH, which is 30% of that found in intact liver (Paine and Hockin, 1980). Methionine (1 mM) in the medium allows maintenance of the concentration of both GSH and cytochrome P-450 (Allen et al., 1981). Remaining to be resolved is the question of whether a causal relationship exists between the concentration of GSH and the maintenance of cytochrome P-450. The presence of 0.25 mM methionine in the medium resulted in GSH concentrations significantly lower than those found in vivo in liver, whereas 0.5, 1.0, and 2.0 mM methionine in the medium eliminated the difference. Further studies are needed to resolve these important interrelationships between GSH and cytochrome P-450 levels.

2. Kidney Cells

Methodology developed for the preparation of freshly isolated hepatocytes has been extended to the preparation of freshly isolated kidney cells. Although some modifications have been necessary, the method described by Jones et al. (1979a) and Ormstad et al. (1980) incorporated all the essential elements of the recirculation perfusion method of hepatocyte preparation (Moldeus et al., 1978a). The kidney cells obtained by the collagenase digestion are characterized as being of tubular origin and exhibit high viability (85–95% trypan blue excluding) and good yield (about 30×10^6 cells per two kidneys). This represents a significant improvement, particularly in yield, over previously published methods of kidney cell preparation (Rasmussen, 1975; Michelakis, 1975). Comparison of the biochemical properties of isolated kidney cells with those of the intact kidney or isolated hepatocyte (Jones and Mason, 1978; Jones et al., 1978) indicated that these cells are representative and useful models for the evaluation of certain aspects of kidney function.

Evaluation of the GSH biosynthetic capacity of the isolated kidney cell (Ormstad et al., 1980; Moldeus et al., 1981) revealed that, unlike isolated hepatocytes, methionine would not serve to support synthesis. This indicates that the cystathionine pathway for the incorporation of methionine sulfur into cysteine (Reed and Orrenius, 1977) is not sufficiently active to support synthesis in kidney cells. Resynthesis of GSH after DEM depletion of GSH was best supported by supplementing the buffered salt medium with a combination of glycine, glutamate, and cystine, although the rate of cysteine uptake by the isolated kidney cells was greater than the uptake of cystine.

Inclusion of methionine with glycine, glutamate, and cysteine caused a significant inhibition in the rate of resynthesis. Substitution of glycylglycine for methionine caused even greater inhibition of synthesis, although neither depressed synthesis is below the limit of cystine alone. Both are known γ-glutamyl acceptors in the transpeptidation reaction of γ-glutamyl transpeptidase, and availability of intracellular GSH as a γ-glutamyl donor was suggested (Ormstad et al., 1980). However, experiments with serine borate, an inhibitor of the transpeptidase, to demonstrate the involvement of γ-glutamyl transpeptidase in the rate of depression were not undertaken.

Due to the high levels of glutathione S-transferase, GSH conjugation reactions are generally considered in the context of hepatic function. Studies with the isolated kidney cell system have shown not only the high levels of conjugate metabolism but also significant conjugate formation. Jones et al. (1979a) found that addition of acetaminophen to isolated kidney cells resulted in the production of numerous metabolites as well as a decrease in cellular GSH levels. With cells prepared from control animals, 15% of the acetaminophen metabolites were sulfhydryl conjugates (i.e., glutathione cysteine or N-acetylcysteine). Rats pretreated with 3-methycholanthrene yielded cells producing sulfhydryl conjugates as 27% of total conjugate formation. The major metabolites of acetaminophen, identified by high-performance liquid chromatography, were the glucuronide and sulfate conjugates, accounting for about 50−25% respectively, of total conjugate formation. During the incubation period, GSH levels were reduced slightly by the presence of acetaminophen, but the number of cells excluding trypan blue was unchanged.

Further studies of the metabolism of GSH and its acetaminophen conjugate (Jones et al., 1979b) noted the contribution of γ-glutamyl transpeptidase to the interorgan metabolism of glutathione. Glutathione at a high concentration (2 mM) was found to be oxidized rapidly to GSSG by isolated kidney cells in an O_2-dependent, KCN-inhibited reaction. In addition, incubation of kidney cells with borate and serine, reported to be a specific inhibitor of γ-glutamyl transpeptidase (Revel and Ball, 1959), did not interfere with the disulfide formation but did prevent further degradation of the oxidized glutathione (Jones et al., 1979b). When the metabolism of the acetaminophen conjugate of glutathione was examined, it was found that kidney cell suspensions produced an intermediate metabolite coeluting with the putative acetaminophen cysteinylglycine conjugate produced by microsomal preparations. As with GSSG, addition of serine-borate inhibited further metabolism of conjugate by blocking transpeptidase activity. More recent experiments have shown glutathione oxidase activity (now termed thiol oxidase) to be separable from kidney γ-glutamyl transpeptidase by column chromatography. AT-125 has been shown to inhibit both γ-glutamyl transpeptidase activity and thiol oxidase activity of chromatocally resolved protein fractions from kidney membrane preparations (Ashkar et al., 1981).

Isolated kidney cells have been used to demonstrate the dramatic effects of AT-125 on glutathione and GSH-conjugate metabolism through γ-glutamyl transpeptidase (Jayaram et al., 1975; Allen et al., 1980). When incubated without AT-125, isolated kidney cells degraded about 90% of added GSH within 30 min. In the presence of AT-125, greater than 95% of the exogenous GSH remained in the medium (Reed et al., 1980a,b). Additionally, HPLC analysis of metabolites derived from GSH, GSSG, the mixed disulfide of cysteine and GSH, or cystinyl bisglycine demonstrated that removal of the γ-glutamyl moiety is inhibited by AT-125, leaving unaffected subsequent peptidase reactions. The fact that the GSH and the other substrates were metabolized to cysteine as the major product clearly shows that isolated kidney cells retain the ability to degrade GSH. This supposition is further confirmed by the finding (Reed and Ellis, 1982) that S-methylglutathione is rapidly removed from the kidney cell incubation medium in the absence of AT-125. The loss of this glutathione conjugate is prevented by AT-125, indicating that release of the γ-glutamyl group is a prerequisite to further metabolism.

Another compelling piece of evidence of the acceptability of the isolated liver and kidney cells as conjugate metabolizing model systems was presented by Moldeus et al. (1978b). In experiments using a combination of isolated kidney and liver cells, it was shown that acetaminophen, when added to the culture medium, was recovered as the mercapturic acid. Formation of the glutathione conjugate was carried out primarily by the isolated hepatocytes, as would be expected from the relatively higher levels of GSH S-transferase in the liver. Only the formation of the cysteine and N-acetylcysteine conjugates could be attributed to the kidney cells, presumably derived from the GSH conjugates effluxed into the medium by the hepatocytes. The slowest step in the pathway was the N-acetylation of the cysteine conjugate. The presence of cysteinyl-S-acetaminophen in urine has been attributed to a slow rate of mercapturic acid formation relative to glycine hydrolysis, producing the cysteine conjugate (Howie et al., 1977).

3. Intestinal Cells

Manipulation of cells in culture has attracted considerable interest with
regard to intestinal mucosa metabolism. Absorption capacity as well as
the efficiency of transport of sugars and amino acids (Fisher and Parsons, 1953; Crane and Mandelstam, 1960) and some drug metabolism
(Hoench et al., 1975) has been shown to be a function of position in
the intestine, proximal segments being most efficient. The spatial element of activity distribution has made the homogeneity of cells in intestinal culture very advantageous. Numerous attempts have been made
to prepare intestinal epithelial cells relying on mechanic and/or enzymatic disruption (Perris, 1966; Stern and Reilly, 1965; Stern, 1966)
and by citrate-stimulated dissociation (Stern and Jensen, 1966; Weisner, 1973a,b).

The citrate dissociation method has the added advantage of yielding
only epithelial cells, excluding interstitial and serosal cells. Additionally, variation of incubation time releases a gradient of cell types, villus tip cells appearing first and crypt zone cells last, making possible
examination of cell population at progression stages of differentiation.
Hoench et al. (1975) have shown that cytochrome P-450 and benzopyrene hydroxylase are found in highest concentration in villus tip cells
and lowest in crypt cells.

More recent enzymatic methods of dissociation, hyaluronidase in conjunction with collagenase, have produced intestinal cells from chickens
(Kimmich, 1970) and rats (Stohs et al., 1976) that are morphologically
undamaged and metabolically competent. Both systems exhibit linear
oxygen uptake for at least 2 hr, as well as receptor control and sensitivity to inhibitors of oxidative phosphorylation. However, only in
the rat system has glutathione metabolism been studied in detail.

Grafström et al. (1980) reported that intestinal mucosa cells oxidize
exogenous high concentrations of GSH to GSSG prior to further degradation. Oxidation was independent of serine-borate and methionine,
but hydrolytic cleavage of glutamate was stimulated by methionine as
well as glycylglycine and inhibited by serine-borate, suggesting the
involvement of γ-glutamyl transpeptidase. The isolated mucosal cells
were found to be about one-fifth as efficient as kidney cells in γ-
glutamyl hydrolysis. The presence of a peptidase for the cleavage of
cystinyl-bis-glycine has previously been confirmed for small intestine
tissue (Kim et al., 1976). The relatively high rates of transpeptidation
by these cells indicate a significant role in glutathione degradation.

Presented in vivo by way of blood and bile, glutathione conjugates
have also been shown to be metabolized in vitro by isolated intestinal
cells. Paracetamol (acetaminophen) was found to be metabolized in isolated perfused liver primarily to its glucuronide and sulfate conjugate
(Grafström et al., 1979). However at concentrations above 5 mM, the
level at which glucuronide formation was saturated, glutathione-para-
cetamol conjugates were formed. Incubation of the preformed para-

cetamol glutathione conjugate resulted in rapid formation of paracetamol-cysteine. Formation of the premercapturic acid was inhibited by serine-borate and stimulated by methionine, confirming the participation of γ-glutamyl transpeptidase in conjugate metabolism in the epithelial cells of the small intestine.

In a slower reaction, detected by administration of preformed paracetamol-S-cysteine, the N-acetyl derivative was formed. However, when paracetamol was contained in intestinal segments in situ (Grafström et al., 1979), paracetamol-S-glutathione (or paracetamol-S-cysteine) was detected only in the bile. The sulfate and glucuronide were both found in the plasma of the portal and caval venous blood, the bile, and the intestinal lumen. The appearance of the glutathione conjugate of paracetamol as only 1% of the biliary excretion of the drug suggests that the intestinally formed mercapturic acid is not a significant excretion product of this compound.

4. Red Blood Cells

Glutathione has long been recognized as the predominant acid-soluble thiol in the red blood cell, and the extensive literature has been reviewed in detail (Beutler, 1980). High concentration of GSH, 2–3 mM, ease of isolation, and cellular integrity have made the erythrocyte an attractive system in which to investigate the metabolism of GSH and GSSG. GSH is synthesized in situ in the erythrocyte, as the cell is not penetrated by GSH or GSSG (Horejsi and Micevova, 1964), although a report of the red blood cell acting as a carrier of GSH to the peripheral tissues from the liver has appeared (Eluyn et al., 1968). Jackson (1969) described assays and erythrocyte levels of the GSH-synthesizing enzymes as well as a spectral assay for γ-glutamyl transpeptidase which indicate that the erythrocyte is capable of both synthesizing and degrading GSH. Later studies (Minnich et al., 1971) confirmed that the erythrocyte could synthesize GSH from its constituent amino acids and that synthesis is completely inhibitable by fluoride, indicating that glycolysis is the exclusive source of ATP for synthesis (Rathbun, 1980). In both studies it was noted that γ-glutamyl cysteine synthetase activity was present at levels far in excess of glutathione synthetase. The low K_m for cysteine, 0.3 mM, of γ-glutamyl cysteine synthetase, as well as the large enzyme concentration support the contention that the rate of cysteine transport, and thus availability, is the rate-limiting step in erythrocyte GSH synthesis (Heinle et al., 1976; Smith et al., 1980).

It has been suggested that the γ-glutamyl cycle functioned in the red cell as a transport mechanism (Pelchar et al., 1974). However, the demonstration that the apparent transpeptidase activity measured was derived from contaminating leukocytes (Board and Smith, 1975; Lunn et al., 1979), as well as evidence of stable GSH pools during amino acid transport (Young et al., 1975), made this position untenable. Recently (Kilra et al., 1981), experiments were performed using red blood cells fused with dipalmitoyl phosphatidylcholine vesicles containing γ-glutamyl transpeptidase purified from hog kidney. Transport of glutamate and alanine, amino acids not readily transported by the erythrocyte, was markedly stimulated in these in plated cells and inhibitable by serine-borate, clearly indicating the participation of the newly acquired transpeptidase. However, it was not shown whether the γ-glutamyl alanine accumulated intracellularly or was further metabolized.

The absence of participation by γ-glutamyl transpeptidase in removing GSH raised questions concerning the mechanism of GSH turnover within the red blood cell. Early experiments with glycine labeling of the red cell GSH pool found the thiol to be synthesized in situ with a $t_{1/2}$ value of about 4 days, with some species variation (Dimant et al., 1955; Smith. 1974). More recent studies (Griffith, 1981) have shown that glutathione synthetase catalyzes an exchange reaction, substituting for glycine for the glycine moiety of preformed GSH, thus explaining the dependence of the measured half-life of red cell GSH on the amino acid used to label the pool.

Srivastava and Beutler (1968) showed that the red cells released GSSG in an energy-dependent process. This observation was later confirmed and the movement of GSSG shown to be unidirectional. Efflux of GSSG was proposed to be the major mechanism of glutathione elimination from the erythrocyte, accomplished with the expenditure of ATP (or other high-energy compound) (Srivastava and Beutler, 1969). The active transport of GSSG was demonstrated in red cell ghosts and the maximum transport velocity calculated to be 0.27 μmol GSSG/ml packed ghosts per hour (Prchal et al., 1975).

GSSG efflux with intact erythrocytes occurs at a rate of 6.7 nmol/hr per nanoliter of red blood cells (Lunn et al., 1979). The calculated half-life of GSH was 4.6 days, a value in agreement with that observed previously.

Factors controlling the half-life of red cell GSH are as yet unclear. Furthermore, participation of the erthrocyte in metabolism of exogenous compounds through GSH-dependent reactions has not been clearly demonstrated. The presence of GSH S-transferase f_1, a distinctive red blood cell isozyme (Marcus et al., 1978), as well as the rapid rate of depletion of GSH by diethyl maleate (Richardson and Murphy, 1975), indicates the availability of this large pool of GSH for reaction with exogenous electrophiles. However, to date, the only such reaction known to take place in the erythrocyte is the conjugation of the leukotriene A_4 with GSH (Cagen et al., 1976). More recently, the conjugation of the leukotriene A_4 with GSH has been shown to precede kidney and leukocyte transpeptidase hydrolysis in the synthesis of leukotriene D_4 (Örning, et al., 1980; Anderson et al., 1982).

III. ENZYMES IN GLUTATHIONE CONJUGATE FORMATION

A. Glutathione S-transferase

Colorfully and correctly labeled "the triple-threat in detoxification" (Jakoby and Keen, 1977), glutathione S-transferases initiate the process of detoxification of electrophilic compounds (Jakoby, 1978). In addition, these enzymes bind and sequester (ligandin) potentially toxic materials such as bilirubin (Habig et al., 1974a). A review of the ligandin activity of GSH S-transferase has been published (Smith et al., 1977). The transferases have been purified from a wide variety of organisms (Jakoby, 1978; Jakoby and Habig, 1980) and shown to exist within each organism as a family of closely related proteins with overlapping but distinct substrate specificities. As early studies of GSH S-transferase developed, primarily with rat liver, it became clear that the spectrum of substrates was broad. Designation as alkyl-, aryl-, alkene, epoxide, and aralkyl-transferase has given way to the single title, but demonstrates the variety of substrates, and ultimately the variety of compounds entering the glutathione conjugation pathway. Despite the variety of substrate classes, glutathione S-transferase produced conjugates share several common features. As summarized by Dauterman (1980) and Mathews (1980), glutathione conjugates are derived from electrophilic compounds, are anionic in nature, are generally produced from electrophiles of over 300 molecular weight, and exhibit the detergent qualities typical of biliary excreted compounds.

Glutathione S-transferase has been detected in organisms ranging from numerous marine species representing teleosts, crustacians, and elasmobranchs (Bend and Fouts, 1973) to a large number of vertebrate species (Grover and Sims, 1964). Insect transferases have been studied, with major emphasis placed on the house fly and cockroach (Clark et al., 1973; Shishido et al., 1972; Motoyama et al., 1978; Oppenoorth et al., 1979), with regard to the role of glutathione conjugation in insecticide resistance. The data collected indicate that pesticide resistance can be traced directly to the enhanced ability to resistant strains to conjugate administered compounds, particularly organophosphorous insecticides (Oppenoorth et al., 1979) in GSH S-transferase-catalyzed reactions.

Although yeast have no transferase activity (Jakoby, 1978), considerable effort has gone into examination of plant GSH S-transferase. The herbicide atrazine has been shown to be metabolized by corn and crop grasses (Frear and Swanson, 1970; Shimabukuro et al., 1970, 1971; Lamoureux et al., 1973) as the glutathione conjugate. In addition to rapid dealkylation in leaf, but not in root or shoot tissue, tolerant plants exhibited high rates of conversion of atrazine to a water-soluble metabolite identified as the glutathione conjugate. Glutathione conjugation was identified as the major detoxification mechanism in studies examining the atrazine-susceptible strain of maize GT 112. Shimabukuro et al. (1971) showed the presence of active hydroxylation systems in both susceptible and resistant corn strains, but only susceptible strains were deficient in transferase activity. Additionally, GSH S-transferase activity has been shown to be increased in corn by administration of antidotes to the thiocarbamate herbicide (Lay and Casida, 1976), suggesting that transferase activity is inducible in plants.

The GSH S-transferase levels have been measured in mammalian species including monkey, guinea pig, rabbit, humans, and most extensively in the rat. Rat liver is the source of transferase enzymes with the highest specific activity. Six transferases have been identified from the liver and kidney, and intestinal mucosa have also been identified as transferase-containing organs (Arias et al., 1976; Fleishner et al., 1976). All are dimeric proteins ranging in molecular weight from 40 to 45,000. Named in reverse order of elution from a CM-cellulose column, transferases AA, A, B, C, D, and E have been found to have similar but distinctly different amino acid compositions (Habig et al., 1976, 1974b).

In all tissues examined with the exception of the red blood cell (Marcus et al., 1978), more than one form of GSH S-transferase has been found. Transferase B has been shown to be the most plentiful in rat, about 5−10% of the total soluble protein (Jakoby et al., 1976) in rat liver; however, other transferases are also presented in significant quantity. In decreasing order of concentration, transferases C, A, AA, E, and D represent an additional 5−10% of liver protein (Jakoby, 1978). In rats treated with phenobarbital, liver transferase B level is increased about twofold (Arias et al., 1976; Pinkus et al., 1977; Bass et al., 1977), making glutathione transferase about 20−30% of the total soluble liver protein. Induced enzyme activity was dependent on new enzyme synthesis, as measured by increasing amounts of immunoreactive protein (Bass et al., 1977; Pinkus et al., 1977). Kidney and intestinal mucosa levels are only slightly elevated. Increases in transferase levels are due to enhanced synthesis at the translational level. No increase in transferase B mRNA was found after phenobarbital induction (Daniel et al., 1977), nor was an alteration of the 2- to 3-day half-life of hepatic transferase B noted (Arias et al., 1976). Additionally, t-butyl-4-hydroxyanisole (BHT) inclusion in the diet of rats and mice increases hepatic transferase (Benson et al., 1978) as well as epoxide hydrase levels (Cha et al., 1978). As yet, no reports of induction of transferases other than B have been published.

Five transferases have been purified from human liver (Kamisaka et al., 1975) and found to be immunologically cross-reactive (Fleishner et al., 1976). Like the rat liver enzymes, these transferases are composed of two apparently identical subunits of molecular weight about 24,000; however, they are not as readily resolved by cation exchange chromatography. Amino acid analysis (Kamisaka et al., 1975) showed essentially identical composition, and these charged isomers were separated by isoelectric focusing. By analogy with the rat liver enzymes,

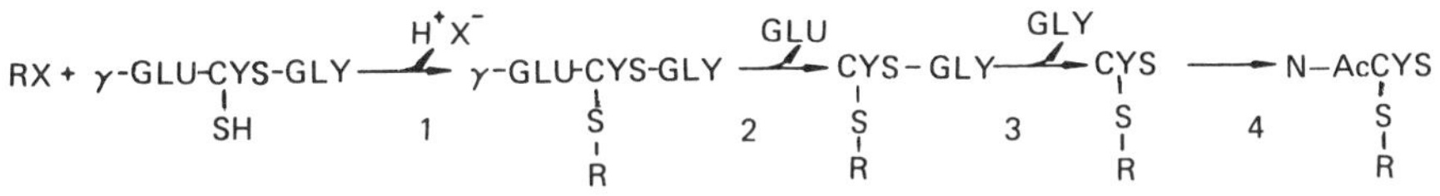

$$RX + \gamma\text{-GLU-CYS-GLY} \xrightarrow{\underset{1}{\overset{H^+X^-}{\longrightarrow}}} \underset{1}{\overset{\gamma\text{-GLU-CYS-GLY}}{\underset{\underset{R}{\overset{|}{S}}}{}}} \xrightarrow{\underset{2}{\overset{GLU}{\longrightarrow}}} \underset{\underset{R}{\overset{|}{S}}}{\overset{CYS\text{-}GLY}{}} \xrightarrow{\underset{3}{\overset{GLY}{\longrightarrow}}} \underset{\underset{R}{\overset{|}{S}}}{CYS} \xrightarrow{4} \underset{\underset{R}{\overset{|}{S}}}{N\text{-AcCYS}}$$

Figure 1 Mercapturic acid synthesis. 1, Glutathione S-transferase; 2, γ-glutamyl transpeptidase; 3, peptidase(s); 4, N-acetyltransferase.

the human liver transferases were named in order of increasing iso-electric point, from α (pI = 7.8) through ε (pI = 8.8). Production of the charged isozyme group by deamination of glutamine and asparagine residues, as has been observed for some other proteins (Midelfort and Mehler, 1972), supports considerable speculation about the maturation process of these proteins. It is interesting to note the presence of a non-cross-reactive transferase, ρ, in the erythrocyte, with pI = 4.7 (Marcus et al., 1978). The long half-life and low rate of protein turn-over in the erythrocyte could account for reduced deamination of red cell transferase, thus yielding the observed low pI value. Further details of purification and physical properties of the numerous puri-fied transferases are given in recent reviews published elsewhere (Jakoby, 1978; Jakoby and Habig, 1980).

IV. ENZYMES IN GLUTATHIONE CONJUGATE DEGRADATION

Mercapturic acids, S-derivatized N-acetylcysteine compounds, are formed from a wide variety of electrophilic agents and the tripeptide glutathione (GSH). As seen in Figure 1, the sequence of reactions is initiated by the GSH S-transferase-catalyzed production of the gluta-thione electrophile conjugate. The pioneering work of Binkley (1961) demonstrated that kidney enzymes could catalyze a first step in GSH hydrolysis to glutamate and cysteinylglycine, which was further hy-drolyzed to glycine and cysteine. Suga et al. (1966) were one of the first groups to synthesize various glutathione conjugates and examine the kidney glutathione hydrolysis products of these conjugates. They concluded that glutathione participates in the formation of mercapturic acids. We now know that steps in the degradation of GSH, GSSG, and glutathione conjugates involve an initial cleavage of the γ-glutamyl bond by glutathionase, which is also known as γ-glutamyl transferase (trans-peptidase), and release of glycine through the action of a broad class of exopeptidases (McDonald and Schwabe, 1977; Hughey et al., 1977), and finally acetyl group transfer from acetyl coenzyme A by N-acetyl-transferase, yielding the mercapturic acid (Hughey et al., 1977). An alternative metabolic route for cysteine conjugations, resulting in the formation of electrophile thiols and methylthio ethers, is provided by the recently discovered enzyme cysteine conjugate β-lyase (Tateishi et al., 1978). These enzymes, which are responsible for catalysis of the degradation of glutathione conjugates, are the subject of this section.

A. γ-Glutamyl Transpeptidase

As the only enzyme known to catalyze the removal of the γ-glutamyl moiety of GSH, considerable study has been devoted to the metabolism of GSH and GSH conjugates by γ-glutamyl transpeptidase (γ-glutamyl-transferase, glutathionase). This membrane-bound enzyme catalyzes two reactions involving γ-glutamyl compounds (including glutamine) of the following general form:

$$\gamma\text{-Glu-R} + \text{acceptor-H} \longrightarrow \gamma\text{-Glu} - \text{acceptor} + \text{RH} \qquad (1)$$

where -R represents the cysteinylglycine moiety of glutathione, and the acceptor varies with the reaction. The hydrolytic reaction uses water as the acceptor to yield cysteinylglycine and glutamate (Elce and Broxmeyer, 1976). The second and most thoroughly studied reaction, transpeptidation, utilizes numerous amino acids and small peptides as γ-glutamyl acceptors (Tate and Meister, 1974). This reaction and the proposed role in amino acid transport have been extensively reviewed elsewhere (Meister et al., 1976; Meister, 1973,1978; Meister and Tate, 1976). In addition, the transpeptidase was thought to be capable of oxygen-dependent conversion of GSH to GSSG (Tate and Orlando, 1979; Tate et al., 1979); but later experiments showed this sequence to be nonenzymatic, with transpeptidase supplying cysteinylglycine to perform essentially a catalytic role in a disulfide interchange reaction (Griffith and Tate, 1980).

In contrast to rat liver, human liver has a high level of γ-glutamyl-transferase activity. γ-Glutamyltransferase activity has been reported to be about 10-fold that in rat liver, whereas human kidney is about 10-fold lower than in rat kidney (Shaw, 1978; Shaw and Newman, 1979). These workers suggest that serious consideration be given to the role of γ-glutamyltransferase in human liver. Postmortem levels of acid-soluble thiols have been found low in GSH content and high in cysteine, suggesting a rapid cleavage of GSH in human liver (Rollins et al., 1981). Fetal liver appears to develop the capability of rapid GSH synthesis and degradation by early in the first trimester (Rollins et al., 1981). This is an important point since conjugation of GSH with the reactive intermediate of acetaminophen has been demonstrated in human fetal liver cells (Rollins et al., 1979).

Purification of the rat kidney of γ-glutamyl transpeptidase by Tate and Meister (1975) by bromelin or detergent solubilization showed the enzyme to be heavily glycosylated. However, proteolytic solubilization produced a small protein, of molecular weight 69,000, versus a "heavy" detergent-derived enzyme, of molecular weight 250,000, composed presumably of transpeptidase and other membrane proteins. Hughey and Curthoys (1976) produced papain and Triton X-100-solubilized enzymes of molecular weights 69,000 and 250,000. The unusual physical behavior of the "heavy" form with a Stokes radius of 70 Å, indicating a molecular weight of 250,000 and a molecular weight of 70,000 when determined by ultracentrifugation ($s_{20,w} = 4.155$), was shown to be due to aggregation of the protein with detergent micelles. Electrophoretic analysis (Horiuchi et al., 1978) found both protease and detergent-solubilized transpeptidases to possess a smaller subunit, of molecular weight about 25,000, on which the γ-glutamyl binding site was located. However, the Triton-purified enzyme contained a large subunit of molecular weight 66,000, 19,000 larger than the papain-derived transpeptidase. Treatment of Triton-solubilized enzyme with papain produces an enzyme identical in subunit size to the protease-solubilized protein that has lost its ability to bind to lecithin vesicles (Hughey et al., 1979). Therefore, a major function of the large subunit of γ-glutamyl transpeptidase may be to bind the enzyme to the brush border membrane.

Although the great majority of total body γ-glutamyl transpeptidase activity is located in the kidneys (Goldberg et al., 1960), enzyme activity has been found in the liver, spleen, reproductive tract, and pancreas (acinar and erythrocytes) (Goldberg et al., 1960; Jackson, 1969; Delap et al., 1976). Histochemical studies (Albert et al., 1961, 1964; Greenberg et al., 1967) have demonstrated areas of highest transpeptidase activity to be those areas most actively involved in absorption or secretory processes (i.e., the epithelial cells of the bile duct and the jejunal mucosa). Numerous studies (Tsao and Curthoys, 1980; Horiuchi et al., 1978) have shown the distribution of transpeptidase in the kidney to follow this pattern, being located primarily on the luminal surface of the brush border membrane of the renal proximal tubules, both convoluted and straight. The remaining kidney transpeptidase is distributed throughout the cortex and medulla (Meister et al., 1976; Marathe et al., 1979).

The significance of the luminal surface location of γ-glutamyl transpeptidase, and the implied availability of only extracellular glutathione and S-substituted conjugate, have been emphasized by recent experiments examining the relative importance of the hydrolytic and transpeptidation reaction. Elce and Broxmeyer (1976) have shown by simultaneous assays of transpeptidation and hydrolysis of glutathione using rat kidney transpeptidase that at physiological acceptor concentrations as well as pH, hydrolysis is the dominant reaction. Demonstration of a 10-fold-lower Michaelis constant for glutathione in the hydrolysis versus transpeptidation also suggests that hydrolysis is the favored reaction. In more detailed kinetic studies, using plasma levels of GSH and GSSG,

McIntyre and Curthoys (1979) reported a dramatic effect of pH on the transpeptidation reaction. Whereas hydrolysis was only slightly altered over the pH range 6.0–9.0, transpeptidation reached significant levels only above pH 8.0, reaching maximum activity at pH 8.5. However, even at the pH optimum, at plasma levels of alanine (0.5 mM) as an acceptor, the rate of transpeptidation was only half that of hydrolysis. Kinetic constants K_m and V_{max}, determined for the hydrolysis reaction of S-substituted GSH compounds (including GSSG), showed that not only were these conjugates substrate for γ-glutamyl transpeptidase, but that the kinetic parameters varied only slightly from those of GSH. Examination of S-modified GSH derivatives in the transpeptidation reaction (Tate and Meister, 1974; Tate, 1975) showed that the conjugates were, in general, metabolized at rates equal to, and often greater than, GSH. The recent demonstration that kidney transpeptidase (Anderson et al., 1982) is capable of hydrolyzing leukotriene C_4 to D_4 is further proof of the physiological significance of the hydrolysis reaction.

Several inhibitors have been used to investigate the metabolic role of γ-glutamyl transpeptidase. Aside from the sulfophthalein derivatives (Binkley, 1961), inhibitors have been compounds proported to mimic the structural features of γ-glutamyl amino acids. Tate and Meister (1974) reported significant, although incomplete inhibition of purified rat liver enzyme by a variety of L-γ-glutamyl hydrazones of the keto acids. Further studies by the same group (Griffith et al., 1979; Tateishi et al., 1978; Griffith and Meister, 1979b) employed D-γ-glutamyl-(o-carboxy)phenylhydrazide to produce nearly complete inhibition of transpeptidase in rat kidneys to demonstrate the apparent transport of γ-glutamyl amino acids in the absence of GSH synthesis. Within the same class of inhibitors is the amino acid analog 6-diazo-5-oxonorleucine (DON). Known to inhibit strongly amide transfer reactions of glutamine (Prusiner and Stadtman, 1973), DON was found to inhibit γ-glutamyl transpeptidase, as was azaserine, although with a lower affinity, by covalently binding to the active site on the small subunit (Griffith and Meister, 1979a). Inhibition was prevented by γ-glutamyl substrates, but not γ-glutamyl acceptors, and was stimulated by maleate, a compound since proposed to induce a conformational change enhancing exposure of the donor binding site (Thompson and Meister, 1979). L-serine in the presence of borate has also been proposed to be a transition-state analog inhibitor of γ-glutamyl transpeptidase (Tate and Meister, 1978).

In addition to its antitumor and antibiotic activity (Hanka and Dietz, 1973), AT-125 [L-(αS,5S)-α-amino-3-chloro-4,5-dihydro-5-isoxazole acetic acid; NSC-176324] has been shown to be a potent, irreversible inhibitor of γ-glutamyl transpeptidase (Allen et al., 1980) as well as asparagine synthetase (Goldberg et al., 1960). Although structurally similar to histidine, AT-125 acts as a glutamine antagonist (Cooney et at., 1974; Jayaram et al., 1975), inhibiting transfer of the amide group by modification of an active-site cysteine (Tso et al., 1980). In addition to in vitro inactivation of transpeptidase (Allen et al., 1980; Griffith and Meister, 1980), the use of AT-125 permits accurate evaluation of the role of transpeptidase in metabolism of not only GSSG and GSH, but also of γ-glutamyl-containing fragments of GSH as well as GSH conjugates (Reed and Ellis, 1982).

B. Cysteinylglycine Hydrolyzing Peptidases

To date, the enzyme(s) responsible for cleavage of the glutathione-derived dipeptide, cysteinylglycine (or the S-substituted mercapturic acid precursor), has not been definitely identified. Considering the large number of peptidases eligible for such a role (Kenny, 1977; Tate, 1980), it is unlikely that a single enzymatic species exists. Evaluation of aminopeptidases in the physiological context of mercapturic acid synthesis is complicated by the fact that seldom has cysteinylglycine been used as a test substrate. Although cytoplasmic peptidases from intestinal mucosa (Das and Radhakrishnan, 1972;1973) and hog (DeLange and Smith, 1971) and human kidney (Stetson, 1975) have been suggested as possible catalytic participants, the most compelling data have been presented for a class of membrane-bound peptidases.

Booth and Kenny (1976) identified five kidney microvilli membrane proteins, including dipeptidyl peptidase III, neutral endopeptidase, and aminopeptidase M. Analysis of samples separated by sodium dodecyl sulfate polyacrylamide gel suggests that these glycoproteins comprised 5, 9, and 5%, respectively, of total membrane protein. Although all three enzymes will hydrolyze glycine-containing peptides (Kerr and Kenny, 1973; Kenny et al., 1976), only aminopeptidase M produced N-terminal glycine products, predicting significant participation in mercapturic acid synthesis. The presence of a cysteinylglycine-hydrolyzing peptidase in the kidney was later confirmed (Hughey et al., 1977). At physiologically competent rates, a partially purified enzyme (200-fold) was shown to hydrolyze not only cysteinylglycine but also cysteinyl-bis-glycine and S-benzylcysteinylglycine, a mercapturic acid presursor. Heat-inactivation studies suggested the presence of only a single enzymatic species, which was later identified as aminopeptidase M (Rankin et al., 1980). As would be expected, peptidase activity was found by serial sectioning to be localized in the outer-stripe region of the kidney, together with γ-glutamyl transpeptidase and N-acetyltransferase activity. Further support was provided by immunological studies (Tsao and Curthoys, 1980) demonstrating peptidase activity, as well as γ-glutamyl transpeptidase, to be exclusively positioned on the luminal surface of the brush border membrane of the rat kidney proximal tubules. The rat intestinal mucosa brush border membrane has also been shown to contain aminopeptidase M bound, like the kidney enzyme, to microsomal membranes (Kenny, 1977) and containing 2 g-atoms of

Zn^+ per 240,000 of protein. This enzyme was also found to be heavily glycosylated (Maroux et al., 1973) and released from the membrane by papain digestion.

Two peptidases of molecular weight 280,000, like aminopeptidase M, composed of identical subunits of 140,000, have been purified from rat intestinal mucosa (Kim and Brophy, 1976; Kim et al., 1976). Peptidase F and S are glycoproteins immunologically identical and differing slightly in carbohydrate content and activation by divalent cations. Peptides with C-terminal glycine residues are readily hydrolyzed (Kim and Brophy, 1976), and like other membrane-bound peptidases exhibit a preference for substrates with hydrophobic NH_2-terminal amino acids (Kenny, 1977). Although the intestinal and kidney proteases have physical properties and substrate preferences in common, it is not known whether they cross-react immunologically, and earlier studies (Kim et al., 1972) demonstrated different electrophoretic mobilities. The physiological role of peptidases F and S relative to aminopeptidase M has not been investigated, nor has the immunological cross-reactivity. Despite the numerous points of identity between these proteins, there is sufficient variation in substrate specificity and reaction characteristic to support designation as nonidentical proteins (Kenny, 1977; McDonald and Schwabe, 1977).

A dipeptidase distinct from aminopeptidase M has been purified from the microvillus membranes of rat kidney jejunum and epididymis (Kozak and Tate, 1982). Smaller than other dipeptidases ($M_r = 105,000$, two subunits $M_r = 50,000$), this dipeptidase is further distinguished by its inhibition by thiol compounds. L-cysteinylglycine, the product of glutathione transpeptidation, was the most effective inhibitor tested ($K_i = 20$ μM) of the dipeptidase, while it was only mildly inhibitory toward aminopeptidase M. Although aminopeptidase M is more abundant, 5% versus about 0.2% of total kidney and jejunal microvillus membrane proteins, the thiol-sensitive dipeptidase was shown to catalyze hydrolysis of the model substrate with much lower K_m and V_{max} values, two to three orders of magnitude greater than those of aminopeptidase M (Kozak and Tate, 1982).

Although specific peptidases have not been extensively characterized from liver, significant enrichment of leucylnaphthalamine hydrolysis has been shown with plasma membrane purification (Coleman and Finean, 1966). Liver peptidase activity has been attributed to a single enzyme species exhibiting characteristics similar to kidney and intestine aminopeptidase M (Emmelot and Visser, 1971). Liver peptidase activity is capable of hydrolyzing glycine-containing peptides, with the notable exception of glycylglycine and glutathione. However, a strong argument is made for liver peptidase involvement in mercapturic acid synthesis by the observation that the enzyme is concentrated in the bile canalicular membrane (Nachlas et al., 1960).

As yet, peptidases capable of hydrolyzing the premercapturic acids have not been investigated in the variety of tissues covered by transpeptidase research. However, the presence of such peptidase is not a generalized plasma membrane phenomenon. Purification of plasma membranes from guinea pig erythrocytes and brain tissue did not yield enrichment of peptidase activity compared to the significant enhancement observed with liver, kidney, and intestinal mucosa (Coleman and Finean, 1966). Evidence presently available indicates that, like γ-glutamyl transpeptidase (Meister et al., 1976), dipeptidases and aminopeptidases which contribute to mercapturic acid synthesis are extensively localized on those membranes participating in either absorption or secretion.

C. N-Acetyltransferase

The N-acetyltransferase reaction of mercapturic acid synthesis has been separated from other N-acetyltransferases by its absolute requirement for acetylcoenzyme A. This requirement provides a sensitive, specific radioactive assay which measures transfer of [^{14}C] acetate. L-cysteine will act as an acceptor, but S-substituted derivatives are preferred, S-benzyl-L-cystine being approximately 10-fold more effective than L-cysteine. As would be expected, rat kidney and liver exhibit the highest tissue activities, with kidney specific activity being twice that of liver (Green and Elce, 1975).

Serial sectioning of kidney showed that like γ-glutamyl transpeptidase and peptidase (assayed with S-benzylcysteinyl p-nitroaniline), N-acetyltransferase is located in the outer stripe region of the kidney medulla. However, when a microsomal fraction was prepared with isopycnically separated, N-acetyltransferase banded with NADPH-cytochrome P-450 reductase, an endoplasmic reticulum marker enzyme. Peptidase and γ-glutamyl transpeptidase were found with the brush border fraction (Hughey et al., 1977). The conclusion that the peptidase and γ-glutamyl transpeptidase occupy a different intracellular location than N-acetyltransferase was earlier implied by the inability to solubilize N-acetyltransferase with detergents. The inactivating effects of phospholipases A and C, but not D (Green and Elce, 1975), show an obligate lipid interaction which is characteristic of many membrane-bound enzymes, including several endoplasmic reticulum proteins (Coleman, 1973).

D. Cysteine Conjugate β-Lyase

Although the majority of xenobiotic compounds are metabolized to the corresponding mercapturic acid, numerous reports showed the formation and excretion of methylthio (CH_3S-) derivatives. This was particularly true of aromatic compounds (Lotlikar et al., 1966; Chatfield a and Hunter, 1973), phenacetin (Focella et al., 1972; Calder et al., 1974) and acetaminophen (Wong et al., 1976) being typical examples.

Metabolic alternatives for cysteine conjugates beyond mercapturic acid
formation were unknown until Tateishi et al. (1978) reported a rat liver
enzyme, cysteine conjugate β-lyase, capable of cleaving the S-C bond
of cysteine moiety, producing the thiol derivative of the original conjugated compound, ammonia, and pyruvate in equimolar amounts
(Tateishi et al., 1978).

In tissues, the enzyme is found in significant concentrations only in
the liver and kidney, with liver containing about 65% of the body total.
In the five rodent species examined, activities ranged from 0.2 to 0.5
nmol/min per milligram of protein, and no consistent variation was observed due to sex (Tateishi and Shimizu, 1980). Purified 500-fold from
rat liver cytosol, the enzyme has a molecular weight of 170,000 and a
pH optimum at 7.5. No cofactor addition was required for reaction and
a marked substrate preference for S-2,4-dinitrophenol-cysteine versus
DNP-glutathione, or S-bromophenylcysteine was observed (Tateishi
et al., 1978).

Although unreactive with cystathionine (Tateishi and Shimizu, 1980),
cysteine conjugate β-lyase has many properties in common with γ-cysta-
thionase. In addition to being primarily liver cytoplasmic components,
both have pyridoxal phosphate dependency and are moderately heat
stable (Tateishi et al., 1978; Tateishi and Shimizu, 1980). Also, the
production of pyruvate instead of serine or alanine, the expected products of hydrolytic or hydrogenolytic cleavage of the conjugate thioether, suggests an α,β-elimination mechanism, as proposed for γ-cysta-
thionase.

The most thoroughly studied example of metabolism through the apparent cysteine conjugate pathway is propachlor (2-chloro-N-isopro-
pylacetanilide). By identification of excretion products, it was shown
that chlorine is replaced by cysteine or a methylsulfonyl group, with
cysteine as the sulfur source (Larsen and Bakke, 1979; Bakke and
Price, 1979). Additionally, the methylthiol glucuronides of propachlor
(Bakke and Price, 1979) were identified. Bakke and Price (1979) proposed a course of metabolism beginning with glutathione conjugation
(Lamoureux and Davidson, 1975) and proceeding through the cysteine
conjugate and mercapturic acid to the glucuronide, with products of
glutathione conjugation being available for urinary excretion. Bakke
et al. (1981c) have reported evidence for cysteine conjugate β-lyase
being present in intestinal flora. This activity appears to have substrate specificity different from that activity in the liver.

The physiological significance of the methylthiolation pathway for the
biotransformation of xenobiotic compounds has not been fully established. However, the recent discovery of deacylase activity capable of
removing the N-acetyl group of mercapturic acids (Tateishi and Shimizu, 1980) and a microsomol thiol S-methyltransferase which can produce the methyl thiol derivative of the original mercapturic acid
(Weisiger and Jakoby, 1980) establish a complete in vivo pathway.

The presence of a premercapturate-metabolizing enzyme in liver cytosol and intestinal microflora raises numerous questions not only about

the physiological role of cysteine conjugate β-lyase but concerning formation and disposition of the cysteine and ultimately glutathione conjugates. Transport of glutathione-derived cysteine conjugates into kidney cells has been postulated for substrate supply of the microsomal N-acetyltransferase (Green and Elce, 1975), also providing potential substrates for the kidney cysteine conjugate β-lyase. However, the intracellular presence of these compounds in the liver has not been convincingly demonstrated. Involvement of hepatic cysteine conjugate β-lyase in methylthiol derivative production is also questioned by evidence showing the requirement for enterohepatic circulation (Bakke et al, 1980, 1981c) as well as intestinal microflora (Bakke et al., 1980, 1981c) for complete propachlor metabolism.

V. GLUTATHIONE STATUS IN ORGANS

In a recent review, the relationships between nutrition and toxicology were identified in three major categories: (1) the effect of nutritional status on the toxicity of drug and environmental chemicals (xenobiotics), (2) the additional nutritional demands that result from exposure to drugs and environmental chemicals, and (3) the presence of toxic substances in foods (Parke and Ioannides, 1981). Cellular detoxification processes often transform biologically inert molecules into chemically reactive intermediates. An optimal nutritional status is needed to maximize cellular protection against reactive intermediates. Such protection appears to be derived primarily from the maintenance of maximal intracellular concentration of glutathione. Therefore, in this section emphasis has been placed on the status of glutathione in organs as well as the formation and fate of glutathione conjugates.

The intracellular concentration of glutathione is maintained in the range of 0.5–10 mM, depending on the cell type (Kosower and Kosower, 1978). Nearly all of the glutathione is present as GSH, with less than 5% of the total present as GSSG, due to the thiol redox status maintained by intracellular glutathione reductase and NADPH. Continual endogenous production of reduced oxygen species, including hydrogen peroxide and lipid peroxide, creates a constant production of GSSG.

The GSH content in various organs and tissues represents at least 90% of the total nonprotein low-molecular-weight thiols present. Measurement of GSH depletion due to chemical intoxification is most conveniently conducted with Ellman's reagent, as illustrated in Table 1. Liver GSH content is nearly twice that found in kidney and testes and over threefold greater than in the lung. Intraperitoneal injection of 1,2-dibromoethane, an excellent substrate for glutathione-S-transferase activity, at doses up to and including twice the LD_{50} dose indicates the enormous protective role of liver GSH against chemical binding in other organs and tissues.

Table 1 Typical Experiment of Acute Depletion of Tissue Thiols by a Glutathione S-Transferase Substrate, 1,2-Dibromoethane

Dose (mg/kg body weight)	Thiols[a] (mg/g wet weight tissue) $\overline{X} \pm SD$			
	0	58	117	234
Liver	1.33 ± 0.14	0.97 ± 0.20 (72)[b]	0.50 ± 0.03 (38)	0.24 ± 0.08 (18)
Kidney	0.66 ± 0.03	0.61 ± 0.07 (92)	0.47 ± 0.05 (70)	0.33 ± 0.01 (50)
Testis	0.78 ± 0.01	0.78 ± 0.6 (100)	0.67 ± 0.02 (86)	0.58 ± 0.02 (75)
Lung	0.24 ± 0.02	0.24 ± 0.01 (100)	0.25 ± 0.01 (105)	0.18 ± 0.02 (73)

[a]Analysis by Ellman method (Ellman, 1959)
[b]Numbers in parentheses expressed as percent of control values.
Source: Unpublished data of P. Beatty and D. J. Reed, 1982.

New information about the status of glutathione in mammalian tissues continues to be reported. Boyd et al. (1979) found an exceedingly high concentration (up to 7—8 mM) of GSH in the glandular gastric tissue compared to those of the squamous portion of the stomach or other portions of the gastrointestinal tract. These workers speculated that the resistance of glandular stomach to certain carcinogens may be due in part to the high GSH content compared to the squamous portion, which is highly susceptible to polycyclic aromatic hydrocarbons.

A nutritional relationship between methionine and cystine was first reported as a sparing effect of cystine on the methionine requirement of the rat (Womack et al., 1937). Part of the dietary requirement for methionine can be replaced on a mole basis by cysteine. This observation is in agreement with the unidirectional process of transsulfuration, in which methionine sulfur and serine carbon are utilized in cysteine biosynthesis via the cystathionine pathway [for a review of this pathway, see Reed and Beatty (1980)].

The cystathionine pathway is of major importance to phase II reactions of drug metabolism that involve glutathione and/or cysteine. Rapid glutathione conjugate formation can cause GSH synthesis at rates up to 2—3 μmol/hr per gram of wet liver tissue (White, 1976). At such rates the liver cysteine pool, which is about 0.2 μmol/g, has a half-life of 2—3 min. While the cystathionine pathway is highly responsive to cellular need for cysteine, the mechanism(s) of control of the enzymes in this pathway remains poorly understood. Recent evidence indicates that the level of enzymic activities associated with this pathway may be less important than the regulation of cysteine degradation.

Liver cysteine content of rats has been shown to be controlled tightly even during dietary excess of either cystine or methionine. The maximum change in cysteine content is from 0.1 to 0.25 μmol/g wet tissue (Kohashi et al., 1978; Hosokawa et al., 1978). Utilization of excess dietary methionine or cystine does not result in great increases in cystathionine pathway enzymes (Stipanuk, 1979). The activity of cystathionine synthase is not rate limiting for methionine sulfur incorporation into cysteine under usual dietary conditions (Stipanuk and Benevenga, 1977).

In contrast, cysteine dioxygenase activity in vivo responded dramatically to the dietary level of cystine or methionine. Increasing the intake levels of these amino acids by feeding 2-40% protein diets increases the level of cysteine dioxygenase as much as 10- to 20-fold (Kohashi et al., 1978). The magnitude of effect of dietary methionine upon cystathionine pathway enzymes and cysteine dioxygenase may be influenced by many parameters, including diet composition and temporal effects (Stipanuk, 1979). For example, a diet containing 0.54% methionine when fed to rats resulted in ^{35}S derived from methionine being incorporated into proteins, glutathione, and taurine in preference to cysteine (Tateishi et al., 1981). Concomitantly, cysteine dioxygenase was induced to a maximum extent (M. Tateishi, private communication, 1982).

While the cystathionine pathway appears to be highly responsive to the need for cysteine biosynthesis in the liver, the organ distribution of the pathway may be quite limited. Evidence is emerging which indicates that in mammals, such as rats, liver may be the main site of cysteine biosynthesis which occurs via the cystathionine pathway. Maintenance of high glutathione content in liver in association with a very dynamic rate of secretion into plasma followed by extensive extracellular degradation of both GSH and GSSG supports the concept of liver glutathione being a physiological reservoir of cysteine. This concept, which was originally proposed by Tateishi et al. (1977) and Higashi et al. (1977), involves two glutathione pools, which are separate in that one has fast (2 hr) and another a slow (30 hr) turnover in the liver.

Meredith and Reed (1981) have observed with freshly isolated rat hepatocytes that the mitochondrial pool of glutathione, which is about 10% of the total cellular pool, has a half-life of 30 hr while the half-life of the cytoplasmic pool is 30 hr. They concluded that the mitochondrial pool may represent the stable pool of glutathione observed in whole animals.

Fasting and refeeding of rats led Cho et al. (1981) to the conclusion that liver and intestine glutathione serves as cyst(e)ine reservoirs during fasting. From their data they concluded, in agreement with Higashi et al. (1977), that two pools of glutathione exist in the liver.

Liver GSH content has been shown to be altered in rats by diurnal
or circadian variations, starvation, and chemical treatments including
certain metal ions. Diurnal variation of hepatic GSH content has been
shown to result in highest GSH levels at night and early morning and
lowest levels in the late afternoon, with maximum variation being as
much as 25–30% (Beck et al., 1958; Calcutt and Ting, 1969; Boyd et
al., 1979). Starvation of rats for 1 or 2 days decreases the level of
liver glutathione to between two-thirds and one-half of the normal level
(Leaf and Neuberger, 1947; Maruyama et al., 1968; Tateishi et al.,
1974).

Fasting has been shown to enhance the hepatoxicity of several chemicals. One of the earliest reports (Davis and Whipple, 1919) compared
fasting and various diets on chloroform hepatoxicity. Such increased
hepatotoxicity has been extended to carbon tetrachloride (Davis, 1924;
Campbell and Kosterlitz, 1948; Krishman and Stenger, 1966; McLean
and McLean, 1966; Highman et al., 1973; Diaz Gomez et al., 1975;
Strubelt et al., 1981), 1,1-dichloroethylene (Jaeger et al., 1974),
paraetamol (Pessayre et al., 1979,1980; Strubelt et al., 1981), bromobenzene (Pessayre et al., 1979,1980; Strubelt et al., 1981), and thioacetamide (Strubelt et al., 1981). Since fasting decreases liver GSH
content in mice (Strubelt et al., 1981) and rats (Maruyama et al., 1968;
Jaeger et al., 1974; Pessayre et al., 1979, 1980), such a decrease may
account for an enhanced toxicity of many of these chemicals. In several instances, workers have demonstrated enhanced toxicity by treatment with diethylmaleate. Such has been reported for paracetamol,
bromobenzene, carbon tetrachloride, and allyl alcohol (Mitchell et al.,
1973; Siegers et al., 1977). Interestingly, thioacetamide, a substrate
for microsomal monoamine oxidase (Vadi and Neal, 1981), has enhanced
hepatotoxicity with fasting (Strubelt et al., 1981) but not with diethyl
maleate (Siegers et al., 1977) treatment.

Alterations or the lack thereof of chemical hepatotoxicity by either
fasting or diethylmaleate treatment and (thus possibly related to GSH
content) now must be viewed from the standpoint of compartmentalization
of intracellular GSH. Meredith and Reed (1982) recently reported that
about 10–12% of GSH content of hepatocytes is a separate pool from the
pool of cytosol GSH. This pool is confined to the mitochondrial matrix
and is resistant to diethylmaleate depletion. Further, preliminary evidence suggests that chemical-induced lipid peroxidation in some instances may correlate better with depletion of mitochondrial GSH than
with cytosolic GSH (Meredith and Reed, 1982).

Since the mitochondrial pool of GSH has a half-life of about 30 hr
(Meredith and Reed, 1982), it is expected that fasting does not deplete
this GSH pool. Fasting did not increase the spontaneous or the carbon
tetrachloride-induced lipid peroxidation. Thus it is interesting to
speculate that lipid peroxidation events are closely related to the status
of the mitochondrial GSH pool in liver. Further, one can speculate that

certain proteins in the mitochondria may participate with GSH in the prevention of lipid peroxidation.

VI. INTERORGAN RELATIONSHIPS OF GLUTATHIONE

Apart from formation of glutathione conjugates, the initial step of liver GSH turnover appears to be efflux of GSH into blood plasma. Metabolism of plasma GSH is characterized by an extremely rapid extracellular hydrolysis which is catalyzed by γ-glutamyl transpeptidase [for a review of the interorgan metabolism of GSH, see McIntyre and Curthoys (1980)]. In humans, the turnover of plasma GSH is very rapid and the GSH half-life has been estimated as 1.6 min (Wendel and Cikryt, 1980). Both GSH and GSSG are rapidly metabolized, and liver efflux of total glutathione appears to be about 80—90% to the blood plasma and 10-20% to the bile (Reed et al., 1980b; Reed and Ellis, 1981,1982).

The rate of glutathione release from perfused rat liver into effluent perfusate has been estimated to be 0.3% of total glutathione per minute (Bartoli and Sies, 1978). According to this group, the total GSH content of the liver is 5.28 μmol/g (Sies et al., 1972).

The reason for a highly dynamic state of glutathione may be to ensure rapid degradation not only of GSH and GSSG, but also of glutathione conjugates and nonprotein mixed disulfides of glutathione. Further, rapid plasma turnover of GSH may occur in mammals to provide the cysteine needed to maintain intracellular GSH for cellular protection against chemical-mediated cellular damage. Certain cell types have an absolute requirement for cyst(e)ine for GSH biosynthesis (Brodie et al., 1981,1982). The cysteine released from extracellular degradation of plasma GSH derived from the liver not only is important to maintain plasma cysteine levels, but also a substantial fraction of the cysteine may return to the liver for GSH synthesis (Meredith and Reed, 1982). This process allows methionine sulfur to be utilized by the liver and in turn to be readily available to all cell types in the body as cysteine and/or cystine for maintenance of intracellular GSH content. In this regard, the liver may be unique among mammalian organs in its ability to utilize extensively the cystathionine pathway for the biosynthesis of L-cysteine from the carbon of serine and the sulfur of methionine (Figure 2) (Reed and Beatty, 1980;1978; Beatty and Reed, 1980,1981; Brodie et al., 1981; Moldeus et al., 1981; Meredith and Reed, 1982).

Several observations support a hypothesis of a highly dynamic relationship which may exist between the status of cysteine, cystine, and glutathione in the liver and the kidney. Efflux of GSH by the liver into the plasma compartment of adult rats occurs at a rate of about 10 μmol/hr (Reed and Ellis, 1982). Rapid degradation of GSH, GSSG, and

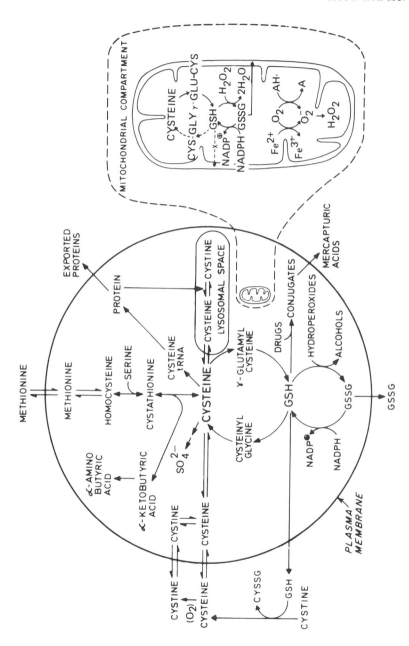

Figure 2 Interrelationships between sulfur-containing amino acids and glutathione in hepato-cytes.

CYSSG by the kidney and possibly by organs other than the liver is an extracellular process that results in cysteine and cystine formation [for a recent review, see Reed and Ellis, (1981)].

The high affinity of the kidney for glutathione in the plasma was first described in vivo by Binkley et al. (1951). Later, Fonteles et al. (1976) revealed that isolated rabbit kidney during perfusion became depleted of glutathione in the renal cortical and medullary regions unless GSH was added to the perfusate. Renal extraction of GSH was not only efficient but capable of extraction of large quantities of GSH.

The oxidation of cysteine to cystine in plasma, with cystine being the predominate form together with the mixed disulfide of cysteine and glutathione (CYSSG), requires that some organ be capable of efficient utilization of cystine. Isolated hepatocyte studies (Reed and Beatty, 1978) reveal that the liver is much more efficient in cysteine utilization than in cystine. Isolated kidney cell studies (Moldeus et al., 1981) provided evidence that the kidney may preferentially utilize cystine over cysteine for uptake and GSH biosynthesis. Further, these studies (Moldeus et al., 1981) demonstrate rapid formation of intracellular cysteine during cystine uptake. Interestingly, the rate of incorporation of ^{35}S into GSH did not correspond to the uptake of [^{35}S]-cystine, and [^{35}S]cysteine was observed to accumulate intracellularly and in a 95% O_2:5% CO_2 atmosphere, whereas CYSSG accumulated in the medium (Moldeus et al., 1981). Therefore, the evidence suggests that the kidney reduces cystine to cysteine by an intracellular process that can cause intracellular accumulation of cysteine. Preliminary evidence suggests efflux of cysteine into the medium (P. Moldeus and D. J. Reed, unpublished data, 1982). Glutathione oxidase activity, which is now shown to be a more general thiol oxidase, exists in kidney tissue and is capable of oxidizing GSH to GSSG and cysteine to cystine. However, this enzyme appears to have a very low affinity for thiol substrates (the K_m value for GSH is 2.2 mM), which suggests that only at high substrate concentration will appreciable conversion of thiol to disulfide occur with this enzyme (Ashkar et al., 1981).

Starvation, which limits the availability of methionine for GSH biosynthesis in the liver, causes the liver GSH content to decrease to about 50% of the level in fed animals (Beck et al., 1958; Jaeger et al., 1973; Lauterburg et al., 1980). Assuming that GSH is a physiological reservoir for plasma cysteine (Higashi et al., 1977), during starvation GSH efflux will continue to occur and the cysteine released will help maintain GSH levels in other organs, including the kidney. A decreased return of cysteine to the liver for GSH synthesis should also cause the liver GSH content to decrease during starvation.

A similar explanation can be made for the marked diurnal variation in liver glutathione concentration. The nadir occurs in the later afternoon, whereas the early morning peak is shortly after the animals normally feed (Beck et al., 1958; Jaeger et al., 1973; Lauterburg et al.,

1980). Efflux of liver GSH and metabolism of the resulting plasma GSH and GSSG appears to help ensure a continuous supply of plasma cysteine. This cysteine pool in turn should minimize the degree of fluctuation of GSH content within the various body organs and cell types that require only cysteine and/or cystine rather than methionine for GSH synthesis. It should be noted, however, that virtually nothing is known about the relationship of plasma GSH to the intracellular GSH status in many organ and cell types, including those of the reproductive system, lungs, and central nervous systems.

Total parenteral nutrition is not well established for the normal development of infants, particularly preterm patients (Driscoll et al., 1972; Anderson et al., 1979). During total parenteral nutrition of beagle pups, cerebral methionine and cystathionine concentrations increase but liver concentrations do not increase (Malloy et al., 1981). Because methionine is metabolized further than cystathionine in the liver, cyst(e)ine content is maintained, whereas cerebral cysteine concentration decreases. Parenterally administered methionine increases the cerebral concentration of methionine, possibly as a result of bypassing the modulating metabolic effects of the gastrointestinal tract and liver (Malloy et al., 1981).

VII. INTERORGAN RELATIONSHIPS OF GLUTATHIONE CONJUGATES

One of the most challenging aspects of the study of glutathione conjugation and metabolism is the role of such a pathway in the oxidative metabolism of hydrocarbons after phase I metabolism mediated by the cytochrome P-450 dependent monooxygenase system (Daly, 1971). Formation of epoxides presents phase II metabolic consequences that are highly dependent on the nutritional status of the metabolizing organism. For example, much remains to be understood about the distribution of metabolites that can result from the epoxide intermediates. The genetic consequences of "multiple-pass" metabolites, particularly those of polycyclic hydrocarbons, appear dependent on the consequences of sequential metabolic events occurring, for example, in the liver, bile, gut, blood, kidney, and possibly again the liver after enterohepatic circulation. The metabolic patterns depicted in Figure 3 only serve to convey the complexity of the combined functions of activation, conjugation, conjugation degradation, excretion, or reactivation of conjugate metabolites. Superimposed on this very general scheme are the stereospecificity and regioselectivity of the reaction of epoxides with GSH.

Unfortunately, the mercapturic acid pathway for xenobiotic metabolism has been investigated primarily as either an initial event catalyzed by GSH-S-transferases (generally liver with some interest in biliary secretion) or as a final step of glutathione conjugate hydrolysis and acetyla-

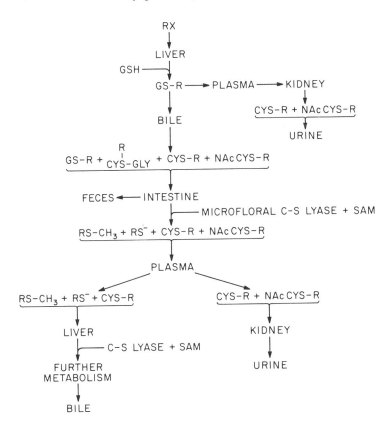

Figure 3 Possible routes of metabolism of glutathione conjugates.

tion to the final product in the kidney with subsequent urinary excretion. Recent studies by several workers, including Bakke et al.
(1980,1981a-c) and Horning et al. (1981a,b), show clearly the need for
a careful investigation of other routes of metabolism. Thus the identity and stability of premercapturate intermediates continue to be investigated and support the conclusion that a mercapturate is often an
artifact created by acidic isolation procedures (Horning et al.,
1981a,b). Possible routes of metabolism of glutathione conjugates are
shown in Figure 3.

The presence of γ-glutamyl transpeptidase activity in canalicular
plasma membrane (Rutenburg et al., 1969), plasma membrane of biliary
duct epithelial cells (Tanaka, 1974), and even bile itself (Rosalki,
1975) is in agreement with observed mercapturic acid pathway intermediates in bile collected from bile duct-cannulated animals.

The importance of gut microflora in the formation of metabolites of GSH conjugates is clearly indicated (Bakke et al., 1980,1981a-c). Such metabolic transformations have important health implications for polycyclic aromatic hydrocarbon metabolism, especially for those hydrocarbons capable of causing human cancers.

Knight and Young (1958) examined the metabolism of a series of hydrocarbons, including benzene, naphthalene, and anthracene, in rats and concluded that unacidified urine contained a mercapturic acid metabolite of each hydrocarbon. However, upon exposure of these intermediates to strong acid, mercapturic formation occurred. They speculated that mercapturic acid formation, when observed was an artifact. A similar suggestion was made by Chasseaud (1973a,b). Horning et al. (1981a,b) have confirmed this observation and shown that for naphthalene the premercapturic acid which is found in urine is a 1,2-dihydro-1-hydroxy-2-N-acetylcysteinylthiol ether. Upon acidification and elimination of water, the N-acetylcysteinylthiol moiety migrates from the 2-position to the 1-position (Horning et al., 1981a,b).

Recent evidence also supports the concept that polycyclic hydrocarbon metabolism results in the formation of dihydromercapturic acids with a hydroxy group in an adjacent ring position. Boyland and Sims (1958) proposed that such an intermediate, 1-naphthylpremercapturic acid, was formed during naphthalenes metabolism and could, during breakup, yield both 1- and 2-naphthol as well as 1-mercapturic acid.

Certain polycyclic hydrocarbons epoxides which are poor substrates for epoxide hydrolase have been examined by Horning et al. (1981a,b). Methylthio and mercaptoacetic derivatives were found to be far more common metabolites of epoxides than was previously thought. In addition, mercapturic acid metabolites in urine samples were largely artifactural, due to elimination of water from precursor metabolites by mild heating of the samples during acidification. Careful acidification permitted identification of the N-acetylcysteinylthiol ether dihydro ortho hydroxy derivatives with elimination of water to rearomatize the ring of such derivatives.

Glutathione conjugates appear to penetrate the hepatocyte with difficulty when delivered intravenously (D. J. Reed and W. W. Ellis, unpublished, 1982) or to the perfusion medium during isolated perfused liver studies (Steele et al., 1981).

Systemic metabolism of styrene oxide glutathione conjugates has been examined in isolated perfused rat lung, liver, and kidney and compared to metabolism in the intact rat. The lung had a minor role in metabolism, whereas metabolism of these conjugates in kidney was a rapid and almost exclusively an extracellular process, the major urinary product being the cysteine conjugate. Liver was the only organ examined that displayed a marked induction of conjugate metabolism by prior treatment of rats with phenobarbital. Untreated livers showed a slow production of styrene oxide cysteine (40% of dose in 2.5 hr), whereas phenobarbital-treated liver showed almost total conversion (90%) of

styrene oxide GSH conjugate to the cysteine conjugate within 30 min
(Steele et al., 1981). These results would be in agreement with the observation that phenobarbital treatment increases the γ-glutamyltrans-
ferase activity in rat liver (Whitfield et al., 1972; Kauffman et al.,
1980). In contrast to this observation, Kaplowitz et al. (1980) observed an increase in liver glutathione content after treatment of rats
with phenobarbital. They concluded that glutathione level underwent
a selective increase of that glutathione noncovalently bound to macromolecules, which may have been induced by phenobarbital.

Brombenzene-induced cytotoxicity is one of the best examples of cytochrome P-450-catalyzed formation of a reactive intermediate that can
be highly destructive to cellular integrity. As remarkable is the high
degree of efficiency of intracellular GSH as the principal protective
agent against such damage. The reactive intermediate, presumably
bromobenzene-3,4-epoxide (Jollow et al., 1974), may nonenzymically
be converted to the corresponding phenol form, trans-dihydrodiol, by
action of epoxide hydrolase, or react enzymically and nonenzymically
with GSH to form the corresponding conjugate.

The status of the cytochrome P-450 system and auxiliary enzymes is
of paramount importance to the degree of bromobenzene-induced cytotoxicity, because the rate of formation of the epoxide determines the
extent to which GSH protection is adequate during bromobenzene metabolism. As expected, the rate of GSH depletion and GSH synthesis is
critical in the steady-state processes of metabolic activation and GSH
detoxification. Sustained GSH protection requires de novo GSH synthesis, requiring the cysteine pool to be replaced every 2−3 min.

A new pathway for mercapturic acid formation has been described by
Doorn et al. (1980b) for o-xylene metabolism. Formation of the o-
methylbenzyl mercapturic acid and excretion into the urine occurred
following administration of o-xylene in the rat. In vitro studies demonstrated that a metabolite of o-xylene, rather than o-xylene, reacts
with GSH. This metabolite has been identified as o-methylbenzyl sulfate (Doorn et al., 1980b). Enzymic attack of the sulfate ester by GSH
leads to formation of the glutathione thiol ether and sulfate anion.
Far less of the corresponding mercapturic acids were formed with m-
or p-xylene (Doorn et al., 1980b).

Some evidence exists which suggests that humans may not convert
cysteine thiol ethers to the N-acetylated or mercapturic acid derivatives. Doorn et al. (1980a) observed S-methylcysteine in the urine of
workers exposed to methyl chloride at concentrations ranging up to
12 mM. Methylmercaptan was not detectable; the concentrations were
stated as being less than 1 µM. In contrast, Sklan and Barnsley
(1968) administered S-methyl-L-cysteine subcutaneously to black
hooded rats and observed no S-methyl-L-cysteine in the urine. Major
urinary products were inorganic sulfate, methylsulfonylacetate, 2-hy-
droxy-3-methylsulfonylpropionate, and N-acetyl-S-methyl-L-cysteine
S-oxide.

VIII. CONCLUSIONS

As the story unfolds on cytochrome P-450-dependent bioactivation of chemicals, the relationships to cellular protection by the main intracellular thiol, GSH, become more apparent. Both enzymatic and nonenzymatic reactions with reactive intermediates occur, leading to the formation of thiol ether conjugates of GSH. Acute chemical intoxification with certain chemicals can cause severe depletion of intracellular cytosolic GSH, and GSH replenishment fails to maintain normal protective levels of GSH. Lack of sufficient cysteine biosynthesis and dependence on extracellular cysteine and/or cystine is a major factor for all types of cells examined thus far except for hepatocytes. Hepatocytes have an enormous capacity to utilize the sulfur atom of methionine and the carbon atoms of serine to synthesize cysteine at a very rapid rate via the cystathionine pathway.

The unique feature of GSH formation in the liver is the evidence that the liver is an important organ for the maintenance of interorgan GSH and GSSG. Interorgan GSH and GSSG plus mixed disulfides of GSH represent an interorgan physiological reservoir for interorgan and presumably intracellular cysteine. Extracellular enzymatic degradation of GSH and related substances containing a γ-glutamyl moiety by the kidney is an essential component of the interorgan status of GSH, GSH conjugates, and cysteine.

A major metabolic pathway for GSH conjugates is their formation in the liver followed by excretion into bile. Enzymatic degradation of GSH conjugates starts in the bile duct and appears to be completed by intestinal cells and microflora, yielding both cysteine conjugates and thiols after cysteine conjugates are further degraded by microflora C-S lyase activity. Thiols of the parent chemicals can undergo either glucuronidation or methylation, with the methyl thiol ethers undergoing oxidation to sulfonyl derivatives. Enterohepatic circulation can return these metabolites to the plasma for further metabolism, such as acetylation in the kidney and excretion. In addition, some of these metabolites are returned to the liver for "second-pass" metabolism. The consequences of further metabolism is of importance relative to chemicals such as the carcinogenic polycyclic aromatic hydrocarbons, and possibly those chemicals capable of causing chemical hepatitis. Nutrition influences may be expressed not only in the status of cytochrome P-450 enzymes but also in the status of intracellular glutathione and glutathione-related enzyme, and even with regard to the nature of the intestinal microflora.

ACKNOWLEDGMENTS

This chapter was aided by grants from the NIEHS (ES-01978) and the American Cancer Society (CH-109).

REFERENCES

Akerboom, T. P. M., and Sies, H. (1981). *Methods Enzymol. 77:* 373.

Albert, Z., Orlowski, M., and Szewczuk, A. (1961). *Nature 191:* 767.

Albert, Z., Orlowski, J., Orlowski, M., and Szewczuk, A. (1964). *Acta Histochem. 18:*78.

Allen, C. M., Hockin, L. J., and Paine, A. J. (1981). *Biochem. Pharmacol. 30:*2739.

Allen, L., Meck, R., and Yunis, A. (1980). *Res. Commun. Chem. Pathol. Pharmacol. 27:*175.

Anders, M. W. (1978). *Biochem. Pharmacol. 27:*1098.

Anderson, M. E., Allison, R. D., and Meister, A. (1982). *Proc. Natl. Acad. Sci. USA 79:*1088.

Anderson, M. E., Bridges, R. J., and Meister, A. (1980). *Biochem. Biophys. Res. Commun. 96:*848.

Anderson, T. L., Muttart, C., Bieber, M. A., Nicholson, J. F., and Heird, W. C. (1979). *J. Pediatr. 94:*951.

Arias, I. M., Fleishner, G., Kirsch, R., Mishkin, S., and Gatmaitan, S. (1976). In *Glutathione: Metabolism and Function,* W. B. Jakoby, Ed., Raven Press, New York, p. 175.

Ashkar, S., Binkley, F., and Jones, D. P. (1981). *FEBS Lett. 124:*166.

Babson, J. R., Abell, N. S., and Reed, D. J. (1981). *Biochem. Pharmacol. 30:*2299.

Babson, J. R., and Reed, D. J. (1978). *Biochem. Biophys. Res. Commun. 83:*754.

Bakke, J. E., Feil, V. J., and Price, C. E. (1976). *Biomed. Mass Spectrom. 3:*226.

Bakke, J. E., and Price, C. E. (1979). *J. Environ. Sci. Health B14:*427.

Bakke, J. E., Gustafsson, J.-A., and Gustafsson, B. E. (1980). *Science 210:*433.

Bakke, J. E., Rafter, J., Larsen, G. L., Gustafsson, J. A., and Gustafsson, B. E. (1981a). *Drug Metab. Dispos. 9:*525.

Bakke, J. E., Aschbacher, P. W., Feil, V. J., and Gustafsson, B. E. (1981b). *Xenobiotica 11:*173.

Bakke, J. E., Larsen, G. L., Aschbacher, P. W., Rafter, J., Gustafsson, J. A., and Gustafsson, B. E. (1981c). In *Sulfur In Pesticide Action and Metabolism,* J. D. Rosen, P. S. Magee, and J. E. Casida, Eds., ACS Symposium Series 158, American Chemical Society, Washington, D. C., p. 165.

Bakke, J. E., Rafter, J., Lindeskog, P., Feil, V. J., Gustafsson, J.-A., and Gustafsson, B. E. (1981d). *Biochem. Pharmacol. 30:*1839.

Bartoli, G. M., and Sies, H. (1978). *FEBS Lett.* 86:89.

Bass, N. M., Kirsh, R. E., Tuff, S. A., and Saunders, S. J. (1977). *Biochim. Biophys. Acta* 494:131.

Beatty, P., and Reed, D. J. (1980). *Arch. Biochem. Biophys.* 204:80.

Beatty, P., and Reed, D. J. (1981). *Biochem. Pharmacol.* 30:1227.

Beck, L. V., Riecls, V. D., and Duncan, B. (1958). *Proc. Soc. Exp. Biol. Med.* 97:229.

Bend, J., and Fouts, J. R. (1973). *Bull. Mt. Desert Isl. Lab.* 13:4.

Benson, A. M., Batzinger, R. P., Ou, S.-Y. L., Beuding, E., Cha, Y.-N., and Talahay, P. (1978). *Cancer Res.* 38:4486.

Berry, M. N., and Friend, D. S. (1969). *J. Cell. Biol.* 43:506.

Beutler, E. (1980). In *Red Cell and Lens Metabolism,* S. S. Srivastava, Ed., Elsevier /North-Holland, Amsterdam, p. 71.

Beutler, E., and West, C. (1977). *Anal. Biochem.* 81:461.

Binkley, F. (1961). *J. Biol. Chem.* 236:1075.

Binkley, F., Christiansen, G. M., and Wu, F. (1951). *J. Biol. Chem.* 192:29.

Board, P. G., and Smith, J. E. (1975). *Blood* 49:667.

Booth, A. G., and Kenny, A. J. (1976). *Biochem. J.* 153:5.

Boyd, S. C., Sesame, H. A., and Boyd, M. R. (1979). *Science* 205:1010.

Boyland, E., and Chausseaud, L. F. (1969). *Adv. Enzymol.* 32:173.

Boyland, E., and Chasseaud, L. F. (1970). *Biochem. Pharmacol.* 19:1526.

Boyland, E., and Sims, P. (1958). *Biochem. J.* 68:440.

Brodie, A., Potter, J., Ellis, W. W., Evenson, M. C., and Reed, D. J. (1981). *Biochem. Biophys.* 210:437.

Brodie, A., Potter, J., and Reed, D. J. (1982). *Eur. J. Biochem.,* 123:159.

Burk, R. F., and Correia, M. A. (1979). *Res. Commun. Chem. Pathol. Pharmacol.* 24:205.

Cagen, L. M., Fales, H. M., and Pisano, J. J. (1976). *J. Biol. Chem.* 251:6550.

Calcutt, G., and Ting, M. (1969). *Naturwissenschaften* 56:419.

Calder, I. C., Creek, M. J., and Williams, P. J. (1974). *Chem.-Biol. Interact.* 8:87.

Campbell, R., and Kosterlitz, H. (1948). *Br. J. Exp. Pathol.* 29:149.

Cha, Y.-N., Marty, F., and Beuding, E. (1978). *Cancer Res.* 38:4496.

Chapman, G. S., Jones, A. C., Meyer, U. A., and Montgomery-Bissell, D. (1973). *J. Cell. Biol.* 59:735.

Chasseaud, L. F. (1973a). *Drug Metab. Rev.* 2:185.

Chasseaud, L. F. (1973b). *Biochem. J.* 131:765.

Chasseaud, L. F. (1979). *Adv. Cancer Res.* 29:175.

Chatfield, D. H., and Hunter, W. H. (1973). *Biochem. J. 134*:879.

Chaung, A. H. L., Mukhtar, H., Bresnick, G. (1978). *J. Natl. Cancer Inst. 60*:321.

Cho, E. S., Sahyoun, N., and Stegink, L. D. (1981). *J. Nutr. 111*:914.

Clark, A. G., Smith, J. N., and Speir, T. W. (1973). *Biochem. J. 135*:385.

Cohn, V. H., and Lyle, J. (1966). *Anal. Biochem. 14*:434.

Coleman, R. (1973). *Biochim. Biophys. Acta 300*:1.

Coleman, R., and Finean, J. B. (1966). *Biochim. Biophys. Acta 125*:197.

Cooney, D. S., Jayaram, H. N., Ryan, J. A., and Bono, V. H. (1974). *Cancer Chemother. Rep. 58*:793.

Crane, R. K., and Mandelstam, P. (1960). *Biochim. Biophys. Acta 45*:460.

Daly, J. W. (1971). In *Handbook of Experimental Pharmacology: Concepts in Biochemical Pharmacology,* B. B. Brodie and J. R. Gillette, Eds., Springer-Verlag, New York, p. 285.

Daniel, V., Smith, G. J., and Litwak, G. (1977). *Proc. Natl. Acad. Sci. USA 74*:1899.

Das, M., and Radhakrishnan, H. N. (1972). *Biochem. J. 128*:463.

Das, M., and Radhakrishnan, H. N. (1973). *Biochem. J. 195*:609.

Dauterman, W. C. (1980). In *Introduction to Biochemical Toxicology.* E. Hodgson and F. E. Guthrie, Eds., Elsevier, New York, p. 101.

Davis, N., and Whipple, C. (1919). *Arch. Intern. Med. 23*:612.

Davis, N. C. (1924). *J. Med. Res. 44*:601.

DeLange, R. J., and Smith, E. L. (1971). In *The Enzymes,* 3rd ed., Vol. 3, P. D. Boyer, Ed., Academic Press, New York, p. 82.

Delap, L. W. Tate, S. S., and Meister, A. (1976). *Life Sci. 20*:673.

Diaz Gomez, M. I., DeCastro, C. R., DeFerreyra, E. C., D'Acosta, N., DeFenos, O. M., and Castro, J. A. (1975). *Toxicol. Appl. Pharmacol. 32*:101.

Dimant, E., Landberg, E., and London, I. M. (1955). *J. Biol. Chem. 213*:769.

Doorn, R. V., Borm, P. J. A., Leijdekkers, C. M., Henderson, P. T., Reuvers, J., and Van Bergen, T. J. (1980a). *Int. Arch. Occup. Environ. Health 46*:99.

Doorn, R. V., Bos, R. P., Brouns, R. M. E., Leijdekkers, C. M., and Henderson, P. T. (1980b). *Arch. Toxicol. 43*:293.

Driscoll, J. M., Jr., Heird, W. C., Schullinger, J. N., Gongaware, R. D., and Winters, R. W. (1972). *J. Pediatr. 81*:145.

Elce, J. S., and Broxmeyer, B. (1976). *Biochem. J. 153*:223.

Ellman, G. L. (1959). *Arch. Biochem. Biophys. 82*:70.

Eluyn, D. H., Parikh, H. C., and Shoemaker, W. C. (1968). *Am. J. Physiol. 215*:1260.

Emmelot, P., and Visser, A. (1971). *Biochim. Biophys. Acta 241*: 273.

Fahey, R. C., Newton, G. L., Dorian, R., and Kosower, E. M. (1980). *Anal. Biochem. 107*:1.

Fahey, R. C., Newton, G. L., Dorian, R., and Kosower, E. M. (1981). *Anal. Biochem. 111*:357.

Fisher, R. B., and Parsons, D. S. (1953). *J. Physiol. 119*:210.

Fleishner, G., Kamisaka, K., and Arias, I. M. (1976). In *Glutathione: Metabolism and Function*, I. M. Arias and W. B. Jakoby, Eds., Raven Press, New York, p. 259.

Focella, A., Heslin, P., and Teitel, S. (1972). *Can. J. Chem. 50*: 2025.

Fonteles, M. C., Pillion, D. J., Jeske, A. H., and Leibach, F. H. (1976). *J. Surg. Res. 21*:169.

Frear, D. S., and Swanson, H. R. (1970). *Phytochemistry 9*:2123.

Goldberg, J. A., Freedman, O. M., Peneda, E. P., Smith, E. E., Chatterji, R., Stein, E. H., and Rutenburg, A. M. (1960). *Arch. Biochem. Biophys. 91*:61.

Grafström, R., Ormstad, K., Moldeus, P., and Orrenius, S. (1979). *Biochem. Pharmacol. 28*:3573.

Grafström, R., Stead, A. H., and Orrenius, S. (1980). *Eur. J. Biochem. 106*:571.

Green, R. M., and Elce, J. S. (1975). *Biochem. J. 197*:238.

Greenberg, E., Walloeger, E. E., Fleishner, G. A., and Engström, G. W. (1967). *Clin. Chem. Acta 16*:79.

Griffith, O. W. (1980). *Anal. Biochem. 106*:207.

Griffith, O. W. (1981). *J. Biol. Chem. 256*:4900.

Griffith, O. W., and Meister, A. (1979a). *Proc. Natl. Acad. Sci., USA 76*:268.

Griffith, O. W., and Meister, A. (1979b). *Proc. Natl. Acad. Sci., USA 76*:5606.

Griffith, O. W., and Meister, A. (1980). *Proc. Natl. Acad. Sci., USA 77*:3384.

Griffith, O. W., and Tate, S. S. (1980). *J. Biol. Chem. 255*:5011.

Griffith, O. W., Bridges, R. J., and Meister, A. (1979). *Proc. Natl. Acad. Sci. USA 76*:6319.

Gronow, M., and Todd, P. (1969). *Anal. Biochem. 28*:450.

Grover, P. C., and Sims, P. (1964). *Biochem. J. 90*:603.

Habig, W. H., Pabst, M. J., Fleishner, G., Gatmaitan, F., Arias, I. M., and Jakoby, W. B. (1974a). *Proc. Natl. Acad. Sci. USA 71*:3879.

Habig, W. H., Pabst, M. J., and Jakoby, W. B. (1974b). *J. Biol. Chem. 249*:7130.

Habig, W. H., Pabst, M. J., and Jakoby, W. B. (1976). *Arch. Biochem. Biophys. 175:*710.

Hanka, L. J., and Dietz, A. (1973). *Antimicrob. Agents Chemother. 3:*425.

Heinle, H., Sawatzhi, G., and Wendel, A. (1976). *Hoppe-Seyler's Z. Physiol. Chem. 357:*1451.

Hernandez, O., Walker, M., Cox, R. H., Foureman, G. L., Bend, J. R., and Smith, B. R. (1980a). *Biochem. Biophys. Res. Commun. 96:*1494.

Hernandez, O., Yagen, B., Cox, R. H., Bend, J. R., and McKinney, J. D. (1982). *J. Liq. Chromatogr., in press.*

Higashi, T., Tateishi, N., Naruse, A., and Sakamoto, Y. (1977). *J. Biochem. 82:*117.

Highman, B., Cyr, W. H., and Streett, R. P., Jr. (1973). *Radiat. Res. 54:*444.

Hissin, P. J., and Hilf, R. (1976). *Anal. Biochem. 74:*214.

Hoench, H., Woo, C. H., and Schmid, R. (1975). *Biochem. Biophys. Res. Commun. 65:*399.

Högberg, J., and Kristoferson, A. (1977). *Eur. J. Biochem. 74:* 77.

Högberg, J., and Kristoferson, A. (1978). *Acta Pharmacol. Toxicol. 42:*271.

Högberg, J., Orrenius, S., and Larson, R. (1975). *Eur. J. Biochem. 50:*595.

Horejsi, T., and Micevova, J. (1964). *Acta Biochem. Pol. 11:*107.

Horiuchi, S., Inoue, M., and Morino, Y. (1978). *Eur. J. Biochem. 78:*609.

Horning, M. G., Nakatsu, K., Lertrataninkoon, K., Halpaap-Wood, K., and Stillwell, W. G. (1981a). *Toxicologist 1:*142.

Horning, M. G., Hugenroth, S., and Lertrataninkoon, K. (1981b). *Pharmacologist 23:*211.

Hosokawa, Y., Yamaguchi, K., Kohashi, N., Kori, Y., and Ueda, I. (1978). *J. Biochem. 84:*419.

Howard, R. B., Christensen, A. K., Gibbs, F. A., and Pesch, L. A. (1967). *J. Cell Biol. 35:*676.

Howie, D., Adriaenssens, P. I., and Prescott, L. F. (1977). *J. Pharm. Pharmacol. 29:*235.

Hughey, R. P., and Curthoys, N. P. (1976). *J. Biol. Chem. 257:* 7863.

Hughey, R. P., Rankin, B. B., Elce, J. S., and Curthoys, N. P. (1977). *Arch. Biochem. Biophys. 186:*212.

Hughey, R. P., Coyle, P. J., and Curthoys, N. P. (1979). *J. Biol. Chem. 254:*1124.

Jackson, R. C., (1969). *Biochem. J. 111:*309.

Jacob, S. T., and Bhavova, P. M. (1962). *Exp. Cell. Res. 27:* 453.

Jaeger, R. J., Connolly, R. B., and Murphy, S. D. (1973). *Res. Commun. Chem. Pathol. Pharmacol.* 6:465.

Jaeger, R. J., Connolly, R. B., and Murphy, S. D. (1974). *Exp. Mol. Pathol.* 20:187.

Jakoby, W. B. (1978). *Adv. Enzymol.* 46:383.

Jakoby, W. B., and Habig, W. H. (1980). In *Enzymatic Basis of Detoxification*, Vol. 2, Academic Press, New York, p. 63.

Jakoby, W. B., and Keen, J. H. (1977). *Trends Biochem. Sci.* 2:229.

Jakoby, W. B., Ketley, J. N., and Habig, W. H. (1976). In *Glutathione: Metabolism and Function*, I. M. Arias and W. B. Jakoby, Eds., Raven Press, New York.

Jayaram, H. N., Corney, D. A., Ryan, J. A., Neil, G., Dion, R. L., and Bono, V. (1975). *Cancer Chemother. Rep.* 59:481.

Jollow, D. J., Mitchell, J. R., Zampaglione, N., and Gillette, J. R. (1974). *Pharmacology* 11:151.

Jones, D. P., and Mason, H. S. (1978). *J. Biol. Chem.* 253:4874.

Jones, D. P., Thor, H., Andersson, B., and Orrenius, S. (1978). *J. Biol. Chem.* 253:6031.

Jungerman, K., and Sasse, D. (1978). *Trends Biochem. Sci.* 3: 198.

Kamisaka, K., Habig, W. H., Ketley, J. N., Arias, I. M., and Jakoby, W. B. (1975). *Eur. J. Biochem.* 60:153.

Kaplowitz, N., Kuhlenkamp, J., Goldstein, L., and Reeve, J. (1980). *J. Pharmacol. Exp. Ther.* 212:240.

Kauffman, F. C., Evans, R. K., Reinke, L. A., and Thurman, R. G. (1980). Abstracts, *19th Annu. Meet. Soc. Toxicol.*, Mar.

Kenny, A. J., (1977). In *Proteinases in Mammalian Cells and Tissues*, A. J. Barrett, Ed., Elsevier, New York, p. 393.

Kenny, A. J., Booth, A. G., George, S. G., Ingram, J., Kershaw, D., Wood, E. J., and Young, A. R. (1976). *Biochem. J.* 157: 169.

Kerr, M. A., and Kenny, A. J. (1973). *Biochem. J.* 137:477.

Kilra, V., Sikka, S. C., and Sethi, G. (1981). *J. Biol. Chem.* 256:5567.

Kim, Y. S., and Brophy, E. J. (1976). *J. Biol. Chem.* 251:3199.

Kim, Y. S., Bartwhistle, W., and Sethi, G. (1972). *J. Clin. Invest.* 51:1419.

Kim, Y. S., Brophy, E. J., and Nicholson, J. A. (1976). *J. Biol. Chem.* 251:3206.

Kimmich, G. A. (1970). *Biochemistry* 9:3659.

Knight, R. H., and Young, L. (1958). *Biochem. J.* 70:111.

Knox, J. H., and Jurand, J. (1978). *J. Chromatogr.* 149:297.

Kohashi, N., Yamaguchi, K., Hosokawa, Y., Kori, Y., Fujii, O., and Ueda, I. (1978). *J. Biochem.* 84:159.

Kosower, N. S., and Kosower, E. M. (1978). *Int. Rev. Cytol.* 54: 109.

Kozak, E. M., and Tate, S. S. (1982). *J. Biol. Chem.* 257:6322-6327.

Krishman, N., and Stenger, R. J. (1966). *Am. J. Pathol.* 49: 239.

Lamoureux, G. L., and Davison, K. L. (1975). *Pest. Biochem. Physiol.* 5:497.

Lamoureux, G. L., Stafford, L. E., Shimabukuro, R. H., and Zaylishie, R. G. (1973). *J. Agric. Food. Chem.* 21:1020.

Larsen, G. L., and Bakke, J. E. (1979). *J. Environ. Sci. Health* B14:495.

Lauterburg, B. H., Vaishnov, Y., Stillwell, W. G., and Mitchell, J. R. (1980). *J. Pharmacol. Exp. Ther.* 213:54.

Lay, M. M., and Casida, J. E. (1976). *Pestic. Biochem. Physiol.* 6:442.

Leaf, G., and Neuberger, A. (1947). *Biochem. J.* 41:280.

Lotlikar, P. D., Scribner, J. D., Miller, J. A., and Miller, C C. (1966). *Life Sci.* 5:1263.

Lunn, G., Dale, G. L., and Beutler, E. (1979). *Blood* 54:238.

Malloy, M. H., Rassin, D. K., Heird, W. C., and Gaull, G. E. (1981). *Am. J. Clin. Nutr.* 34:1520.

Marathe, G. V., Nash, G., Naschemeyer, R. H., and Tate, S. S. (1979). *FEBS Lett.* 107:436.

Marcus, C. J., Habig, W. H., and Jakoby, W. B. (1978). *Arch. Biochem. Biophys.* 188:287.

Maroux, S., Lauvard, D., and Baratti, J. (1973). *Biochim. Biophys. Acta* 321:282.

Maruyama, E., Kojuma, J., Higashi, T., and Sakamoto, Y. (1968). *J. Biochem.* 63:398.

Mathews, H. B. (1980). In *Introduction to Biochemical Toxicology,* E. Hodgson and F. E. Guthrie, Eds., Elsevier, New York, p. 167.

McDonald, J. K., and Schwabe, C. (1977). In *Proteinases in Mammalian Cells and Tissue,* R. J. Barret, Ed., American Elsevier, New York, p. 393.

McIntyre, T. M., and Curthoys, N. P. (1979). *J. Biol. Chem.* 254:6499.

McIntyre, T. M., and Curthoys, N. P. (1980). *Int. J. Biochem.* 12:545.

McLean, A. E. M., and McLean, E. K. (1966). *Biochem. J.* 100:564.

Meister, A. (1973). *Science* 180:33.

Meister, A. (1978). In *Functions of Glutathione in Liver and Kidney,* H. Sies and A. Wendel, Eds., Springer-Verlag, New York.

Meister, A., and Tate, S. S. (1976). *Annu. Rev. Biochem.* 45: 559.

Meister, A., Tate, S. S., and Ross, L. L. (1976). In *The En-zymes of Biological Membranes*, Vol. 3, A. Martenosi, Ed., Plenum Press, New York, p. 315.

Meredith, M. J., and Reed, D. J. (1981). *Toxicol. Appl. Pharma-col., in press.*

Meredith, M. J., and Reed, D. J. (1982). *J. Biol. Chem.* 257:3747.

Michelakis, A. M. (1975). *Methods Enzymol.* 39:20.

Midelfort, C. F., and Mehler, A. H. (1972). *Proc. Natl. Acad. Sci. USA* 69:1816.

Minnich, V., Smith, M. B., Brauner, M. G., and Majerus, P. W. (1971). *J. Clin. Invest.* 50:507.

Mitchell, J. R., Jollow, D. J., Potter, W. Z., Gillette, J. R., and Brodie, B. B. (1973) *J. Pharmacol. Exp. Ther.* 187:185-194.

Moldeus, P., Högberg, J., and Orrenius, S. (1978a). *Methods Enzymol.* 52:60.

Moldeus, P., Jones, D. P., Ormstad, K., and Orrenius, S. (1978b). *Biochem. Biophys. Res. Commun.* 83:195.

Moldeus, P., Ormstad, K., Reed, D. J. (1981). *Eur. J. Biochem.* 116:13.

Motoyama, N., Kulkarni, A. P., Hodgson, E., and Dauterman, W. C. (1978). *Pestic. Biochem. Physiol.* 9:255.

Nachlas, M. M., Manis, B., Rosenblatt, D., and Seligman, A. M. (1960). *J. Biophys. Biochem. Cytol.* 7:261.

Oppenoorth, F. J., Van der Pas, L. J. T., and Haux, N. W. H. (1979). *Pestic. Biochem. Physiol.* 11:176.

Ormstad, K., Jones, D. P., and Orrenius, S. (1980). *J. Biol. Chem.* 255:175.

Örning, L., Hammarström, J., and Samuelsson, B. (1980). *Proc. Natl. Acad. Sci. USA* 77:2014.

Paine, A. J., and Hockin, L. (1980). *Biochem. Pharmacol.* 29:3215.

Paine, A. J., and Legg, R. F. (1978). *Biochem. Biophys. Res. Commun.* 81:672.

Parke, D. V., and Ioannides, C. (1981). *Annu. Rev. Nutr.* 1: 207.

Pelchar, A. G., Tate, S. S., and Meister, A. (1974). *Proc. Natl. Acad. Sci. USA* 71:293.

Perris, A. D. (1966). *Can. J. Biochem.* 44:687.

Perry, T. L., and Hansen, S. (1981). *Clin. Chim. Acta* 117:7.

Pessayre, D., Dolder, A., Artigou, J.-Y., Wandscheer, J.-C., Descatoire, V., Degott, C., and Benhamou, J. P. (1979). *Gastroenterology* 77:264.

Pessayre, D., Wandscheer, J.-C., Cobert, B., Level, R., Degott, C., Batt, A. M., Martin, N., and Benhamou, J. P. (1980). *Biochem. Pharmacol.* 29:2219.

Pinkus, L. M., Kelley, J. N., and Jakoby, W. B. (1977). *Biochem. Pharmacol.* 26:2359.

Plummer, J. L., Smith, B. R., Sies, H., and Bend, J. R. (1981). *Methods Enzymol.* 77:50.

Prchal, J., Srivastava, S. K., and Beutler, E. (1975). *Blood 46:* 111.

Prusiner, S., and Stadtman, E. R., Eds. (1973). *The Enzymes of Glutamine Metabolism,* Academic Press, New York, p. 605.

Rankin, B. B., McIntyre, T. M., and Curthoys, N. P. (1980). *Biochem. Biophys. Res. Commun.* 96:991.

Rappaport, C., and Howze, G. B. (1966). *Proc. Soc. Exp. Biol. Med.* 121:1010.

Rasmussen, H. (1975). *Methods Enzymol.* 39:11.

Rathbun, W. B. (1980). In *Glutathione in the Lens and Erythrocyte,* S. S. Srivastava, Ed., Elsevier/North Holland, Amsterdam, p. 169.

Reed, D. J., and Beatty, P. W. (1978). In *Functions of Glutathione in Liver and Kidney,* H. Sies and A. Wendel, Eds., Springer-Verlag, Berlin, p. 13.

Reed, D. J., and Beatty, P. W. (1980). In *Reviews in Biochemical Toxicology,* E. Hodgson, J. R. Bend, and R. M. Philpot, Eds., Vol. 2, Elsevier, New York, p. 213.

Reed, D. J., and Ellis, W. W. (1981). *Pharmacologist* 23:167.

Reed, D. J., and Ellis, W. W. (1982). In *Biological Reactive Intermediates 2,* Part A, R. Synder, D. V. Parke, J. J. Kocsis, and D. J. Jollow, Eds., Plenum Press, New York, p. 75.

Reed, D. J., and Orrenius, S. (1977). *Biochem. Biophys. Res. Commun.* 77:1257.

Reed, D. J., Babson, J. R., Beatty, P. W., Brodie, A. E., Ellis, W. W., and Potter, D. W. (1980a). *Anal. Biochem.* 106:55.

Reed, D. J., Ellis, W. W., and Meck, R. A. (1980b). *Biochem. Biophys. Res. Commun.* 94:1273.

Revel, J. P., and Ball, E. G. (1959). *J. Biol. Chem.* 234:577.

Richardson, R. J., and Murphy, S. D. (1975). *Toxicol. Appl. Pharmacol.* 31:505.

Rollins, D., Von Bahr, C., Glaumann, H., Moldeus, P., and Rane, A. (1979). *Science* 205:1414.

Rollins, D., Larsson, A., Steen, B., Krishnaswamy, K., Hagenfeldt, L., Moldeus, P., and Rane, A. (1981). *J. Pharmacol. Exp. Ther.* 217:697.

Rosalki, S. B. (1975). *Adv. Clin. Chem.* 17:53.

Rutenburg, A. M., Kim, H., Fischbein, J. W., Hanker, J. S., Wasserkrug, H. L., and Seligman, A. M. (1969). *J. Histochem. Cytochem.* 17:517.

Saville, B. (1958). *Analyst* 83:670.

Seglen, P. O. (1973). *Exp. Cell Res.* 82:391.

Seligman, A. M. (1969). *J. Histochem. Cytochem.* 17:517.

Shaw, L. M. (1978). In *Evaluation of Liver Function; A Multi-*

faceted Approach to Clinical Diagnosis, L. Demers and L. M. Shaw, Eds., Urban & Schwarzenberg, Baltimore.

Shaw, L. M., and Newman, D. A. (1979). *Clin. Chem. 25:75.*

Shimabukuro, R. H., Swanson, H. R., and Walsh, W. C. (1970). *Plant. Physiol. 46:103.*

Shimabukuro, R. H., Frear, H. R., Swanson, H. R., and Walsh, W. C. (1971). *Plant Physiol. 47:10.*

Shishido, T., Usui, K., Sato, M., and Fukami, J.-I. (1972). *Pestic. Biochem. Physiol. 2:51.*

Siegers, C.-P., Schütt, A., and Strubelt, O. (1977). *Proc. Eur. Soc. Toxicol. 18:160.*

Sies, H., Gerstenecker, C., Menzel, H., and Flohe, L. (1972). *FEBS Lett. 27:171.*

Sirica, A. E., and Pitot, H. C. (1980). *Pharmacol. Rev. 31:205.*

Sklan, N. M., and Barnsley, E. A. (1968). *Biochem. J. 107:217.*

Smith, J. E. (1974). *J. Lab. Clin. Med. 83:444.*

Smith, G. L., Sapico-Ohl, V., and Litwach, G. (1977). *Cancer Res. 37:8.*

Smith, J. E., Moore, K., and Board, P. G. (1980). *Enzyme 25:* 236.

Srivastava, S. K., and Beutler, E. (1968). *Lancet 2:23.*

Srivastava, S. K., and Beutler, E. (1969). *Biochem. J. 114:833.*

Steele, J. W., Yagen, B., Hernandez, O., Cox, R. H., Smith, B. R., and Bend, J. R. (1981). *J. Pharmacol. Exp. Ther. 219:35.*

Stern, B. K. (1966). *Gastroenterology 51:855.*

Stern, B. K., and Jensen, W. E. (1966). *Nature 209:789.*

Stern, B. K., and Reilly, R. W. (1965). *Nature 205:563.*

Stetson, P. (1975). *Fed. Proc. Fed. Am. Soc. Exp. Biol. 34:557.*

Stipanuk, M. H. (1979). *J. Nutr. 109:2126.*

Stipanuk, M. H., and Benevenga, N. J. (1977). *J. Nutr. 107:* 1455.

Stohs, S. J., Grafstrom, R. C., Burke, M. D., and Orrenius, S. (1976). *Arch. Biochem. Biophys. 179:71.*

Strubelt, O., Dost-Kempf, E., Siegers, C. -P., Younes, M., Völpel, M., Preuss, U., and Dreckmann, J. G. (1981). *Toxicol. Appl. Pharmacol. 60:66.*

Suga, T., Kumaoha, H., and Akagi, M. (1966). *J. Biochem. 60:* 133.

Tager, J. M., Söling, H. D., and Williamson, J. R., Eds. (1976). *The Use of Isolated Liver Cells and Kidney Tubules in Metabolic Studies,* North-Holland, Amsterdam.

Tanaka, M. (1974). *Acta Pathol. Jap. 24:651.*

Tate, S. S. (1975). *FEBS Lett. 54:319.*

Tate, S. S. (1980). In *Enzymatic Basis of Detoxification,* Vol. 2, W. B. Jakoby, Ed., Academic Press, New York, p. 95.

Tate, S. S., and Meister, A. (1974). *J. Biol. Chem.* 249:7593.
Tate, S. S., and Meister, A. (1975). *J. Biol. Chem.* 250:4619.
Tate, S. S., and Meister, A. (1978). *Proc. Natl. Acad. Sci. USA* 75:4806.
Tate, S. S., and Orlando, J. (1979). *J. Biol. Chem.* 254:5573.
Tate, S. S., Grau, E. M., and Meister, A. (1979). *Proc. Natl. Acad. Sci. USA* 76:2715.
Tateishi, N., and Shimizu, H. (1980). In *Enzymatic Basis of Detoxification*, Vol. 2, W. B. Jakoby, Ed., Academic Press, New York, p. 121.
Tateishi, N., Higashi, T., Shinya, S., Naruse, A., and Sakamoto, Y. (1974). *J. Biochem.* 75:93.
Tateishi, N., Higashi, T., Naruse, A., Nakashimo, K., Shiozaki, H., and Sakamoto, Y. (1977). *J. Nutr.* 107:51.
Tateishi, M., Suzuki, S., and Shimizu, H. (1978). *J. Biol. Chem.* 253:8854.
Tateishi, N., Higashi, T., Naruse, A., Hikita, K., and Sakamoto, Y. (1981). *J. Biochem.* 90:1603.
Thompson, G. A., and Meister, A. (1979). *J. Biol. Chem.* 254:2956.
Thor, H., Moldeus, P., Högberg, J., Hermanson, R., Reed, D. J., and Orrenius, S. (1978a). *Toxicol. Aspects Food Safety Arch. Toxicol. Suppl.* 1:107.
Thor, H., Moldeus, P., Kristoferson, A., Högberg, J., Reed, D. J., and Orrenius, S. (1978b). *Arch. Biochem. Biophys.* 188:114.
Thor, H., Moldeus, P., Hermanson, R., Högberg, J., Reed, D. J., and Orrenius, S. (1978c). *Arch. Biochem. Biophys.* 188:122.
Thor, H., Moldeus, P., and Orrenius, S. (1979). *Arch. Biochem. Biophys.* 192:405.
Tietze, F. (1969). *Anal. Biochem.* 27:502.
Todd, P., and Gronow, M. (1969). *Anal. Biochem.* 28:369.
Tsao, B., and Curthoys, N. P. (1980). *J. Biol. Chem.* 255:7708.
Tso, J. Y., Bower, S. G., and Zalkin, H. (1980). *J. Biol. Chem.* 255:6734.
Vadi, H. V., and Neal, R. A. (1981). *Chem.-Biol. Interact.* 35:25.
Wagle, S. R., and Ingebretsen, W. R. (1975). *Methods Enzymol.* 35:579.
Weisiger, R. A., and Jakoby, W. B. (1980). In *Enzymatic Basis of Detoxification*, Vol. 2, W. B. Jakoby, Ed., Academic Press, New York, p. 131.
Weisner, M. M. (1973a). *J. Biol. Chem.* 248:2536.
Weisner, M. M. (1973b). *J. Biol. Chem.* 248:2542.
Wendel, A., and Cikryt, P. (1980). *FEBS Lett.* 120:209.
White, I. N. H. (1976). *Chem.-Biol. Interact.* 13:333.

Whitfield, J. B., Pounder, R. E., Neale, G., and Moss, D. W. (1972). *Gut* 13:702.

Womack, M., Kremmer, K. S., and Rose, W. C. (1937). *J. Biol. Chem.* 121:403.

Wong, L. T., Solomonraj, G., and Thomas, B. H. (1976). *Xenobiotica* 6:575.

Young, J. D., Ellory, J. C., and Wright, P. C. (1975). *Biochem. J.* 152:713.

7
Ascorbic Acid in Drug Metabolism

David E. Holloway* and Francis J. Peterson†
Cornell University, Ithaca, New York

I. INTRODUCTION

Ascorbic acid, a unique chemical entity that functions both as an essential nutrient and as an active reducing agent, commands an important role in the metabolism and detoxification of many endogenous and foreign compounds. The ever-increasing volume of published research concerning ascorbic acid and drug biotransformation attests to the vitamin's central involvement in the organismal response to pharmacologic agents. Much of this work has focused on the role of ascorbic acid in maintaining normal rates of drug metabolism in species that require a dietary source of this vitamin, studied most commonly in the vitamin C-deficient guinea pig. Other investigators have demonstrated that many drugs which induce the mixed-function oxidase system also, in ascorbate-synthesizing species, accelerate the rate of ascorbate biosynthesis. Yet another line of investigation has been study of the protection that vitamin C affords against the toxicities of a wide variety of biologically active chemicals, including drugs. This review focuses on these areas of inquiry into the interaction between ascorbic acid and drugs, after first examining important methodological considerations in the design of drug-ascorbic acid studies.

Present affiliation: University of Miami School of Medicine, Miami, Florida
†*Present affiliation*: James Ford Bell Technical Center, General Mills, Inc., Minneapolis, Minnesota

II. METHODOLOGICAL CONSIDERATIONS IN DRUG-ASCORBIC ACID STUDIES

The vast majority of experimental studies on the role of ascorbic acid in drug metabolism have utilized the model of acute ascorbic acid deficiency in the guinea pig, although other experimental models (Peterson et al., 1983a) and animals (Omaye et al., 1980), including humans (Section III.B), have been employed. Recent findings raise a number of important questions concerning experimental details of such studies, and new information provides alternative experimental models for future experiments investigating the role of ascorbic acid in drug metabolism.

In the design of experimental studies of ascorbate function in cytochrome P-450-mediated reactions, a number of methodological questions must be addressed prior to the actual initiation of experimental work:

1. What species is to be employed?
2. What experimental diet will be used?
3. How will vitamin C be administered?
4. What nutritional model is to be employed (i.e., acute deficiency, chronic deficiency, vitamin overdosage)?
5. What index of cytochrome P-450-mediated function is to be studied (e.g., total cytochrome P-450 levels, isozymes of cytochrome P-450, microsomal drug metabolism) and how is it to be monitored (e.g., in vivo versus in vitro, or hepatic versus extrahepatic measures of drug metabolism)?

Each of these questions is addressed in turn in the following sections.

A. Choice of Species

Ascorbic acid function in drug metabolism can be studied in either ascorbate-synthesizing or ascorbate-requiring species. Naturally, the types of questions addressed often differ depending on whether or not the species under study produces its own ascorbic acid. Studies in ascorbate-synthesizing species have largely involved use of the rat as the experimental animal. One major route of inquiry has been to ascertain the effects of drug treatment on the rate of synthesis of ascorbic acid in the rat (discussed in Section III.A.4). Drug-induced acceleration of ascorbate synthesis raises intriguing questions about the potential role of ascorbic acid in protection of the organism against injury by foreign compounds.

Another possible use of ascorbate-synthesizing species is in the examination of effects of massive vitamin overdosage on biological functions, including rates of drug metabolism. For example, vitamin C overdose has been reported to alter rates of drug conjugation (Houston and Levy, 1976a) and to elevate mixed-function oxidase (MFO) activity in the rat (Kachole et al., 1978). In the conduct of such studies, it is

important that the investigator be aware of the differences between
species that synthesize ascorbic acid and those that require a dietary
supply.

Ascorbic acid absorption in the rat occurs by passive diffusion
(Spencer et al., 1963; Stevenson and Brush, 1969). In contrast, the
guinea pig (Stevenson and Brush, 1969; Mellors et al.,1977; Siliprandi
et al., 1979) and humans (Stevenson, 1974; Toggenburger et al., 1979)
absorb ascorbic acid by a Na^+-dependent, energy-requiring, carrier-
mediated mechanism. By this means, ascorbic acid, when present in
low concentration in the intestinal lumen, is much more rapidly absorbed than is possible by passive diffusion alone. However, intestinal
absorption by passive diffusion has also been demonstrated in the
guinea pig (Mellors et al., 1977). Absorption by passive diffusion becomes quantitatively important when large amounts of ascorbic acid are
consumed, thereby saturating the active transport carrier. Any ascorbic acid that is unabsorbed in the proximal intestine is unlikely to
be absorbed at all, due to its rapid degradation by microflora of the
colon and cecum (Young and James, 1942; Young and Rettger, 1943).

Because ascorbate-synthesizing species maintain tissue levels of ascorbic acid at a high level, the response of tissue ascorbate levels to
increasing dietary ascorbate differs markedly between, for example,
rats and guinea pigs. Table 1 demonstrates that a diet containing
500 mg of ascorbic acid per kilogram, which markedly increases hepatic
ascorbate concentration in the guinea pig relative to levels in guinea
pigs on a marginal vitamin C intake (50 mg/kg diet), has little effect
on hepatic ascorbate levels in the rat. Further increase in dietary ascorbate level to 20,000 mg/kg diet did not significantly increase plasma
ascorbate concentration but did raise hepatic ascorbate levels in the
rat. However, this effect is much smaller than the effect seen in the
guinea pig.

Another animal model in which the role of ascorbic acid in drug metabolism has been studied is the monkey (Chadwick et al., 1971; Omaye
et al., 1980). Omaye et al. reported that ascorbic acid depletion of
the Cynomolgus monkey for 5 weeks to a mean plasma ascorbic acid
level of 0.04 mg/dl did not alter the rate of metabolism of either antipyrine or theophylline. A similar finding has been reported in human
subjects (Holloway et al., 1982a). These results contrast with the
demonstration by Axelrod et al. (1954) of prolonged antipyrine half-
life in guinea pigs deprived of ascorbic acid for 16—20 days.

An additional animal model of potential value for study of ascorbic acid
function in drug metabolism is the fish, which like the guinea pig, develops scurvy in the absence of a dietary source of ascorbic acid (Halver et al., 1975). Ascorbic acid deficiency in trout has been shown to
result in elevation of plasma cholesterol levels (John et al., 1979).
Elevation of cholesterol levels in ascorbic acid-deficient guinea pigs is
a result of decreased activity of the cytochrome P-450-dependent enzyme cholesterol 7α-hydroxylase (Holloway and Rivers, 1981; Holloway

Table 1 Comparison of Tissue Response to Dietary Ascorbic Acid in the Guinea Pig and Rat[a]

Dietary ascorbic acid (mg/kg diet)	Guinea pig		Rat	
	Plasma (mg/dl)	Liver (mg/100 g)	Plasma (mg/dl)	Liver (mg/100 g)
0	–	–	1.54 ± 0.18*	22.5 ± 1.6*
50	0.10 ± 0.01*	1.6 ± 0.1*	–	–
500	0.61 ± 0.05[†]	13.7 ± 0.6[†]	1.65 ± 0.22*	25.8 ± 1.4*
20,000	2.07 ± 0.22[‡]	28.0 ± 1.1[‡]	2.05 ± 0.23*	34.4 ± 1.0[†]

[a]Data expressed as mean ± SEM of 8–10 animals per group. Means not followed by the same superscript symbol are significantly different. $P < 0.05$.

Source: Guinea pig ascorbate concentrations from Peterson et al. (1983a); rat ascorbate concentrations from D. E. Holloway's group (unpublished results).

et al., 1981b), raising the possibility that altered cytochrome P-450-dependent function may account for similar alterations in fish.

Also of interest are animals in the "gray zone" that lies between the ascorbate-requiring and the ascorbate-synthesizing species. Thus the young willow ptarmigan, despite an active ascorbate-synthesizing capability, nevertheless develops scurvy and dies unless its diet is supplemented with additional ascorbic acid (Hanssen et al., 1979). Hamsters fed a fat-free, high-glucose diet exhibit a relative vitamin C deficiency compared to controls, as indicated by lower tissue ascorbate levels and depressed ascorbate-requiring function such as conversion of cholesterol to bile acid (Ginter and Mikus, 1977). These animal models suggest additional experimental approaches by which the interaction between ascorbic acid nutriture and drug metabolism might profitably be explored.

B. Choice of Experimental Diet

The study of the role of ascorbic acid in drug metabolism in vivo necessitates the use of a scorbutigenic (scurvy-producing) test diet to permit control of the amount of ascorbic acid ingested by the experimental animals. Scorbutigenic diets are of two forms: cereal-based and semipurified. Little information is presently available concerning the relative merits of these diets in the conduct of experimental studies using guinea pigs. For the study of acute ascorbic acid deficiency, the choice of experimental diet may be of secondary importance owing to the short-term nature of such experiments as a result of the rapid development of scurvy in the guinea pig. For longer-term experiments (e.g., chronic ascorbic acid deficiency), choice of diet assumes greater importance.

Two commonly used guinea pig test diets are the cereal-based formulation of Krehl and the semipurified formulation of Reid and Briggs (both diets available from Teklad Mills, Madison, Wisconsin). Diet compositions are presented elsewhere (Holloway et al., 1982b). Use of a semipurified diet confers the obvious advantage that the nutritional composition is precisely known. Clearly, this factor is of supreme importance if dietary factors other than ascorbic acid are to be experimentally manipulated. However, attendant on the use of semipurified diets are several problems. The first is that a fraction of the animals will refuse to eat the diet at all and must therefore be excluded from the experiment, introducing a bias of unknown proportion into the experimental design. One approach that has been employed successfully to increase acceptance of semipurified diets by guinea pigs is preparation of the diet in the form of a gel, which is more readily accepted by guinea pigs than the diet in dry form (Navia and Lopez, 1973). Second, although animals fed cereal-based and semipurified diets grow at the same rate (Reid and Briggs, 1953), altered gastrointestinal morphology and function are a consequence of prolonged consumption of semipurified diet by the guinea pig. Thus Holloway et al. (1982b) demonstrated that relative to Krehl-fed guinea pigs, guinea pigs fed the Reid-Briggs diet exhibited distension and increased weight of the gut, with loss of typical haustral markings, greatly increased bile volume, decreased fecal output, and decreased bile acid turnover rate. These findings suggest that there are important differences in gastrointestinal function between guinea pigs fed cereal-based diets and those fed semipurified diets. The metabolic consequences of such alterations are largely unknown, although the study of Holloway and co-workers documented different responses of bile acid metabolism to large doses of ascorbic acid in guinea pigs fed Krehl versus Reid-Briggs diets. This finding raises the prospect that experimental results may be dependent on the type of experimental diet fed. Thus careful attention to the type of diet employed, especially in comparisons among experiments, appears warranted.

A problem in the use of cereal-based diets which is avoided through use of semipurified diets is the presence in natural foods of both exogenous and endogenous biologically active compounds, including compounds with pharmacologic activity. For example, the halogenated hydrocarbon insecticides are potent inducers of hepatic MFO activity (Azarnoff, 1977), as are certain indoles present in cruciferous vegetables (Loub et al., 1975). Rats fed Purina rat chow exhibit higher aryl hydrocarbon hydroxylase activity in lung and intestine than did rats fed semipurified diets; this effect is due to the vegetable component of the diet—alfalfa meal (Wattenberg, 1971). However, there is no difference in *hepatic* MFO activity (including benzo[a]pyrene hydroxylation) between rats fed chow versus semipurified diets (Abbott et al., 1976). Thus, in the choice of an experimental diet for use in studies with guinea pigs, possible interferences from pharmacologically active compounds or other potential contaminants in cereal-based diets must be weighed against problems associated with the use of semipurified diets.

C. Mode of Vitamin C Administration

1. Ascorbic Acid Stability

Central to any discussion of methods to administer ascorbic acid to experimental animals is the well-known lability of the vitamin under nonacidic conditions. Simply dissolving ascorbic acid in water initiates the destruction of the vitamin, which is oxidized by atmospheric oxygen present in solution. This process is markedly accelerated by heat and by the presence of metal ion catalysts such as copper or iron (Tsuhako et al., 1981). Oxidation occurs in a two-stage process: ascorbic acid is reversibly oxidized to dehydroascorbic acid, which then spontaneously undergoes irreversible hydrolysis of the γ-lactone ring to form 2,3-diketogulonic acid.

Ascorbic acid in solution is self-protective, in that with increasing ascorbate concentration, the solution is rendered increasingly acidic, thereby stabilizing the vitamin. Thus, when ascorbic acid (10 mg/liter) is dissolved in tap water at room temperatures, no ascorbate remains after 1 hr; while at a concentration of 100 mg/liter, approximately 50% remains; and at 500 mg/liter, approximately 80% remains at 1 hr and 50–60% at 24 hr (Hornig and Moser, 1981). Ascorbate stability is greatly enhanced through the use of distilled water and/or refrigeration of the ascorbate solution (Tsuhako et al., 1981). Care must be exercised to assure that oxidation of vitamin C is minimized in any experiment in which accurate knowledge of vitamin intake is required.

2. Ascorbic Acid Administration and Retention

Commonly employed methods to administer ascorbic acid to experimental animals in nutrition experiments include (1) mixing the vitamin in the diet, which may then either be fed as a powder or pelleted prior to use; (2) dissolving the vitamin in the animals' drinking water; (3) oral administration in solution; and (4) parenteral administration. Each method has its advantages and disadvantages, and selection of a method depends on the design and objectives of a particular study. A summary of method comparisons is presented in Table 2.

Administration of a given amount of ascorbic acid by each of these four methods will not result in identical amounts of ascorbic acid retained by the guinea pig nor, consequently, in similar tissue ascorbate concentrations. For the most part, this is simply a reflection of the guinea pig's limited ability to absorb vitamin C (Penney and Zilva, 1946; Holloway et al., 1981a; Holloway, 1981). The amount of ascorbic acid retained by the guinea pig depends on the route of vitamin C administration, the size of the dose, and the frequency of dosing.

Grollman and Firor (1934) demonstrated that intraperitoneally administered ascorbic acid is more efficiently utilized by the guinea pig than is vitamin C given orally. When guinea pigs fed a scorbutigenic diet were given daily intraperitoneal injections of 0.25 mg of ascorbate, they maintained body weight and survived to the end of the experiment (40 days); however, guinea pigs given this dose orally died within 30–40 days with marked signs of scurvy. More efficient utilization of parenteral ascorbate is also evident at considerably higher dosages. Penney and Zilva (1946) demonstrated that intramuscular administration of 25 mg of ascorbic acid resulted in tissue ascorbate concentrations averaging 2.8-fold higher than those in animals given an identical oral dose.

The difference in tissue levels attained between parenterally and orally administered ascorbic acid is dependent on at least two factors:

Table 2 Comparison of Different Methods of Administering Ascorbic Acid to Guinea Pigs[a]

	Mode of ascorbic acid administration			
	Mixed in diet (powdered)	Mixed in drinking water	Oral administration[b]	Parenteral administration[b]
Ease of preparation and administration	+++	++	+/−	+
Stability of vitamin	+++	++[c]	++	++
Interanimal variability in amount ingested	++	+/−	+++	+++
Usefulness in study of chronic deficiency	++	+/−	+++	+++
Usefulness in study of excessive intake	+++	+++	+/−	+/−
Efficiency of method[d]	+++	+++	+	+++
Suggested vitamin C dosages	200-500[e]	1%	0.5-2.0[f]	0.5-2.0[f]

[a]Rating of methods: +++, excellent; ++, good; +, fair; +/−, poor.
[b]Ascorbate dose administered once per day.
[c]Depends on concentration used (see the text).
[d]Efficiency = amount retained/amount ingested.
[e]mg/kg diet.
[f]mg/100 g body weight per day.

(1) the frequency of oral dosing, and (2) the age of the animals. When 25 mg of vitamin C was given orally in 0.5-mg doses every 10 min, tissue levels were similar to those observed in animals receiving a single intraperitoneal dose of 25 mg of vitamin C (Penney and Zilva, 1946). Jacobsen (1935) demonstrated that tissue vitamin C levels were 40% greater in guinea pigs receiving two divided oral doses of 25 mg of ascorbate than in animals given a single daily dose of 50 mg. In older animals (500 days), intramuscular ascorbate injection raised tissue levels 108–127% above the respective tissue levels resulting from oral dosing with the same amount of vitamin C; this increase was only 35–50% in animals 60 days of age (Hughes and Jones, 1971). The authors concluded that the efficiency of ascorbate absorption declines with age in the guinea pig. The highest reported tissue ascorbate concentrations attained (liver, 50–90 mg per 100 g) have resulted from repeated intraperitoneal injections of large doses of sodium ascorbate (5 × 100 mg per 12 hr) to guinea pigs (Degkwitz and Kim, 1973).

Continuous provision of a given amount of ascorbic acid in the guinea pig's diet or drinking water results in higher tissue ascorbate levels than would occur if the same amount of the vitamin were given as a single oral dose. This is the natural result of consumption of ascorbic acid throughout the day, thereby maximizing intestinal absorption of the vitamin. In contrast, a single oral dose may be only partially absorbed. Table 3 presents data from Holloway (1980) in which guinea pigs were fed for 131–145 days either a scorbutigenic diet supplemented with 500 mg of ascorbate/kg, or the unsupplemented diet plus a daily oral dose of 2.0 mg per 100 g body weight six times per week, resulting in nearly identical vitamin C intakes on a weekly basis (105 mg and 108 mg, respectively). Presentation of ascorbic acid mixed in the diet resulted in tissue ascorbate concentrations that were 60% higher, on the average, than the respective ascorbate levels in guinea pigs fed vitamin C as a single daily oral dose.

Available evidence suggests that similar ascorbate levels are attained when a given dose of ascorbic acid is continuously available (as when given in frequent small doses, or mixed in the diet) or given parenterally (Penney and Zilva, 1946). This probably reflects a similar extent of vitamin loss by both routes of administration: parenteral ascorbate doses of 20 mg or more result in urinary loss of the vitamin (Zilva, 1936), while ingested ascorbate is incompletely absorbed (Holloway, 1981).

3. Ascorbic Acid Administration: Technical Aspects

Perhaps the simplest method of administering ascorbic acid is to mix the vitamin into the animal's diet. Powdered diets that are essentially free of ascorbic acid can either be purchased preformulated or prepared from basic ingredients by the investigator. Cereal-based or

Table 3 Influence of Mode of Ascorbic Acid Administration on Tissue Ascorbate Concentrations in Guinea Pigs[a]

| | Mode of ascorbic acid administration | | |
Parameter	Oral[b] (2.0 mg/100 g BW/day)	Mixed in diet (500 mg/kg diet)	Difference
Final average body weight (g)	905	881	
Food intake (g/day)	30.5	29.9	
Actual ascorbic acid intake (mg/day)	18	15	
Ascorbic acid concentrations:			
Plasma (mg/dl)	0.31	0.49	+58%
Liver (mg/100 g)	11.2	20.3	+81%
Spleen (mg/100 g)	24.7	35.7	+45%
Adrenal (mg/100 g)	65.1	98.5	+51%

[a]Number of observations: oral administration, 5–10; mixed in diet, 11.
[b]Administered once per day, six times per week. From Holloway (1980).

semipurified diets are available from a number of suppliers in either powder or pellet form and with or without the addition of a specified level of ascorbic acid.

Best control of the actual amount of ascorbic acid in the diet is obtained by mixing the ascorbic acid into the powdered diet in the animal facility diet kitchen. The diet is then stored under refrigeration in sealed plastic bags within suitable containers and used within 3 weeks. Under these conditions little loss of ascorbic acid occurs. By this means, diets with varying amounts of ascorbic acid can readily be prepared as needed for experimental studies. Good uniformity in tissue ascorbate levels is obtained when ascorbic acid is mixed into the diet despite the usual variation in food intake that occurs among animals. This method is quite useful both for induction of chronic ascorbic acid deficiency and for provision of excessive dietary ascorbate.

Pelleted diets are more readily accepted by guinea pigs than are powdered diets, and use of such diets confers the additional benefit of decreased waste due to less scattering of the diet by the animals. Unfortunately, the heat and moisture generally employed in the pelleting process result in considerable destruction of added ascorbic acid, rendering the pelleted form of diet unsuitable for use in experiments in which rigorous control of dietary ascorbate level is required. However, successful pelleting of diets with different levels of ascorbate has been achieved by some investigators (Sikic et al., 1977a). Pelleted diets are quite useful when ascorbic acid is administered by extra-dietary means.

Administration of vitamin C in the animals' drinking water, often at a level of 1%, is a method frequently used to assure tissue vitamin C saturation (Hughes and Jones, 1970). Very high tissue ascorbate levels due to continuous ascorbate ingestion throughout the day are attained even when much lower ascorbate concentrations are employed (e.g., 0.033−0.1%) (Kuenzig et al., 1977; Rikans et al., 1978). While vitamin C is unstable in water at low concentrations (as discussed above), considerable stability over a 24-hr period is to be expected at concentrations of 0.05% or more (Hornig and Moser, 1981). Since variation in water consumption among guinea pigs can be quite large, this method may result in considerable interanimal variation in vitamin C intake. The method is of little value for inducing chronic ascorbate deficiency because vitamin C, at the concentrations required, would be rapidly oxidized and lost.

Best control of actual vitamin C dosage is achieved by oral or parenteral administration of the vitamin. Dosing solutions should be prepared immediately before use to minimize oxidative loss of vitamin C. For oral dosing, ascorbic acid is generally dissolved in a 5−20% solution of sucrose or glucose (to improve acceptance of the acid solution) and

1 ml is administered to the animals by means of a syringe with a blunted needle. Moderate doses of vitamin C (e.g., 25 mg or less) are readily accepted by the animals; however, problems with acceptance are encountered when large doses of ascorbic acid are administered in this manner. In such a case, stomach tubing may be employed, but this procedure is quite stressful to the guinea pig (Ohno and Myoga, 1981). Oral dosing with 0.5 mg of ascorbate per day is the standard method devised by Ginter et al. (1968) to induce chronic ascorbic acid deficiency in the guinea pig. Somewhat higher dosages (0.15 mg per 100 g body weight per day) have been similarly employed by other investigators (Holloway, 1980). Several authors have found that guinea pigs can be adequately maintained when ascorbic acid is given orally every other day rather than daily (Zilva, 1941; Ginter et al., 1968).

Parenteral ascorbate administration is generally achieved through the intraperitoneal injection of approximately 1 ml of an ascorbate solution prepared with distilled water or isotonic saline. Less time is required to dose the animals intraperitoneally than orally; however, this procedure may be more stressful to the guinea pig. Although not widely used for this purpose, parenteral ascorbate administration would be expected to provide the good control of intake necessary to induce chronic ascorbic acid deficiency. Subcutaneous injections of large doses of ascorbic acid (2 × 200 mg/kg body weight per day) have been reported to cause inflammation in guinea pigs (Alleva et al., 1976). Intraperitoneal doses larger than 835 mg/kg body weight cause convulsions in the guinea pig (Fujita et al., 1982). Parenteral ascorbate injections find special application in preventing undesirable interactions between vitamin C and other nutrients in the gastrointestinal tract; for example, when studying the effects of mineral consumption on ascorbate metabolism.

D. Choice of Nutritional Model

In the design of drug-ascorbic acid studies, it is essential to distinguish between the normal biochemical role of vitamin C in the organism and the pharmacologic effects of the vitamin. Biochemical effects of ascorbic acid are generally analyzed through the study of ascorbic acid-deficient guinea pigs. In this way, vitamin C-dependent functions are isolated for analysis. Two models for the study of deficiency are acute vitamin C deficiency and chronic, or marginal, vitamin C deficiency. The pharmacologic range of ascorbic acid intake can be defined as dosages greater than the requirement for optimal biologic function. Of course, the amount of vitamin C required for optimal health is unknown, and even for the guinea pig, estimates vary widely (Mannering, 1949; Veen-Baigent et al., 1975; Yew, 1973; Rokosova and Chvapil, 1974; Holloway et al., 1982b).

1. Vitamin C Deficiency

Vitamin C effects on drug metabolism have been studied most often through use of the model of acute ascorbic acid deficiency. Guinea pigs are placed on a scorbutigenic diet and are usually studied after 10–21 days of vitamin C depletion. Studies of acute vitamin C deficiency can easily be compromised by secondary sequelae of scurvy. For the first 10–14 days on a scorbutigenic diet, guinea pigs gain weight and appear normal (Collins and Elvehjem, 1958; Sikic et al., 1977b). During this period, tissue ascorbate concentrations decline precipitously to very low levels (Penney and Zilva, 1946; Sikic et al., 1977b; Ginter, 1978). The first signs of scurvy are inanition and weight loss; these changes occur within 10–21 days on the scorbutigenic diet. Previous consumption of large doses of ascorbic acid does not delay the initiation of scurvy (Zilva, 1936). Additional signs of scurvy (hemorrhage, weakness, painful joints) are evident after 21 days, and death due to scurvy or secondary infection usually occurs by 28–30 days (Holst and Frohlich, 1907; Sikic et al., 1977b). The time course of scurvy depends on the age of the animal: very young animals (< 200 g) will exhibit signs of scurvy more rapidly, and older animals (> 500–600 g) more slowly. In addition to the gross changes associated with scurvy are negative nitrogen balance (Ginter, 1958) and disruption of the tricarboxylic acid cycle (Banerjee et al., 1959). It is clear, then, that acute scurvy is a metabolically unstable state, and that, depending on the degree of scurvy induced, the parameters investigated may be altered by secondary consequences of scurvy rather than uncomplicated ascorbic acid depletion.

To avoid metabolic changes that occur in scorbutic guinea pigs, most studies of drug metabolism have concentrated on changes in MFO activity in the early stages of vitamin C deficiency (10–21 days). Nevertheless, as indicated above, even at this stage of scurvy, such changes as inanition and weight loss are regularly observed, and may confound interpretation of data. Despite these shortcomings of the method, a great deal of useful information has resulted from the study of drug metabolism in guinea pigs with acute vitamin C deficiency.

Acute ascorbic acid depletion has also been studied in the monkey (Section II.A) and in humans (Section III.B). Vitamin C depletion occurs more slowly in primates than in guinea pigs: Maintenance on a liquid diet devoid of ascorbic acid results in the development of scurvy in the monkey after 70–105 days (Baker et al., 1975; Machlin et al., 1976; Machlin et al., 1979). Human subjects on an ascorbate-free liquid diet exhibit early signs of scurvy (petechiae and bruising) after 29–103 days of depletion and more advanced scorbutic symptoms (joint pain and joint effusions) after 67–103 days (Hodges et al., 1971). Human subjects fed scorbutigenic diets composed of normal foods first exhibit signs of scurvy after 4–5 months (Crandon et al., 1940; Pijoan and Lozner, 1944; Krebs et al., 1948).

Ginter has pioneered in the development of the model of chronic ascorbic acid deficiency in the guinea pig (Ginter et al., 1968). This model has been successfully utilized for investigations into the effect of vitamin C deficiency on lipid metabolism (Ginter, 1978; Holloway and Rivers, 1981) and, more recently, drug metabolism (Peterson et al., 1983a). Use of this model confers the following advantages: (1) guinea pigs receive sufficient ascorbic acid to maintain normal growth rates and normal non-ascorbate-dependent metabolism, thereby avoiding the secondary complications of scurvy; (2) guinea pigs can be maintained in this state of chronic deficiency for as long as 1 year (Ginter, 1978), providing a greatly expanded time frame for experimental studies; and (3) the model more closely duplicates the state of indigenous human ascorbic acid deficiency, which rarely progresses to clinical scurvy (Ten State Nutrition Survey, 1972; Burr et al., 1974).

The state of chronic ascorbic acid deficiency provides sufficient dietary ascorbic acid to maintain most normal body functions, so that any changes observed can be clearly attributed to vitamin C insufficiency. The influence of chronic ascorbate deficiency on the MFO system is discussed in Section III.A.2. Chronic ascorbic acid deficiency, as induced by Ginter et al., involves placing guinea pigs on an unsupplemented scorbutigenic diet for 2 weeks, followed by administration of a maintenance dose of 0.5 mg of ascorbate per day; controls receive 5 mg of ascorbate daily (Ginter et al., 1968). Since this procedure produced symptoms of scurvy in guinea pigs in our laboratory (Simpson, 1971), guinea pigs were either fed the unsupplemented Krehl scorbutigenic diet for 1 week followed by daily oral dosing (six times per week) with 0.15 mg of ascorbate per 100 g body weight (Holloway, 1980), or were fed the Krehl diet supplemented with a low dietary level (50 mg/kg diet) of ascorbic acid (Peterson et al., 1983a). The latter procedure is preferred due to time savings in animal care. Caution is advised, however, in selection of a dietary level of vitamin C which will induce chronic deficiency yet maintain a normal rate of growth. Conditions should be individually established for each laboratory (e.g., based on strain of guinea pig, diet employed, etc.). Cereal-based diets should be analyzed for ascorbic acid prior to use. Alfalfa, which is an important component of these diets, is a good source of vitamin C (Fox and Levy, 1936), necessitating treatment to remove or destroy the ascorbic acid present prior to inclusion of alfalfa in the diet. Oven drying is a good method to reduce the ascorbate content of alfalfa to an acceptable level (Singh et al., 1968).

2. Excessive Ascorbic Acid Administration

In contrast to the wide variety of MFO components which are altered by ascorbic acid deficiency in the guinea pig (Section III.A.1 and 2), the only cytochrome P-450-dependent enzyme shown to be responsive to the chronic consumption of excessive ascorbic acid is cholesterol 7α-hydroxylase, the rate-limiting enzyme in bile acid biosynthesis (Peterson et al., 1983a). However, a recent report (Sutton et al., 1982) indicates that short-term administration of large doses of ascorbic acid to guinea pigs (2 × 150 mg for 4 days) does decrease activities of a variety of MFO components. Excessive ascorbate administration has been shown to elevate glutathione S-aryltransferase activity in the guinea pig (Sikic et al., 1977a), and large doses of ascorbic acid are reported to alter rates of drug conjugation and, consequently, drug half-life in humans (Section III.B). Study of the metabolism of drugs as yet untested may reveal additional metabolic pathways altered by dietary excess of ascorbic acid. Such questions are of potential clinical significance in view of the presently popular consumption of pharmacologic doses of vitamin C (Baker et al., 1981).

Large doses of ascorbic acid are most easily administered by means of the guinea pigs' drinking water or diet, the latter route providing the best control of actual intake. The influence of dietary ascorbate at levels up to 20 g/kg diet on the MFO system has been reported (Section III. A.3). Animals fed such massive intakes of vitamin C for 7—21 weeks grow normally and appear healthy in all respects (Holloway, 1980).

E. Indices of Drug Metabolism

Numerous approaches to the study of drug metabolism in vitamin C deficiency have been employed. Additional avenues available to the investigator have not yet been utilized specifically for the study of ascorbic acid's role in drug metabolism. Methods for the study of drug metabolism can be classified according to the classical hierarchy of biologic level of organization: (1) organismal, (2) system, (3) organ, (4) cellular, (5) subcellular, and (6) molecular.

1. Organismal Level

Methods to study drug metabolism in vivo include measurement of the duration of drug effectiveness, pharmacokinetic analysis, and quantitation of drug metabolites and conjugates in the excreta. The first indication of impaired drug metabolism in vitamin C deficiency was the demonstration by Richards et al. (1941) that ascorbate-deficient guinea pigs have longer pentobarbital-induced sleeping times than those of controls. More recently, mixed-function oxidase activity as affected by vitamin C deficiency has been studied in humans (Holloway et al., 1982a; Trang et al., 1982), the monkey (Omaye et al., 1980), and the guinea pig (Axelrod et al., 1954) through measurement of the in vivo kinetics (pharmacokinetics) of drug metabolism. Drugs that have been studied by this means include acetanilide, aniline, antipyrine, caffeine, and theophylline. In pharmacokinetic studies, sequential samples (usually blood) are collected following drug administration, permitting measurement of alteration in drug concentration over time. In the simplest case, that of a drug such as antipyrine, which distributes in the body according to a one-compartment model, construction of a semi-logarithmic plot of drug concentration versus time permits determination of the disposition rate constant and extrapolated zero-time drug concentration. From these values, drug half-life, metabolic clearance rate, and apparent volume of distribution can easily be calculated (Gibaldi and Perrier, 1975). Subjects and animals in pharmacokinetic studies may serve as their own controls, before and/or after a period of vitamin C depletion, thereby minimizing experimental variability.

The aminopyrine breath test relies on measurement of $^{14}CO_2$ excretion following administration of [^{14}C]aminopyrine as a means to measure drug metabolism in vivo. This test has been utilized to study the effects of diverse conditions and diseases on aminopyrine metabolism in man and animals (Hepner and Vesell, 1974; Lauterburg and Bircher, 1976). Rather than measuring the overall rate of drug metabolism, it is possible to measure the rate of formation and excretion of specific drug metabolites. For example, the metabolism of antipyrine to its major metabolites is under the control of more than one enzyme system in animals and humans (Danhof et al., 1979, 1982). Measurement of rates of metabolite formation under different nutritional states would be expected to provide knowledge concerning dietary effects on specific cytochrome P-450-dependent enzyme systems. Neither the aminopyrine breath test nor measurement of antipyrine metabolites have yet been employed in the study of vitamin C effects on drug metabolism.

2. System Level

Mediation of ascorbate's role in drug metabolism via the endocrine system cannot be ruled out at the present time. The fact that phenobarbital administration induces MFO activity to the same extent in control and ascorbate-deficient guinea pigs (Zannoni et al., 1972; Kuenzig et al., 1977) raises the possibility that the locus of ascorbate action may not be at the level of enzyme synthesis, but may perhaps be at some higher control point in the regulation of hepatic function. In this regard, it is intriguing that ascorbic acid deficiency is known to alter thyroid (Kassouny and Rivers, 1972) and adrenal function (Encarnacion et al., 1974; Fordyce and Kassouny, 1977). As is well known, the MFO system is influenced by both thyroid hormone (Kato and Takahashi, 1968) and the adrenocortical hormones (Castro et al., 1970). Investigation of possible hormonal mediation of ascorbic acid effects on drug metabolism may provide important new information concerning drug-ascorbic acid interactions.

3. Organ Level

Use of the isolated perfused liver permits study of hepatic drug metabolism in a situation resembling that in vivo, yet eliminates extrahepatic factors which may affect the rate of drug metabolism. This technique has been used in numerous studies of drug metabolism (Garattini et al., 1973), but has not been utilized to date as a method to examine the influence of vitamin C in this process.

4. Cellular Level

A single report relates ascorbic acid to the mixed-function oxidase system in the isolated hepatocyte. Bissell and Guzelian (1979) demonstrated that addition of ascorbic acid to cultured rat hepatocytes results in higher levels of cytochromes b5 and P-450 and NADPH-cytochrome c reductase than are observed in the absence of the vitamin. Although rat hepatocytes normally synthesize ascorbic acid, culture of the cells results in ascorbic acid loss as well as reduced synthetic capacity, resulting in a much lower cellular ascorbate concentration than is observed in vivo. Synthesis and degradation of heme were unaffected by the addition of ascorbic acid. To date no studies have documented the influence of exogenous ascorbic acid on the rate of drug metabolism in isolated hepatocytes; this technique offers an exciting approach to the study of vitamin C-drug interactions, free of interposing factors which are unavoidable in more complex systems.

5. Subcellular Level

By far the greatest part of present knowledge of drug-ascorbate interactions has resulted from the study of enzyme activity in hepatic microsomes. These are vesicles that are formed from fragments of endoplasmic reticulum by means of differential centrifugation and resuspension of liver homogenates. A summary of ascorbate-induced alterations in components of the microsomal mixed-function oxidase system is presented in Section III (Table 4). A variety of techniques have been employed in the investigation of this system, including (1) measurement of individual components of the MFO system, (2) measurement of drug-metabolizing enzyme activities, (3) determination of the kinetics of MFO enzyme activity, (4) analysis of cytochrome P-450 binding spectra, and (5) reconstitution studies with purified components of the MFO system. Limited information is also available concerning the influence of ascorbate deficiency on extrahepatic MFO activity (Degkwitz et al., 1974; Kuenzig et al., 1977; Sikic et al., 1977b).

Components of the MFO System. The MFO system embedded in the endoplasmic reticulum consists of the following: NADPH-cytochrome P-450 (c) reductase, a flavoprotein that transfers electrons from NADPH to cytochrome P-450; cytochrome P-450, the heme-containing terminal oxidase of the system, which binds the substrate and oxygen, intro-

ducing one atom of oxygen into the substrate and reducing the other
to water; cytochrome b_5, a hemoprotein that binds neither substrate
nor oxygen but transfers electrons to cytochrome P-450; and NADH-
cytochrome b_5 reductase, a flavoprotein that reduces cytochrome b_5
(Peterson and Holtzman, 1980). All of these components but the last
have been studied in vitamin C-deficient guinea pigs, in which both
of the cytochromes, but not NADPH-cytochrome P-450 (c) reductase,
are decreased (Section III.A.1). The major nonprotein component of
the endoplasmic reticulum is phospholipid, nutritional alteration of
which might be expected in turn to alter enzyme activity. However,
this does not appear to be the mechanism of the vitamin C effect on MFO
activity (Sato and Zannoni, 1976).

Numerous reports in recent years have characterized multiple forms
of cytochrome P-450 isolated from liver microsomes (Lu and West, 1980).
Multiplicity of forms of the terminal oxidase account, at least in part,
for the wide range of substrates metabolized by this system as well as
differential effects of inducing agents and other factors on the metabolism of various drugs (Lu et al., 1976). Rikans et al. (1978) demonstrated quantitative differences in the forms of cytochrome P-450 which
are separable by polyacrylamide gel electrophoresis between control and
ascorbate-deficient guinea pigs. This is an exciting avenue for future
study of the effect of vitamin C deficiency on drug metabolism.

Drug-metabolizing enzyme activity. The metabolism of a wide variety
of drugs has been studied in microsomes from ascorbate-deficient
guinea pigs. Drugs studied and the effect of vitamin C deficiency on
their metabolism are summarized in Table 4 (Section III).

Kinetics of drug-metabolizing enzymes. The kinetics of microsomal
MFO enzymes are studied by measuring product formation in incubations
with microsomes over a wide range of substrate concentrations and plot-
ting the rate of product formation versus substrate concentration by
standard methods (Gillette, 1971). From such plots, V_{max}, the maximal reaction rate, and the apparent K_m, the substrate concentration
that gives half-maximal reaction rate, are determined. For those enzyme activities reduced by ascorbic acid deficiency V_{max} is of course
reduced. Available evidence indicates that the apparent K_m is not
affected by vitamin C deficiency (Section III.A.1).

Cytochrome P-450 binding spectra. The addition of substrate to hepatic microsomal suspensions results in a characteristic cytochrome P-
450 binding spectrum which differs depending on the specific substrate
used (Peterson and Holtzman, 1980). The observed spectrum is a result of a shift in the absolute spectrum of the oxidized form of cytochrome P-450 when the substrate binds to cytochrome P-450. Addition
of substrate to one of two identical cuvettes containing the microsomal
suspension in a dual-beam spectrophotometer produces the binding
spectrum. Zannoni et al. (1972) found that the aniline-cytochrome
P-450 binding spectrum was shifted in microsomes from guinea pigs de-

prived of ascorbic acid for 21 days. A normal spectrum was observed after 10, but not 3 or 6, days of vitamin C resupplementation of the deficient animals.

Reconstitution experiments. Intensive research in recent years has led to the purification of individual components of the microsomal mixed-function oxidase system. Three components have been found necessary for enzymatic activity: NADPH-cytochrome P-450 reductase, cytochrome P-450, and phospholipid (Lu and West, 1978). Although not essential for activity of the system, cytochrome b_5 stimulates the metabolism of various substrates presumably via transfer to cytochrome P-450 of the second electron necessary for the reduction of oxygen in the mixed-function oxidase reaction (Imai, 1981; Bösterling and Trudell, 1982). A single report has described reconstitution of MFO components from control and ascorbic acid-deficient guinea pigs (Bjorkhem and Kallner, 1976). In this experiment, the cytochrome P-450-dependent hydroxylation of cholesterol, but not lauric acid, was reduced when partially purified cytochrome P-450 from ascorbate-deficient animals was studied. The severity of the ascorbic acid deficiency induced in this experiment, however, raises the question of whether this result was due to uncomplicated ascorbic acid depletion. The metabolism of other substrates (e.g., drugs) by reconstituted MFO systems from ascorbate-deficient guinea pigs has not yet been studied.

6. *Molecular Level*

Recent studies have extended knowledge of cytochrome P-450 to the molecular level through improved understanding of the mechanism of cytochrome induction and its genetic control (Nebert et al., 1981) as well as isolation and study of specific mRNAs which direct cytochrome P-450 synthesis (Bresnick et al., 1981; Negishi and Nebert, 1981; Pickett et al., 1982). The new knowledge and techniques developed in these studies provide new avenues for research and raise provocative questions concerning drug-ascorbate interactions.

Nebert et al. (1981) have identified a cytosolic receptor that very tightly binds certain xenobiotics which induce cytochrome P-450 synthesis. Following translocation to the nucleus, the inducer-receptor complex provides the signal that initiates the synthesis of specific monooxygenases capable of metabolizing the inducer as well as other foreign compounds. Knowledge of this system provides new insight into the contrast in response of the MFO system to the administration of phenobarbital or pesticides to ascorbate-deficient guinea pigs. As discussed above (Section II.E.2), administration of phenobarbital to ascorbate-deficient guinea pigs results in stimulation of MFO activity to the same extent as in control animals. In contrast, induction of MFO activity by dieldrin is rapidly and progressively impaired in guinea pigs fed a scorbutigenic diet (Wagstaff and Street, 1971). Similarly, induction of MFO activity by DDT and lindane is impaired in both guinea pigs and monkeys fed ascorbic acid-deficient diets (Chadwick et al., 1973;1971). These results raise the possibility that dietary restriction of ascorbic acid may in some way disrupt the receptor-mediated control of certain monooxygenase activities, although other explanations are, of course, possible.

An interesting question for future study is whether impairment of monooxygenase induction in ascorbate deficiency reflects the same or a different biochemical defect as the overall depression in noninduced MFO activity in ascorbic acid deficiency. Since defective heme synthesis in ascorbate deficiency cannot explain reduced MFO activity (Section III.A.1), it may be that less cytochrome P-450-coding mRNA is produced, thereby accounting for decreased apocytochrome synthesis. Alternatively, the ascorbate-induced defect may come at a later point (e.g., incorporation of ferrous iron into the apocytochrome molecule) (Section III.A.1). Improved understanding of cytochrome P-450 biosynthesis and its regulation signifies that possibilities such as these are now more amenable to experimental investigation.

III. PRESENT KNOWLEDGE OF INTERACTIONS BETWEEN ASCORBIC ACID AND FOREIGN COMPOUNDS

A. Ascorbic Acid and Drug Metabolism in Animal Models

1. *Influence of Acute Ascorbic Acid Deficiency*

Richards et al. (1941) first demonstrated an influence of ascorbic acid deficiency on drug metabolism when they discovered that the pentobarbital-induced sleeping time was significantly longer in scorbutic guinea pigs than in control animals. Subsequent studies (Axelrod et al., 1954) demonstrated that the prolonged half-lives of such drugs as antipyrine and acetanilide in scorbutic guinea pigs could be returned to normal by repleting the animals with vitamin C. Conney et al. (1961) were able to correlate the prolonged duration of drug action in vivo in vitamin C deficiency with a decrease in the in vitro hepatic microsomal biotransformation of the parent drug. The duration of zoxazolamine-induced paralysis in acutely vitamin C-deficient guinea pigs was increased twofold over vitamin C-supplemented animals, while the in vitro hepatic metabolism of this muscle relaxant was decreased 67% in the ascorbic acid-deficient group.

Since these early studies, a number of investigations have documented alterations in the hepatic monooxygenase system due to vitamin C deprivation. Results from different laboratories are in good agreement with respect to the effects of vitamin C deficiency on hepatic monooxygenase activities. Table 4 summarizes the effects of ascorbic acid deficiency on components and activities of the hepatic monooxygenase system in the guinea pig. Acute ascorbic acid deficiency does not result in a decrease in all monooxygenase activities simultaneously. For example,

Kato et al. (1969) found hydroxylase activity but neither cytochrome levels nor N-demethylase activity depressed in hepatic microsomes from 12-day-deficient guinea pigs. This finding most likely reflects the degree of ascorbate depletion induced since Zannoni et al. (1972) found that microsomal cytochrome content and drug-metabolizing enzyme activity in guinea pigs were reduced after 21, but not 10, days on a scorbutigenic diet.

Although the model employed in most of the drug metabolism studies to date is that of acute ascorbic acid deficiency, the results appear to reflect ascorbate deficiency per se rather than the sequelae of acute scurvy. Alterations of cytochrome content and MFO activity are generally observed before the occurrence of the inanition and weight loss which accompany scurvy (Sikic et al., 1977b). In addition, pair-fed controls do not exhibit the alterations in microsomal cytochromes or enzyme activity observed in the ascorbate-deficient animals (Avenia, 1972; Degkwitz et al., 1973). Resupplementation of ascorbate-deficient guinea pigs with ascorbic acid results in a return of cytochrome concentration and MFO activity to control levels in 3−10 days (Wade et al., 1972; Zannoni et al., 1972; Degkwitz and Staudinger, 1974; Sikic et al., 1977b). The time to achieve normalization of microsomal components appears to be related to the amount of vitamin C supplied to the animal. Administration of 100 mg of vitamin C by stomach tube five times per day led to the return of cytochromes P-450 and b_5 to control levels in 3 days (Degkwitz and Staudinger, 1974), which is the most rapid rate of normalization reported.

While ascorbic acid deficiency clearly results in lower V_{max} values for the microsomal metabolism of a variety of drugs, the apparent K_m values of hepatic microsomal biotransformations are not altered by vitamin C deprivation (Wade et al., 1972; Sato and Zannoni, 1976; Sikic et al., 1977a). These data suggest that the overall decrease in drug metabolism caused by acute vitamin C deficiency is probably not due to qualitative changes in enzyme protein.

Attempts to elucidate the mechanism by which vitamin C alters drug-metabolizing enzyme activity have served to rule out several possibilities. The in vitro addition of ascorbic acid does not stimulate drug-metabolizing enzyme activity, ruling out a cofactor role for vitamin C in drug metabolism (Conney et al., 1961; Sikic et al., 1977b). Lipid peroxidation is known to decrease drug metabolism, and antioxidants, such as N,N'-diphenyl-p-phenylenediamine, have been shown to protect drug enzyme activities from inactivation through peroxidative mechanisms (Carpenter, 1972). The possibility that microsomes from ascorbic acid-deficient guinea pigs are more susceptibile to peroxidative destruction was investigated by Sato and Zannoni (1976). They found that the rate of lipid peroxidation, as indicated by oxygen consumption and malonaldehyde formation, was actually somewhat lower in microsomes from deficient animals than in microsomes from controls.

Table 4 Influence of Acute Ascorbic Acid Deficiency on Hepatic Components and Activities in the Guinea Pig

Component/activity	Effect	References[a]
Metabolism in vivo:		
Acetanilide	↓	1
Aniline	↓	1
Antipyrine	↓	1
Components of MFO system:		
Cytochrome P-450	↓	4,6-14,16-18,20,21 23-28,30-33
Cytochrome P-420	→	21,23
Cytochrome b_5	↓ or →	(↓): 4,6,7,9-11,14, 16,17,26,28,33 (→): 12,13,20,30
NADPH-cytochrome P-450 (c) reductase	→(or ↓)	(→): 10,11,23,24 (↓): 13,18
Phospholipid	→ or ↓	(→): 21; (↓): 7
Microsomal activities:		
NADPH oxidation	→ or ↓	(→): 4; (↓): 20,21
Oxygen consumption	↓	21
Microsomal mixed function oxidases:		
Acetanilide hydroxylase	↓(or →)	(↓): 3,6,10,19 (→): 8
Aminopyrine N-demethylase	↓	6,9,10,13,18,22,23, 27,30
Aniline hydroxylase	↓	5,11,13,20,30
Cholesterol 7α-hydroxylase	↓	29
Coumarin hydroxylase	↓	4
Ethoxycoumarin O-dealkylase	↓	24
Hexobarbital hydroxylase	↓	5,11,15
p-Nitroanisole O-demethylase	↓	13,18,21
Zoxazolamine hydroxylase	↓(or →)	(↓): 2,5; (→): 11
Benzo[a]pyrene hydroxylase	→	24
Epoxide hydrase	→	24
Ethylmorphine N-demethylase	→	11
Transferases:		
Glutathione S-aryltransferase	↓	23
p-Aminobenzoic acid N-acetyl-transferase	→	23

Table 4 (Continued)

Component/activity	Effect	References[a]
Transferases:		
UDP-glucuronyltransferase (native)	↑	23
UDP-glucuronyltransferase ("activated")	→	23
Enzymes of heme metabolism:		
δ-Aminolevulinic acid synthetase	→	25
δ-Aminolevulinic acid dehydratase	→	25
Ferrochelatase	→	25
Microsomal heme oxygenase	↓ (or ↑)	(↓): 27,32 (21-day depletion) (↑): 32 (14-day depletion)

[a](1) Axelrod et al. (1954); (2) Conney et al. (1961); (3) Degkwitz and Staudinger (1965); (4) Degkwitz et al. (1968); (5) Kato et al. (1969); (6) Leber et al. (1969); (7) Schulze and Staudinger (1970); (8) Degkwitz et al. (1970); (9) Leber et al. (1970); (10) Degkwitz et al. (1972); (11) Wade et al. (1972); (12) Luft et al. (1972); (13) Zannoni et al. (1972); (14) Degkwitz et al. (1973); (15) Gundermann et al. (1973); (16) Degkwitz and Kim (1973); (17) Degkwitz et al. (1974); (18) Sato and Zannoni (1974); (19) Fielding and Hughes (1975); (20) Dow and Goldberg (1975); (21) Sato and Zannoni (1976); (22) Sikic et al. (1977a); (23) Sikic et al. (1977b); (24) Kuenzig et al. (1977); (25) Rikans et al. (1977); (26) Rikans et al. (1978); (27) Omaye and Turnbull (1979a); (28) Omaye and Turnbull (1979b); (29) Harris et al. (1979); (30 Turnbull and Omaye (1980); (31) Walsch and Degkwitz (1980a); (32) Walsch and Degkwitz (1980b); (33) Milne and Omaye (1980). Negative findings of Kato et al. (1969) were excluded from table as they are most likely due to insufficient degree of ascorbate depletion.

Further, no increase in cytochrome P-420 levels, the cytochrome species often increased when lipid peroxidation occurs, was found in microsomes from vitamin C-deficient guinea pigs (Sikic et al., 1977b).

These studies suggest that ascorbic acid does not act solely as an anti-oxidant in maintaining the capacity of the monooxygenase system to metabolize drugs.

Sato and Zannoni (1976) also studied some physiochemical properties of hepatic cytochrome P-450 in microsomes from ascorbic acid-deficient guinea pigs. They found that cytochrome P-450 from vitamin C-deficient animals was less stable to sonication and dialysis than the cytochrome from control animals. The decrease in cytochrome P-450 due to dialysis treatment was partially blocked by the addition of ascorbic acid. Additionally, an observed decrease in the cytochrome P-450-carbon monoxide spectrum and in aniline hydroxylase activity caused by the ferrous iron chelator α,α'-dipyridyl was prevented by ascorbic acid. The authors suggested that there may be an interaction between ascorbic acid and cytochrome P-450 which involves the reduced form of heme iron.

The consistent demonstration of reduced cytochrome P-450 content in vitamin C-deficient guinea pigs led Luft et al. (1972) to suggest that vitamin C may exert its effect on the MFO system through an alteration in heme biosynthesis. However, more recent studies have demonstrated that vitamin C deficiency does not alter activities of the key enzymes involved in heme synthesis (Rikans et al., 1977;1978). The activities of δ-aminolevulinic acid synthetase, δ-aminolevulinic acid dehydratase, and ferrochelatase were not significantly altered in vitamin C deficiency. Furthermore, the urinary excretion of porphyrins and porphyrin precursors, which are often increased by enzymatic insufficiencies in the heme-biosynthetic pathway, were not increased in vitamin C-deficient guinea pigs (Turnbull and Omaye, 1980). Alternatively, ascorbic acid deficiency could decrease microsomal cytochrome content by accelerating the rate of heme catabolism. However, microsomal heme oxygenase, which catalyzes the enzymatic degradation of cytochrome P-450 (Maines and Kappas, 1977), was not found to be elevated in ascorbic acid-deficient guinea pigs (Omaye and Turnbull, 1979a). Thus an effect of ascorbic acid deficiency on heme synthesis or cytochrome P-450 degradation does not appear to be the mechanism by which vitamin C deficiency alters monooxygenase activity. A recent review discusses the involvement of ascorbic acid in heme metabolism (Omaye and Turnbull, 1980).

Ascorbic acid deficiency could also affect microsomal monooxygenase activity by influencing the availability of ferrous iron for incorporation into heme. Although iron deficiency per se in rats does not alter cytochrome P-450 content (Becking, 1972), a shift in the equilibrium of the hepatic iron pool from the ferrous to the ferric state would make the iron unavailable for incorporation into heme and, ultimately, cytochrome P-450 (Omaye and Turnbull, 1980). Ceruloplasmin, a copper-containing glycoprotein found in blood serum, controls the oxidation of iron from the ferrous to ferric state for subsequent incororation into transferrin (Osaki et al., 1966). Milne and Omaye (1980) found elevated ceruloplasmin activity and decreased cytochrome P-450 levels in ascorbate-deficient guinea pigs, leading the authors to suggest that reduced availability of ferrous iron may account for depressed cytochrome levels in vitamin C deficiency. Further, since ascorbic acid facilitates the absorption of dietary iron (Moore and Dubach, 1951) and participates in the transfer of iron from plasma protein (transferrin) to the liver by reducing ferric iron to the ferrous state (Mazur et al., 1960), a deficiency in ascorbic acid may interfere multifactorially with the availability of iron for heme biosynthesis. This is an exciting possibility requiring further research.

Hepatic ascorbic acid concentration and hepatic cytochrome P-450 content correlate in a highly significant manner (Rikans et al., 1978; Peterson et al., 1983a). Since overall heme metabolism is not influenced significantly by ascorbic acid deficiency, the possibility exists that only specific isozymes of the hemoprotein family may be affected. The presence of multiple forms or isozymes of cytochrome P-450 is now well recognized (Peterson and Holtzman, 1980), and these forms differ in substrate specificities and other physiochemical properties. Guinea pig liver microsomes contain multiple forms of cytochrome P-450, which have been separated by gel electrophoresis into nine heme-containing bands (Rikans et al., 1978). Ascorbic acid-deficient microsomes manifest significant differences in the gel electrophoretic profile when compared to vitamin C-adequate microsomes. These differences suggest that ascorbic acid has a selective effect on specific forms of cytochrome P-450. In support of this concept are the differential effects of ascorbic acid depletion on metabolism by the MFO system (Kuenzig et al., 1977). In addition, chronic ascorbic acid deficiency (see Section III.A.2) decreases the activities of several monooxygenase activities without significantly altering the total content of hepatic cytochrome P-450. These studies suggest that certain isozymes of cytochrome P-450 are significantly reduced by ascorbic acid deficiency and that ascorbate-responsive forms of cytochrome P-450 are responsible for the metabolism of most of the cytochrome P-450 substrates studied to date (Table 4).

2. Chronic Ascorbic Acid Deficiency and Drug Metabolism

Only recently has the influence of chronic ascorbic acid deficiency upon hepatic MFO activity been investigated (Holloway, 1980; Holloway and Rivers, 1981; Peterson et al., 1983a; Ginter et al., 1982). Earlier work documented the influence of acute vitamin C deficiency upon hepatic MFO activity, with the single exception of the report of Bjorkhem and Kallner (1976) discussed above (Section II.E.5). The experimental model of chronic ascorbic acid deficiency has been characterized and used extensively in studies concerning the interaction of ascorbic acid and cholesterol metabolism (Ginter et al., 1968,1973). Advantages of the model over that of acute vitamin C deficiency are discussed in Section II.D.1.

Table 5 presents hepatic ascorbate levels and MFO components and activities in control and chronically deficient guinea pigs. As in acute ascorbic acid deficiency, cytochrome P-420, NADPH-cytochrome c reductase, and ethylmorphine N-demethylase are unaffected by chronic ascorbate deficiency, whereas aniline hydroxylase, ethoxycoumarin O-deethylase, and cholesterol 7α-hydroxylase are decreased. However, the observed reductions in drug-metabolizing enzyme activity in chronic deficiency (9—34%) are less than those commonly observed in acute vitamin C deficiency (e.g., 50—66%; Zannoni et al., 1972). Furthermore, some parameters invariably altered by acute ascorbate deficiency, such as cytochrome P-450 and aminopyrine N-demethylase, are not changed in chronic ascorbic acid deficiency. Such differences in response to these two models of ascorbic acid deficiency occur despite attainment of similar hepatic ascorbate levels by both approaches (Table 6). Ginter et al. (1982) have also recently observed decreased drug-metabolizing enzyme activity in guinea pigs with chronic ascorbic acid deficiency. Aniline hydroxylase and p-nitroanisole O-demethylase activities were reduced 20—80% in deficient animals, in contrast to the smaller changes observed by Peterson et al. (1983a).

One monooxygenase activity which demonstrates exceptional sensitivity to vitamin C deprivation is cholesterol 7α-hydroxylase. The activity of this enzyme is decreased by 46% after only 10 days on an ascorbate-deficient diet (Harris et al., 1979), in contrast to other hepatic monooxygenase activities which are unaffected by this degree of depletion (Zannoni et al., 1972). Chronic ascorbate deficiency caused a further decrease in the activity of this enzyme (60—70%) which was unaccompanied by a decrease in total cytochrome P-450 content (Holloway and Rivers, 1981; Peterson et al., 1983a). The activity of this enzyme shows a marked dependence on hepatic ascorbic acid concentration (Figure 1). These data indicate the unique sensitivity of this cytochrome P-450-dependent activity to vitamin C status and further demonstrates the differing responses of MFO activities to ascorbic acid.

Despite some differences between models, the overall effect of chronic ascorbate deficiency, like that of acute ascorbate deficiency, is a depression in mixed-function oxidase activity. The lack of complicating physiological factors (e.g., inanition, weight loss), the stability of the animals on the chronic-deficient regimen, and similarities of the model to human hypovitaminosis C (Section II.D.1) recommend the chronic-deficient model for future investigation of the drug-ascorbic acid connection.

3. Excessive Ascorbate Intake and Drug Metabolism

Despite a plethora of studies examining the effects of ascorbic acid deficiency on hepatic drug metabolism, there exists a paucity of data concerning the influence of ascorbic acid overdose and drug metabolism. In light of the advocacy of massive intakes of the vitamin for possible

Table 5 Influence of Chronic Ascorbic Acid Deficiency on Ascorbate Content and MFO Activities of Guinea Pig Liver[a]

Parameter	Control (500 mg AA/kg diet)	Deficient (30-50 mg AA/kg diet)
Experiment 1		
Hepatic ascorbic acid (mg/100 g)	16.3 ± 1.4	2.4 ± 0.5[b]
Cytochrome P-450 (nmol/mg protein)	0.80 ± 0.02	0.76 ± 0.02
Cytochrome P-420 (nmol/mg protein)	0.23 ± 0.03	0.21 ± 0.01
Cytochrome b_5 (nmol/mg protein)	0.48 ± 0.03	0.51 ± 0.01
NADPH-cytochrome c reductase (nmol reduced/mg protein/min)	81.3 ± 5.4	85.2 ± 5.1
Cholesterol 7α-hydroxylase (pmol/mg protein/min)	5.06 ± 1.09	2.04 ± 0.41[b]
Experiment 2		
Hepatic ascorbic acid (mg/100 g)	13.7 ± 0.6	1.6 ± 0.1[b]
Cytochrome P-450 (nmol/mg protein)	0.84 ± 0.03	0.76 ± 0.03
Aniline hydroxylase (nmol/mg protein)	0.55 ± 0.03	0.42 ± 0.02[b]
Aminopyrine N-demethylase (nmol/mg protein/min)	4.61 ± 0.12	4.33 ± 0.11
Ethoxycoumarin O-deethylase (pmol/mg protein/min)	0.77 ± 0.02	0.51 ± 0.01[b]
Benzphetamine N-demethylase (nmol/mg protein/min)	4.58 ± 0.14	4.18 ± 0.11[b]
Ethylmorphine N-demethylase (nmol/mg protein/min)	3.39 ± 0.12	3.18 ± 0.16
Cholesterol 7α-hydroxylase (pmol/mg protein/min)	5.21 ± 0.69	1.85 ± 0.19[b]

[a]Data expressed as mean ± SEM of 5–6 observations (Exp. 1) or 9–10 observations (Exp. 2, except cholesterol 7α-hydroxylase where n = 5–6). Experimental period: 7 weeks (Exp. 1); 9 weeks (Exp. 2).
[b]Significantly different from control value, $p < 0.05$.
Source: Data from Holloway and Rivers, 1981 (Exp. 1); Holloway, 1980 (Exp. 1, NADPH-cytochrome c reductase); Peterson et al., 1983a (Exp. 2).

Table 6 Comparison of Hepatic Ascorbic Acid and Cytochrome P-450 Content in Acute and Chronic Vitamin C Deficiency

Model of deficiency	Duration of deficiency (days)	Group	Hepatic ascorbic acid (mg/100 g)	Hepatic microsomal cytochrome P-450 (nmol/mg protein)
Acute[a]	14	Control	16.4 ± 2.3	0.93 ± 0.07
		Deficient	4.6 ± 0.7	0.71 ± 0.07[b]
Acute[c]	20	Control	25 ± 7	0.93 ± 0.19
		Deficient	3 ± 1	0.64 ± 0.15[b]
Acute[d]	25	Control	28.6 ± 12.2	1.22 ± 0.04
		Deficient	1.4 ± 0.3	0.48 ± 0.04[b]
Chronic[e]	67	Control	13.7 ± 0.6	0.84 ± 0.03
		Deficient	1.6 ± 0.1	0.76 ± 0.03

[a]Dow and Goldberg (1975); N = 6; data expressed as mean ± SD.
[b]Significantly different from respective control group.
[c]Kuenzig et al. (1977); N = 6–16; data expressed as mean ± SD.
[d]Omaye and Turnbull (1979b); N = 15–18; data expressed as mean ± SEM.
[e]Peterson et al. (1983a); N = 9–10; data expressed as mean ± SEM.

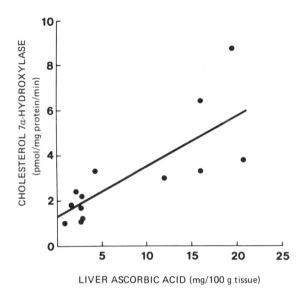

Figure 1 Correlation between hepatic microsomal cholesterol 7α-hydroxylase activity and liver ascorbic acid concentration in guinea pigs (r = 0.79, P < 0.01). (From Holloway and Rivers, 1981.)

health benefits (Pauling, 1970), study of the effects of excessive vitamin C intake on MFO activity appears warranted.

Sato and Zannoni (1974) have reported that supplementation of ascorbic acid in excess of the guinea pig's requirement for the vitamin (approximately 5 mg/day) (National Research Council, 1972) results in a dose-dependent enhancement of hepatic drug metabolism. However, data supporting this conclusion are confounded by the use of different dietary treatments and different routes of vitamin C administration, so that the intake of ascorbic acid was not the only variable. More recent studies, carefully regulating the amount of ascorbic acid in the diet, have failed to demonstrate the existence of a dose-response relationship between drug-metabolizing enzyme activities and ascorbic acid (Sikic et al., 1977a; Peterson et al., 1983a). However, when hepatic microsomal cytochrome P-450 content and hepatic ascorbate concentration were correlated among chronically deficient, control, and excess guinea pigs, a statistically significant relationship was obtained (Figure 2). The biological importance of the increase in cytochrome P-450 between control and excess groups is open to question since it was unaccompanied by any increase in drug-metabolizing enzyme activity.

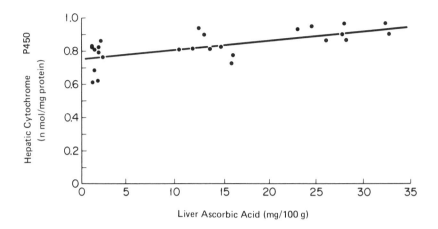

Figure 2 Correlation between hepatic microsomal cytochrome P-450 content and liver ascorbic acid concentration ($r = 0.66$, $P < 0.001$). (From Peterson et al., 1983a.)

Unlike other components of the MFO system, cholesterol 7α-hydroxylase activity was markedly depressed by excessive ascorbate consumption (Holloway and Rivers, 1981; Peterson et al., 1983a). Depressed cholesterol 7α-hydroxylase activity occurred despite the absence of any significant difference in cytochrome P-450 content between control and excess animals. The mechanism of this effect of ascorbic acid is unknown, but it is interesting that another biological antioxidant, vitamin E, when consumed in excess, also depresses cholesterol 7α-hydroxylase activity (Kritchevsky et al., 1980).

In contrast to the chronic consumption of excessive dietary ascorbic acid, which, outside of an effect on cholesterol 7α-hydroxylase, appears to have only a very small effect on the hepatic microsomal MFO system, the acute administration of excessive ascorbic acid is reported to markedly alter various components of this system. Sutton et al. (1982) reported that oral administration of 150 mg of ascorbic acid to guinea pigs twice a day for 4 days significantly reduced levels of cytochromes P-450 and b_5 as well as activity of biphenyl-4-hydroxylase. Metabolism of ethylmorphine and ethoxyresorufin and the activity of NADPH-cytochrome c reductase were unaffected by this treatment. Decreases in microsomal heme occurred despite the fact that excessive ascorbate administration doubled the activity of δ-aminolevulinic acid synthetase and halved the activity of microsomal heme oxygenase.

Since the ascorbic acid intake of guinea pigs in the study of Sutton et al. (300 mg/day) was less than that in our study of excessive ascorbate intake (20 g ascorbate/kg diet or approximately 500 mg/day), it is

apparent that massive vitamin C overdosage does not invariably lead
to reductions in cytochrome content. Furthermore, Sutton et al. did
not report tissue or plasma levels of ascorbic acid, making it difficult
to compare results among studies. In contrast to the findings of Sutton et al. in the guinea pig, Kachole et al. (1978) found that acute
vitamin C administration to rats (250 mg/kg intraperitoneally for 3
days) very markedly raised hepatic microsomal cytochrome levels and
enzyme activities. Holloway's group (unpublished) found no effect of
chronic consumption of excess ascorbic acid (20 g ascorbate/kg diet)
upon cholesterol 7α-hydroxylase activity in the rat. As discussed above,
this enzyme is especially sensitive to excessive dietary ascorbate in the
guinea pig. More work is required to sort out conflicting results among
experiments that differ in species of animal used, amount of vitamin C
administered, route of administration, MFO component(s) studied, and
length of the experimental period.

4. Stimulation of Ascorbic Acid Synthesis by Foreign Compounds

In 1940, Longenecker et al. reported that a wide variety of chemically
unrelated drugs, when administered to rats, caused a marked stimulation of urinary ascorbic acid excretion, presumably as a consequence
of accelerated ascorbate biosynthesis. The authors summarized current
literature demonstrating a protective effect of the vitamin when coadministered with a variety of toxic compounds, and suggested that drug-
induced stimulation of ascorbate synthesis may be "a protective mechanism available to the animal against foreign toxic substances." It is
quite surprising to note, more than 40 years later, that this hypothesis
remains untested despite its obvious potential biochemical and clinical
significance.

Recent studies have provided a new understanding of the control of
drug-metabolizing enzymes, directly relevant to the subject under discussion. Nebert et al. (1981) have characterized the "pleiotypic response" by which means the organism responds to certain foreign compounds that enter the body. This response is best understood for
polycyclic aromatic hydrocarbons (such as 3-methylcholanthrene, benzo[a]pyrene, and 2,3,7,8-tetrachlorodibenzo-p-dioxin) which induce
drug-metabolizing enzyme activities regulated by the Ah locus (Nebert
et al., 1981). Introduction of one of these compounds into the body
causes the activation of multiple structural genes and subsequent induction of diverse metabolic pathways, such as the hepatic microsomal
mixed-function oxidase system (Conney et al., 1957); drug conjugation
with glucuronic acid (Hollman and Touster, 1962); and in animals that
possess the enzyme L-gulonolactone oxidase, ascorbic acid synthesis
(Conney and Burns, 1959). Barbital and phenobarbital, but not 3-
methylcholanthrene or benzo[a]pyrene, also increase glucuronic acid
synthesis and urinary excretion (Touster and Hollman, 1961; Lake et
al., 1976). An intriguing and potentially important question is whether

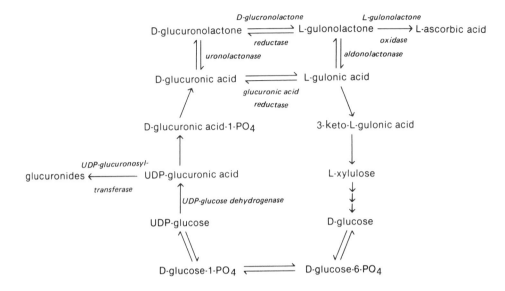

Figure 3 Glucuronic acid pathway.

induction of ascorbate biosynthesis is an *incidental* or *integral* component of the pleiotypic response to drug administration. Does accelerated
ascorbate synthesis serve to protect the organism from harmful effects
of xenobiotics, as do increases in MFO activity and glucuronide formation, which (for the most part) speed the removal of compounds from
the body? For if acceleration of ascorbate synthesis is indeed integral
to the organismal response to potentially dangerous foreign compounds,
then humans and other species dealt decks full but for the absence of
the solitary card, L-gulonolactone oxidase, have a dual genetically
based biological liability—not only the well-known susceptibility to the
disease caused by dietary lack of this vitamin, but also an inability to
respond fully, as can ascorbate-synthesizing species, to environmental
insult in the form of xenobiotic ingestion or administration.

One important component of ascorbic acid's role in drug metabolism
is the effect of inducing agents on the enzymatic pathway leading to ascorbic acid synthesis. Ascorbic acid is synthesized from glucose via
the glucuronic acid pathway, as depicted in Figure 3. In 1961, Conney et al. demonstrated that Chloretone stimulation of glucuronic acid
and ascorbic acid excretion in the rat was due to increased activity of
UDP-glucose dehydrogenase, while other enzyme activities between D-
glucose and L-ascorbic acid were either unchanged or decreased.
Chloretone has also been shown to increase the activity of this enzyme
in the guinea pig (Holloman and Touster, 1962). Horio and Yoshida

(1982) recently confirmed that xenobiotics (PCB,DDT) increase the activity of UDP-glucose dehydrogenase but not L-gulonolactone oxidase in the rat. They further documented a good correlation between hepatic ascorbate concentration and UDP-glucose dehydrogenase activity in rats fed a variety of inducing agents.

In agreement with the findings of Conney et al. (1961), Touster and Hollman (1961) found that Chloretone and barbital pretreatment of rats increased the activity of UDP-glucose dehydrogenase. These investigators further discovered that stimulation of ascorbate synthesis by benzo[a]pyrene and 3-methylcholanthrene was associated with increased activity not of UDP-glucose dehydrogenase but, instead, of UDP-glucuronosyltransferase (Hollman and Touster, 1962). They concluded that there may be two classes of chemicals which induce the synthesis of glucuronic and ascorbic acids. Similarly, Chakraborty et al. (1978b). reported that the increased urinary ascorbic acid excretion resulting from administration of parathion or malathion to rats was associated with an increase in L-gulonolactone oxidase activity; UDP-glucose dehydrogenase was not assayed in this experiment.

If acceleration of ascorbate synthesis is an integral component of the pleiotypic response to drug administration, ascorbate synthesis and mixed-function oxidase activity should be governed by a common regulatory mechanism. Several authors have reasoned, based on the parallel activities of ascorbate synthesis and the MFO system following drug administration, that an inhibitor of one system should similarly affect the other. This has in fact been demonstrated. Hoffman et al. (1966) showed that the alkaloid lycorine, when administered to rats, reduced both drug-metabolizing enzyme activity and ascorbate synthesis. Renton et al. (1979) demonstrated that interferon-inducing agents suppress the induction of both ascorbate synthesis and MFO activity resulting from phenobarbital or 3-methylcholanthrene administration. Additionally, studies by Kato, Yoshida, and co-workers have documented parallel alterations in MFO activity and urinary ascorbic acid excretion with changes in dietary protein level (Kato et al., 1980) and quality (Kato et al., 1981b) and dietary content of sulfur amino acids (Kato et al., 1982).

Thus available evidence suggests that acceleration of ascorbate synthesis following drug administration may be an important rather than an incidental component of the organismal response to environmental challenge. The fact that some drugs (e.g., Chloretone, barbital) stimulate ascorbate synthesis through induction of UDP-glucose dehydrogenase, whereas others (e.g., the organophosphorus insecticides) do so by other means (L-gulonolactone oxidase induction) raises the intriguing possibility that there are separate mechanisms by which drugs stimulate ascorbate synthesis. Extension of present knowledge of regulation of drug metabolism (Nebert et al., 1981) to include drug effects on ascorbic acid synthesis may prove enlightening.

If increased ascorbate synthesis is of value to the rat (and other species) in the face of xenobiotic challenge, the question remains: What function does an increased supply of ascorbic acid serve? Since other components of the pleiotypic response to drug administration tend to protect the organism against potential drug toxicity through increased drug metabolism (MFO system) and conjugation (UDP-glucuronosyl-transferase), thereby hastening drug excretion, it is logical to ask whether increased ascorbic acid biosynthesis also exerts a protective function following drug exposure. Two possible protective mechanisms for ascorbic acid are: (1) acceleration of xenobiotic transformation to more readily excreted metabolites, or (2) chemical interaction with the xenobiotic or its toxic metabolites, thereby preventing damage to cellular macromolecules. The first possibility is clearly true with respect to ascorbic acid administration to ascorbate-deficient guinea pigs (Section III.A.1). However, administration of large doses of vitamin C to guinea pigs adequately supplied with the vitamin does not further increase drug-metabolizing enzyme activity (Section III.A.3). In contrast, large doses of ascorbic acid administered to rats on a short-term basis have been reported to increase markedly hepatic microsomal cytochrome levels and MFO activities (Kachole et al., 1978). This intriguing observation warrants further study. Ascorbic acid protection against the toxicity of foreign compounds is discussed in the following section.

5. Ascorbic Acid as a Chemical Entity in the Detoxification of Foreign Compounds

Perhaps one of the most intriguing ways in which ascorbic acid participates in the detoxification of foreign compounds is through simple chemical interaction with toxic substances in the body. In recent years there has been a tremendous increase in interest in the use of ascorbic acid as a protectant against the toxicities of an extraordinarily wide range of chemical substances. Two approaches to this subject have been employed. A number of studies have investigated the toxicity of chemicals in ascorbic acid-deficient guinea pigs (Table 7), while many more studies have investigated the effects of large doses of ascorbic acid on chemical toxicity in a number of species (Table 8).

From Tables 7 and 8 it is evident that ascorbic acid administration affords protection against the toxicities of many different chemicals. Protective effects of ascorbic acid have been documented both for ascorbate-requiring species (guinea pig) and ascorbate-synthesizing species (rat, mouse, chicken, Japanese quail). Data summarized in Table 7 demonstrate that ascorbate-deficient guinea pigs are much more sensitive to toxic chemicals than are guinea pigs supplied with adequate dietary ascorbate. In addition to the chemicals listed, phenobarbital has also been reported to be more toxic in vitamin C-deficient animals than in controls (Degkwitz and Staudinger, 1974). Although in-

Table 7 Ascorbic Acid Effects on Chemical Toxicity Studied in Vitamin C-Deficient Guinea Pigs

Chemical administered	Ascorbate effect on toxicity	Measured response	Duration of ascorbate deficiency (days)	Ascorbate dose[a] (mg)	Reference
Chloroform	→	Mortality	16	30 (s.c.)	Beyer et al. (1944)
Diethyl ether	→	Mortality	16	30 (s.c.)	Beyer et al. (1944)
Hydrazine sulfate	→	Liver histopathology	20	30 (s.c.)	Beyer (1943)
Theophylline	→	Mortality	16–20	20 (p.o.)	Axelrod et al. (1954)
Vinyl ether	→	Mortality	16	30 (s.c.)	Beyer et al. (1944)

[a]p.o., per os; s.c., subcutaneously.

Table 8 Ascorbic Acid Effects on Chemical Toxicity In Vivo: Super-
Requisite Dosages[a]

Chemical administered	Ascorbate effect on toxicity	Measured response
Drugs:		
Acetaminophen	↓	Mortality
	↓	Hepatotoxicity
Adriamycin	↓	Mortality, cardio-myopathy
	↓	Mortality
Cocaine	↓	Hepatotoxicity
Ethanol	↓	Mortality
	↓	Mortality
Neoarsphenamine	↓	Mortality, renal toxicity
Pentylenetetrazol	→	Mortality
Picrotoxin	→	Mortality
Strychnine	↓	Mortality
Amines, nitrite, nitro-samines:		
Aminopyrine + $NaNO_2$	↓	Hepatotoxicity
	↓	Hepatotoxicity
Dimethylamine + $NaNO_2$	↓	Hepatotoxicity
Dimethylnitrosamine	→	Hepatotoxicity
	→	Hepatotoxicity
Alcohol and tobacco toxi-cants:		
Acetaldehyde	↓	Mortality
	↓	Mortality
Acetaldehyde + caffeine	↓	Mortality
Acetaldehyde + dopamine	↓	Mortality
Acetaldehyde + nicotine	↓	Mortality
Acrolein	↓	Mortality
Cyanide	↓	Mortality
	↓ / →	Mortality
Formaldehyde	↓	Mortality
Nicotine	↓	Mortality
	→	Mortality

Ascorbate dose[b] (mg/kg BW[c])	Species	Reference
200 (i.p.)	Mouse	Raghuram et al (1978)
2 × 1000 (i.p.)	Mouse	Peterson et al. (1983c)
300 mg/kg diet + 143 or 835 (i.p.)	Guinea Pig	Fujita et al. (1982)
200 (i.p.)	Mouse	Fujita et al. (1982)
2 × 1000 (i.p.)	Mouse	Peterson et al. (1983c)
25 mg (i.p.)	Mouse	Yunice and Lindeman (1977)
99 (i.p.)	Rat	Yunice and Lindeman (1977)
39-813 (i.v./i.m.)	Rat	McChesney et al. (1944)
−	Mouse	Dey (1967)
−	Mouse	Dey (1967)
50-2000 (i.p.)	Mouse	Dey (1967)
5-70 mg (p.o.)	Rat	Kamm et al. (1973)
10 and 20 mg (p.o.)	Mouse	Greenblatt (1973)
22-720 (p.o.)	Rat	Cardesa et al. (1974)
20 mg (p.o.)	Mouse	Greenblatt (1973)
360 (p.o.)	Rat	Cardesa et al. (1974)
352 (p.o.)	Rat	Sprince et al. (1975)
176-528 (p.o.)	Rat	Sprince et al. (1977)
176-528 (p.o.)	Rat	Sprince et al. (1981)
176-528 (p.o.)	Rat	Sprince et al. (1981)
176-528 (p.o.)	Rat	Sprince et al. (1981)
176-528 (p.o.)	Rat	Sprince et al. (1979)
18-528 (p.o.)	Rat	Sprince et al. (1982)
18-528 (i.p.)	Rat	Sprince et al. (1982)
176-528 (p.o.)	Rat	Sprince et al. (1979)
200 mg + 200 mg cysteine (diet)	Rat	Hueper (1943)
2 × 20 (i.m.)	Mouse	Taber and Larson (1964)

Table 8 (Continued)

Chemical administered	Ascorbate effect on toxicity	Measured response
Environmental contam- inants: PCB	↓ → / ↓ ↓	Growth rate Growth rate (→); liver histopathology (↓) Growth rate
Insecticides/herbi- cides: Chlordane	↓	Growth rate, mortality, liver and kidney histo- pathology
Malathion	↓	Growth rate
Parathion	↓	Growth rate
Paraquat	↓	Mortality, lung dam- age
Other organic com- pounds, oxygen: Carbon tetrachloride	↓	Gonadal inhibition
Mineral spirits (inhalation)	↓	Mortality
Oxygen, hyperbaric	↓ ↓	Lung damage, pento- barbital-induced pa- ralysis Seizure activity, mor- tality
Tetanus toxin	↓	Mortality
Vitamin A overdose	↑	Mortality
Heavy metals: Cadmium	↓	Growth rate, anemia
	↓	Growth rate, anemia
	↓ ↓	Growth rate anemia Growth rate, anemia, histopathology in testes, bone marrow, duodenum, adrenal, esophagus, heart, RBC
	↓	Growth rate, anemia

Ascorbate dose[b] (mg/kg BW[c])	Species	Reference
50 and 2000 mg/kg diet	Guinea pig	Kato et al. (1977)
200 (p.o.)	Rat	Chakraborty et al. (1978a)
30–2000 mg/kg diet	Guinea pig	Kato et al. (1981a)
200 (p.o.)	Rat	Chatterjee et al. (1981)
200 (p.o.)	Rat	Chakraborty et al. (1978b)
200 (p.o.)	Rat	Chakraborty et al. (1978b)
15 mg	Mouse	Barabas and Suveges (1978)
2 × 1000 (i.m.)	Rat	Chatterjee (1967)
600 and 20,000 mg/kg diet	Guinea pig	Jenkins et al. (1971)
1500 (i.p.)	Rat	Jamieson and van den Brenk (1964)
2112 (i.p.)	Mouse	Schatz and Lal (1980)
2 × 1000 (i.p.)	Rat	Dey (1966)
1-4 × 100 (i.p./p.o.) or 1000 (i.p.)	Rat	George et al. (1978)
0.5-10 g/kg diet	Japanese quail	Fox and Fry (1970)
1-10 g/kg diet	Japanese quail	Fox et al. (1971)
100 (p.o.)	Rat	Chatterjee et al. (1973)
10 g/kg diet	Japanese quail	Richardson et al. (1974)
1 g/kg diet	Chicken	Hill (1979)

Table 8 (Continued)

Chemical administered	Ascorbate effect on toxicity	Measured response
Cobalt	↓	Growth rate, mortality
	↓	Growth rate
Copper	↓	Growth rate
Lead	→	Anemia, kidney weight, and histopathology
	→	Growth rate, anemia
Mercury	→	Growth rate, organ weights
	→	Growth rate, kidney histopathology
	↑/→	Growth rate
Nickel	↓	Growth rate, renal histopathology, liver damage (assessed by SGOT)
Selenium	↓	Growth rate
Vanadium	↓	Mortality
	↓	Growth rate, mortality
	→/↓	(→): Growth rate, anemia; (↓): liver and kidney histopathology
	↓	Growth rate

[a]Super-requisite dosages: ascorbate doses in excess of amount normally required by organism (= any amount of exogenous ascorbate for ascorbate-synthesizing species).
[b]D.W., in drinking water; i.m., intramuscularly; i.p., intraperitoneally; i.v., intravenously; p.o., per os; s.c., subcutaneously.
[c]Unless otherwise noted.

creased toxicity might be anticipated in the face of decreased MFO activity in vitamin C deficiency, slowed drug metabolism and elimination cannot explain the toxic effects of these chemicals. Theophylline is normally metabolized by guinea pigs at the rate of 8% per hour; yet in the study of Axelrod et al. (1954), some scorbutic guinea pigs died within 1 hr following drug administration, before significant quantities of theophylline could have been eliminated from the body of normal animals.

Ascorbate dose[b] (mg/kg BW[c])	Species	Reference
2.5 g/kg diet	Chicken	Olson and Kienholz (1968)
1 g/kg diet	Chicken	Hill (1979)
1-10 g/kg diet	Chicken	Hill (1979)
100 (p.o.)	Rat	Rudra Pal et al. (1975)
10 g/kg diet	Rat	Suzuki and Yoshida (1979)
5 (po) and 1% (D.W.)	Guinea pig	Blackstone et al. (1974)
100 (p.o.)	Rat	Chatterjee and Rudra Pal (1975)
2-10 g/kg diet	Chicken	Hill (1979)
200 (p.o.)	Rat	Chatterjee et al. (1979)
0.02-1.1 g/kg diet	Chicken	Hill (1979)
0.125-1 (i.p.)	Mouse	Mitchell and Floyd (1954)
1.1-4.4 g/kg diet	Chicken	Berg and Lawrence (1971)
200 (p.o.)	Rat	Chakraborty et al. (1977)
0.25-2 g/kg diet	Chicken	Hill (1979)

With respect to the effect of ascorbic acid in ascorbate-synthesizing species, it is interesting to consider that tissue ascorbate levels in these animals are maintained under normal conditions at very high levels (Table 1). Nevertheless, it has repeatedly been demonstrated that ascorbate supplementation to these animals confers marked protection against a wide variety of chemical agents (Table 8). The mechanism(s) by which ascorbic acid exerts its protective effect is, for the most part, poorly understood. For several specific toxic reactions and classes of chemicals, however, recent studies have provided new in-

sight into vitamin C effects in detoxification. Probably the best understood role of ascorbate as a detoxifying agent is in the prevention of nitrosamine formation when nitrite and secondary or tertiary amines are
ingested together. Ascorbic acid very effectively blocks the reaction
but is ineffective against nitrosamines already formed (Table 8).

Fox et al. (1980) have determined that ascorbic acid exerts its major
effect on cadmium through an effect on dietary iron. Ascorbic acid ingestion increases iron absorption (Moore and Dubach, 1951) while iron
is protective against cadmium toxicity (Fox et al., 1971). Another
mechanism by which ascorbate may influence heavy metal toxicity is by
increasing urinary excretion of metals through formation of chelates;
this phenomenon has been documented for lead in the rat (Goyer and
Cherian, 1979).

A fundamental, but little studied, role for ascorbic acid in chemical
detoxification is the reaction of the vitamin with reactive intermediates
formed during the metabolic biotransformation of drugs. These reactive compounds, which can be highly toxic to living cells, are produced
in part by the microsomal MFO system. They include both chemically
modified foreign compounds and toxic metabolites generated through
oxygen activation. Active species of oxygen (e.g., superoxide, hydrogen peroxide) can be formed directly as a product of MFO activity
or through the interaction of oxygen with reactive intermediates generated by mixed-function oxidation of foreign compounds. Since the
reactive metabolites of a number of drugs are extremely labile and have
not been positively identified, it has been difficult to quantitate the
formation of these metabolites. However, the amount of radiolabeled
substrate irreversibly bound to microsomal protein has been used as a
means to measure the formation of these reactive intermediates. The
tissue damage that results from reactive intermediates appears to correlate well with the amount of covalently bound metabolite. For example, hepatic damage from a reactive metabolite of acetaminophen correlates well with the extent of covalent binding of the labeled parent
compound to hepatic microsomal protein (Potter et al., 1974).

Endogenous systems designed to protect the cell against such toxic
compounds include glutathione, glutathione peroxidase, catalase,
superoxide dismutase, epoxide hydrase, and glucuronosyltransferase,
all of which are capable of inactivating and accelerating the elimination
of these toxic metabolites. However, the capacity of these systems to
detoxify and eliminate foreign compounds and active oxygen can be
overwhelmed by the rapid and continuous production of reactive metabolites, with tissue injury or death the ultimate outcome. The protection afforded by ascorbic acid treatment against the toxicity of compounds that form reactive intermediates (e.g., acetaminophen, chloroform; see Table 8) suggests that ascorbic acid may play an important
role in the detoxification of these compounds. A number of experimental approaches have been utilized in the effort to determine the mechanism of this effect of vitamin C.

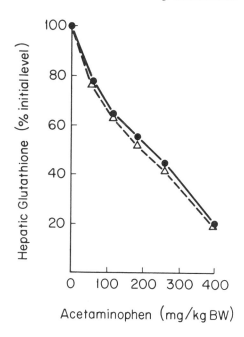

Figure 4 Acetaminophen-induced hepatic glutathione depletion in saline treated (circles) and ascorbic acid-treated (triangles) male CD-1 mice. Acetaminophen in basic saline and ascorbic acid (2000 mg/kg in saline) or saline were injected intraperitoneally in rapid succession. Mice were killed 2 hr later and hepatic glutathione levels quantitated. (From F. J. Peterson et al., 1983b).

In an attempt to elucidate the mechanism by which drugs stimulate urinary ascorbic acid excretion, Longenecker et al. (1940) searched for, but did not find, stable urinary conjugates of ascorbic acid and previously administered toxic agents. Studies with the analgesic agents phenacetin (Mulder et al., 1978) and acetaminophen (Corcoran et al., 1980) have confirmed that stable drug-ascorbate conjugates are not biologically synthesized. Thus conjugation with ascorbate has been ruled out as the mechanism by which ascorbic acid detoxifies reactive intermediates of foreign compounds.

An alternative approach to elucidation of the mechanism of ascorbate protection against chemical toxicity has been to compare the action of ascorbic acid with that of the important cellular nucleophile, glutathione. The central importance of reduced glutathione for cellular protection

against the reactive metabolites and peroxides resulting from administration of certain drugs is well established (Reed and Beatty, 1980).
A number of studies have demonstrated that ascorbic acid, like reduced
glutathione, is an effective protectant against drug-induced cell damage. Ascorbic acid exerts a protective effect against acetylphenylhydrazine-induced red cell destruction (Winterbourn, 1979; Williamson
and Winterbourn, 1980) and the covalent binding of reactive intermediates generated by MFO activation of a number of drugs (Mulder et al.,
1978; Andrews et al., 1979; Thorgeirsson et al., 1980; Nelson et al.,
1981; Lake et al., 1981). However, recent studies suggest that ascorbic acid and glutathione protect the cell by different mechanisms.
If these two compounds had similar modes of action, it would be expected that ascorbic acid supplementation prior to or at the time of
drug treatment would spare hepatic glutathione. As demonstrated in
Figure 4, however, depletion of glutathione by acetaminophen is not
altered by ascorbate treatment of the animals. Thus it appears that
ascorbic acid and glutathione contribute to drug detoxification in different ways.

Another possible mechanism of ascorbate detoxification is that ascorbate reduces reactive drug metabolites to less-reactive compounds,
thereby preventing reactions with cellular macromolecules and resultant cellular damage. Andrews et al. (1979) demonstrated that the addition of ascorbic acid to microsomal incubations with 2-acetylamino-
fluorene prevented the covalent binding of this compound to microsomal

Table 9 Effect of Ascorbic Acid on Serum Glutamate-Pyruvate Transaminase (SGPT) and Histological Score in Mice Treated with Acetaminophen[a]

Ascorbic acid (mg/g BW)	SGPT (IU /liter)	Histological score
0	7449 ± 754	3.7 ± 0.21
0.5	538 ± 115	—
1.0	215 ± 34	—
2.0	108 ± 19	0.83 ± 0.30

[a]Mice received an intraperitoneal injection of acetaminophen (425 mg/kg
body weight) in basic saline and a simultaneous intraperitoneal injection of ascorbic acid in saline. Mice receiving injections of saline without ascorbate plus basic saline without acetaminophen had SGPT activities of 68 ± 21. Data represent mean ± SEM of seven mice per group.
Severity of liver injury was scored 0 (normal) to 4 (most severe) on
coded and randomized liver sections from each animal.
Source: Peterson et al. (1983b).

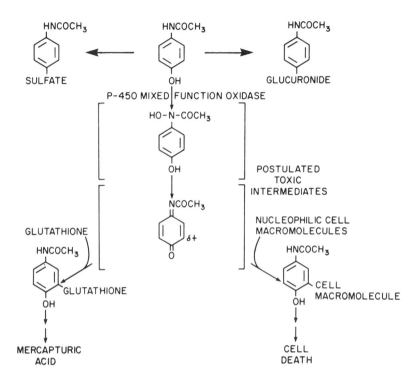

Figure 5 Proposed pathways of acetaminophen metabolism in vivo. Shown are the major routes of detoxification—sulfation and glucoronidation, and the minor pathway leading to the suggested toxic intermediate(s) of acetaminophen. (From Potter et al., 1974.)

protein. It was demonstrated that ascorbate reduces the reactive intermediate formed back to the parent compound. Similarly, Corcoran et al. (1980) showed that ascorbic acid inhibited the in vitro covalent binding of acetaminophen to microsomal protein by reducing the reactive intermediate of acetaminophen back to the parent compound. These in vitro studies provide strong evidence for the mechanism by which ascorbic acid limits the toxicity of drugs that generate reactive intermediates in vivo.

Recently, it has been demonstrated that the hepatic damage produced by acetaminophen and cocaine can be dramatically reduced by ascorbic acid (Peterson's group, unpublished results). As seen in Table 9, the administration of ascorbic acid, close to the time when the liver is exposed to the toxic influence of acetaminophen, confers significant protection against the activated parent compound. Furthermore,

Table 10 Effect of Ascorbic Acid on the Urinary Disposition of a Non-Toxic Dose of Acetaminophen in the Mouse[a]

	Total urinary metabolites (%)		
	Acetaminophen glucuronide	Acetaminophen sulfate	Acetaminophen (free)
Saline-treated mice	45.1 ± 4.0	28.1 ± 1.9	12.2 ± 2.0
Ascorbate-treated mice	53.5 ± 2.7	11.4 ± 1.8	28.9 ± 3.7

[a]A nontoxic dose of acetaminophen (50 mg/kg and 100 μCi/kg) was administered intraperitoneally in basic saline. Urinary metabolites were collected over dry ice and separated by thin-layer chromatography. Values are mean ± SEM for five mice in each group. Recovery of administered acetaminophen was >80%.
Source: Data from Peterson et al. (1983b).

ascorbic acid decreases acetaminophen-induced hepatotoxicity in a dose-dependent fashion. The hepatic damage from an overdose of acetaminophen is postulated to be the result of a reactive intermediate, N-acetyl-p-benzoquinoneimine, which is produced by the microsomal MFO system (Jollow et al., 1974). As represented schematically in Figure 5, the major portion of acetaminophen is detoxified and eliminated as a conjugate of glucuronic acid or sulfate, but a small quantity of the parent drug is metabolized by the cytochrome P-450 system to the reactive intermediate. Once this reactive intermediate has depleted the available stores of glutathione, the toxic metabolite binds to cellular macromolecules, causing cell damage and, ultimately, cell death. Ascorbic acid is postulated to interact with the toxic metabolite of acetaminophen sometime after glutathione is depleted but before the metabolite can bind to tissue macromolecules.

In their study of the interaction between acetaminophen and ascorbic acid in humans, Houston and Levy (1976b) suggested that ascorbic acid competes with acetaminophen for available sulfate in the body (with the consequent formation of ascorbate sulfate) and thereby decreases an important detoxification cofactor for acetaminophen inactivation and excretion. However, data from this study also demonstrate a significant increase in the amount of urinary free acetaminophen as well as an increase in the apparent half-life of the drug in ascorbate-treated subjects. These findings, together with previous in vitro data, raise the possibility that ascorbic acid functions by reducing reactive intermediates of acetaminophen back to the parent drug, thus increasing urinary excretion of the unmetabolized compound and prolonging acetaminophen's half-life in vivo. Recent studies in the mouse support this mechanism of ascorbate action (Peterson et al., 1983b). The data in Table 10 demonstrate that ascorbate treatment in mice dosed with acetaminophen markedly increases the excretion of free drug, supporting the hypothesis that ascorbate functions in vivo by reducing reactive intermediates of acetaminophen to the parent compound.

Ascorbic acid is also known to be an effective scavenger of superoxide, the toxic species produced by one-electron reduction of oxygen. Superoxide can be generated from the MFO system following the dissociation of the oxycytochrome P-450 complex (Peterson and Holtzman, 1980) or by the reduction of molecular oxygen by a free radical intermediate of drugs such as α-methyldopa (Dybing et al., 1976). Nishikimi (1975) has shown that ascorbic acid effectively reduces superoxide and may thus function as a defense against superoxide toxicity.

Recent in vivo studies in mice and guinea pigs have demonstrated that ascorbic acid significantly protects against the cardiotoxic effect of acute adriamycin administration (Fujita et al., 1982). Although the exact mechanism of adriamycin toxicity is unknown, it is thought that either a free radical intermediate of adriamycin or superoxide generated through interaction of a reactive intermediate and oxygen may be responsible (Mason, 1979). Ascorbate protection against adriamycin-induced cardiotoxicity is not easily explained by the latter mechanism, however. Mouse heart contains very little catalase and adriamycin administration decreases glutathione peroxidase activity (Doroshow et al., 1980); these enzymes are necessary to break down the hydrogen peroxide (also toxic) which is generated following reduction of superoxide. This makes it unlikely that ascorbate could *decrease* adriamycin toxicity by reducing superoxide to hydrogen peroxide in the mouse heart. A more likely mechanism of ascorbate action is through reduction of the reactive intermediate of adriamycin back to the parent compound.

Despite considerable progress in understanding the role of ascorbic acid in reducing the toxicities of some foreign compounds, very much remains to be learned about this exciting and important interaction. New information on this subject may well reveal important facets of ascorbic acid's biological function in vivo. On a more practical level, exploration of the use of ascorbate as a detoxifying agent in human medicine may lead to a simple, safe, and effective means to decrease toxicities associated with a wide spectrum of drugs and other foreign compounds.

B. Ascorbic Acid and Drug Metabolism in Man

Although a substantial body of information has accumulated in the literature exploring the effects of ascorbic acid nutriture on drug metabolism in the guinea pig, much less is known of the effects of ascorbic acid intake on drug metabolism in humans. Alteration of the rate of drug metabolism in humans by vitamin C deficiency may be of considerable clinical importance. Prolonged elevation of drug levels and prolonged drug effects would be anticipated if vitamin C-deficient humans, like vitamin C-deficient guinea pigs, have reduced rates of drug metabolism. Since symptomatic vitamin C deficiency (scurvy) is rare in industralized nations, the major problem of potential clinical significance is whether prolonged dietary inadequacy of vitamin C short of the scorbutic state (subclinical ascorbic acid deficiency) has important effects on drug metabolism in humans. The recent demonstration (Peterson et al., 1983a) that chronic marginal ascorbic acid deficiency, like acute ascorbic acid deficiency, depresses drug metabolism in guinea pigs raises the possibility of a similar effect in humans.

Three reports have, in fact, documented lower rates of drug metabolism in subjects with low vitamin C status. Beattie and Sherlock (1976) reported that four patients with liver disease having white blood cell ascorbate levels less than 100 nmol per 10^8 cells or (17.6 µg per 10^8cells) had greater antipyrine half-lives than 16 similar patients with higher white blood cell ascorbate levels. Smithard and Langman (1978) reported that vitamin supplementation of nine elderly subjects with low initial leukocyte ascorbate levels (mean 94.3 nmol per 10^8 cells or 16.6 µg per 10^8 cells) resulted in a 15% decrease in antipyrine half-life and a 24% increase in antipyrine clearance rate, whereas vitamin supplementation of 10 elderly subjects with higher leukocyte ascorbate levels (mean 213.4 nmol per 10^8 cells or 37.6 µg per 10^8 cells) did not alter the rate of antipyrine metabolism. Subjects were first studied shortly after admission to an acute geriatric ward and then 2 weeks after supplementation with a multivitamin preparation providing large doses of B vitamins and ascorbic acid (300 mg/day). Consequently, alteration of drug metabolism in the study of Smithard and Langman cannot be attributed conclusively to improved ascorbate status.

Ginter and Vejmolova (1981) studied the effect of ascorbic acid supplementation on antipyrine metabolism in diabetics with low initial serum ascorbate levels. The patients received either vitamin C (500 mg/day) or placebo for a period of 1 year, at which time antipyrine pharmacokinetics were determined. Vitamin C administration significantly increased serum vitamin C levels ($0.5-0.6$ mg/dl, placebo-treated; $1.3-1.4$ mg/dl, ascorbate-treated), and the vitamin C-treated group had significantly shorter antipyrine half-lives than did the placebo-treated group.

Two recent studies of experimental vitamin C depletion in healthy volunteers (Holloway et al., 1982a; Trang et al., 1982) have failed to demonstrate an effect of dietary vitamin C restriction on drug metabolism. Holloway et al. (1982a) studied antipyrine metabolism in five volunteers (ages 31–61) maintained on a controlled diet providing 3–4 mg of ascorbic acid per day. The subjects lived on a hospital metabolic ward for the duration of the study and antipyrine metabolism was measured during an initial control period (75 mg of supplemental ascorbate per day), after 28 and 63 days of vitamin C depletion (no ascorbate supplement given), and during a second control period (75 mg of supplemental ascorbate per day). Antipyrine metabolism was unaltered by vitamin C depletion despite attainment of a mean (± SEM) plasma ascorbate level of 0.12 ± 0.01 and a mean leukocyte level of 8.1 ± 0.6 µg per 10^8 cells at the conclusion of the depletion period. As discussed above (Section III.A.1), antipyrine half-life has previously been shown to be prolonged in ascorbic acid-deficient guinea pigs.

Similarly, Trang et al. (1982) failed to observe any change in caffeine pharmacokinetics in 10 elderly subjects (ages 66–86) who consumed diets containing approximately 15 mg ascorbic acid per day for 4 weeks. Plasma vitamin C levels (± SEM) at the end of the depletion period were 0.27 ± 0.04 mg/dl and leukocyte ascorbate levels were 10.0 ± 1.9 µg per 10^8 cells. The effect of vitamin C deficiency on caffeine metabolism in experimental animals has not been documented.

Controlled studies of vitamin C depletion in humans thus have not confirmed earlier reports (Beattie and Sherlock, 1976; Smithard and Langman, 1978; Ginter and Vejmolova, 1981) which suggest that human drug metabolism is ascorbate dependent. A possible explanation of this discrepancy is that acute depletion studies, despite attainment of low plasma and tissue ascorbate levels, do not duplicate the physiological effect of prolonged inadequate vitamin C intake (chronic marginal vitamin C deficiency). It is possible that long-term marginal vitamin C deficiency, with leukocyte ascorbate levels in the range 6–10 µg per 10^8 cells may result in impairment of drug metabolism, whereas attainment of similar ascorbate status in an acute depletion study is without effect. Further study of this clinically important question appears warranted.

Two studies have documented the effects of large doses of ascorbic acid upon antipyrine metabolism in normal human subjects (Wilson et al., 1976; Houston, 1977). Wilson et al. (1976) reported that administration of 0.3–4.8 g of ascorbic acid per day for 7–14 days did not alter the rate of antipyrine metabolism in healthy volunteers. In contrast, Houston (1977) reported that administration of 1 g of ascorbate acid per day for 7 days resulted in a 21% decrease in antipyrine half-life and a 25% increase in the total body clearance of antipyrine. No data on the ascorbic acid levels before or after supplementation were presented in either study.

Alternative mechanisms by which ascorbic acid may alter drug metabolism and disposition have also been investigated. Hansten and

Hayton (1980) studied the effect of ascorbic acid supplementation (3 g/ day) on the renal clearance and plasma plateau level of salicylate, since alteration of urinary pH changes the clearance and blood levels of this drug. Ascorbic acid at the dosage tested did not significantly alter urine pH, nor did it affect renal excretion or blood levels of salicylate. Houston and Levy (1975) have shown that ascorbic acid (3/g dose) alters the metabolism of salicylamide. Ascorbate supplementation decreased excretion of the drug as the sulfate conjugate, with a corresponding increase in salicylamide glucuronide excretion. These authors have documented a similar phenomenon when acetaminophen and ascorbic acid (3 g) are administered concomitantly (Houston and Levy 1976b). It is clear from this work that ascorbic acid administration can alter rates of drug metabolism quite independently of its effect on the hepatic microsomal mixed-function oxidase system.

IV. OVERVIEW: ASCORBIC ACID ROLE IN XENOBIOTIC METABOLISM AND TOXICITY

In the day-to-day challenge of surviving in modern environments, the ancient (Visser, 1980), ubiquitous, and poorly understood molecule ascorbic acid cuts a swath through drugs, heavy metals, environmental contaminants, and other foreign compounds as a double-edged sword, functioning both to maintain normal rates of drug metabolism and to protect against the toxicities that result from many of these chemical substances. In fact, these two functions are intimately linked in ascorbate-synthesizing species which are capable of responding to xenobiotic insult not only with induction of hepatic drug-metabolizing enzyme activity, but also with acceleration of an already rapid pace of ascorbate biosynthesis (Burns et al., 1954), the latter response potentially conferring additional protection against toxic chemicals and their metabolites.

Unfortunately, humans are not numbered among the ranks of the ascorbate synthesizers. As a consequence, we must prepare to face the prospect that the biochemical flaw which is responsible has compromised our safety in the present-day chemical environment. How ironic to think that we, who are founders of cities, builders of machines, and inventors of compounds not before known, we alone of the myriad denizens of the urban landscape may be unable to respond fully to the environmental assault of potentially toxic compounds which we ourselves have largely created. Mercifully, this judgment must await future research. Much remains to be done, much to be learned, in establishing fully the interaction between vitamin C and foreign compounds. Why do rats respond to certain chemicals with increased ascorbate synthesis? Is this response beneficial to the organism? Are guinea pigs protected more fully against inducers of the pleiotypic response when ascorbate is coadministered? An additional aspect of the problem not dealt with in this review is the potential role of ascorbic acid in the prevention of cancer and/or birth defects. This relationship comes to light when one considers that many inducers of MFO activity and ascorbate synthesis (e.g., 3-methylcholanthrene, benzo[a]-pyrene, TCDD) are carcinogenic, mutagenic, or teratogenic. Would we have greater immunity to these life-threatening conditions were we, like the rat, capable of synthesizing ascorbate and responding to environmental challenge with acceleration of this process? If so, currently recommended intakes for vitamin C, based on the amount of ascorbate necessary to prevent scurvy and maintain adequate reserves (National Research Council, 1980), may fall short of the amount required for optimal health in a chemically complex environment.

Optimal health for humans would appear to require, among other things, intake of an optimal amount of vitamin C. Unfortunately, just what this optimal intake might be is unknown even for the guinea pig, much less for us. Nevertheless, with advancing knowledge of vitamin C requirements and functions, a better understanding of the biologic effects of ascorbic acid over a wide range of dietary intakes is developing. At least two aspects of vitamin C requirements must be considered: (1) the requirement for normal or optimal functioning of the organism, and (2) the requirement for vitamin C in the face of environmental challenge (e.g., xenobiotic ingestion).

A. Ascorbic Acid Requirement for Normal Function

A wide variety of biologic parameters have been examined in the effort to quantitate the guinea pig's requirement for vitamin C. Early work, reviewed by Mannering in 1949, focused on the minimum amount of vitamin C necessary to prevent all signs of scurvy in the guinea pig. While 0.5 mg/day was sufficient to prevent macroscopic scurvy, dosages of 2−3 mg/day were found necessary to prevent signs of microscopic scurvy (especially evident in tooth formation) and to promote normal rates of wound healing (Mannering, 1949). Veen-Baigent et al. (1975) studied the influence of ascorbate intake on a variety of biologic parameters over a much wider dosage range than was employed in these early studies. Guinea pigs were maintained for 6−8 weeks on ascorbic acid intakes ranging from 0.05 to 100 mg/per 100 g body weight per day. Maximal growth rates were observed in guinea pigs fed 50 or 100 mg of ascorbate per 100 g body weight, although the differences among groups were not significant by the statistical test employed at intakes greater than 0.15 mg per 100 g body weight. Additional parameters studied by these authors included organ weights, hematocrit, hemoglobin, serum iron and trace elements, serum lipids, wound healing, and the proline, hydroxyproline, and glycine content of regenerated skin. Based on the results of this study, the authors concluded

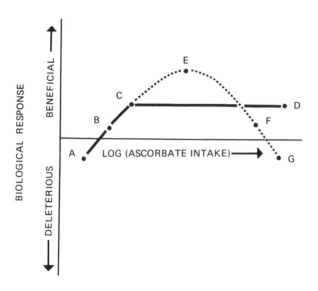

Figure 6 Hypothetical schema representing two possible biological response patterns to increasing ascorbic acid intake: plateau response
(A-B-C-D) and parabolic response (A-B-C-E-F-G). Influence of ascorbate intake on biological function: A, clinical disease (overt deficiency); B, low-normal function (subclinical deficiency); C and D,
maximal response of parameter 1 (optimal intake   and excessive intake, respectively); E, maximal response of parameter 2 (optimal intake); F, low-normal function (excessive intake); G, clinical disease
(excessive intake). (Modified from Holloway, 1980.)

that an ascorbic acid intake of 0.5 mg per 100 g body weight per day
supported maximal response of the wide variety of parameters studied.
Higher intakes were considered to confer no additional benefit. Yew
(1973), in contrast, demonstrated improved recovery time following
anesthesia and increased levels of proline and hydroxyproline in scar
tissue in guinea pigs fed 5.0 versus 0.5 mg of ascorbate per 100 g
body weight per day. Growth rates also were higher at the higher
dosage level but not significantly so. No further improvement was observed when the ascorbate dosage was increased to 50 mg per 100 g
body weight.
    Recent studies relevant to the question of the guinea pig's require-
ment for vitamin C include investigation of biologic functions dependent on the hepatic microsomal mixed-function oxidase system (e.g.,
drug metabolism, bile acid synthesis). How do these systems respond
to increasing ascorbic acid intake? Response of drug-metabolizing en-

zyme activity to increasing dietary ascorbate is straightforward: both acute and chronic vitamin C deficiency depress MFO activity; control animals (e.g., those fed 2 mg of ascorbate per 100 g body weight or 500 mg of ascorbate/kg diet) have significantly higher activity; and further increase in ascorbate intake (15–50 mg/100 g body weight or 20,000 mg/kg diet) does not further raise drug-metabolizing enzyme activity (Peterson et al., 1983a). This response is represented by curve A-B-C-D in Figure 6.

In contrast, a much more complex dependence of cholesterol 7α-hydroxylase activity and bile acid synthesis on ascorbate has been described. As is true for drug-metabolizing enzyme activity, both acute and chronic vitamin C deficiency depress cholesterol 7α-hydroxylase activity and bile acid synthesis; higher activities are observed in guinea pigs fed control amounts of ascorbic acid (e.g., 500 mg/kg diet) (Section III.A.1 and 2). In contrast to ascorbate effects on drug-metabolizing enzymes, however, a further increase in dietary ascorbate to 20 mg per 100 g body weight (Holloway et al., 1982b) or 5000 mg/kg diet (Ginter et al., 1979) results in further acceleration of the rate of bile acid synthesis. Continued increase in ascorbate intake into the range of massive vitamin C overdose—65 mg per 100 g body weight (Holloway et al., 1982b) or 20,000 mg/kg diet (Holloway and Rivers, 1981; Holloway et al., 1981b)—paradoxically causes a marked inhibition of cholesterol 7α-hydroxylase activity and bile acid synthesis in guinea pigs fed the Krehl cereal-based, scorbutigenic diet. This response is represented in Figure 6 by curve A-B-C-E-F-G, in which point E represents maximal activity at a hypothetical optimal vitamin C dosage.

Presently available evidence thus suggests that these two systems—the drug-metabolizing enzyme system and the bile acid synthetic pathway—have very different vitamin C requirements for maximal activity. The large difference between vitamin C requirements for maximal activities of these two systems—both localized in hepatic microsomes—provides a graphic example of the difficulty involved in accurately assessing an optimal intake of vitamin C for the guinea pig (or any other species). Clearly, the parameter measured has a crucial effect on the "optimal intake" established.

B. Influence of Xenobiotics on Ascorbic Acid Requirement

Tables 7 and 8 listed a host of chemicals whose toxicities are decreased by administration of vitamin C. Thus, when challenged by many foreign chemicals, organisms have an increased need for vitamin C to prevent or minimize chemical toxicity. This relationship has been examined in PCB-fed guinea pigs by Kato et al. (1981a). Guinea pigs not fed PCB exhibited similar growth rates over the 10- to 12-day experimental period whether fed 30, 200, 800, or 2000 mg of ascorbate/kg diet. However, PCB-fed guinea pigs required 800 mg/kg diet to attain the maximal growth rate. This intake is fourfold higher than the NRC recommendation of 200 mg/kg diet for guinea pigs, a level adequate for maximal growth in normal guinea pigs (National Research Council, 1972). Similarly, a dietary level of 800 mg of ascorbate/kg was found necessary to minimize lipid peroxidation in PCB-fed guinea pigs, whereas the extent of lipid peroxidation was similar in non-PCB-fed guinea pigs given diets containing 50 or 2000 mg of ascorbate/kg. These results demonstrate the protection afforded by administration of large doses of ascorbic acid to guinea pigs fed toxic compounds, and suggest that increased amounts of ascorbic acid are required in these circumstances for normal functions such as growth. From these data, it may be inferred that rats given foreign compounds also have an increased requirement for ascorbic acid. However, this requirement is simply met through acceleration of ascorbate biosynthesis. Humans and the guinea pig may be at a disadvantage compared to rats due to an inability to respond to xenobiotic challenge in this manner.

What are the implications for human health? It is possible that drugs and other xenobiotics which increase ascorbic acid synthesis in the rat increase the requirement for vitamin C following ingestion or administration to humans. The protective capability of ascorbic acid against drugs and foreign compounds as a means to improve human health remains to be explored and exploited.

ACKNOWLEDGMENT

The secreterial assistance of Ms. Lynn M. Povinelli is much appreciated.

REFERENCES

Abbott, V., Deloria, L., Guenthner, T., Jeffery, E., Kotake, A., Nerland, D., and Mannering, G. (1976). Comparison of hepatic microsomal drug-metabolizing systems from rats fed crude and purified diets. *Drug Metab. Dispos.* 4:215-222.

Alleva, F. R., Alleva, J. J., and Balazs, T. (1976). Effect of large daily doses of ascorbic acid on pregnancy in guinea pigs, rats, and hamsters. *Toxicol. Appl. Pharmacol.* 35:393-395.

Andrews, L. S., Fysh, J. M., Hinson, J. A., and Gillette, J. R. (1979). Ascorbic acid inhibits covalent binding of enzymatically generated 2-acetylaminofluorene-N-sulfate to DNA under conditions in which it increases mutagenesis in *Salmonella TA-1538*. *Life Sci.* 24:59-64.

Avenia, R. W. (1972). Studies on the role of ascorbic acid in the metabolism of drugs by the guinea pig hepatic microsomal mixed-function oxidase system. Ph.D. thesis, Cornell University, Ithaca, N. Y.

Axelrod, J., Udenfriend, S., and Brodie, B. B. (1954). Ascorbic acid in aromatic hydroxylation. III. Effect of ascorbic acid on hydroxylation of acetanilide, aniline and antipyrine in vivo. *J. Pharmacol. Exp. Ther. 111*:176-181.

Azarnoff, D. L. (1977). Insecticides: effect on drug metabolism. *Clin. Pharmacol. Ther. 22*:817-822.

Baker, E. M., Halver, J. E., Johnsen, D. O., Joyce, B. E., Knight, M. K., and Tolbert, B. M. (1975). Metabolism of ascorbic acid and ascorbic-2-sulfate in man and the subhuman primate. *Ann. N. Y. Acad. Sci. 258*:72-79.

Baker, H., Pauling, L., and Frank, O. (1981). Mega-ascorbate taken with other vitamins permits elevation of circulating vitamins including B_{12} in humans. *Nutr. Rep. Int. 23*:669-677.

Banerjee, S., Biswas, D. K., and Singh, H. D. (1959). Dehydrogenase activity of the tissues in scurvy. *J. Biol. Chem. 234*: 405-408.

Barabas, K., Suveges, G. (1978). The effect of reductant substances on the toxicity of paraquat. *Proc. Hung. Annu. Meet. Biochem. 18*:95-96.

Beattie, A. D., and Sherlock, S. (1976). Ascorbic acid deficiency in liver disease. *Gut 17*:571-575.

Becking, G. C. (1972). Influence of dietary iron levels on hepatic drug metabolism in vivo and in vitro in the rat. *Biochem. Pharmacol. 21*:1585-1593.

Berg, L. R., and Lawrence, W. W. (1971). Cottonseed meal, dehydrated grass and ascorbic acid as dietary factors preventing toxicity of vanadium for the chick. *Poult. Sci. 50*:1399-1404.

Beyer, K. H. (1943). Protective action of vitamin C against experimental hepatic damage. *Arch. Intern. Med. 71*:315-324.

Beyer, K. H., Stutzman, J. W., and Hafford, B. (1944). The relation of vitamin C to anesthesia. *Surg. Gynecol. Obstet. 79*: 49-56.

Bissel, D. M., and Guzelian, P. S. (1979). Ascorbic acid deficiency and cytochrome P-450 in adult rat hepatocytes in primary monolayer culture. *Arch. Biochem. Biophys. 192*:569-576.

Bjorkhem, I., and Kallner, A. (1976). Hepatic 7α-hydroxylation of cholesterol in ascorbate-deficient and ascorbate-supplemented guinea pigs. *J. Lipid Res. 17*:360-365.

Blackstone, S., Hurley, R. J., and Hughes, R. E. (1974). Some interrelationships between vitamin C (L-ascorbic acid) and mercury in the guinea pig. *Food Cosmet. Toxicol. 12*:511-516.

Bösterling, B., and Trudell, J. R. (1982). Association of cytochrome b5 and cytochrome P-450 reductase with cytochrome P-450 in the membrane of reconstituted vesicles. *J. Biol. Chem. 257*: 4783-4787.

Bresnick, E., Brosseau, M., Levin, W., Reik, L., Ryan, D. E., and Thomas, P. E. (1981). Administration of 3-methylcholanthrene to rats increases the specific hybridizable mRNA coding for cytochrome P-450c. *Proc. Natl. Acad. Sci. USA 78*:4083-4087.

Burns, J. J., Mosbach, E. H., and Schulenberg, S. (1954). Ascorbic acid synthesis in normal and drug-treated rats, studied with L-ascorbic-1-C^{14} acid. *J. Biol. Chem. 207*:679-687.

Burr, M. L., Elwood, P. C., Hole, D. J., Hurley, R. J., and Hughes, R. E. (1974). Plasma and leukocyte ascorbic acid levels in the elderly. *Am. J. Clin. Nutr. 27*:144-151.

Cardesa, A., Mirvish, S. S., Haven, G. T., and Shubik, P. (1974). Inhibitory effect of ascorbic acid on the acute toxicity of dimethylamine plus nitrite in the rat. *Proc. Soc. Exp. Biol. Med. 145*:124-128.

Carpenter, M. P. (1972). Vitamin E and microsomal drug hydroxylations. *Ann. N. Y. Acad. Sci. 203*:81-92.

Castro, J. A., Green, F. E., Gigon, P. L., Sasame, H., and Gillette, J. R. (1970). Effect of adrenalectomy and cortisone administration on components of the liver microsomal mixed function oxygenase system of male rats which catalyze ethylmorphine metabolism. *Biochem. Pharmacol. 19*:2461-2467.

Chadwick, R. W., Cranmer, M. F., and Peoples, A. J. (1971). Metabolic alterations in the squirrel monkey induced by DDT adminstration and ascorbic acid deficiency. *Toxicol. Appl. Pharmacol. 20*:308-318.

Chadwick, R., Peoples, A., and Cranmer, M. (1973). The effect of protein quality and ascorbic acid deficiency on stimulation of hepatic microsomal enzymes in guinea pigs. *Toxicol. Appl. Pharmacol. 24*:603-611.

Chakraborty, D., Bhattacharyya, A., Majumdar, K., and Chatterjee, G. C. (1977). Effects of chronic vanadium pentoxide administration on L-ascorbic acid metabolism in rats: influence of L-ascorbic acid supplementation. *Int. J. Vitam. Nutr. Res. 47*:81-87.

Chakraborty, D., Bhattacharyya, A., Chatterjee, J., Chatterjee, K., Sen, A., Chatterjee, S., Majumdar, K., and Chatterjee, G. C. (1978a). Biochemical studies on polychlorinated biphenyl toxicity in rats: manipulation by vitamin C. *Int. J. Vitam. Nutr. Res. 48*:22-31.

Chakraborty, D., Bhattacharyya, A., Majumdar, K., Chatterjee, K., Chatterjee, S., Sen, A., and Chatterjee, G. C. (1978b). Studies on L-ascorbic acid metabolism in rats under chronic toxicity due to organophosphorus insecticides: effects of supplementation of L-ascorbic acid in high doses. *J. Nutr. 108*:973-980.

Chatterjee, A. (1967). Role of ascorbic acid in the prevention of gonadal inhibition by carbon tetrachloride. *Endokrinologie 51*: 319-322.

Chatterjee, G. C., and Rudra Pal, D. (1975). Metabolism of L-ascorbic acid in rats under in vivo administration of mercury: effect of L-ascorbic acid supplementation. *Int. J. Vitam. Nutr. Res. 45*:284-292.

Chatterjee, G. C., Banerjee, S. K., and Rudra Pal, D. (1973). Cadmium administration and L-ascorbic acid metabolism in rats: effect of L-ascorbic acid supplementation. *Int. J. Vitam. Nutr. Res. 43*:370-377.

Chatterjee, K., Chakraborty, D., Majumdar, K., Bhattacharyya, A., and Chatterjee, G. C. (1979). Biochemical studies on nickel toxicity in weanling rats—influence of vitamin C supplementation. *Int. J. Vitam. Nutr. Res. 49*:264-275.

Chatterjee, K., Banerjee, S. K., Tiwari, R., Majumdar, K., Bhattacharyya, A., and Chatterjee, G. C. (1981). Studies on the protective effects of L-ascorbic acid in chronic chlordane toxicity. *Int. J. Vitam. Nutr. Res. 51*:254-265.

Collins, M., and Elvehjem, C. A. (1958). Ascorbic acid requirement of the guinea pig using growth and tissue ascorbic acid concentrations as criteria. *J. Nutr. 64*:503-511.

Conney, A. H., and Burns, J. J. (1959). Stimulatory effect of foreign compounds on ascorbic acid biosynthesis and on drug-metabolizing enzymes. *Nature 184*:363-364.

Conney, A. H., Miller, E. C., and Miller, J. A. (1957). Substrate-induced synthesis and other properties of benzpyrene hydroxylase in rat liver. *J. Biol. Chem. 228*:753-766.

Conney, A. H., Bray, G. A., Evans, C., and Burns, J. J. (1961). Metabolic interactions between L-ascorbic acid and drugs. *Ann. N. Y. Acad. Sci. 92*:115-127.

Corcoran, G. B., Mitchell, J. R., Vaishnav, Y. N., and Horning, E. C. (1980). Evidence that acetaminophen and N-hydroxy-acetaminophen form a common arylating intermediate, N-acetyl-p-benzoquinone. *Mol. Pharmacol. 18*:536-542.

Crandon, J. H., Lund, C. C., and Dill, D. B. (1940). Experimental human scurvy. *N. Engl. J. Med. 223*:353-369.

Danhof, M., Krom, D. P., and Breimer, D. D. (1979). Studies on the different metabolic pathways of antipyrine in rats: influence of phenobarbital and 3-methylcholanthrene treatment. *Xenobiotica 9*:695-702.

Danhof, M., Verbeek, R., Van Boxtel, C. J., Boeijinga, J. K., and Breimer, D. D. (1982). Differential effects of enzyme induction on antipyrine metabolite formation. *Br. J. Clin. Pharmacol. 13*:379-386.

Degkwitz, E., and Kim, K. S. (1973). Comparative studies on the influence of L-ascorbate, D-arabino-ascorbate and 5-oxo-D-gluconate on the amounts of cytochromes P-450 and b5 in liver microsomes of guinea pigs. *Hoppe-Seyler's Z. Physiol. Chem.* 354:555-561.

Degkwitz, E., and Staudinger, H. (1965). Untersuchungen zur Hydroxylierung von Acetanilid mit Lebermikrosomen normaler und skorbutischer Meerschweinchen. *Hoppe-Seyler's Z. Physiol. Chem.* 342:63-72.

Degkwitz, E., and Staudinger, H. (1974). Role of vitamin C on microsomal cytochromes. In *Vitamin C: Recent Aspects of its Physiological and Technological Importance*, G. S. Birch and K. J. Parker, Eds., Wiley, New York, pp. 161-178.

Degkwitz, E., Luft, D., Pfeiffer, U., and Staudinger, H. (1968). Untersuchungen über mikrosomale Enzymaktivitäten (Cumarinhydroxylierung, NADPH-Oxydation, Glucose-6-phosphatase und Esterase) und Cytochromgehalte (P-450 und b5) bei normalen, skorbutischen und hungernden Meerschweinchen. *Hoppe-Seyler's Z. Physiol. Chem.* 349:465-471.

Degkwitz, E., Leber, H. -W., Kaufman, L., and Staudinger, H. (1970). Studies on the apparent Michaelis constant of acetanilide during its p-hydroxylation in the liver microsomes of scorbutic guinea pigs. *Hoppe-Seyler's Z. Physiol. Chem.* 351:397-400.

Degkwitz, E., Hochli-Kaufmann, L., Luft, D., and Staudinger, H. (1972). Decrease of cytochrome contents and changes in the kinetics of the monooxygenase in liver microsomes of guinea pigs at different stages of L-ascorbic acid deficiency. *Hoppe-Seyler's Z. Physiol. Chem.* 353:1023-1033.

Degkwitz, E., Walsch, S., Dubberstein, M., and Winter, J. (1973). Influence of L-ascorbate on the contents of cytochromes P-450 and b5 in several organs of guinea pigs. *Enzyme* 16:237-245.

Degkwitz, E., Walsch, S., and Dubberstein, M. (1974). Influence of L-ascorbate on the concentrations of microsomal cytochrome P-450 and cytochrome b5 in adrenals, kidneys and spleen of guinea pigs. *Hoppe-Seyler's Z. Physiol. Chem.* 355:1152-1158.

Dey, P. K. (1966). Efficacy of vitamin C in counteracting tetanus toxin toxicity. *Naturwissenschaften* 53:310.

Dey, P. K. (1967). Protective action of ascorbic acid and its precursors on the convulsive and lethal actions of strychnine. *Indian J. Exp. Biol.* 5:110-112.

Doroshow, J. H., Locker, G. Y., and Myers, C. E. (1980). Enzymatic defenses of the mouse heart against reactive oxygen metabolites. *J. Clin. Invest.* 65:128-135.

Dow, J., and Goldberg, A. (1975). Ethanol metabolism in the vitamin C deficient guinea-pig. *Biochem. Pharmacol.* 24:863-866.

Dybing, E., Nelson, S. D., Mitchell, J. R., Sasame, H. A., and Gillette, J. R. (1976). Oxidation of α-methyldopa and other catechols by cytochrome P-450-generated superoxide anion: possible mechanism of methyldopa hepatitis. *Mol. Pharmacol.* 12: 911-920.

Encarnacion, D., Devine, M. M., and Rivers, J. M. (1974). Influence of vitamin C nutriture and inanition on ACTH stimulated release of adrenal corticosteroids in guinea pigs. *Int. J. Vitam. Nutr. Res.* 44:309-318.

Fielding, A. M., and Hughes, R. E. (1975). The absence of an inhibitory effect of metyrapone (2-methyl-1,2-di(3-pyridyl)propan-1-one) on hepatic microsomal hydroxylation in scurvy. *Experientia* 31:1394-1395.

Fordyce, M. K., and Kassouny, M. E. (1977). Influence of vitamin C restriction on guinea pig adrenal calcium and plasma corticosteroids. *J. Nutr.* 107:1846-1851.

Fox, F. W., and Levy, L. F. (1936). Experiments confirming the antiscorbutic activity of dehydroascorbic acid and a study of its storage and that of ascorbic acid by the guinea pig at different levels of intake. *Biochem. J.* 30:211-217.

Fox, M. R. S., and Fry, B. E., Jr. (1970). Cadmiun toxicity decreased by dietary ascorbic acid supplements. *Science* 169:989-991.

Fox, M. R. S., Fry, B. E., Jr., Harland, B. F., Schertel, M. E., and Weeks, C. E. (1971). Effect of ascorbic acid on cadmiun toxicity in the young coturnix. *J. Nutr.* 101:1295-1306.

Fox, M. R. S., Jacobs, R. M., Jones, A. O. L., Fry, B. E., Jr., and Stone, C. L. (1980). Effects of vitamin C and iron on cadmium metabolism. *Ann. N. Y. Acad. Sci.* 355:249-261.

Fujita, K., Shinpo, K., Yamada, K., Sato, T., Niimi, H., Shamoto, M., Nagatsu, T., Takeuchi, T., and Umezawa, H. (1982). Reduction of adriamycin toxicity by ascorbate in mice and guinea pigs. *Cancer Res.* 42:309-316.

Garattini, S., Guaitani, A., and Bartosek, I. (1973). Use of isolated perfused liver in the study of drug metabolism. In *Isolated Liver Perfusion and Its Applications*, I. Bartosek, A. Guaitani, and L. L. Miller, Eds., Raven Press, New York. pp. 225-234.

George, T., Bai, N. J., and Krishnamurthy, S. (1978). Ascorbic acid effect on hypervitaminosis A in rats. *Int. J. Vitam. Nutr. Res.* 48:233-239.

Gibaldi, M., and Perrier, D. (1975). *Pharmacokinetics*, Marcel Dekker, New York, pp. 1-17.

Gillette, J. R. (1971). Techniques for studying drug metabolism in vitro. In *Fundamentals of Drug Metabolism and Drug Disposition*, B. W. LaDu, H. G. Mandel, and E. L. Way, Eds., Williams & Wilkins, Baltimore, Md., pp. 400-418.

Ginter, E. (1958). L-ascorbic acid in protein metabolism. II. Nitrogen balance in the early stages of guinea pig avitaminosis. *Biologia (Bratislava)* *13*:45-52.

Ginter, E. (1978). Marginal vitamin C deficiency, lipid metabolism, and atherogenesis. *Adv. Lipid Res.* *16*:167-220.

Ginter, E., and Mikus, L. (1977). Reduction of gallstone formation by ascorbic acid in hamsters. *Experientia* *33*:716-717.

Ginter, E., and Vejmolova, J. (1981). Vitamin C-status and pharmacokinetic profile of antipyrine in man. *Br. J. Clin. Pharmacol.* *12*:256-258.

Ginter, E., Bobek, P., and Ovecka, M. (1968). Model of chronic hypovitaminosis C in guinea-pigs. *Int. J. Vitam. Nutr. Res.* *38*:104-113.

Ginter, E., Nemec, R., Cerven, J., and Mikus, L. (1973). Quantification of lowered cholesterol oxidation in guinea pigs with latent vitamin C deficiency. *Lipids* *8*:135-141.

Ginter, E., Bobek, P., and Vargova, D. (1979). Tissue levels and optimum dosage of vitamin C in guinea pigs. *Nutr. Metab.* *23*:217-226.

Ginter, E., Kosinova, A., Hudecova, A., and Madaric, A. (1982). Synergism between vitamin C and E: effect on microsomal hydroxylation in guinea pig liver. *Int. J. Vitam. Nutr. Res.* *52*:55-59.

Goyer, R. A., and Cherian, M. G. (1979). Ascorbic acid and EDTA treatment of lead toxicity in rats. *Life Sci.* *24*:433-438.

Greenblatt, M. (1973). Ascorbic acid blocking of aminopyrine nitrosation in NZO/B1 mice. *J. Natl. Cancer Inst.* *50*:1055-1056.

Grollman, A., and Firor, W. M. (1934). Studies on the adrenal. VII. The relation of the adrenal cortical hormone to the vitamins. *J. Nutr.* *8*:569-582.

Gundermann, K., Degkwitz, E., and Staudinger, H. (1973). Mixed function oxygenation of (+) and (−)-hexobarbital and spectral changes of cytochrome P-450 in the liver of guinea pigs fed without L-ascorbic acid. *Hoppe-Seyler's Z. Physiol. Chem.* *354*:238-242.

Halver, J. E., Smith, R. R., Tolbert, B. M., and Baker, E. M. (1975). Utilization of ascorbic acid in fish. *Ann. N. Y. Acad. Sci.* *258*:81-101.

Hanssen, I., Grav, H. J., Steen, J. B., and Lysnes, H. (1979). Vitamin C deficiency in growing willow ptarmigan (*Lagopus lagopus lagopus*). *J. Nutr.* *109*:2260-2278.

Hansten, P. D., and Hayton, W. L. (1980). Effect of antacid and ascorbic acid on serum salicylate concentration. *J. Clin. Pharmacol.* *20*:326-331.

Harris, W. S., Kottke, B. A., and Subbiah, M. T. R. (1979). Bile acid metabolism in ascorbic acid-deficient guinea pigs. *Am. J. Clin. Nutr.* *32*:1837-1841.

Hepner, G. W., and Vesell, E. S. (1974). Assessment of aminopyrine metabolism in man after oral administration of ^{14}C-aminopyrine. Effects of phenobarbital, disulfiram, and portal cirrhosis. *N. Engl. J. Med.* *291*:1384-1388.

Hill, C. H. (1979). Studies on the ameliorating effect of ascorbic acid on mineral toxicities in the chick. *J. Nutr.* *109*:84-90.

Hodges, R. E., Hood, J., Canham, J. E., Sauberlich, H. E., and Baker, E. M. (1971). Clinical manifestations of ascorbic acid deficiency in man. *Am. J. Clin. Nutr.* *24*:432-443.

Hoffman, D. G., Bousquet, W. F., and Miya, T. S. (1966). Lycorine inhibition of drug metabolism and ascorbic acid biosynthesis in the rat. *Biochem. Pharmacol.* *15*:391-393.

Hollman, S., and Touster, O. (1962). Alterations in tissue levels of uridine diphosphate glucose dehydrogenase, uridine diphosphate glucuronic acid pyrophosphatase and glucuronyl transferase induced by substances influencing the production of ascorbic acid. *Biochim. Biophys. Acta* *62*:338-352.

Holloway, D. E. (1980). The influence of ascorbic acid nutriture upon bile acid metabolism and bile composition in the guinea pig. Ph. D. thesis, Cornell University, Ithaca, N. Y.

Holloway, B. A. (1981). Kinetic analysis of ascorbic acid in the guinea pig. Master's thesis, Cornell University, Ithaca, N. Y.

Holloway, D. E., and Rivers, J. M. (1981). Influence of chronic ascorbic acid deficiency and excessive ascorbic acid intake on bile acid metabolism and bile composition in the guinea pig. *J. Nutr.* *111*:412-424.

Holloway, B. A., Holloway, D. E., and Rivers, J. M. (1981a). Influence of ascorbic acid intake upon kinetic parameters of ascorbate metabolism in the guinea pig. *Fed. Proc.* *40*:915.

Holloway, D. E., Peterson, F. J., Prigge, W. F., and Gebhard, R. L. (1981b). Influence of dietary ascorbic acid upon enzymes of sterol biosynthesis in the guinea pig. *Biochem. Biophys. Res. Commun.* *102*:1283-1289.

Holloway, D. E., Hutton, S. W., Peterson, F. J., and Duane, W. C. (1982a). Lack of effect of subclinical ascorbic acid deficiency upon antipyrine metabolism in man. *Am. J. Clin. Nutr.* *35*:917-924.

Holloway, D. E., Peterson, F. J., and Rivers, J. M. (1982b). Effects of dietary ascorbic acid on bile acid metabolism in guinea pigs fed Krehl or Reid-Briggs diets. *Nutr. Rep. Int.* *25*:941-951.

Holst, A., and Frohlich, T. (1907). Experimental studies relating to ship beriberi and scurvy. II. On the etiology of scurvy. *J. Hygiene* 7:634-671.

Horio, F., and Yoshida, A. (1982). Effects of some xenobiotics on ascorbic acid metabolism in rats. *J. Nutr.* 112:416-425.

Hornig, D. H., and Moser, U. (1981). The safety of high vitamin C intakes in man. In *Vitamin C (Ascorbic Acid)*, J. N. Counsell and D. H. Hornig, Eds., Applied Science Publishers, Englewood, N. J., pp. 225-248.

Houston, J. B. (1977). Effect of vitamin C supplement on antipyrine disposition in man. *Br. J. Clin. Pharmacol.* 4:236-239.

Houston, J. B., and Levy, G. (1975). Modification of drug biotransformation by vitamin C in man. *Nature* 255:78-79.

Houston, J. B., and Levy, G. (1976a). Effect of route of administration on competitive drug biotransformation interaction: salicylamide-ascorbic acid interaction in rats. *J. Pharmacol. Exp. Ther.* 198:284-294.

Houston, J. B., and Levy, G. (1976b). Drug biotransformation interactions in man. VI. Acetaminophen and ascorbic acid. *J. Pharm. Sci.* 65:1218-1221.

Hueper, W. C. (1943). Experimental studies in cardiovascular pathology. VII. Chronic nicotine poisoning in rats and in dogs. *Arch. Pathol.* 35:846-856.

Hughes, R. E., and Jones, P. R. (1970). D-Araboascorbic acid and guinea pig scurvy. *Nutr. Rep. Int.* 1:275-279.

Hughes, R. E., and Jones, P. R. (1971). The influence of sex and age on the deposition of L-xyloascorbic acid in tissues of guinea pigs. *Br. J. Nutr.* 25:77-83.

Imai, Y. (1981). The roles of cytochrome b_5 in reconstituted monooxygenase systems containing various forms of hepatic cytochrome P-450. *J. Biochem.* 89:351-362.

Jacobsen, E. (1935). On the storage of ascorbic acid in the organs of guinea pigs given crystalline ascorbic acid with a vitamin C-free diet. *Skand. Arch. Physiol.* 72:259-264.

Jamieson, D., and van den Brenk, H. A. S. (1964). The effects of antioxidants on high pressure oxygen toxicity. *Biochem. Pharmacol.* 13:159-164.

Jenkins, L. J., Jr., Coon, R. A., Lyon, J. P., and Siegel, J. (1971). Effect on experimental animals of long-term inhalation exposure to mineral spirits. II. Dietary, sex and strain influences in guinea pigs. *Toxicol. Appl. Pharmacol.* 18:53-59.

John, T. M., George, J. C., Hilton, J. W., and Slinger, S. J. (1979). Influence of dietary ascorbic acid on plasma lipid levels in the rainbow trout. *Int. J. Vitam. Nutr. Res.* 49:400-405.

Jollow, D. J., Thorgeirsson, S. S., Potter, W. Z., Hashimoto, M., and Mitchell, J. R. (1974). Acetaminophen-induced hepatic necrosis. VI. Metabolic disposition of toxic and nontoxic doses of acetaminophen. *Pharmacology* 12:251-271.

Kachole, M. S., Makhija, S. J., and Pawar, S. S. (1978). Stimulation of mixed function oxidase system by ascorbic acid. *Indian J. Exp. Biol.* 16:695-696.

Kamm, J. J., Dashman, T., Conney, A. H., and Burns, J. J. (1973). Protective effect of ascorbic acid on hepatotoxicity caused by sodium nitrite plus aminopyrine. *Proc. Natl. Acad. Sci. USA* 70:747-749.

Kassouny, M. E., and Rivers, J. M. (1972). Vitamin C depletion and in vitro uptake and organification of ^{131}I by guinea pig thyroid tissue. *J. Nutr.* 102:797-804.

Kato, R., and Takahashi, A. (1968). Thyroid hormone and activities of drug-metabolizing enzymes and electron transport systems of rat liver microsomes. *Mol. Pharmacol.* 4:109-120.

Kato, R., Takanaka, A., and Oshima, T. (1969). Effect of vitamin C deficiency on the metabolism of drugs and NADPH-linked electron transport system in liver microsomes. *Jap. J. Pharmacol.* 19:25-33.

Kato, N., Okada, T., Takenaka, Y., and Yoshida, A. (1977). Ameliorative effect of dietary ascorbic acid on PCB toxicity in guinea pigs. *Nutr. Rep. Int.* 15:125-130.

Kato, N., Tani, T., and Yoshida, A. (1980). Effect of dietary level of protein on liver microsomal drug-metabolizing enzymes, urinary ascorbic acid and lipid metabolism in rats fed PCB-containing diets. *J. Nutr.* 110:1686-1694.

Kato, N., Kawai, K., and Yoshida, A. (1981a). Effect of dietary level of ascorbic acid on the growth, hepatic lipid peroxidation, and serum lipids in guinea pigs fed polychlorinated biphenyls. *J. Nutr.* 111:1727-1733.

Kato, N., Tani, T., and Yoshida, A. (1981b). Effect of dietary quality of protein on liver microsomal mixed function oxidase system, plasma cholesterol and urinary ascorbic acid in rats fed PCB. *J. Nutr.* 111:123-133.

Kato, N., Mochizuki, S., Kawai, K., and Yoshida, A. (1982). Effect of dietary level of sulfur-containing amino acids on liver drug-metabolizing enzymes, serum cholesterol and urinary ascorbic acid in rats fed PCB. *J. Nutr.* 112:848-854.

Krebs, H. A., Peters, R. A., Coward, K. H., Mapson, L. W., Parsons, L. G., and Platt, B. S. (1948). Vitamin C requirements of human adults. *Lancet* 1:853-858.

Kritchevsky, D., Nitzsche, C., Czarnecki, S. K., and Story, J. A. (1980). Influence of vitamin E supplementation on cholesterol metabolism in rats. *Nutr. Rep. Int.* 22:339-342.

Kuenzig, W., Tkaczevski, V., Kamm, J. J., Conney, A. H., and Burns, J. J. (1977). The effect of ascorbic acid deficiency on

extrahepatic microsomal metabolism of drugs and carcinogens in
the guinea pig. *J. Pharmacol. Exp. Ther. 201*:527-533.

Lake, B. G., Longland, R. C., Gangolli, S. D., and Lloyd, A. G.
(1976). The influence of some foreign compounds on hepatic
xenobiotic metabolism and the urinary excretion of D-glucuronic
acid metabolites in the rat. *Toxicol. Appl. Pharmacol. 35*:113-
122.

Lake, B. G., Harris, R. A., Phillips, J. C., and Gangolli, S. D.
(1981). Studies on the effects of L-ascorbic acid on acetaminophen-induced hepatotoxicity. I. Inhibition of the covalent binding
of acetaminophen metabolites to hepatic microsomes in vitro.
Toxicol. Appl. Pharmacol. 60:229-240.

Lauterburg, B. H., and Bircher, J. (1976). Expiratory measurement of maximal aminopyrine demethylation in vivo: effect of
phenobarbital, partial hepatectomy, portacarval shunt and bile
duct ligation in the rat. *J. Pharmacol. Exp. Ther. 196*:501-
509.

Leber, H.-W., Degkwitz, E., and Staudinger, H. (1969). Studies
on the effect of ascorbic acid on the activity and biosynthesis
of mixed function oxygenases and on the concentration of haemo-
proteins in the microsome fraction of guinea pig liver. *Hoppe-
Seyler's Z. Physiol. Chem. 350*:439-445.

Leber, H.-W., Degkwitz, E., and Staudinger, H. (1970). Effect
of ascorbic acid on the induction of monooxygenase in rat liver
microsomes. *Hoppe-Seyler's Z. Physiol. Chem. 351*:995-1001.

Longenecker, H. E., Fricke, H. H., and King, C. G. (1940). The
effect of organic compounds upon vitamin C synthesis in the
rat. *J. Biol. Chem. 135*:497-510.

Loub, W. D., Wattenberg, L. W., and Davis, D. W. (1975). Aryl
hydrocarbon hydroxylase induction in rat tissues by naturally
occurring indoles of cruciferous plants. *J. Natl. Cancer. Inst.
54*:985-988.

Lu, A. Y. H., and West, S. B. (1978). Reconstituted mammalian
mixed function oxidases: requirements, specificities and other
properties. *Pharmacol. Ther. Part A 2*:337-358.

Lu, A. Y. H., and West, S. B. (1980). Multiplicity of mammalian
microsomal cytochromes P-450. *Pharmacol. Rev. 31*:277-295.

Lu, A. Y. H., Kuntzman, R., and Conney, A. H. (1976). The
liver microsomal hydroxylation enzyme system. *Front. Gastro-
intest. Res. 2*:1-31.

Luft, D., Degkwitz, E., Hochli-Kaufmann, L., and Staudinger, H.
(1972). Effect of δ-aminolevulinic acid on the content of cytochrome P-450 in the liver of guinea pigs fed without ascorbic
acid. *Hoppe-Seyler's Z. Physiol. Chem. 353*:1420-1422.

Machlin, L. J., Garcia, F., Kuenzig, W., Richter, C. B., Spiegel,
H. E., and Brin, M. (1976). Lack of antiscorbutic activity of

ascorbate 2-sulfate in the rhesus monkey. *Am. J. Clin. Nutr.* 29:825-831.

Machlin, L. J., Garcia, F., Kuenzig, W., and Brin, M. (1979). Antiscorbutic activity of ascorbic acid phosphate in the rhesus monkey and the guinea pig. *Am. J. Clin. Nutr.* 32:325-331.

Maines, M. D., and Kappas, A. (1977). Metals as regulators of heme metabolism. *Science 198:*1215-1221.

Mannering, G. J. (1949). Vitamin requirements of the guinea pig. *Vitam. Horm.* 7:201-221.

Mason, R. P. (1979). Free radical metabolites of foreign compounds and their toxicological significance. In *Reviews in Biochemical Toxicology*, Vol. 1, E. Hodgson, J. R. Bend, and R. E. Philpot, Eds., Elsevier/North-Holland, Amsterdam, pp. 151-200.

Mazur, A., Green, S., and Carleton, A. (1960). Mechanism of plasma iron incorporation into hepatic ferritin. *J. Biol. Chem.* 235:595-603.

McChesney, E. W., Barlow, O. W., and Klinck, G. H., Jr. (1944). The detoxification of neoarsphenamine by means of various organic acids. *J. Pharmacol. Exp. Ther.* 80:81-92.

Mellors, A. J., Nahrwold, D. L., and Rose, R. C. (1977). Ascorbic acid flux across mucosal border of guinea pig and human ileum. *Am. J. Physiol. 233:*E374-E379.

Milne, D. B., and Omaye, S. T. (1980). Effect of vitamin C on copper and iron metabolism in the guinea pig. *Int. J. Vitam. Nutr. Res.* 50:301-308.

Mitchell, W. G., and Floyd, E. P. (1954). Ascorbic acid and ethylene diamine tetraacetate as antidotes in experimental vanadium pcsioning. *Proc. Soc. Exp. Biol. Med.* 85:206-208.

Moore, C. V., and Dubach, R. (1951). Observations on the absorption of iron from foods tagged with radioiron. *Trans. Assoc. Am. Physicians 64:*245-256.

Mulder, G. J., Hinson, J. A., and Gillette, J. R. (1978). Conversion of the N-O-glucuronide and N-O-sulfate conjugates of N-hydroxyphenacetin to reactive intermediates. *Biochem. Pharmacol.* 27:1641-1649.

National Research Council (1972). *Nutrient Requirements of Domestic Animals: 10. Nutrient Requirements of Laboratory Animals,* National Academy of Sciences, Washington, D. C., pp. 9-19.

National Research Council (1980). *Recommended Dietary Allowances,* 9th ed., National Academy of Sciences, Washington, D. C., pp. 72-82.

Navia, J. M., and Lopez, H. (1973). A purified gel diet for guinea pigs. *Lab. Anim. Sci.* 23:111-114.

Nebert, D. W., Eisen, H. J., Negishi, M., Lang, M. A., Hjelmeland, L. M., and Okey, A. B. (1981). Genetic mechanisms con-

trolling the induction of polysubstrate monooxygenase (P-450)
activities. *Annu. Rev. Pharmacol. Toxicol.* 21:431-462.

Negishi, M., and Nebert, D. W. (1981). Structural gene products
of the Ah complex: increases in large mRNA from mouse liver
associated with cytochrome P-450 induction by 3-methylcholan-
threne. *J. Biol. Chem.* 256:3085-3091.

Nelson, S. D., Forte, A. J., Vaishnav, Y., Mitchell, J. R., Gillette, J. R., and Hinson, J. A. (1981). The formation of arylating and alkylating metabolites of phenacetin in hamsters and
hamster liver microsomes. *Mol. Pharmacol.* 19:140-145.

Nishikimi, M. (1975). Oxidation of ascorbic acid with superoxide
anion generated by the xanthine-xanthine oxidase system. *Biochem. Biophys. Res. Commun.* 63:463-468.

Ohno, T., and Myoga, K. (1981). The possible toxicity of vitamin
C in the guinea pigs. *Nutr. Rep. Int.* 24:291-294.

Olson, J. D., and Kienholz, E. W. (1968). Cobalt and vitamin C
for chicks. *Poult. Sci.* 47:1704.

Omaye, S. T., Green, M. D., Turnbull, J. D., Amos, W. H., and
Sauberlich, H. E. (1980). Influence of ascorbic acid and ery-
thorbic acid on drug metabolism in the cynomolgus monkey. *J.
Clin. Pharmacol.* 20:172-183.

Omaye, S. T., and Turnbull, J. D. (1979a). Heme oxygenase activity, drug metabolism, and ascorbic acid distribution in the
livers of ascorbic acid-deficient guinea pigs. *Biochem. Pharmacol.* 28:1415-1419.

Omaye, S. T., and Turnbull, J. D. (1979b). Degradation of cytochrome P-450 heme in ascorbic acid-deficient guinea pigs. *Biochem. Pharmacol.* 28:3651-3657.

Omaye, S. T., and Turnbull, J. D. (1980). Effect of ascorbic acid
on heme metabolism in hepatic microsomes. *Life Sci.* 27:441-
449.

Osaki, S., Johnson, D. A., and Frieden, E. (1966). The possible
significance of the ferrous oxidase activity of ceruloplasmin in
normal human serum. *J. Biol. Chem.* 241:2746-2751.

Pauling, L. (1970). *Vitamin C and the Common Cold,* W. H. Freeman, San Francisco.

Penney, J. R., and Zilva, S. S. (1946). The fixation and retention
of ascorbic acid by the guinea-pig. *Biochem. J.* 40:695-706.

Peterson, F. J., and Holtzman, J. L. (1980). Drug metabolism in
the liver—a perspective. In *Extrahepatic Metabolism of Drugs
and Other Foreign Compounds,* T. E. Gram, Ed., SP Medical
and Scientific Books, New York, pp. 1-123.

Peterson, F. J., Holloway, D. E., Duquette, P. H., and Rivers,
J. M. (1983a). Dietary ascorbic acid and hepatic mixed function

oxidase activity in the guinea pig. *Biochem. Pharmacol.* 32: 91-96.

Peterson, F. J., Holloway, D. E., Lindemann, N. J., and Niewoehner, D. E., (1983b). Studies on the mechanism of ascorbic acid protection against acetaminophen-induced hepatic damage in mice. Submitted for publication.

Pickett, C. B., Telakowski-Hopkins, C. A., Donohue, A. M., Lu, A. Y. H., and Hales, B. F. (1982). Differential induction of rat hepatic cytochrome P-448 and glutathione S-transferase B messenger RNAs by 3-methylcholanthrene. *Biochem. Biophys. Res. Commun.* 104:611-619.

Pijoan, M., and Lozner, E. L. (1944). Vitamin C economy in the human subject. *Bull. Johns Hopkins Hosp.* 75:303-314.

Potter, W. Z., Thorgeirsson, S. S., Jollow, D. J., and Mitchell, J. R. (1974). Acetaminophen-induced hepatic necrosis. V. Correlation of hepatic necrosis, covalent binding and glutathione depletion in hamsters. *Pharmacology* 12:129-147.

Raghuram, T. C., Krishnamurthi, D., and Kalamegham, R. (1978). Effect of vitamin C on paracetamol hepatotoxicity. *Toxicol. Lett.* 2:175-178.

Reed, D. J., and Beatty, P. W. (1980). Biosynthesis and regulation of glutathione: toxicological implications. In *Reviews in Biochemical Toxicology*, Vol. 2, E. Hodgson, J. R. Bend, and R. M. Philpot, Eds., Elsevier/North-Holland, New York, pp. 213-241.

Reid, M. E., and Briggs, G. M. (1953). Development of a semi-synthetic diet for young guinea pigs. *J. Nutr.* 51:341-354.

Renton, K. W., Keyler, D. E., and Mannering, G. J. (1979). Suppression of the inductive effects of phenobarbital and 3-methylcholanthrene on ascorbic acid synthesis and hepatic cytochrome P-450-linked monooxygenase systems by the interferon inducers, poly rI · rC and tilorone. *Biochem. Biophys. Res. Commun.* 88:1017-1023.

Richards, R. K., Kueter, K., and Klatt, T. J. (1941). Effects of vitamin C deficiency on action of different types of barbiturates. *Proc. Soc. Exp. Biol. Med.* 48:403-409.

Richardson, M. E., Fox, M. R. S., and Fry, B. E., Jr. (1974). Pathological changes produced in Japanese quail by ingestion of cadmium. *J. Nutr.* 104:323-338.

Rikans, L. E., Smith, C. R., and Zannoni, V. G. (1977). Ascorbic acid and heme synthesis in deficient guinea pig liver. *Biochem. Pharmacol.* 26:797-799.

Rikans, L. E., Smith, C. R., and Zannoni, V. G. (1978). Ascorbic acid and cytochrome P-450. *J. Pharmacol. Exp. Ther.* 204: 702-713.

Rokosova, B., and Chvapil, M. (1974). Relationship between the dose of ascorbic acid and its structural analogs and proline hydroxylation in various biological systems. *Connect. Tissue. Res.* 2:215-221.

Rudra Pal, D., Chatterjee, J., and Chatterjee, G. C. (1975). Influence of lead administration on L-ascorbic acid metabolism in rats: effect of L-ascorbic acid supplementation. *Int. J. Vitam. Nutr. Res.* 45:429-437.

Sato, P. H., and Zannoni, V. G. (1974). Stimulation of drug metabolism by ascorbic acid in weanling guinea pigs. *Biochem. Pharmacol.* 23:3121-3128.

Sato, P. H., and Zannoni, V. G. (1976). Ascorbic acid and hepatic drug metabolism. *J. Pharmacol. Exp. Ther.* 198:295-307.

Schatz, R. A., and Lal, H. (1980). Protection against hyperbaric oxygen toxicity by pargyline, succinic acid and ascorbic acid: role of brain GABA and brain ammonia. *Brain Res. Bull.* 5 (*Suppl.* 2):781-788.

Schulze, H. -U., and Staudinger, H. (1970). Changes in the phospholipid content of liver microsomes following various pretreatments of rats and guinea pigs. *Hoppe-Seyler's Z. Physiol. Chem.* 351:184-193.

Sikic, B. I., Mimnaugh, E. G., and Gram, T. E. (1977a). Effects of dietary ascorbic acid supplementation on hepatic drug-metabolizing enzymes in the guinea pig. *Biochem. Pharmacol.* 26: 2037-2041.

Sikic, B. I., Mimnaugh, E. G., Litterst, C. L., and Gram, T. E. (1977b). The effects of ascorbic acid deficiency and repletion on pulmonary, renal, and hepatic drug metabolism in the guinea pig. *Arch. Biochem. Biophys.* 179:663-671.

Siliprandi, L., Vanni, P., Kessler, M., and Semenza, G. (1979). Na^+-dependent, electroneutral L-ascorbate transport across brush border membrane vesicles from guinea pig small intestine. *Biochim. Biophys. Acta* 552:129-142.

Simpson, R. C. (1971). The relationship between chronic ascorbic acid deficiency and lipid metabolism. Master's thesis, Cornell University, Ithaca, N. Y.

Singh, K. D., Morris, E. R., Regan, W. O., and O'Dell, B. L. (1968). An unrecognized nutrient for the guinea pig. *J. Nutr.* 94:534-542.

Smithard, D. J., and Langman, M. J. S. (1978). The effect of vitamin supplementation upon antipyrine metabolism in the elderly. *Br. J. Clin. Pharmacol.* 5:181-185.

Spencer, R. P., Purdy, S., Hoeldtke, R., Bow, T. M., and Markulis, M. A. (1963). Studies on intestinal absorption of L-ascorbic acid-1-C^{14}. *Gastroenterology* 44:768-773.

Sprince, H., Parker, C. M., Smith, G. G., and Gonzales, L. J. (1975). Protective action of ascorbic acid and sulfur compounds against acetaldehyde toxicity: implications in alcoholism and smoking. *Agents Actions* 5:164-173.

Sprince, H., Parker, C. M., and Smith, G. G. (1977). L-Ascorbic acid in alcoholism and smoking: protection against acetaldehyde toxicity as an experimental model. *Int. J. Vitam. Nutr. Res.* (Suppl. 16):185-217.

Sprince, H., Parker, C. M., and Smith, G. G. (1979). Comparison of protection by L-ascorbic acid, L-cysteine, and adrenergic-blocking agents against acetaldehyde, acrolein, and formaldehyde toxicity: implications in smoking. *Agents Actions* 9:407-414.

Sprince, H., Parker, C. M., and Smith, G. G. (1981). Lethal synergy of acetaldehyde with nicotine, caffeine, or dopamine in rats: protection by ascorbic acid, cysteine, and anti-adrenergic agents. *Nutr. Rep. Int.* 23:43-54.

Sprince, H., Smith, G. G., Parker, C. M., and Rinehimer, D. A. (1982). Protection against cyanide lethality in rats by L-ascorbic acid and dehydroascorbic acid. *Nutr. Rep. Int.* 25:463-470.

Stevenson, N. R. (1974). Active transport of L-ascorbic acid in the human ileum. *Gastroenterology* 67:952-956.

Stevenson, N. R., and Brush, M. K. (1969). Existence and characteristics of Na^+-dependent active transport of ascorbic acid in guinea pig. *Am. J. Clin. Nutr.* 22:318-326.

Sutton, J. L., Basu, T. K., and Dickerson, J. W. T. (1982). Effect of large doses of ascorbic acid on the mixed function oxidase system in guinea pig liver. *Biochem. Pharmacol.* 31:1591-1594.

Suzuki, T., and Yoshida, A. (1979). Effect of dietary supplementation of iron and ascorbic acid on lead toxicity in rats. *J. Nutr.* 109:982-988.

Taber, R. I., and Larson, P. S. (1964). In vivo and in vitro studies on the question of a biologic relationship between nicotine and ascorbic acid. *Arch. Int. Pharmacodyn.* 151:243-259.

Ten State Nutrition Survey, 1968-1970 (1972). U.S. DHEW Publ. (HSM) 72-8132, Centers for Disease Control, Atlanta, Ga., pp. 177-215.

Thorgeirsson, S. S., Sakai, S., and Wirth, P. J. (1980). Effect of ascorbic acid on in vitro mutagenicity and in vivo covalent binding of N-hydroxy-2-acetylaminofluorene in the rat. *Mutat. Res.* 70:395-398.

Toggenburger, G., Landoldt, M., and Semenza, G. (1979). Na^+-dependent, electroneutral L-ascorbate transport across brush border membrane vesicles from human small intestine: inhibition by D-erythorbate. *FEBS Lett.* 108:473-476.

Touster, O., and Hollman, S. (1961). Nutritional and enzymatic studies on the mechanism of stimulation of ascorbic acid synthesis by drugs and carcinogenic hydrocarbons. *Ann. N. Y. Acad. Sci. 92*:318-323.

Trang, J. M., Blanchard, J., Conrad, K. A., and Harrison, G. G. (1982). The effect of vitamin C on the pharmacokinetics of caffeine in elderly men. *Am. J. Clin. Nutr. 35*:487-494.

Tsuhako, M., Matsuo, T., Nariai, H., Motooka, I., and Kobayashi, M. (1981). Effects of various phosphates on the stability of ascorbic acid. *Yakugaku Zasshi 101*:404-409.

Turnbull, J. D., and Omaye, S. T. (1980). Synthesis of cytochrome P-450 heme in ascorbic acid-deficient guinea pigs. *Biochem. Pharmacol. 29*:1255-1260.

Veen-Baigent, M. J., Ten Cate, A. R., Bright-See, E., and Rao, A. V. (1975). Effects of ascorbic acid on health parameters in guinea pigs. *Ann. N. Y. Acad. Sci. 258*:339-354.

Visser, C. M. (1980). Role of ascorbate in biological hydroxylations: origin of life considerations and the nature of the oxenoid species in oxygenase reactions. *Bioorg. Chem. 9*:261-271.

Wade, A. E., Wu, B., and Smith, P. B. (1972). Effects of ascorbic acid deficiency on kinetics of drug hydroxylation in male guinea pigs. *J. Pharm. Sci. 61*:1205-1208.

Wagstaff, D. J., and Street, J. C. (1971). Ascorbic acid deficiency and induction of hepatic microsomal hydroxylative enzymes by organochlorine pesticides. *Toxicol. Appl. Pharmacol. 19*:10-19.

Walsch, S., and Degkwitz, E. (1980a). Influence of L-ascorbate deficiency on the metabolism of hepatic microsomal cytochrome P-450 in guinea pigs. *Hoppe-Seyler's Z. Physiol. Chem. 361*: 79-83.

Walsch, S., and Degkwitz, E. (1980b). Activity of microsomal heme oxygenase in liver and spleen of ascorbic acid-deficient guinea pigs. *Hoppe-Seyler's Z. Physiol. Chem. 361*:1243-1249.

Wattenberg, L. W. (1971). Studies of polycyclic hydrocarbon hydroxylases of the intestine possibly related to cancer: effect of diet on benzpyrene hydroxylase activity. *Cancer 28*:99-102.

Williamson, D., and Winterbourn, C. C. (1980). Effect of oral administration of ascorbate on acetylphenylhydrazine-induced Heinz body formation. *Br. J. Haematol. 46*:319-321.

Wilson, J. T., Van Boxtel, C. J., Alvan, G., and Sjoqvist, F. (1976). Failure of vitamin C to affect the pharmacokinetic profile of antipyrine in man. *J. Clin. Pharmacol. 16*:265-270.

Winterbourn, C. C. (1979). Protection by ascorbate against acetylphenylhydrazine-induced Heinz body formation in glucose-6-phosphate dehydrogenase deficient erythrocytes. *Br. J. Haematol. 41*:245-252.

Yew, M. S. (1973). "Recommended daily allowances" for vitamin C. *Proc. Natl. Acad. Sci. USA 70*:969-972.

Young, R. M., and James, L. H. (1942). Action of intestinal micro-organisms on ascorbic acid. *J. Bacteriol. 44*:75-84.

Young, R. M., and Rettger, L. F. (1943). Decomposition of vitamin C by bacteria. *J. Bacteriol. 46*:351-363.

Yunice, A. A., and Lindeman, R. D. (1977). Effect of ascorbic acid and zinc sulfate on ethanol toxicity and metabolism. *Proc. Soc. Exp. Biol. Med. 154*:146-150.

Zannoni, V. G., Flynn, E. J., and Lynch, M. (1972). Ascorbic acid and drug metabolism. *Biochem. Pharmacol. 21*:1377-1392.

Zilva, S. S. (1936). Vitamin C requirements of the guinea pig. *Biochem. J. 30*:1419-1429.

Zilva, S. S. (1941). The influence of intermittent consumption of vitamin C on the development of scurvy. *Biochem. J. 35*:1240-1245.

Part II
EFFECTS OF DRUGS ON NUTRITION

8

Drug–Nutrient Interactions in Teratogenesis

Robert M. Hackman* and Lucille S. Hurley
University of California, Davis, California

I. INTRODUCTION

The occurrence of birth defects has been noted since the earliest human records, but the factors that predispose or initiate abnormal embryonic development are not well understood. The early Babylonians thought that defective infants were messages from the gods, while the ancient Greeks connected congenital malformations with mythological figures. Some cultures attributed monstrous offspring to the interbreeding of humans and animals. A popular view in Europe during the Middle Ages was that congenital anomalies resulted from cohabitation of humans with witches and demons. Emergence of scientific inquiry in the sixteenth and seventeenth centuries led to the idea that birth defects were due to interruptions in developmental processes, narrowness of the uterus, faulty maternal posture, or external physical violence. After Mendel's fundamental principles of genetics were rediscovered in 1900, it was generally assumed that abnormal development was under genetic control, and purely genetic explanations were accepted for a variety of biological phenomena, including birth defects. The importance attributed to genetics resulted in little consideration of other factors that could influence development (Wilson, 1973a,b; Warkany, 1979).

Genetic background is indeed an important determinant of fetal outcome. General studies on the inheritance of harelip in mice found that

Present affiliation: College of Human Development and Performance, University of Oregon, Eugene, Oregon

approximately 17% of the variation in response was attributable to hereditary factors, with 83% of the variance attributed to environmental influences (Reed, 1936). The author states that "the variation in the
expression of harelip was due in small part to sex, litter size and age
of the mother, etc., but in the major portion to intangible factors
working from within the mother but not correlated with her activities."
    When Hale (1933) showed that sows fed a ration deficient in vitamin
A prior to and during pregnancy produced piglets with no eyeballs,
theories of abnormal development were modified to incorporate environmental influences such as nutrient deficiencies as risk factors in teratogenesis. Maternal dietary deficiencies in rats were also found to produce anomalies in fetuses (Warkany and Schraffenberger, 1944). Experimental teratology in the 1950s continued to demonstrate the teratogenicity produced by a variety of environmental factors, such as drugs and
toxins, radiation, and severe nutritional deficiences. However, these
animal studies were not considered by many to be relevant to human
birth defects. A clear demonstration that drugs could seriously damage
the human embryo occurred in the early 1960s. Almost 8000 pregnant
women taking a presumably nontoxic sedative, thalidomide, produced
severely malformed infants (McBride, 1961). There was no longer any
doubt that drugs could affect the unborn.
    Experimental teratologists have continued to identify a variety of
environmental factors that result in abnormal fetal development. In
addition to single agents that can cause abnormal development, a clear
body of evidence shows the importance of multiple environmental and
genetic variables as risk factors. One of the earliest examples demonstrated that genetic strain, varying amounts of cortisone, different
maternal weight categories, and type of commercial diet all influenced
the frequency of cortisone-induced cleft palate in mice (Warburton et
al., 1962). The authors state that "no satisfactory account of the results could be given without assuming that every one of the four factors interacted with one or more of the others." They conclude that
"both genetic and nutritional factors influence the embryo's response
to cortisone, and genetic factors influence the influence of the nutritional factors." This and other evidence has led to a current working
hypothesis regarding production of birth defects. It states that a majority of malformations arise not from a single genetic or a single extrinsic factor, but rather are the result of a complex interaction among
genetics and a set of environmental conditions (Fraser et al., 1954;
Kalter, 1965). Current and future research will continue to refine models
assessing fetal risk to identify and incorporate such interactions. The
number of possible interacting factors is extensive, but relatively few
attempts have been made to assess clearly the relationships among the
multifactorial causes of abnormal development. There seems not only
to be a paucity of research studies, but also limited understanding by

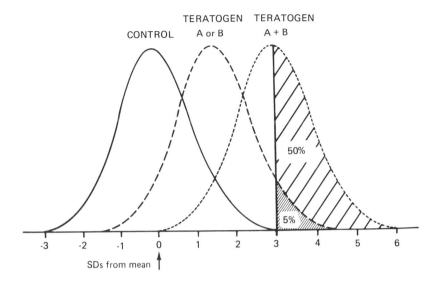

Figure 1 Hypothetical diagram illustrating apparent synergism between two teratogens that interact additively. (From Fraser, 1977.)

many teratologists as well as policymakers of the potential importance of considering interacting factors as determinants of fetal outcome.

Runner (1967) reviewed numerous examples of interactions of drugs, nutritional factors, and genetics in development and proposed four general models to accommodate the existing experimental information. (1) An additive effect occurs when two treatments affect unrelated pathways, but the disruption of the pathways causes the same or similar malformations. (2) A nonadditive effect would result when separate steps in a common enzymatic pathway are affected by two different treatments. Results of concomitant treatment would show no greater response than that produced by the single treatment having the larger affect. (3) In a synergistic effect, the same or similar steps in a common pathway are influenced by two treatments which act additively on each other. This is the most commonly reported type of interaction. (4) The final model is that of interference or protection. One treatment could provide a substrate or reduce the requirement for a metabolic intermediate, providing a bypass to a block imposed by another treatment. Metabolic balance is thus restored.

The model of synergism proposed by Fraser (1965; 1977) employs a multifactorial threshold concept (see Figure 1). Two treatments may appear additive or synergistic, depending on the (hypothetical) threshold level beyond which a malformation is expressed, and on the magnitude of shift in the distribution curve describing the frequency of the malformation. Suppose that two treatments act additively. If one teratogen shifts the distribution curve by 1.5 standard deviations, then 5% of the population will fall beyond the threshold and be affected. If another treatment has the same effect, the curve shifts three standard deviations and 50% of the population is affected. Fraser (1977) states that "deductions about the synergism of teratogens should be made only if synergism is still present after a statistical transformation of the data that results in linear dose-response curves."

Both models discussed above provide a useful framework for conceptualizing the interaction between two factors such as nutritional status and drugs. However, fetal risk is more likely influenced by a multitude of factors, some exogenous and some endogenous. Perhaps a multidimensional model is needed to accommodate the interactions among three or more factors, or the interactions among interactions. Nonetheless, study of the interactions between two factors such as nutrients and drugs is a useful means toward formulating a more complete model of influences on fetal outcome.

Evidence has been accumulating for the past 30 years indicating the importance of the effect of nutritional status on the ability of drugs to induce malformations. These interactions between nutrients and drugs are reviewed in this chapter. While teratogenic drugs can interact with protein, lipids, and carbohydrates, we have limited our discussion to research involving the interaction between drugs and vitamins or minerals. The interaction between certain vitamins and their structural analogs has also not been included in the discussion.

II. DRUG-VITAMIN INTERACTIONS

A. Vitamin A

1. Animal Studies

Hypervitaminosis A has been used extensively as a tool to probe the biochemical and morphological development of the embryo, both separately and in conjunction with a variety of other agents. A complete review of such research will not be presented here. A good example of the interaction between two teratogens involves vitamin A and trypan blue (Wilson, 1962). After establishing the minimally effective dose (3% malformed young) of vitamin A and trypan blue given individually to pregnant rats, the two teratogens were administered in combination. Simultaneous administration of subliminal doses of vitamin A and trypan blue (doses which by themselves produced no terata) resulted in 1.3% malformed young. Using a minimally effective dose of one agent combined with a subminimum dose of the other agent produced a frequency of malformed fetuses of approximately 20% in each case. This example underscores the potential significance of interactions of compounds which by themselves may appear either weakly teratogenic or not teratogenic at all.

2. Human Studies

Women taking steroidal oral contraceptives displayed significantly higher plasma vitamin A levels than did controls (Gal et al., 1971). Although none of the women taking oral contraceptives had plasma vitamin A levels approaching toxicity, the authors expressed concern regarding the occurrence of moderate hypervitaminosis A in certain susceptible individuals in the event of conception shortly after discontinuing oral contraceptive use. These findings were again reported in subsequent studies (Gal and Parkinson, 1973), with the advice that a treatment-free interval of oral contraceptive use occur prior to pregnancy. The report of higher plasma vitamin A levels in women taking oral contraceptives than in nonusers was confirmed by others (Briggs et al., 1972), but these authors questioned the possibility of teratogenic risk. The plasma vitamin A concentration of oral contraceptive users was well below that reached in hypervitaminosis A; it was proposed that in risk assessment, the plasma constituents that bind vitamin A be considered as well as the absolute amounts of the vitamin. In fact, women taking oral contraceptives were found to have increased concentrations of retinol binding protein (Briggs, 1974). Although no measurement of vitamin A was made in these subjects, the author maintains that the risk of unbound vitamin A accumulating in the mother is small.

B. B Vitamins

1. Riboflavin

Research designed specifically to examine drug-nutrient interactions in development was first conducted by Landauer in the late 1940s. Nutritional manipulation was a technique used to study potential modes of action of a variety of teratogens. Attempts to modify the incidence of insulin-induced teratogenesis in chicken embryos led to research on the potential sparing effect of riboflavin. When riboflavin at conventional doses was not effective in diminishing insulin-induced teratogenesis, boric acid was used to solubilize riboflavin for administration of a more concentrated solution. It was soon found that boric acid itself was teratogenic and that the response could be modified by riboflavin (Landauer, 1952). Groups that received riboflavin either 4 hr before or 4 hr after boric acid administration had almost twice the number of normal embryos than did groups given boric acid alone. However, the defects were never totally eliminated by riboflavin. Livers of boric acid treated embryos had a lower riboflavin content than did untreated em-

bryos. Boric acid inhibition of riboflavin-containing enzymes was proposed as an hypothesis to explain the observations. Supplemental riboflavin was thought to complex with boric acid and reduce the amount of
biologically active toxin available to the embryo.

A riboflavin-boric acid interaction was also found using riboflavin-5-
phosphate, which has a higher solubility than riboflavin. The vitamin
supplement substantially lowered the teratogenic effects of boric acid
in chicken embryos (Landauer and Clark, 1964). Riboflavin-5-phos-
phate dissolved in boric acid and used immediately was only marginally
effective, but preparation of the riboflavin-boric acid solution 1 week
prior to injection markedly reduced the teratogenic response compared
to groups receiving boric acid alone.

Methophenazine is a phenothiazine derivative with tranquilizing and
antihistaminic properties, and was used during human pregnancy in the
late 1950s. The flavin moiety of the drug is similar to the flavin rings
of riboflavin. In pregnant rats given 400 mg/kg methophenazine in a
single dose per os on day 14 of gestation, 57% of fetuses were malformed
and 21% of implantation sites were resorbed (Horvath and Druga, 1971).
Intraperitoneal injection of riboflavin 2 hr after drugging decreased
the resorption rate to 14% when given at 10 mg/kg and to 7% when given
at 100 mg/kg. The malformation response was unchanged by riboflavin
supplementation. The mechanism of fetal death may be due to the
structural similarity of methophenazine with riboflavin, perhaps producing a critically low flavin adenine dinucleotide (FAD) content in the
embryo. However, the disturbance of morphogenesis by the drug appears to occur in a manner independent of riboflavin metabolism.

2. Niacin

Landauer (1948) found that nicotinamide or α-ketoglutaric acid administered to chicken eggs reduced the frequency of insulin-induced malformations. In the group that was given nicotinamide plus insulin at
96 hr of development, there were almost twice as many normal embryos
on day 17 as there were in those that received insulin alone. The micromelia induced by insulin appeared most responsive to nicotinamide
supplementation, while other types of malformations, such as abnormal
beak, abnormal eyes, and rumplessness, showed an inconsistent pattern in responsible to supplementation (see Table 1).

Landauer and Rhodes (1952) later showed that the proper combination of insulin and nicotinamide gave complete protection against micromelia and beak defects caused by insulin alone. However, a different
type of beak defect was noted with the combination treatment that did
not occur from insulin alone. Also, nicotinamide offered only minor
protection against rumplessness induced by insulin, and this amount
of nicotinamide was often toxic by itself. Such results, while interesting, appeared inconsistent and difficult to interpret. Adequate

Table 1 Effect of Injecting Nicotinamide (18.9 mg), Insulin (2 units), or the Same Amounts of Insulin and Nicotinamide Simultaneously in White Leghorn Embryos After 96 Hr of Incubation

	Nicotinamide	Insulin	Insulin and nicotinamide
Survivors to day 17 (N)	72	72	51
Normal (%)	95.8 ± 2.4	45.8 ± 6.0	82.4 ± 5.4
Micromelia (%)	0	41.7 ± 5.6	5.9 ± 3.3
Abnormal beak (%)	0	19.4 ± 4.7	5.9 ± 3.3
Abnormal eyes (%)	2.8 ± 2.0	13.9 ± 4.1	2.0 ± 2.0

Source: Landauer (1948).

statistical models had not been formulated, adding to the lack of research interest in studying interactions. Nevertheless, a summary of Landauer's findings led him to conclude that the principal lesion in the embryonic system caused by insulin was a disruption in carbohydrate metabolism which could be influenced by nicotinamide supplementation. The time of maximum effectiveness of nicotinamide protection from various structural defects varied. Landauer suggested that the variable effects represented interference at different links of a common metabolic chain. Damage at different links in the chain produced different terata, but damage to the chain was repairable to different degrees by identical supplementation (of nicotinamide). This hypothesis has never been confirmed.

Micromelia in chick embryos was also produced with sulfanilamide and was eliminated by nicotinamide (Zwilling and DeBell, 1950). However, there were 10--50% fewer survivors than in the group receiving sulfanilamide alone, suggesting that nicotinamide might have killed the abnormal fetuses and left the normal ones intact.

Studies were also conducted in chicken eggs which demonstrated a teratogenic interaction between the nicotinamide analogs 3-acetylpyridine (3-AP) and 6-aminonicotinamide (6-AN) (Landauer and Clark, 1962) and between 3-AP and sulfanilamide (Landauer and Clark, 1964). Although not directly involving nicotinamide, these studies indicated that disruptions of a possibly similar metabolic chain involving insulin, nicotinamide, and a variety of drugs interacting with these compounds could influence embryo development. They also underscored the importance of genetic background of the embryo as a component of fetal outcome. Over a span of almost 30 years, Landauer studied the interactions of various metabolites and drugs altering carbohydrate metabolism. This led to his hypothesis that certain teratogens might exert their effects by reducing the energy available to the normally developing embryo (Landauer and Salam, 1974) (see also Section II.C).

The teratogenicity of 6-AN was also demonstrated in rats (Chamberlain and Nelson, 1963). Single injections of 6-AN (8 mg/kg) to pregnant rats on day 10 of gestation produced resorption of 75% of the implantation sites and malformations in 85% of the fetuses. Simultaneous injection of nicotinamide (8 mg/kg) prevented all the effects of 6-AN treatment. Doses of nicotinamide administered between 2 and 24 hr after drug treatment had no effect on modulating the fetal response to 6-AN. Intraamniotic injection of nicotinamide or its coenzyme forms (NAD or NADH) in addition to 6-AN reduced the frequency of skeletal and brain anomalies well below that produced by 6-AN treatment (Chamberlain and Goldyne, 1970). The coenzyme treatment also appeared to correct the depressed fetal and placental weight observed in 6-AN treated fetuses.

The interaction of genetic factors with niacin and 6-AN has been shown to influence fetal outcome in mice. The frequency of cleft palate caused by 6-AN given on day 13.5 was higher in A/J than in C57BL/6J mouse fetuses. The frequency of cleft palate in C57BL/6J fetuses was reduced when dams were fed a high-niacin diet throughout gestation, while the response to 6-AN in the A strain was not greatly affected by the niacin level (Verrusio et al., 1968). When C57BL/6J dams were fed a high-niacin diet for as short a period as 1–12 hr, or as long as 1–30 days prior to 6-AN injection, the frequency of cleft palate was 50% lower than in C57BL/6J dams fed a low-niacin diet and the drug (Pollard and Fraser, 1973). A/J mice showed a 30% reduction in cleft palate when a high-niacin diet was fed for 1 hr to 1 week prior to 6-AN treatment, but little difference was seen between the low- and high-niacin groups fed for 2–4 weeks prior to drug treatment. The authors postulated the existence of an extrachromosomal genetic system that could control the activity of certain regulatory enzyme systems, and could be induced by niacin. The two strains appeared to differ in the degree that this extrachromosomal enzyme system was influenced by niacin. Perhaps a product of this enzyme system protects against the effects of 6-AN, and some type of feedback inhibition on this system exists in the A/J strain. However, in no instance was such an enzyme system identified or characterized.

The teratogen 2-amino-1,3,4-thiadiazole (ATDA) is an antagonist of nicotinamide. In pregnant rats given ATDA on day 11 of gestation, 95% of fetuses were malformed and their weight was abnormally low (2.5 g)

(Beaudoin, 1973). Dams given ATDA on day 11 followed by a dose of 50 mg of nicotinamide or 50 mg of NAD or 100 mg of nicotinic acid showed no malformations and a fetal weight closer to normal (approximately 4.2 g). The hypothesis was developed that ATDA disrupts pathways of energy metabolism required for normal development and growth, and that any substance capable of being converted to NAD may protect embryos from this disruption.

The organophosphate insecticide Bidrin is teratogenic to chicken embryos. Nicotinic acid analogs (nicotinic acid, nicotinamide, NAD, and NADP) given alone with Bidrin produced a high frequency of normal-appearing chicks at the end of incubation, although hatching was usually unsuccessful (Rogers et al., 1964). In general, organophosphorous and methyl carbamate compounds administered to chicken eggs produced teratogenesis, and the incidence of malformation was found to be correlated with fetal NAD levels (Proctor and Casida, 1975). The teratogenic compounds appear to block a step in the metabolic pathway(s) leading to production of embryonic NAD. This block can apparently be bypassed by direct administration of NAD precursors, leading to reduction in teratogenesis. Compounds not serving as NAD precursors were ineffective (Proctor et al., 1976).

3. *Pyridoxine*

Alterations in pyridoxine metabolism have been reported in studies with isonicotinic acid hydrazide (INH). In chick embryos INH was found to increase the extractability of bone collagen (Levene, 1961). Pyridoxal, but not pyridoxine, given 1 day after INH injection in an amount equimolar to the drug reduced collagen solubility by 25%. Pyridoxal alone was quite toxic, but when given with INH, pyridoxal toxicity was reduced by 10—80%. The author suggests that the interaction involves the aldehyde moiety of pyridoxal combining with INH to form a Schiff's base. INH or the INH-pyridoxal complex inhibit pyridoxal kinase and decrease synthesis of pyridoxal phosphate. Pyridoxine reduced chick embryo mortality by 50% and lowered the frequency of malformed embryos by 66% when given concurrently with INH, compared to groups receiving INH alone (Castellano et al., 1973). The authors suggest that INH toxicity was due to its anti-vitamin B_6 activity, especially impairing amino acid metabolism. INH is used clinically as a tuberculostatic agent. In humans with active tuberculosis, use of INH, streptomycin, or p-aminosalicylic acid, the three major tuberculostatic drugs, has been associated with a higher frequency (two to three times) of malformations than in a control group taking no drugs and with inactive tuberculosis (Varpela, 1964). Interpretation of these data is difficult, however, because one cannot distinguish between the effects of drug use and the effects of active tuberculosis and its associated factors. The data also do not distinguish between possible different effects of the three different drugs. However, the combined use of these three drugs is no longer the preferred treatment in tuberculosis.

Hydrazine toxicity in pregnant rats was also partially reversed by pyridoxine supplementation (Lee and Aleyassine, 1970). Dams receiving hydrazine from days 11 to 20 of gestation failed to deliver pups. Pyridoxine given at a site distant from the drug injection resulted in the delivery of pups 50% of the time. When hydrazine was given from days 11 to 20, only 37% of implantation sites yielded live fetuses at term and fetal weight was significantly lower than normal. Pyridoxine given with hydrazine improved fetal survival and body weight. Edema and pallor of fetuses from dams receiving the drug were not eliminated by pyridoxine, leading the authors to suggest that a mechanism other than an interaction with pyridoxine might be involved in explaining these effects of hydrazine.

4. Folic Acid

Aminopterin and methotrexate: *Animal studies* Early research with vitamins involved in single-carbon metabolism showed that the feeding of 4-aminopteroylglutamic acid (aminopterin), an antagonist of folic acid, resulted in reduced growth and toxicity in mice (Franklin et al., 1948). Supplemental feeding of folic acid was generally ineffective in counteracting the toxic effects of the antogonist. Aminopterin also inhibited development of chick embryos (Karnofsky et al., 1949) and high levels of folic acid (20 mg per egg) did not counteract the effects. The embryotoxicity of aminopterin could not be reversed by folic acid, but the injection of thymidine together with the antagonist partially reversed embryotoxicity in frog eggs (Grant, 1960) and chick eggs (Snell and Cravens, 1950). Pregnant rats injected with aminopterin showed complete resorption of their litters (Thiersch and Phillips, 1950).

Aminopterin was also found to reduce embryo DNA levels when given to rats on day 10 of gestation (Kinney and Morse, 1964). Folic acid injected at 75–150 mg/kg 1 hr prior to aminopterin injection partially reversed the effect of the drug on embryo DNA, but high doses (225 mg/kg folic acid) had no effect on the low DNA levels caused by the drugs.

Human studies The ability of aminopterin to cause total resorption of rat litters (Thiersch and Phillips, 1950) led to its use as a human abortifacient. Thiersch (1952) reported 12 cases of therapeutic abortion using aminopterin. Spontaneous abortion was achieved in 10 cases. Two women failed to abort and their fetuses were removed. In both cases the fetuses were malformed, one with hydrocephalus and the other with cleft lip and palate. In another study, 6 of 12 women receiving aminopterin did not abort (Thiersch, 1956). One of the fetuses went to term and was born with anencephaly. Other studies also detail malformations found in fetuses from mothers taking aminopterin and failing to abort (Meltzer, 1956; Goetsch, 1962). Warkany et al. (1959) described a grossly malformed infant from a mother who developed signs of folic acid deficiency after taking aminopterin for self-induced abortion.

Methotrexate, a methyl derivative of aminopterin and an inhibitor of folate reductase, has also produced congenital malformations when used unsuccessfully as an abortifacient (Milunsky et al., 1968; Powell and Ekert, 1971).

Phenytoin. Phenytoin (diphenylhydantoin, Dilantin) is one of three drugs commonly used to treat epilepsy. The frequency of congenital malformations is two to three times higher in epileptic women than in the normal population. In patients, epilepsy begins by the age of 20, so that epileptic women commonly require prolonged drug treatment during the reproductive years. Distinguishing the effect of drug treatment from the effect of the epilepsy producing abnormalities themselves is important when assessing the teratogenic potential of phenytoin, but is difficult to accomplish. Some animal and human studies (described below) have suggested that the teratogenicity of phenytoin may be mediated by interference with folic acid metabolism (Richens, 1976).

Animal studies The teratogenicity of phenytoin has been clearly shown in rats and mice. The incidence of phenytoin-induced malformations in rat fetuses varied according to the time during gestation that the drug was given; day 8 of gestation was the most sensitive (Mercier-Parot and Tuchmann-Duplessis, 1974). The teratogenicity of phenytoin in mice has been correlated with the concentration of phenytoin in maternal serum, but not with maternal or fetal genotype or with the presence or absence of a seizure disorder (Finnell, 1981). High doses of phenytoin during organogenesis did not produce congenital malformations in a small number of rhesus monkeys (Wilson, 1973b).

A favored hypothesis to explain the teratogenicity of phenytoin was that it induces folic acid deficiency. This idea is based on the observation that phenytoin lowers blood folic acid levels in the epileptic women (Hoffbrand and Necheles, 1968). Twelve-day-old mouse embryos from dams treated with phenytoin on day 10 of gestation contained 40% less folate than did fetuses from dams treated as vehicle controls (Netzloff et al., 1979). However, because of the small size of the embryos, this study did not distinguish malformed from normal embryos. The effect of folic acid supplementation on phenytoin teratogenesis was studied in pregnant mice (Mercier-Parot and Tuchmann-Duplessis, 1974). Compared to animals receiving the drug alone, those given folic acid simultaneously with phenytoin showed a higher frequency of resorptions and an equal or higher incidence of cleft palate (Table 2). The authors conclude that "it seems unlikely that folic acid supplements would be effective in reducing the incidence of congenital malformations in epileptic women treated with phenytoin during pregnancy."

Human studies The use of phenytoin has been associated with an increased incidence of malformations in humans (Monson et al., 1973), although the existence and the strength of such an association varies among different studies (reviewed by Speidel and Meadow, 1974).

Table 2 Effects of Intraperitoneal Injections of Phenytoin (75 mg/kg) and Folic Acid During Days 12, 13, and 14 of Gestation in Mice

Treatment	Number females injected	Percentage mortality in pregnant females	Percent resorbed	Average number fetuses	Percentage with gross malformations	Percentage with cleft palate
Control	13	0	0	0.4	0	0
Phenytoin	29	13	4	1.9	2.6	20
Phenytoin + folic acid (0.5 mg/female)	27	22	33	1.5	1.1	34
Phenytoin + folic acid (1 mg/female)	40	12	28	2.7	3.4	18
Folic acid (0.5 mg/female)	16	0	6	0.6	0	0

Source: Mercier-Parot and Tuchmann-Duplessis (1974).

Meyer (1973) has estimated that 1850 children from treated and untreated mothers would have to be assessed to determine the risk associated with phenytoin use. Since few epileptics are untreated, such a study is difficult, if not impossible. Risk assessment of phenytoin is also complicated by additional factors which can influence fetal outcome. For example, phenytoin is most often given with other anticonvulsant drugs in various combinations and concentrations, and drug-drug interactions could be important. Genetic factors must also be considered. Genetic factors have been proposed to influence the relationship between epilepsy and cleft lip and palate in humans (Dronamraju, 1970). In mice, genetic factors are known to influence the rate of biotransformation of certain drugs (Nebert, 1980); such a phenomenon might be relevant to understanding differences in phenytoin sensitivity in humans. The interaction of phenytoin and folic acid metabolism is also an important consideration.

Phenytoin has been reported to impair the absorption of folate polyglutamates, but not folic acid, in humans (Hoffbrand and Necheles, 1968). Patients taking phenytoin for over a year also showed impaired jejunal folate conjugase activity in vitro, suggesting that phenytoin impairs the breakdown of folate polyglutamates. Plasma folic acid levels at 7 months of gestation were found to be 55—70% lower than normal in two women bearing malformed fetuses who had been taking phenytoin in combination with other drugs for a number of years (Biale et al., 1975). However, in general, plasma folate levels in women taking phenytoin are not as low as those seen in patients with overt megaloblastic folate-responsive anemia and are not associated with malformed infants (Pritchard et al., 1971).

It should be remembered that gross malformations are not the only index of abnormal development. Postnatal behavioral defects resulting from prenatal exposure to certain drugs affecting the central nervous system have been well documented in animals (Vorhees et al., 1979). Assessment of possible postnatal effects of phenytoin exposure in utero might also be made and could be one means of assessing potential interactions between phenytoin and folic acid. Phenytoin could reduce the bioavailability of folic acid to the central nervous system, which could be manifested in behavioral abnormalities as the central nervous system completes development postnatally. For example, phenytoin interactions with folic acid has been reported on a behavioral level, although not directly relating to perinatal development. Folic acid supplementation improved the mental state of 22 of 26 chronic epileptics who took anticonvulsants for 1—3 years and exhibited folic acid deficiency (Reynolds, 1967). It has been suggested that folic acid and its derivatives have significant convulsant properties, partially reversing the action of epileptic drugs, including phenytoin (Reynolds, 1973).

There is no evidence that folic acid supplementation affects blood folate levels in women taking anticonvulsant drugs during pregnancy.

Furthermore, no studies show that folic acid supplementation reduces the incidence of birth defects in infants of mothers taking antiepileptic drugs. Further research is obviously needed before folate supplementation is recommended to pregnant women taking anticonvulsant drugs.

Hydrazine. The involvement of single-carbon metabolism in hydrazine teratogenicity has been suggested from in vitro chick culture studies (Telang and Mulherkar, 1974). Hydrazine malformations were greatly ameliorated by folic acid (77% reversal), glycine, and p-aminobenzoic acid (85% each). Reversal was moderate with vitamin B_{12}, choline, histidine, and ascorbic acid. Little reversal was attained from serine. The inhibition of amino acid conversions involving folic acid was proposed as a mechanism for hydrazine teratogenesis.

Thalidomide. A metabolite of thalidomide, N-phthaloyl-DL-glutamic acid, was found to increase the solubility of folic acid in vitro (Eckert and Dörr, 1971). The change in folate solubility was suggested as an explanation for the teratogenic effect of thalidomide. However, no in vivo measurements of folic acid in response to thalidomide were made to extend this hypothesis to the whole animal. Furthermore, the proposed hypothesis assumes that high folate concentrations are teratogenic, an assumption for which there is no evidence.

5. B-Vitamin Supplementation

Some investigators have reported that folic acid and/or pyridoxine supplementation may modify the incidence of cortisone-induced cleft palate. In albino mice the frequency of cleft palate decreased from 85% in five litters receiving cortisone alone to 26% in nine litters injected with 10 mg of folic acid plus cortisone (Peer et al., 1958a). A protective effect was also reported for pyridoxine but not with riboflavin. These findings were not confirmed when mice were injected with cortisone and fed supplemental folic acid or riboflavin during gestation (Kalter, 1959); in no instance did the vitamin supplementation reduce the incidence of cortisone-induced cleft palate. The author suggested that differences between these studies might be explained by the different genetic strains of mice, the different routes of administration of the drug and nutrients, and the differences in the number of animals in each experimental group.

The apparent amelioration of cleft palate development by folic acid and pyridoxine supplementation led to the suggestion that women who had given birth to children with cleft lip or palate should take supplemental B vitamins and vitamin C (Peer et al., 1958b). In such a study, 1.9% of the children of 176 women given these supplements during pregnancy had cleft lip or palate, compared to 4.7% in a matched control population receiving no supplements (Peer et al., 1964). In contrast, other investigators have found no association between the occurrence of cleft lip and palate and the lack of prenatal vitamin supplement during pregnancy in humans (Fraser and Warburton, 1964). It is possible that the low but apparently meaningful changes in the rate of cleft lip and palate reported after supplementation could actually be due to random variability. A summary of the 19-year project initiated by Peer in 1964 adds weight to this argument (Briggs, 1976). Females with prior histories of cleft lip and palate infants were given a multiple B-vitamin preparation with ascorbic acid and additional amounts of folic acid. Of the 176 women in the initial study by Peer et al. and the 228 women in the subsequent clinical trial who took the vitamin supplements, the incidence of cleft lip and palate in their young was approximately 2%. In a matched control group of women not taking vitamin supplements, the incidence of cleft lip and palate was 4—5%. The results do not disagree with Peer's initial hypothesis, but they place much less emphasis on the significance of reducing cleft lip and palate through vitamin supplementation. However, it is difficult to evaluate these findings without knowledge of the dietary intake of the women. If their usual intake of these vitamins was adequate, additional supplementation would not be expected to overcome the abnormal development of their infants. However, if their intake of these vitamins was low or marginal, supplementation could have an effect.

C. Ascorbic Acid

Extensive studies on the interaction of ascorbic acid and certain teratogenic drugs were made by Landauer. Based on his findings that ascorbate or ascorbic acid reduced the teratogenic response to 3-AP, 6-AN, and sulfanilamide in chicken embryos, Landauer proposed that ascorbate acts as an antiteratogen (Landauer and Sopher, 1970). 3-AP, 6-AN, and sulfanilamide were used extensively by Landauer to study the interacting effects of nicotinamide, α-ketoglutarate, and other metabolic intermediates. Ascorbate mixed with 3-AP, 6-AN, or sulfanilamide and administered at 96 hr of incubation to chick embryos resulted in approximately twice the number of normal survivors at term as in groups receiving any of the drugs alone. However, in no instance did ascorbate offer complete protection from the teratogens. The reduced incidence of teratogenesis from these three drugs also occurred to varying degrees by supplementation with succinate and glycerophosphate. Similar responses were found when ascorbic acid was used instead of ascorbate. In contrast, the combination of ascorbate with insulin was more teratogenic than when insulin was given separately.

These results, combined with previous work on the protective effects of nicotinamide, α-ketoglutarate, glucose, pyruvate, tryptophan, and ADP against 3-AP, 6-AN, and sulfanilamide led to the proposal of a unifying hypothesis (Landauer and Sopher, 1970). If high-energy intermediates of the TCA cycle or respiratory chain could alleviate the frequency and severity of malformations produced by specific teratogens, then energy metabolism would play a central role in the normal processes of development. The importance of energy metabolism in cellular and organismal biology is well recognized, but Landauer's studies present no direct evidence linking metabolic intermediates and the three teratogens he used to fetal energy metabolism. Measurements of fetal cellular respiration were never reported. If cellular respiration were reduced by the teratogens and restored by metabolic intermediates such as ascorbate or nicotinamide, and if the trends in cellular respiration were consistent with an alleviation of teratogenicity, the concept of "antiteratogens" would be much stronger. In addition, the effects observed may be nonspecific; perhaps any chemical compound that can be metabolized will provide energy or intermediates to facilitate energy production. Finally, a direct interaction between the drugs and alleviating agents must also be considered. For example, do the intermediates inhibit uptake or transport of the drug?

A protective effect of ascorbic acid on nitrite toxicosis has also been reported in guinea pigs and rats. When challenged with sodium nitrite, pregnant guinea pigs with low plasma ascorbic acid levels had significantly more aborted litters than did dams adequate in ascorbate (Kociba and Sleight, 1970). The increased fetotoxic effects of sodium nitrite in the ascorbic acid-deficient guinea pigs was associated with elevated maternal methemoglobin levels leading to anoxia. Ascorbic acid provides reducing equivalents for methemoglobin conversion to hemoglobin. Levels of methemoglobin in fetuses did not differ significantly between those from dams deficient or adequate in ascorbic acid, further implicating maternal anoxia as the primary mechanism to explain the response.

Rats given sodium nitrite or methylurea orally on day 9 of gestation showed a greatly reduced incidence of resorptions and fewer malformed fetuses when ascorbic acid was given orally following drug treatment (Ivankovic et al., 1973). The capacity of ascorbic acid to inhibit endogenous synthesis of nitroso compounds probably explains these results.

III. DRUG-MINERAL INTERACTIONS

A. Calcium

The drug 6-azauridine (6-AzUR) is an antimetabolite of pyrimidine bases and has been used to treat cancer, psoriasis, and rheumatic conditions. 6-AzUR is teratogenic to chick and rat embryos. Compared to controls, chicken embryos exposed to 6-AzUR during development had significantly higher dry weight, ash content, and calcium content of bone, and lower plasma calcium levels. The authors speculate that 6-AzUR might reduce resorption of bone calcium or enhance calcium utilization from the shell.

B. Potassium

The teratogenicity of acetazolamide was first shown in rats when fed at 0.6% in a stock diet throughout gestation (Layton and Hallesy, 1965). Acetazolamide inhibits carbonic anhydrase activity (Maren, 1967), resulting in acidosis and depletion of body potassium. The teratogenic activity of acetazolamide can be modified by manipulation of maternal potassium metabolism (Ellison and Maren, 1972a). Pregnant rats fed acetazolamide throughout gestation had 38% abnormal fetuses at term; maintenance of normal maternal plasma and tissue potassium concentrations with potassium salts in the diet and drinking water to equal approximately 12 mEq/kg per day from day 6 until term, in combination with acetazolamide in the diet, resulted in 8% malformed young. The effectiveness of potassium supplementation was reversed when very high levels of potassium were given; approximately 21 mEq/kg per day in addition to the drug resulted in 66% of the young being malformed. A significant observation was that a potassium-retaining agent fed in the diet together with acetazolamide completely eliminated the teratogenicity of acetazolamide. The fetal potassium concentration after 20 days of the 0.6% acetazolamide diet was higher in abnormal fetuses (82.7 ± 1.1 mEq/kg) than in normal fetuses from dams fed a control diet (62.0 ± 1.4 mEq/kg). Maternal potassium depletion or acidosis alone had no deleterious effects on the rat fetuses (Ellison and Maren, 1972b). Future research is needed to determine if the acetazolamide-induced defects arise primarily from disturbances in potassium metabolism or from alteration in carbonic anhydrase activity, which may then secondarily affect potassium levels and may also have a specific role in fetal development, although there is little information available.

C. Zinc

Animal studies Interactions of zinc nutrition and drugs have been studied with several compounds. The teratogenicity of ethylenediaminetetraacetic acid (EDTA), a chelator of divalent cations, was prevented by supplementary dietary zinc in pregnant rats (Swenerton and Hurley, 1971). A purified diet containing 2% EDTA and 100 μg/g zinc fed to pregnant rats produced malformations in 7% of the fetuses; rats receiving the same diet and no EDTA had no malformed young. When the rats were given 3% dietary EDTA from days 6 to 14 or days 6 to 21 of gestation, 40% and 54% of their implantation sites were resorbed, and 87% and 100% of the fetuses were malformed, respectively. The types and frequencies of malformations induced by EDTA treatment were strikingly similar to those caused by zinc deficiency during prenatal development (Hurley, 1980). A diet containing 3% EDTA and 1000 μg/g zinc fed from days 6 to 21 resulted in resorptions of 8% and no malformations, demonstrating the protective nature of supplemental zinc (Table 3). The mechanism of the protective effect of zinc is unknown.

Table 3 Incidence of Congenital Malformations in Rats Fed 3% Dietary
EDTA and Two Levels of Dietary Zinc

	Dietary zinc (μg/g)	
	100	1000
Number of litters	11	7
Number of fetuses	83	81
Malformations (percent of fetuses)		
Cleft lip	1.2	0
Cleft palate	57	0
Brain abnormalities	44	0
Micro- or anophthalmia	18	0
Micro- or agrathia	63	0
Clubbed legs	92	0
Fused or missing digits	57	0
Curly, short, or missing tail	98	0

Source: Swenerton and Hurley (1971).

but it is possible that zinc could bind EDTA in the intestine, blood, or
at the tissue level, thus reducing or eliminating the teratogenicity of
the chelator. Additional studies by others supported the hypothesis
that EDTA acts by producing zinc deficiency (Kimmel and Sloan, 1975).
The zinc-EDTA interaction was one of the first illustrations that the
nutritional requirements of trace elements may be modified and increased
by other substances in the environment.

An interaction has also been demonstrated between zinc and 6-mer-
captopurine (6-MP). The teratogenic effect of 6-MP is due to interference with DNA synthesis. Teratogenicity may be increased with marginal dietary zinc intake and reduced with supplemental dietary zinc
(Hirsch and Hurley, 1978). 6-MP injected on day 11 of gestation in rats
fed throughout gestation diets containing 9, 100, or 1000 μg/g zinc
caused 41, 30, and 8% resorptions, respectively. The frequency of malformed fetuses was 58% in the 1000-μg/g zinc group compared to 94% in
groups fed 9 or 100 μg/g zinc. The DNA content and incorporation of
[3H]thymidine into fetuses was affected by 6-MP treatment, but was not
markedly altered by dietary zinc intake. Placentas from 6-MP-treated
dams displayed a greatly reduced labyrinth area as a proportion of placental area compared to nontreated controls. The proportion of labyrinth area rose significantly as dietary zinc increased from 9 to 100 to
1000 μg/g (Schrader et al., 1978).

An intriguing interaction has been suggested between zinc and thalidomide. Pregnant rats fed 10 g per day of a diet containing less than

1 μg/g zinc and injected with a thalidomide analog, EM_{12}, showed malformations similar to those resulting from EM_{12} administration to pregnant rabbits, a species sensitive to teratogenic effects of thalidomide
(Jackson and Schumacher, 1979). In contrast, thalidomide and EM_{12}
do not produce malformations in rats fed a zinc-adequate diet. Unfortunately, the control group in this experiment was fed a stock (natural ingredient) diet and was thus not an adequate control for the
zinc-deficient group, who were fed a purified diet. The authors speculate that the chelating ability of EM_{12} might alter normal zinc metabolism and reduce the zinc available to the fetus. In addition, zinc deficiency may alter the pharmacokinetics of EM_{12} clearance by impairing
biotransformation of the drug.

A possible interaction between zinc and salicylate, another chelator
of divalent cations, was first explored in rats by measuring isotopic
zinc activity in the urine and various maternal and fetal tissues after
salicylate or aspirin injection (Koshakji and Schulert, 1972). Salicylate-treated dams did not differ from controls in urinary output of ^{65}Zn
24 h after drug treatment. However, measurement of urinary output of
zinc might not reflect changes in plasma zinc levels or shifts of zinc
between different metabolic pools in the body. Salicylate could also
cause reduced bioavailability of zinc to the fetus which may not be expressed as an increase in urinary output of the element by the mother.
Salicylate given on day 16 also did not alter the specific activity of the
isotope incorporated into fetal or placental tissue, but did cause an increase in the specific activity of the zinc isotope in the maternal liver.
However, distribution of zinc in 16-day fetuses may not reflect biochemical mechanisms during organogenesis, the period of susceptibility of
malformation. The kinetics of salicylate binding and transport to the
rat fetus on day 16 of gestation are also likely to be different from
those earlier in gestation, affecting isotope uptake in fetal and placental tissues.

Other evidence suggesting an interaction between zinc and salicylate
is more convincing, however. The teratogenic response to salicylate
given on day 9 was higher in pregnant rats fed a diet marginal in zinc
concentration than it was in those fed an adequate diet (Kimmel et al.,
1972). It has also been noted that zinc deficiency and aspirin toxicity
produce very similar effects in pregnant rats (O'Dell et al., 1977).
Rats fed a diet containing less than 0.4 μg/g zinc throughout gestation
had a significantly longer than normal gestation period, and significantly lower rectal temperature and blood pressure. Dams fed diets containing 100 μg/g zinc and given 100, 150, or 200 mg/kg aspirin twice
daily by gavage from day 19 of gestation until delivery also had a significantly longer than normal gestation period. The rats given 200
mg/kg aspirin also had low rectal temperature and blood pressure, similar to those seen in the zinc-deficient group. It is interesting to note
that salicylate has been reported to inhibit the activity in vitro of a
number of metalloenzymes that require zinc (Grisolia et al., 1968,1970),

but alterations in zinc metalloenzymes have not been related to the common pathologies of zinc deficiency and salicylate toxicity.

The interaction between zinc and salicylate has recently been studied in relation to genetic interactions as well (Hackman and Hurley, 1981a). Pregnant rats were fed throughout gestation a purified diet containing 0.4, 4.5, 9, 100, or 1000 μg/g zinc and were given a single oral dose of saline or 250, 500, or 750 mg/kg salicylate on day 9 of gestation. Two strains of rats, Sprague-Dawley and Wistar, were studied. The teratogenic effect of salicylate increased as the concentration of dietary zinc decreased. The two strains showed different responses to the diet-drug treatment.

Statistical analysis of the factors affecting fetal outcome indicated significant effects due to the single variables dietary zinc, salicylate dose, and genetic background. Beyond the influence of the single factors, however, a significant adjustment to the litter response was caused by the two-way interactions between zinc and salicylate, zinc and genetic background, and salicylate with the genetic background. Equally important was the finding that the three-way interactions between zinc, salicylate, and genetic background significantly adjusted the teratogenic response after the single- and two-factor interactions had been accounted for (Hackman and Hurley, 1981a). The exact mechanism(s) by which dietary zinc interacts with salicylate is still unknown. However, the importance of considering the interaction between various environmental factors such as nutrients and drugs, and the interaction between environmental factors and the genetic background of the organism when assessing fetal risk, is clearly demonstrated.

The influence of genetic factors on drug-nutrient interactions is also exemplified with acetazolamide (Figure 2). The teratogenicity of this drug, a carbonic anhydrase inhibitor, has recently been shown to vary as a function of dietary zinc intake (Hackman and Hurley, 1981b, 1983). Acetazolamide produces postaxial forelimb ectrodactyly (missing digits on the forepaws) in CBA mouse fetuses, whereas SWV fetuses are generally resistant (Biddle, 1975a). Pregnant CBA and SWV females were fed purified diets throughout gestation containing 0.4, 4.5, 9, 100, or 1000 μg/g zinc and given teratogenic doses of acetazolamide on day 10 of gestation. The incidence of resorptions, malformations, and total abnormal sites from litters receiving the drug decreased as maternal dietary zinc increased. The magnitude of the response was strongly influenced by the strain. The incidence of forelimb ectrodactyly in live fetuses in the sensitive (CBA) strain was 100% when dams were fed 0.4 μg/g dietary zinc and declined steadily as dietary zinc increased to 100 μg/g, the amount of zinc used as the control level. Supplemental zinc above the control level did not further reduce or eliminate the malformation.

The SWV strain was also found to be sensitive to acetazolamide if the diet was inadequate in zinc. In dams fed the 0.4- or 4.5-μg/g zinc

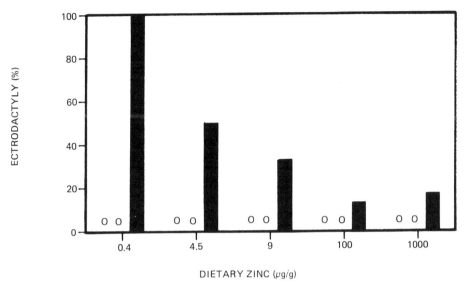

Figure 2 Frequency of fetuses with postaxial forelimb ectrodactyly in mice fed various levels of dietary zinc and given acetazolamide, in percent of live fetuses with ectrodactyly. No response was found in fetuses from dams in blank or vehicle-treated groups. (From Hackman and Hurley, 1981b.)

diet, 8% and 5% of their live fetuses had ectrodactyly. Dietary zinc of 9 $\mu g/g$ or more eliminated the malformation.

The mechanism of the acetazolamide-zinc interaction is unknown. The results must be viewed in the context of the reported acetazolamide-potassium interaction (see above), as well as possibly a more direct interaction with zinc. This study further illustrates the importance of the genetic component in fetal outcome; the drug-nutrient interaction was greatly modified by the genetic background of the animal. Genetic studies of acetazolamide teratogenicity have been used as a tool to probe the underlying biochemical mechanism of acetazolamide teratogenicity (Biddle, 1975b). Such approaches may offer valuable information regarding the multiplicity and strength of factors influencing prenatal development.

Human studies A small study has shown an association between low plasma zinc in pregnant alcoholic women and the number of birth defects in their newborns (Flynn et al., 1981). No clear correlation was found between the incidence of malformations and fetal cord plasma zinc or quantity of alcohol consumed. Low maternal plasma zinc levels might be a clue helping to explain the mechanism of the fetal alcohol syndrome. More research is needed to confirm these important findings relating to alcohol and zinc metabolism during pregnancy. Research examining the possible role of alcohol in altering the metabolism of other nutrients besides zinc may also provide useful clues regarding alcohol-induced birth defects.

D. Copper

D-Penicillamine (dimethylcysteine), a drug used in the treatment of Wilson's disease, cystinuria, and rheumatoid arthritis, has the capacity to bind divalent cations such as copper and zinc and increase their excretion from the body. The possible deleterious effect of D-penicillamine (DP) during pregnancy has been debated (Hurley and Keen, 1979). The potential teratogenicity of DP in humans was suggested by Mjølnerød et al. (1971) and Solomon et al. (1977), who described infants with abnormalities resembling those of copper deficiency born to two women taking DP. Other investigators have questioned the teratogenicity of DP (Scheinberg and Sternlieb, 1975; Walshe, 1977), but the apparent absence of serious drug effects in fetuses of patients with Wilson's disease could be due to the extremely high copper concentration in the tissues of these women. Keen et al. (1981a,b) have recently shown that DP is teratogenic in rats and that its administration during pregnancy produced low copper and zinc levels in maternal and fetal tissues.

In this experiment, rats were mated and were fed throughout pregnancy a complete purified diet containing either no DP or one of three different levels of the drug. At term, the frequency of resorbed implantation sites was slightly higher in the drug-treated rats than in the controls, but there was a very high frequency of malformed fetuses in the rats fed the two higher levels of DP (an amount equivalent to that used clinically for human patients). Most of the fetuses showed cutis laxa (lax skin). One of the most striking malformations was spina bifida occulta. DP produced a dramatic decrease in the copper concentration of maternal plasma and liver, in fetal liver, and in whole fetus. These results suggest that the teratogenic effect of DP may be mediated through its effect on tissue and plasma copper.

Another drug used for the removal of copper in patients with Wilson's disease is triethylenetetraamine (TETA). This drug has been suggested for use in cases of Wilson's disease in which treatment by DP is contraindicated because of a toxic response by the patient. Like DP, TETA is known to interact with divalent cations such as copper and nickel by increasing the excretion of these elements in the urine, presumably in the chelate form. Experiments in which TETA was fed to pregnant rats showed that this drug also produced significantly lower than normal levels of copper in maternal plasma and maternal and fetal liver (Cohen et al,, 1982). However, no malformations were seen in these fetuses except for lax skin. Another difference between DP and TETA was the high concentration of iron in tissues of DP-treated animals which did not appear with TETA. In contrast, however, the fetal liver of TETA treated rats showed a very high concentration of zinc (Keen et al., 1982).

The physiological significance of these differences and the mechanisms bringing them about are unknown and are under investigation at the present time. The binding of divalent cations by these two drugs is, however, very different, suggesting that their impact on copper metabolism will be different, in time of effect, interaction with other copper binding compounds, including metalloproteins, and concomitant influence on other divalent cations. Thus studies of the interactions between drugs and copper may be useful as probes in elucidating the role of copper in development and the effect of its deficiency as well as providing effects of such interactions (Keen et al., 1882).

E. Manganese and Iron

Studies of a possible interaction between manganese or iron and salicylate during prenatal development have not provided clear evidence of such an association. The distribution of tracer doses of manganese or iron in maternal, fetal, or placental tissues was the same in controls and in rats injected with ^{54}Mn or ^{59}Fe following aspirin or salicylate injection on day 9 of gestation (Koshakji and Schulert, 1972). Salicylate-treated dams were also not different from controls in urinary output of isotopes 24 h after drug treatment. Furthermore, salicylate given on day 16 and followed by isotope tracers did not alter the specific activity of metal isotopes incorporated into maternal, fetal, or placental tissues. However, urinary output and isotope uptake may not reflect changes in bioavailability at the tissue level, and chelation of trace elements by salicylate cannot be rejected from these studies.

Parenteral injection of manganous sulfate or ferrous gluconate on days 8−10 of gestation in rats, together with oral salicylate treatment on day 9, was found to potentiate the teratogenicity of salicylate (Kimmel et al., 1977). The metal treatment increased salicylate levels in maternal plasma and embryo above those caused by the drug alone. Postnatal effects of prenatal salicylate-metal exposure were assessed in 40-day-old pups from dams receiving 125 mg/kg aspirin orally on day 9 and ferrous gluconate injections on days 8−10. Relative to vehicle controls, both the aspirin and iron-aspirin groups had increased exploratory activity, but only the iron-aspirin group had impaired maze learning.

IV. CONCLUDING REMARKS

The research that we have reviewed demonstrates clearly that drugs
may interact with nutrients in affecting prenatal development. The teratogenic effects of certain drugs may be exacerbated or alleviated by altering the dietary concentration of specific elements.

This principle has relevance for problems of human teratology, most
specifically, for the potential prevention of human birth defects. The
literature reviewed here suggests that women who have marginal deficiencies of essential nutrients may be more susceptible to the teratogenic effects of drugs than are those in good nutritional status. One
approach for research on prevention of malformations in infants thus
presents itself—evaluation of nutritional status for critical nutrients
and subsequent supplementation. Carefully controlled human studies
are needed.

We have also shown that drug-nutrient interactions may be influenced
by genetic factors. Thus, in assessing fetal risk, the interactions
among nutrients, drugs, and genetic factors should be considered.
Furthermore, such multivariate approaches may provide not only new
concepts and information in research on teratology, but may also serve
as probes for the understanding of biochemical mechanisms of fetal development. Such approaches may also be fruitful in other areas of nutrition research as well.

REFERENCES

Beaudoin, A. R. (1973). NAD precursors as antiteratogens against
    aminothiadiazole. *Teratology 13*:95-100.
Biale, Y., Lewenthal, H., and Ben-Adereth, N. (1975). Congenital
    malformations due to anticonvulsive drugs. *Obstet. Gynecol.
    45*:439-441.
Biddle, F. G. (1975a). Teratogenesis of acetazolamide in the CBA/J
    and SWV strains of mice. I. Teratology. *Teratology 11*:31-36.
Biddle, F. G. (1975b). Teratogenesis of acetazolamide in the CBA/J
    and SWV strains of mice. II. Genetic control of the teratogenic
    response. *Teratology 11*:37-46.
Briggs, M. H. (1974). Vitamin A and the teratogenic risks of oral
    contraceptives. *Br. Med. J. 3*:170-171.
Briggs, R. M. (1976). Vitamin supplementation as a possible factor in
    the incidence of cleft lip/palate deformities in humans. *Clin.
    Plast. Surg. 3*:647-652.
Briggs, M. H., Briggs, M., and Bennun, M. (1972). Steroid contra-
    ceptives and plasma carotenoids. *Contraception 6*:275-280.
Castellano, M. A., Tortora, J. L., Germino, N. I., Rama, F., and
    Ohanian, C. (1973). The effects of isonicotinic acid hydrazide

on the early chick embryo. *J. Embryol. Exp. Morphol.* 29:209-219.

Chamberlain, J. G., and Goldyne, M. E. (1970). Intra-amniotic injection of pyridine nucleotides or adenosine triphosphate as countertherapy for 6-aminonicotinamide (6-AN) teratogenesis. *Teratology* 3:11-16.

Chamberlain, J. G., and Nelson, M. N. (1963). Congenital abnormalities in the rat resulting from single injections of 6-aminonicotinamide during pregnancy. *J. Exp. Zool.* 153:285-298.

Cohen, N. L., Keen, C. L., Lonnerdal, B., and Hurley, L. S. (1982). Low tissue copper and teratogenesis in triethylenetetramine-treated rats. *Fed. Proc.* 41:944.

Dronamraju, K. R. (1970). Epilepsy and cleft lip and palate. *Lancet* 2:876-877.

Eckert, T., and Döor, N. W. (1971). Intermolekulare Wechselwirkungen der Folsaure mit N-Phthaloyl-DL-glutaminsaure. *Experientia* 27:671-672.

Ellison, A. C., and Maren, T. H. (1972a). The effect of potassium metabolism on acetazolamide-induced teratogenesis. *Johns Hopkins Med. J.* 130:105-115.

Ellison, A. C., and Maren, T. H. (1972b). The effects of metabolic alterations on teratogenesis. *Johns Hopkins Med. J.* 130:87-94.

Finnell, R. H. (1981). Phenytoin-induced teratogenesis: a mouse model. *Science* 211:483-484.

Flynn, A., Martier, S. S., Sokol, R. J., Miller, S. I., Golden, N. L., and Del Villano, B. C. (1981). Zinc status of pregnant alcoholic women: a determinant of fetal outcome. *Lancet* 1:572-575.

Franklin, A. L., Stokstad, E. L. R., and Jukes, T. H. (1948). Observations on the effect of 4-amino-pteroylglutamic acid in mice. *Proc. Soc. Exp. Biol. Med.* 67:398-400.

Fraser, F. C. (1965). Some genetic aspects of teratology. In *Teratology: Principles and Techniques*, J. G. Wilson and J. Warkany, Eds., University of Chicago Press, Chicago, pp. 21-38.

Fraser, F. C. (1977). Interactions and multiple causes. In *Handbook of Teratology*, Vol. 1, J. G. Wilson and F. C. Fraser, Eds., Plenum Press, New York, pp. 445-463.

Fraser, F. C., and Warburton, D. (1964). No association of emotional stress or vitamin supplement during pregnancy to cleft lip or palate in man. *Plast. Reconstr. Surg.* 33:395-399.

Fraser, F. C., Kalter, H., Walker, B. E., and Fainstat, T. D., (1954). The experimental production of cleft palate with cortisone and other hormones. *J. Cell. Comp. Physiol.* 43(Suppl.): 237-259.

Gal, I., and Parkinson, C. E. (1973). Changes in serum vitamin A
    levels during and after oral contraceptive therapy. *Contracep-
    tion* 8:13-25.
Gal, I., Parkinson, C., and Craft, I. (1971). Effects of oral con-
    traceptives on human plasma vitamin-A levels. *Br. Med. J.* 2:
    436-438.
Goetsch, C. (1962). An evaluation of aminopterin as an abortifa-
    cient. *Am. J. Obstet. Gynecol.* 83:1424-1476.
Grant, P. (1960). The influence of folic acid analogs on develop-
    ment and nucleic acid metabolism in *Rana pipiens* embryos.
    Dev. Biol. 2:197-202.
Grisolia, S., Santos, I., and Mendelson, J. (1968). Inactivation of
    enzymes by aspirin and salicylate. *Nature* 219:1252.
Grisolia, S., Mendelson, J., and Diederich, D. (1970). Inactivation
    of metalloenzymes by salicylate. *FEBS Lett.* 11:140-143.
Hackman, R. M., and Hurley, L. S. (1981a). The influence of dietary
    zinc and genetic strain on salicylate teratogenesis in rats. *Tera-
    tology* 23:40A.
Hackman, R. M., and Hurley, L. S. (1981b). The effect of dietary
    zinc and genetic interaction on acetazolamide teratogenesis in mice.
    Teratology 23:39-40A.
Hackman, R. M., and Hurley, L. S. (1983). Interaction of dietary
    zinc, genetic strain and acetazolamide in teratogenesis in mice.
    Teratology, in press.
Hale, F. (1933). Pigs born without eyeballs. *J. Hered.* 24:105.
Hirsch, K. S., and Hurley, L. S. (1978). Relationship of dietary
    zinc to 6-mercaptopurine teratogenesis and DNA metabolism in
    the rat. *Teratology* 17:303-313.
Hoffbrand, A. V., and Necheles, T. F. (1968). Mechanisms of fol-
    ate deficiency in patients receiving phenytoin. *Lancet* 2:528-
    530.
Horvath, C. A., and Druga, A. (1971). Action of the phenothiazine
    derivative methophenazine on prenatal development in rats.
    Teratology 11:325-330.
Hurley, L. S. (1980). *Developmental Nutrition*, Prentice-Hall,
    Englewood Cliffs, N. J.
Hurley, L. S., and Keen, C. L. (1979). Teratogenic effects of cop-
    per. In *Copper in the Environment, Part 2: Health Effects*,
    J. Nriagu, Ed., Wiley, New York, pp. 33-56.
Ivankovic, S., Preussmann, R., Schmahl, D., and Zeller, J. (1973).
    Protection of nitrosamide-induced hydrocephaly by ascorbic acid
    after prenatal administration of ethylurea and nitrite to rats.
    Z. Krebsforsch. 79:145-147.
Jackson, A. J., and Schumacher, H. J. (1979). The teratogenic ac-
    tivity of a thalidomide analogue EM_{12} in rats on a low-zinc diet.
    Teratology 19:341-344.

Kalter, H. (1959). Attempts to modify the frequency of cortisone-induced cleft palate in mice by vitamin, carbohydrate, and protein supplementation. *Plast. Reconstr. Surg.* 24:498-504.

Kalter, H. (1965). Interplay of intrinsic and extrinsic factors. In *Teratology: Principles and Techniques,* J. G. Wilson and J. Warkany, Eds., University of Chicago Press, Chicago, pp. 57-80.

Karnofsky, D., Patterson, P., and Ridgeway, L. (1949). Effects of desoxypyridoxine and vitamin B_6 on development of the chick embryo. *Proc. Soc. Exp. Biol. Med.* 71:73-76.

Keen, C. L., Mark-Savage, P., Lonnerdal, B., and Hurley, L. S. (1981a). Low tissue copper and teratogenesis in rats resulting from D-penicillamine. *Fed. Proc.* 40:917.

Keen, C. L., Mark-Savage, P., Lonnerdal, B., and Hurley, L. S. (1981b). Abnormal copper status resulting from D-penicillamine administered during pregnancy. *Teratology* 23:44A.

Keen, C. L., Lonnerdal, B., Cohen, N. L., and Hurley, L. S. (1982). Drug-induced Cu deficiency: a model for Cu deficiency teratogenicity. *Fed. Proc.* 41:944.

Keen, C. L., Lonnerdal, B., and Hurley, L. S. (1982). Teratogenic effects of copper deficiency and excess. In *Inflammatory Diseases and Copper,* J. R. J. Sorenson (Ed.), Humana Press, Inc., Clifton, N.J., pp. 109-122.

Kimmel, C. A., and Sloan, C. S. (1975). Studies on the mechanism of EDTA teratogenesis. *Teratology* 12:330-331.

Kimmel, C. A., Butcher, R. E., and Schumacher, H. J. (1972). Salicylates and nutrition: pre- and postnatal effects. *Anat. Rec.* 172:345.

Kimmel, C. A., Butcher, R. E., Vorhees, C. V., and Schumacher, H. J. (1977). Metal-salt potentiation of salicylate-induced teratogenesis and behavorial changes in rats. *Teratology* 10:293-300.

Kinney, C. S., and Morse, L. M. (1964). Effect of a folic antagonist, aminopterin, on fetal development and nucleic acid metabolism in the rat. *J. Nutr.* 84:288-294.

Kociba, R. J., and Sleight, S. S. (1970). Nitrite toxicosis in the ascorbic acid deficient guinea pig. *Toxicol. App;. Pharmacol.* 16:424-429.

Koshakji, R. P., and Schulert, A. R. (1972). Biochemical mechanisms of salicylate teratology in the rat. *Biochem. Pharmacol.* 22:407-416.

Landauer, W. (1948). The effect of nicotinamide and α-ketoglutaric acid on the teratogenic action of insulin. *J. Exp. Zool.* 109:283-290.

Landauer, W. (1952). Malformations of chicken embryos produced by boric acid and the probable role of riboflavin in their origin. *J. Exp. Zool.* 120:469-508.

Landauer, W., and Clark, E. M. (1962). The interaction in teratogenic activity of the two niacin analogs 3-acetylpyridine and
6-aminonicotinamide. J. Exp. Zool. 151:253-258.
Landauer, W., and Clark, E. M. (1964). Teratogenic risks of drug
synergism. Nature 203:527-528.
Landauer, W., and Rhodes, M. B. (1952). Further observations on
the teratogenic nature of insulin and its modification by supplementary treatment. J. Exp. Zool. 119:221-261.
Landauer, W., and Salam, N. (1974). The experimental production
in chicken embryos of muscular hypoplasia and associated defects of beak and cervical vertebrae. Acta Embryol. Exp. 1:
51-66.
Landauer, W., and Sopher, D. (1970). Succinate, glycerophosphate
and ascorbate as sources of cellular energy and as antiteratogens. J. Embryol. Exp. Morphol. 24:187-202.
Layton, W. M., and Hallesy, D. W. (1965). Deformity of forelimb
in rats: association with high doses of acetazolamide. Science
149:306-308.
Lee, S., and Aleyassine, H. (1970). Hydrazine toxicity in pregnant
rats. Arch. Environ. Health 21:615-619.
Levene, C. I. (1961). The lathyrogenic effect of isonicotinic acid
hydrazide (INAH) on the chick embryo and its reversal by pyridoxal. J. Exp. Med. 113:795-809.
Maren, T. H. (1967). Carbonic anhydrase: chemistry, physiology
and inhibition. Physiol. Rev. 47:595-781.
McBride, W. G. (1961). Thalidomide and congenital abnormalities.
Lancet 2:1358.
Meltzer, H. (1956). Congenital anomalies due to attempted abortion
with 4-aminopteroglutamic acid. JAMA 161:1253.
Mercier-Parot, L., and Tuchmann-Duplessis, H. (1974). The dysmor-
phogenic potential of phenytoin: experimental observations.
Drugs 8:340-353.
Meyer, J. G. (1973). The teratological effects of anticonvulsants
and the effects on pregnancy and birth. Eur. Neurol. 10:
179-190.
Milunsky, A. J., Graef, J. W., and Gaynor, M. F. (1968). Methotrexate-induced congenital malformations. J. Pediatr. 72:790-
795.
Mjølnerød, O. K., Dommerud, S. A., Rasmussen, K., and Gjeruldsen, S. T. (1971). Congenital connective-tissue defect probably due to D-penicillamine treatment in pregnancy. Lancet
1:673-675.
Monson, R. R., Rosenberg, L., Hartz, S. C., Shapiro, S., Heinon-
en, P. O. P., and Slone, D. (1973). Diphenylhydantoin and
selected congenital malformations. N. Engl. J. Med. 289:1049-
1052.

Nebert, D. W. (1980). Genetic differences in drug metabolism: possible importance in teratogenesis. In *Phenytoin-Induced Teratology and Gingival Pathology*, T. M. Hassel, M. C. Johnston, and K. A. Dudley, Ed., Raven Press, New York, pp. 113-127.

Netzloff, M. L., Streiff, R. P., Frias, J. L., and Rennert, O. M. (1979). Folate antagonism following teratogenic exposure to diphenylhydantoin. *Teratology 19*:45-50.

O'Dell, B. L., Reynolds, G., and Reeves, P. G. (1977). Analogous effects of zinc deficiency and aspirin in the pregnant rats. *J. Nutr. 107*:1222-1228.

Peer, L. A., Bryan, W., Strean, L. P., Walker, J. C., Bernhard, W. G., and Peck, G. C. (1958a). Induction of cleft palate in mice by cortisone and its reduction. *J. Int. Coll. Surg. 30*: 249-254.

Peer, L. A., Strean, L. P., Walker, J. C., Bernhard, W. G., and Peck, G. C. (1958b). Study of 400 pregnancies with birth of cleft lip-palate infants. *Plast. Reconstr. Surg. 22*:442-449.

Peer, L. A., Gordon, H. W., and Bernhard, W. G. (1964). Effect of vitamins on human teratology. *Plast. Reconstr. Surg. 34*: 358-362.

Pollard, D. R., and Fraser, F. C. (1973). Induction of cytoplasmic factor increasing resistance to the teratogenic effect of 6-aminonicotinamide in mice. *Teratology 7*:267-270.

Powell, H. R., and Ekert, H. (1971). Methotrexate-induced congenital malformations. *Med. J. Aust. 2*:1076-1077.

Pritchard, J. A., Scott, D. E., and Whalley, P. J. (1971). Maternal folate deficiency and pregnancy wastage. *Am. J. Obstet. Gynecol. 109*:341-346.

Proctor, N. H., and Casida, J. E. (1975). Organophosphorous and methyl carbamate insecticide teratogenesis: diminished NAD in chicken embryos. *Science 190*:580-581.

Proctor, N. H., Moscioni, A. D., and Casida, J. E. (1976). Chicken embryo NAD levels lowered by teratogenic organophosphorous and methylcarbamate insecticides. *Biochem. Pharmacol. 25*:757-762.

Reed, S. C. (1936). Harelip in the house mouse. I. Effects of the external and internal environment. *Genetics 21*:339-360.

Reynolds, E. H. (1967). Effects of folic acid on the mental status and fit-frequency of drug-treated epileptic patients. *Lancet 1*: 1086-1088.

Reynolds, E. H. (1973). Anticonvulsants, folic acid, and epilepsy. *Lancet 1*:1376-1378.

Richens, A. (1976). *Drug Treatment of Epilepsy*. Henry Kimpton, London, pp. 127-129.

Rogers, J. C., Chambers, H., and Casida, J. E. (1964). Nicotinic acid analogs: effects on response of chick embryos and hens to organophosphate toxicants. *Science 144*:539-540.

Runner, M. N. (1967). Comparative pharmacology in relation to teratogensis. *Fed. Proc.* 26:1131-1136.

Scheinberg, H. I., and Sternlieb, I. (1975). Pregnancy in penicillamine treated patients with Wilson's disease. *N. Engl. J. Med.* 293:1300-1302.

Schrader, R. E., Hirsch, K. S., Levin, J., and Hurley, L. S. (1978). Attenuating effect of zinc on abnormal placental morphology in 6-mercaptopurine treated rats. *Teratology* 17:315-325.

Snell, E. S., and Cravens, W. W. (1950). Reversal of aminopterin inhibition in the chick embryo with deoxyribosides. *Proc. Soc. Exp. Biol. Med.* 74:87-91.

Soloman, L., Abrams, G., Dinner, M., and Berman, L. (1977). Neonatal abnormalities associated with D-penicillamine treatment during pregnancy. *N. Engl. J. Med.* 196:54-55.

Speidel, B. D., and Meadow, S. R. (1974). Epilepsy, anticonvulsants and congenital malformations. *Drugs* 8:354-365.

Swenerton, H., and Hurley, L. S. (1971). Teratogenic effects of a chelating agent and their prevention by zinc. *Science* 173:62-64.

Telang, N. T., and Mulherkar, L. (1974). In vitro studies on the effect of hydrazine on the morphogenesis of chick embryos and the mechanism of its action. *Oncology* 30:529-541.

Thiersch, J. B. (1952). Therapeutic abortions with folic acid antagonist, 4-aminopteroylglutamic acid (4-amino P. G. A.). *Am. J. Obstet. Gynecol.* 63:1298-1304.

Thiersch, J. B. (1956). The control of reproduction in rats with the aid of antimetabolites and early experiences with antimetabolites as abortifacient agents in man. *Acta Endocrinol.* 28:37-49.

Thiersch, J. B., and Phillips, F. S. (1950). Action of 4-aminopteroylglutamic acid on the early pregnancy of rats and mice. *Fed. Proc.* 9:346-349.

Varpela, E. (1964). On the effect exerted by first-line tuberculosis medicines on the foetus. *Acta Tuberc. Scand* 45:53-69.

Verrusio, A. C., Pollard, D. R., and Fraser, F. C. (1968). A cytoplasmically transmitted, diet-dependent difference in response to the teratogenic effect of 6-aminonicotinamide. *Science* 160:206-207.

Vorhees, C. V., Brunner, R. L., and Butcher, R. E. (1979). Psychotropic drugs as behavorial teratogens. *Science* 205:1220-1225.

Walshe, J. M. (1977). Pregnancy in Wilson's disease. *Q. J. Med.* 46:73-83.

Warburton, D., Trasler, D. G., Naylor, A., Miller, J. R., and Fraser, F. C. (1962). Pitfalls in tests for teratogenicity. *Lancet* 2:1116-1117.

Warkany, J. (1979). The medical profession and congenital malformations (1900—1979). *Teratology 20*:201-204.

Warkany, J., Beaudry, P. H., and Hornstein, S. (1959). Attempted abortion with aminopterin (4-aminopteroylglutamic acid). *Am. J. Dis. Child. 97*:274-281.

Warkany, J., and Schraffenberger, E. (1944). Congenital malformations induced in rats by maternal nutritional deficiency. IV. Preventive factor. *J. Nutr. 27*:477-484.

Wilson, J. G. (1962). Teratogenic interaction of minimal doses of hypervitaminosis A and trypan blue in the rat. *Anat. Rec. 142*:292.

Wilson, J. G. (1973a). *Environment and Birth Defects.* Academic Press, New York.

Wilson, J. G. (1973b). Drugs as teratogens in man. *Teratology 7*:3-15.

Zwilling, E., and DeBell, J. T. (1950). Micromelia and growth retardation as independent effects of sulfanilamide in chick embryos. *J. Exp. Zool. 115*:59-81.

9

Human Milk:
A Portal of Drugs from Mother to Infant

Lynn Marie Janas and Mary Frances Picciano
University of Illinois, Urbana, Illinois

I. INTRODUCTION

Human milk is a significant route of drug excretion from the maternal system and of infant drug exposure during lactation which has frequently been ignored in the past. A review of the literature reveals a scarcity of information on this topic, and many conclusions based on single case reports. With the development of the science of pharmacokinetics, studies of drug excretion into human milk may be designed in accord with the properties of the specific drug in question. Without consideration of both drug pharmacokinetics and variability patterns of human milk composition, as lactation advances, within a single day, and even within a single nursing, results of studies of drug excretion into human milk may be misleading and offer little information from which recommendations to the lactating mother may be made. This review will focus on available literature to date concerning drugs excreted in human milk, and on some of the potential and observed effects of infant exposures to these drugs, in an attempt to highlight the dearth of information concerning this portal of drugs to the infant.

II. FACTORS INFLUENCING DRUG TRANSFER

A. Milk Composition and Properties

Human milk is a unique and complex biological fluid containing numerous lipid, protein, carbohydrate, vitamin, mineral, and immune constituents present in quantities ideally suited for the rapid growth and development of the human infant during the first 6 months of life. The composition of colostrum and human milk varies throughout lactation and is influenced by many factors, including biochemical individuality, maternal nutrition, stage of lactation, time of day, and the single nursing period itself. Numerous studies have reported patterns of variation of human milk which are both quantitative and qualitative in nature, which represent the evolutionary fine tuning of this biological fluid to meet the needs of the vulnerable and immature neonate.

1. Biochemical Individuality

Many maternal factors affect human milk constituents. For instance, the age of the mother may influence milk levels of fat, protein, copper, iron, and zinc (Picciano and Guthrie, 1976). Maternal parity and lactation history (i.e., number of previous children and number of previous lactations) have been noted to have an effect on copper, iron, and zinc content of milk, while fat content may be influenced by parity alone (Picciano and Guthrie, 1976). Use of contraceptive agents prior to pregnancy may decrease concentrations of manganese (Kirksey et al., 1979), and also concentrations of fats, proteins, and calcium (Barsivala and Virkar, 1973) in human milk. These are just several of the factors, unique to the individual mother, which influence the nutrient content of her milk.

2. Maternal Nutrition

Maternal nutrition is an important influence on milk composition. For example, the caloric intake and relative amounts and types of fats and carbohydrates in the diet, as well as the fatty acids present in the diet, have been shown to influence the fatty acid profile of the milk (Insull and Ahrens, 1959; Insull et al., 1959). A fat-free diet resulted in increased milk levels of saturated fatty acids (C12:0 and C14:0) and decreased levels of unsaturated fatty acids (C18:2 and C18:3). Another important finding, the increased dietary unsaturated fatty acids which resulted in increased milk levels of unsaturated fatty acids, has been reported by other investigators (Read et al., 1965; Potter and Nestel, 1976). The increased dietary intake of vegetable oils in the American diet, which are high in unsaturated fatty acids, has been associated with increased levels of these fatty acids in the milk of American women (Glass et al., 1967; Guthrie et al., 1977). In contrast, milk from British women revealed fatty acid patterns comparable to those observed 30–40 years ago (Department of Health and Social Security, 1977), reflecting relatively unchanged dietary fatty acid intakes. In addition to fat, protein quality may influence protein and amino acid content of human milk (Wurtman and Fernstrom, 1979), and diets deficient in lysine and methionine have been associated with lowered milk

levels of these amino acids (Lindblad and Rahimtoola, 1974). Human
milk levels of biotin, niacin, pantothenic acid, and vitamin B_6 vary according to maternal intake until a plateau is reached (Coryell et al.,
1945; Deodhar et al., 1964; West and Kirksey, 1976). The fetal endow-
ment of vitamin B_{12} may be compromised in infants of vegetarian
mothers and be an important determinant of adequacy of milk content of
this nutrient (Higginbottom et al., 1978; Jadhav et al., 1962).

3. Stage of Lactation

Human milk exhibits many remarkable changes in composition as lactation is established. Colostrum, the milk produced during the first 5
days postpartum, is particularly rich in nutrient content. Immuno-
globulin levels are highest in colostrum and decrease to a lower level
at about day 6 postpartum (McClelland et al., 1978). Total protein
content of human milk decreases as lactation advances, while nonprotein nitrogen content remains unaltered (Atkinson et al., 1980). Fat
content of human milk increases as lactation advances (Macy et al.,
1953), and lactose content is higher in colostrum than in mature milk
(Macy et al., 1953; Lönnerdal et al., 1976). In general, human milk
levels of minerals and trace elements tend to decrease as lactation progresses. Human milk concentrations of zinc decrease rapidly in early
lactation and more slowly as lactation advances, as do concentrations of
copper (Casey, 1976; Jensen et al., 1972; Picciano and Deering, 1977).
Levels of sodium are roughly twice as high in colostrum as in mature
milk, and levels of chloride also decrease as lactation progresses (Miller
and Jackson, 1951).

4. Diurnal Variation

Marked diurnal variations of certain nutrients in human milk exist within the same women and make it difficult to obtain human milk samples
with representative nutrient contents. The fat content of human milk is
lowest in the morning, reaches its highest level in the middle of the
morning, and then declines throughout the day (Gunther and Stanier,
1949; Hytten, 1954a); and the cholesterol content of human milk increases from midday to evening (Picciano et al., 1978). Protein and
dry weight have been reported to increase from morning to midday
(Picciano, 1978; Hall, 1975). With regard to mineral and electrolyte
variations, calcium has been reported to decrease from morning to evening (Picciano, 1978) and iron and zinc to increase and decrease, respectively, from morning to midday (Picciano and Guthrie, 1976). No
differences in calcium, magnesium, zinc, potassium, and copper were
reported during a single day (Picciano et al., 1978). Chloride concentration in human milk was reported to exhibit diurnal variation, reaching a maximum level at midday (Kermack and Miller, 1951).

5. Variation Within a Single Feeding Period

The composition of human milk exhibits striking variation within a single feeding period. The lipid and protein contents of human milk tend to increase from the beginning to the end of a single nursing (Macy et al., 1931; Hytten, 1954b; Picciano, 1978). Differences in fore- and hind-milk concentrations of cholesterol (Picciano et al., 1978), sodium, potassium, calcium, and iron (Gunther et al., 1965; Picciano, 1978) have also been reported while levels of other minerals such as magnesium, potassium, copper, and zinc were reported to remain relatively constant within the single nursing period (Picciano et al., 1978).

B. Drug Physiochemical Properties

The effect produced by a drug depends on both physiochemical and pharmacokinetic properties of the drug molecule. The physiochemical properties of a drug that influence rate of membrane transport across the gastrointestinal, kidney, as well as mammary gland membranes are the lipophilicity, ionization, and molecular size of the drug molecule (Garrett, 1971). Lipophilic drugs are transported across the mammary gland epithelium and into the milk by simple diffusion processes (Rasmussen, 1966). The transport of weak acidic or basic drugs depends on the pH of the drug medium. Important in this regard is that the pH of human milk (pH 7) is generally lower than that of plasma (pH 7.4). Because of this pH difference, weakly basic compounds are expected to pass into milk with greater ease than weakly acidic compounds. Highly ionized drug molecules may be transported across biological membranes only if they are of low molecular weight (< 100).

C. Maternal Pharmacokinetics

Many metabolic and physiologic processes affect the pharmacokinetics, or fate of drugs in the body. The physiologic states of lactation and infancy impose their own unique effects on the bodily processes of absorption, distribution, metabolism, and elimination. Some of the metabolic and physiologic effects on lactation have been previously reviewed (Peaker, 1976), but pharmacokinetics in the lactating woman have, to a great extent, been ignored and information on this topic is scarce.

The absorption of drugs is influenced by the stability of the drug in the gastrointestinal tract and the state of the gastrointestinal tract at the time of drug ingestion. Both the increased cell size and cell number observed in the gastrointestinal tract of the lactating rat (Fell et al., 1963) and the high blood flow to the gastrointestinal tract relative to other organs except the liver, mammary gland, and skin (Hanwell and Linzell, 1973a,b) suggest an increase in absorptive capacity of the gastrointestinal tract induced by lactation.

Changes in cardiovascular function may alter drug distribution in the lactating woman. An increased cardiac output occurs during the first few days of lactation, which results in an increased blood flow to all organs (Hanwell and Linzell, 1973a,b). This flow is directed more specifically to the gut, mammary gland and skin as lactation is more established. Protein binding, an important determinant of drug distribution in the body, may be different in the lactating woman than in the nonlactating woman if circulating protein levels differ. Free fatty acids present in the serum may induce conformational changes in serum albumin which result in decreased binding affinity of drugs such as salicyclic acid and penicillins for serum albumin. Since standard values of circulating blood compounds such as protein and fatty acids in the lactating woman are not readily available, it is difficult to estimate effects of these compounds on drug kinetic patterns of the lactating woman.

Metabolism of drugs occurs primarily in the liver, but the lung, kidney, blood, and intestine are also involved. The increased blood flow to the liver observed in lactation suggests an increased function of this organ in lactation. Although the lung and kidney are the usual routes utilized in drug excretion, the lactating woman utilizes the mammary glands as an additional significant route of elimination.

D. Infant Pharmacokinetics

Pharmacokinetics in the infant are dramatically different from those of the adult. The infant is not a miniature version of the adult but is very unique, both physiologically and metabolically, and is characterized by a rapid growth rate never again achieved in life. Comprehensive reviews of infant pharmacokinetics are available (Shirkey, 1980; Morselli, 1977; Morselli, 1976), and highlights will be summarized below.

Among the striking changes in morphology of the gastrointestinal tract which occur during the neonatal period are the hyperacidity observed shortly after birth, and the relative achlorhydria that follows (Morselli, 1977). Since pH-dependent diffusion is a major regulator of drug absorption from the gastrointestinal tract, changes in pH may profoundly affect pharmacokinetics. The prolonged gastric emptying observed in the neonate (Smith, 1976) may also influence pharmacokinetics. Since bilary function is immature in the newborn (Watkins et al., 1973; Murphy and Singer, 1974), the fate of drugs involved in enterohepatic circulation may be different in the neonate than in the more mature infant or the adult.

The distribution of drugs is different in the infant than in the adult mainly due to differences in relative sizes of body compartments and in protein binding capacity of the plasma. The infant has more extracellular fluid and total body water and less total body fat relative to total body weight than the adult. Plasma protein levels reach adult levels at 10—12 months of age (Windorfer et al., 1974; Ecobichon and Stephens, 1973). High concentrations of bilirubin and free fatty acids in the plasma are characteristics of the altered protein binding observed in the neonate (Odell, 1973; Spector et al., 1973; Gugler et al., 1974). The developmental stage of the blood-brain barrier in the infant is an important determinant of drug distribution in the brain, and is incomplete in newborn animals (Brown, 1973). The lower blood pH of infant plasma also affects protein binding of drugs.

The capacity to metabolize drugs is undeveloped in the infant. Metabolism of drugs by hepatic conjugation, hepatic microsomal mixed-function oxidation, and plasma esterification reactions is lower in the infant than in the adult (Morselli, 1976). The activities of the hepatic microsomal mixed-function oxidases (Aranda et al., 1974) and of the plasma esterases (Ecobichon and Stephens, 1973) have been reported to increase with age. With regard to conjugation reactions, the newborn has a reduced capacity for glucuronidation reactions (Vest, 1965), but is capable of both sulfation (Levy et al., 1975) and demethylation reactions (Meffin et al., 1973). Drug metabolism by liver microsomal enzymes via both conjugation and mixed oxidations may be reduced in the neonate (Stern et al., 1970; Sereni et al., 1973) and complicate the pharmacokinetic profile of a drug administered to the neonate.

Although elimination of drugs is accomplished primarily by the kidney, this organ is not considered to be mature until at least 1 year of age due to reduced tubular secretion and glomerular filtration (Edelman and Spitzer, 1976). These processes may be stimulated by drug administration to the newborn (Braunlich, 1976). Since the pH of the urine is lower in the newborn than in the adult, an increased reabsorption rate of weakly basic drugs would be expected. It has been suggested (Braunlich, 1976) that the degree of difference between neonatal and adult elimination capacity might be lessened due to the fact that the infant lacks the diurnal variation in renal function observed in the adult (Stanbury and Thomson, 1951; Mills, 1966).

III. DRUGS DETECTED IN HUMAN MILK

A. Analgesics and Anti-Inflammatory Agents

A number of analgesic and anti-inflammatory drugs have been identified in human milk. One such compound is the widely used acetaminophen. Its passage into human milk and the consequence of such milk ingestion in the nursing infant has been investigated (Berlin et al., 1980). Eleven mothers and infants were studied and from analyses of saliva and milk samples collected at defined intervals for 24 hr after a single 650-mg dose of acetaminophen, it was observed that the drug appeared in both saliva and milk within 15 min and peak concentrations were observed at 1—2 hr. The disappearance of acetaminophen in milk ($t_{1/2}$ 1.35—3.5 hr) closely paralled that in saliva ($t_{1/2}$ 1.72—3.3 hr). Analysis of infant urine samples taken 3—5 hr after maternal drug administration revealed neither acetaminophen nor its metabolite in any of the samples, suggesting that the absorption of acetaminophen in the infant is negligible and that this compound may indeed be a safe choice of an analgetic/antipyretic drug for use by the nursing mother. Levy et al. (1975) reported the half-life of acetaminophen in newborns to be approximately 3.5 hr compared to 2.0 hr in the adult, which suggests a well-developed capability for sulfate conjugation of the drug by the infant.

Aspirin, another widely used analgesic and anti-inflammatory agent, has been measured in serum and milk from a woman taking 4 g/day and in serum of her infant (Erickson and Oppenheim, 1979). Maternal plasma concentration was 18 mg per 100 ml, but salicylate was not detected in either her milk (< 0.5 mg per 100 ml) or in the serum of her nursing infant. Upon hydrolysis in the gut, aspirin is present as salicylic acid, and in the plasma is highly protein bound. Because of these physio-chemical properties, minimal passage of this drug into human milk would be expected; however, metabolic acidosis has been reported in a 16-day-old nursing infant whose mother ingested approximately 648 mg every 4 hr for arthritis (Clark and Wilson, 1981). Erickson and Oppenheim (1979) suggest that toxicity symptoms would be unlikely in the normal breast-fed infant, but caution that an infant with a blood-clotting disorder might be at risk from the very low levels of aspirin (< 5 mg per 100 ml) which may be passed to the infant through human milk. The antiplatelet effect of aspirin is observed at doses of 1 mg/kg per day (O'Brien et al., 1970).

The excretion of two other analgesics and anti-inflammatory drugs, mefenamic and flufenamic acid, into human milk has been investigated (Buchanan et al., 1968, 1969). In one study (Buchanan et al., 1968); mefenamic acid, an analgesic agent, was administered to 10 nursing mothers immediately postpartum. The dosage was 250 mg three times a day for 4 days after a loading dose of 500 mg. Maternal plasma and milk specimens were obtained 2 hr after the morning dose on days 2, 3, and 4 postpartum and infant plasma and urine specimens were obtained 1 hr after the midday nursing on day 4 postpartum. Although maternal plasma levels of mefenamic acid averaged 0.95, 0.97, and 0.91 µg/ml on days 2, 3, and 4, respectively, postpartum, only trace levels of this drug were observed in milk, infant plasma, and infant urine specimens. The excretion of flufenamic acid (an analgesic and anti-inflammatory compound) was studied utilizing the same experimental design as that described for mefenamic acid (Buchanan et al., 1969), and findings were similar. Although the mean maternal plasma concentration of free flufenamic acid varied on each day sampled from 2.90 to 6.41 µg/ml, mean milk concentrations only ranged from 0.50 to 0.55 μg/ml on these same days. Free plus conjugated flufenamic acid concentrations in milk on days 3 and 4 were 0.173 and 0.187 μg/ml, respectively, and in infant blood and urine on day 4 were 0.188 and 0.075 μg/ml compared to the control values of 0.043 and 0.022 obtained from cord blood and first voided urine specimens. These results indicated that small quantities of flufenamic acid, like mefenamic acid, are transferred to the nursing infant via human milk.

Although no adverse effects on the infant have been reported for the aforementioned analgesic and anti-inflammatory agents at standard dosages, such may not be the case for the more potent drugs, especially if prescribed at elevated dosages, as suggested by seizure episodes reported on day 7 postpartum in a human milk fed infant whose mother was treated with indomethacin (Eeg-Olofsson et al., 1978). The maternal dosage of 3 mg/kg indomethacin was high relative to the standard dosage of 1–2 mg/kg and administration began on day 4 postpartum.

Cimetidine is an antagonist of hydrochloric acid secretion which has been used successfully in the treatment of peptic ulcers. Its mode of action is thought to be mediated through inhibition of histamine release, secondary to mucosal injury (Clayman, 1977). Controversy surrounds the use of acid-inhibiting drugs, such as cimetidine, since an increased intragastric pH has been positively correlated with increased concentrations on N-nitrosomine compounds, which are powerful carcinogens (Reed et al., 1981). In a single case study of cimetidine excretion into human milk (Somogyi and Gugler, 1979) after both single and chronic dosage regimes, drug concentrations in milk were consistently higher than those in plasma. After a single 400-mg dose, the milk to maternal plasma ratio was approximately 3.4 and this ratio increased threefold after administration of 1 g of cimetidine per day for 3 days. These authors calculated than an infant ingesting 1 liter of milk per day would receive about 6 mg of cimetidine. Since cimetidine is liberally transferred into human milk during chronic dosage and there exists the potential carcinogenic effect of increased intragastric pH, cimetidine usage by the nursing mother is contraindicated.

Another compound used in the treatment of a gastrointestinal disorder is sulfasalazine, which is used in the treatment of ulcerative colitis. This drug has been detected in human milk with no adverse effects on the infant (Khan and Truelove, 1979). Both sulfasalazine and its metabolite sulfapyridine are excreted in human milk in concentrations which are approximately one-third to one-half of those of maternal serum. Since low serum concentrations of these compounds (approximately 1 μg/ml) are typical in patients receiving chronic sulfasalazine therapy, these investigators suggested that levels of the drugs and its metabolites in human milk are likely to be innocuous.

B. Antimicrobial Agents

1. Antibacterial Agents

Many commonly used antibacterial agents are excreted in human milk, and although untoward effects on the infant have not been thoroughly investigated, it has been suggested that use of these drugs may be associated with sensitization of the infant (Criep et al., 1959-1960). Concern has been raised that the intestinal microflora of the infant may be affected by maternal antibiotic therapy. However, results of a study of Borderon et al. (1980) have indicated that contrary to the affect of antibiotic therapy during pregnancy, maternal antibiotic treatment after delivery does not affect the infant microflora to alter resistance to susceptible organisms.

Tetracycline antibiotics are broadly used antibiotic compounds, which have been used in the treatment of women with infections following cesarian deliveries (Posner et al., 1956). Although we are unaware of any studies in which serum or urine of the human milk fed infant were analyzed, human milk levels of doxycycline, a tetracycline antiobiotic, were reported to be 30–40 percent of maternal serum levels (Morganti et al., 1968). Average concentrations of doxycycline in human milk were 0.77 and 0.38 γ/ml at 3 and 24 hr, respectively, after a 100-mg dose which was administered 24 hr following a 200-mg loading dose. Since tetracycline is poorly absorbed when ingested with milk or other foods with high calcium contents, it would be interesting to know the fraction of drug appearing in the milk which is available to the infant.

It has been suggested that in the human milk-fed infant whose mother is treated with penicillin, an allergic reaction or sensitization may be incurred (Criep et al., 1959–1960). The use of penicillin in the treatment of mastitis in cows, and its subsequent transfer into milk, was considered a public health problem in the late 1950s by the American Medical Association Council on Drugs due to the reactions mentioned above (Kautz, 2959). At 2 hr after an intramuscular dose of 100,000–300,000 units per day of penicillin to 11 women during the first postpartum week, 0.015–0.06 unit/ml were detected in the milk of eight women and 0.112–1.92 units/ml were measured in maternal serum (Green et al., 1946). Results of this study are in agreement with those of Rozansky and Brzezinsky (1969) and Rasmussen (1959) who reported milk concentration to be approximately 10–20% of that of maternal serum. Two semisynthetic compounds, cephradine, a cephalosporin, and epicillin, a penicillin, which have both gram-positive and gram-negative antimicrobial activity, have each been measured in the milk of six lactating women at 1, 2, 4, and 6 hr after nine doses of 500 mg every 6 hr, and again a milk/maternal serum ratio of 20% was observed (Mischler et al., 1978). In addition, concentrations remained constant throughout the sampling period, and averaged 0.60 µg/ml for cephradine and 0.25 µg/ml for epicillin. Studies of the presence of two additional cephalosporin antibiotics in human milk have been performed (Kafetzis et al., 1980; Yoshioka et al., 1979). In a study of cefotaxime transport into human milk, a 1-g dose was administered intravenously to 12 nursing mothers on day 3 postpartum (Kafetzis et al., 1980). Milk and maternal blood samples were obtained at regular intervals for 6 hr after the drug was administered. Peak milk concentrations occurred at 2−3 hr and ranged from 0.25 to 0.52 mg/liter, and the milk/maternal serum ratios at 2 and 3 hr averaged 0.091 and 0.17, respectively. It was suggested that cefotaxime in human milk might affect the oropharyngeal flora of the suckling infant. Cefazolin levels were determined in the milk and serum of 20 lactating women (Yoshioka et al., 1979). after a single 2-g intravenous dose of the drug. Analysis of milk samples obtained at 2, 3, and 4 hr after drug administration revealed milk concentrations of 1.25, 1.51, and 1.16 µg/ml, respectively. The milk to maternal serum ratio at 2 hr was approximately 0.023.

Chloramphenicol, an antibiotic commonly used in the treatment of infection in infants and young children, has been studied in infants and young children (Sack et al., 1980) and in low-birth-weight infants (Glazer et al., 1980) and its presence found to be highly variable and consequently unpredictable. In infants and young children 4 months to 4 years old, the half-life of chloramphenicol ranged from 2.1 to 8.3 hr (Sack et al., 1980). In low-birth-weight infants 1−8 days old, the half-life of this drug ranged from 10 to 48 hr, and in infants 11 days to 8 weeks old, ranged from 5.5 to 15.7 hr (Glazer et. al., 1980). In human milk samples analyzed from two groups of women, one receiving 1 g and the other receiving 2 g of chloramphenicol per day, maximum milk levels averaged 1.69 and 3.55 µg/ml of active drug, respectively (Havelka et al., 1968). In all samples analyzed, only 50% of the compound excreted in human milk was the active metabolite as established by the use of two methods of chloramphenicol quantitation, the chemical method, which enables determination of total antiobiotic concentration, and the microbiological method, which enables determination of the antimicrobially effective concentration.

A drug frequently used for treatment of urinary tract infections, nitrofurantoin, is known to cause hemolysis in individuals with glucose-6-phosphate dehydrogenase deficiency. Since this compound has been detected in human milk in concentrations of 0.3−0.5 µg/ml in women 2 hr after receiving 200 mg of nitrofurantoin, following 100 mg every 6 hr the previous day, it has been recommended by Varsano et al. (1973) that nursing mothers use nitrofurantoin with caution in populations where the glucose-6-phosphate dehydrogenase deficiency is common. In the study just mentioned where detection limits were not mentioned, as in a previous study where detection limits were 2 µg/ml (Hosbach and Foster, 1967), no drug was detected in milk samples from women administered continuous doses of 100 mg of nitrofurantoin. With increased sensitivity of methodology, quantification of low concentrations of this drug will be possible and enable the study of its pharmacodynamics in the nursing mother and infant.

Sulfamethoxypyridazine is another antibacterial agent which can produce hemolysis in individuals with glucose-6-phosphate dehydrogenase deficiency. Jaundice and hemolysis have been reported in three infants with this inborn error of metabolism. The mothers of two of the affected infants were treated with sulfamethoxypyridazine prior to delivery (Brown and Cevik, 1965). The mother of the third infant was lactating and treated with this drug for urinary tract infection after delivery (Harley and Robin, 1966). In three women administered a 2-g sulfamethoxypyridazine loading dose followed by a 1-g daily maintenance dose, maternal serum levels ranged from 7.3 to 12.7 mg per 100 ml of milk while levels ranged from 1 to 2.7 mg per 100 ml. Serum and milk concentrations of drug were essentially the same within a single woman at 24 and 48 hr after drug therapy was initiated (Sparr and Pritchard, 1958). Infant serum concentrations of sulfamethoxypyridazine at 48 hr were 0.1 and 0.3 mg per 100 ml in two infants and was undetected in the third infant.

Methenamine, also used in the treatment of urinary tract infection, has been quantified in the milk and plasma of four lactating women 5 hr after a 1-g oral dose (Allgén et al., 1979). Milk concentrations ranged from 48 to 52 μmol/liter and were found to be roughly the same as those of maternal plasma. These investigators concluded that since these milk levels would yield an infant dose which was approximately 1/100 of the adult therapeutic dose, toxic effects in the child would be unlikely. In an early study (Berger, 1941), the excretion of another drug used in the treatment of urinary tract infections, mandelic acid was investigated in the milk of six women. The presence of mandelic acid in milk was quite variable and averaged approximately 0.27 g/day in milk from women administered 12 g/day. Infant urinary mandelic acid excretion per day was estimated from daily urine samples and averaged 0.086 g/kg body weight.

A report of clindamycin in the milk of two nursing mothers who received 600 mg of clindamycin every 6 hr revealed levels of 2.13–3.8 μg/ml in the milk (Smith et al., 1975). When these same women were put on a regimen of 300 mg every 6 hr, clindamycin concentration in the milk dropped accordingly and values ranged from 0.74 to 1.8 μg/ml.

Metronidazole is prescribed in the treatment of *Trichomonas vaginalis* infections and has been studied in the milk of three women treated with a single 2-g dose of the drug (Erickson et al., 1981). Since peak milk concentrations occurred at 2 to 4 hr after administration and declined steadily in the next 24 hr, it was suggested that a single 2-g dose, followed by cessation of nursing for 24 hr, might be a suitable regimen for treatment of trichomoniasis in the lactating women.

Isoniazid, a widely used antitubercular drug, has been analyzed in human milk samples from a woman administered a single oral dose of 300 mg (Berlin and Lee, 1979). Peak milk concentrations of isoniazid and its metabolite, acetylisoniazid, were observed at 3 hr (16.6 μg/ml) and 5 hr (3.76 μg/ml), respectively. The half-lives of isoniazid in milk, maternal saliva, and plasma were 5.9, 5.2, and 4.6 hr, while those of acetylisoniazid were 13.5 hr in milk and 16.1 hr in plasma. It was suggested that the 7 mg/day excretion of isoniazid in milk may represent a significant hazard to nucleic acid synthesis and hepatic function of the infant.

2. Antiparasitic Agents

Praziquantel is an anthelmintic which is currently being heralded as the key to eradication of schistosomiasis, a common and crippling parasitic disease of the Third World (New Scientist, 1981). In milk and maternal plasma of 10 healthy nursing mothers, 5 who received a single 50-mg/kg dose and 5 who received three 20-mg/kg dose of praziquantel at 4-hr intervals, analyses disclosed milk levels of the drug which were roughly one-fourth of those of maternal plasma and whose disappearance pattern paralled that of plasma (Pütter and Held, 1979). Peak milk and plasma levels occurred at 2 hr after a single dose and averaged 0.44 and 1.36 mg/liter, respectively. In women following the multiple-dose regimen, peak milk concentrations occurred at 4 hr (0.25 mg/liter) and 10 hr (0.46 mg/liter), and maternal plasma followed this pattern as well with peak concentrations at 4 hr (1.22 mg/liter) and 10 hr (1.92 mg/liter). Whether protection of the infant may be provided by maternal ingestion of praziquantel, as in the case of pyrimethamine (Clyde, 1960), is yet to be determined.

A study of pyrimethamine excretion in human milk revealed that malaria was eliminated in totally breast-fed infants less than 6 months of age whose mothers ingested two 50- to 75-mg doses of the drug (Clyde and Shute, 1956). In another instance, a Tanganyikan lactating woman from a highly infected area was able to relieve her infant of malaria symptoms and to protect her infant from further attacks by taking 25 mg of pyrimethamine per week (Clyde, 1960). When maternal drug therapy was stopped for 2 weeks, the infant suffered a malaria attack, indicating that the pyrimethamine received from the mother was an adequate treatment for the infant. Since pyrimethamine is known to be a folic acid antagonist, it would be interesting to study the folic acid status in mothers and infants exposed to this drug.

3. Vaccinations

Although early reports claimed that human milk feeding exerted an inhibitory effect on antibody response to oral polio vaccine (Warren et al., 1964; Plotkin et al., 1966), more recent reports dispute this claim. DeForest et al. (1973) reported no difference in antibody response of human milk and formula fed infants after oral polio vaccine. These results are supported by similar findings of John et al. (1976).

The immediate postpartum period has been suggested as a satisfactory time for vaccinating women of childbearing age against rubella (Farquhar, 1972). These researchers reported that in a follow-up study of 18- to 20-month-old infants, there was no detectable antibody response to rubella in formula-fed infants and human milk-fed infants whose mothers were vaccinated immediately postpartum. In a case study of a single maternal-infant dyad after maternal postpartum rubella immunization, virus was isolated from the milk and infant throat swab, but not from the maternal throat swab at 12 days after vaccination (Buimovici-Klein et al., 1977). The lack of serologic response detected in the infant after this exposure may have been the result of protective immune factors of the infant gastrointestinal tract, or of those in the milk itself.

C. Anticoagulants

Anticoagulants prescribed for postpartum phlebitis may pass into human milk, but few studies have examined both their passage into milk, and their effects on the nursing infant. Their potential risk to the infant is profoundly demonstrated in a case report of a 4-week-old infant who developed a huge scrotal hematoma after herniotomy (Eckstein and Jack, 1970). The mother of this infant was taking 75–100 mg of phenindione daily. Although milk levels of phenindione were not measured, the decrease in prothrombin time from 55% to 23% of normal observed in the mother when breast feeding was discontinued suggests that milk is a significant route of excretion of phenindione and that it may be necessary to reduce the maternal dose upon cessation of breast feeding.

Warfarin functions to reduce vitamin K_1-dependent clotting factor synthesis by interrupting the vitamin K_1-epoxide cycle at the level of the epoxide reductase (Leck and Park, 1981). Because it is a weakly acidic and extensively protein-bound drug, its passage into human milk is predicted to be minimal. This has been substantiated in an investigation with 13 lactating women (Orme et al., 1977). Maternal plasma concentrations ranged from 1.2 to 2.6 μg/ml and no warfarin (< 25 ng/ml) was detected in milk or infant plasma samples analyzed. Dicoumarol is another anticoagulant with physiochemical properties similar to warfarin and its use has been demonstrated to be without effect on the prothrombin activity of 125 nursing infants when maternal dosage was 600 mg (Brambel and Hunter, 1950).

A relatively high frequency of hemorrhage in nursing infants of mothers taking ethylbiscoumacetate has been observed (Gostof et al., 1952) and believed to be due to the passage of a metabolite of this drug into human milk. Paradoxically, this unidentified metabolite acts to increase prothrombin formation in the nursing infant while the native drug added to expressed milk and subsequently fed to infants acts to

decrease prothrombin formation. These investigators attribute the observed high frequency of hemorrhage to a lowering of capillary resistance induced by ethylbiscoumacetate or its alleged metabolite.

D. Anticonvulsants

The Committee on Drugs of the American Academy of Pediatrics has
recommended that, at present, there is no evidence to suggest that
women who require anticonvulsant therapy should avoid nursing their
infants or discontinue drug therapy (American Academy of Pediatrics,
1979). However, there remains a paucity of information concerning the
amounts of anticonvulsants conveyed to the infant, and their physiological effects. For instance, methemoglobinemia in a nursing infant
whose mother was treated with phenobarbitone and phenytoin has been
reported to subside when the infant was fed milk from a donor, and
reappeared when nursing was reinitiated (Finch and Lorber, 1954). The
amount of drug in this mother's milk was not determined due to technical difficulties. Sedation of a nursing infant whose mother received
phenobarbitone and primidone regularly was claimed to contribute to
the sudden death of her infant (Juul, 1969). It is possible that maternal drug use was coincidental with the death of the infant; however,
deep slumber and difficulty in waking have been reported in 5% of infants whose mothers were taking phenobarbital (Tyson et al., 1938a).
    The levels of five anticonvulsants have been measured in human milk
and maternal serum of nine women (Kaneko et al., 1979). Primidone and
ethosuximide were reported to have a milk/maternal serum ratio of 0.8
and 0.78, while phenobarbital and carbamazepine ratios were 0.45 and
0.39, respectively. Diphenylhydantoin had a milk/maternal serum ratio
of 0.18, but a higher ratio has been reported for colostral samples
(Mirkin, 1971). A plasma half-life of 60 hr has been calculated for placentally transferred diphenylhydantoin in the newborn (Mirkin, 1971).
Diphenylhydantoin has been reported to be metabolized rapidly in newborn infants, and to display a plasma half-life similar to that of the
adult (Rane, 1974). Therapeutic plasma concentrations of diphenylhydantoin are not achieved by oral administration in the neonate treated
for seizures, but the apparent lack of absorption of an oral dose is unexplained (Painter et al., 1978). Whether diphenylhydantoin ingested
by the breast-fed infant reaches the systemic circulation is unknown.
    Carbamazepine and its active metabolite carbamazepine 10,11-epoxide
have been measured in maternal plasma, milk, and infant plasma at days
2, 3, and 30 postpartum in a single case of chronic drug therapy (Pynnönen and Sillanpää, 1975). Milk concentrations of carbamazepine were
equal to those of infant plasma levels, and about 60% of maternal plasma
concentrations. Levels of the active metabolite were less than one-third
of the levels of carbamazepine in both the milk and maternal plasma, but
no metabolite was found in infant plasma after day 3 postpartum, in-

dicating a capacity of the infant for metabolism and excretion of the 10, 11-epoxide derivative. In another case report, a similar milk/maternal serum ratio (approximately 0.6) of carbamazepine was reported (Niebyl et al., 1979).

E. Antineoplastic Agents

Cyclophosphamide, a synthetic antineoplastic agent, is absorbed from the gastrointestinal tract and from parenteral sites, and has been qualitatively reported in the milk of a woman treated with this drug for lymphosarcoma (Wiernik and Duncan, 1971). A transient neutropenia has been reported in an infant who nursed for 6 days while his mother was treated with 800 mg of cyclophosphamide per day (Amato and Niblett, 1977). It was an oversight on the part of clinicians which resulted in needless exposure of the infant to this toxic compound. Methotrexate levels in maternal plasma, urine, and milk have been qualitatively analyzed in a single patient receiving 22.5 mg of methotrexate/day (Johns et al., 1972). The highest milk/maternal plasma ratio achieved was 0.08 at 10 hr after administration of the drug. After 12 hr, the cumulative maternal urine contained 10,000 times the amount of methotrexate in the collected milk, leading the authors to conclude that the milk was a minor route of excretion of this drug. No volumes of urine or milk were reported.

F. Bronchodilators

Unfortunately, there have been no studies of bronchodilator excretion in human milk to date. There is a single case report in the literature of a 3-month-old nursing infant whose symptoms of irritability and distirbed sleep patterns appeared 1 day after her mother started taking a decongestant containing 120 mg of d-isoephedrine and 6 mg of dexbromphenisamine maleate (Mortimer, 1977). Symptoms ceased within 12 hr after breast feeding was discontinued. Concentrations of the drugs, and their derivatives in the milk, were not determined.

G. Cardiovascular Agents

Propranolol, a β-adrenergic receptor blocking agent which decreases heart rate, cardiac output, and blood pressure, has been measured in milk of two women who received single oral doses of 20, 40, 80, and 160 mg at intervals of several days (Karlberg et al., 1974). With increased dosage, propranolol levels were proportionally increased in milk, and the milk/maternal plasma ratio was one. In a study of a single subject to compare milk levels of propranolol after continuous and single oral doses of propranolol, milk/maternal plasma concentrations ratios were 0.4 after a single dose (40 mg) and 0.64 after continuous doses (40 mg four times a day) (Bauer et al., 1979). Clearly, there is a need for well-executed studies to determine the pharmacokinetics of propranolol excretion in human milk and of the quantity assimilated by the nursing infant.

Although several investigators have reported milk and maternal plasma levels of digoxin, the powerful cardiac glycoside which increases the force of myocardial contraction and increases the refractory period of the atrial valve node, plasma levels have been reported in only three maternal-infant dyads (Loughnan, 1978; Finley et al., 1979). In two maternal-infant dyad where the maternal dose was 0.75 mg, milk levels was detected in infant plasma and digoxin concentrations in milk averaged 85% of those in maternal plasma (Loughnan, 1978). In the third maternal-infant dyad where the maternal dose was 0.75 mg, milk levels were approximately 90% of maternal plasma levels, and infant plasma concentrations were approximately 10% of those of maternal plasma (Finley et al., 1979). Although certain adult gastrointestinal flora may inactivate digoxin (Lindenbaum et al., 1981), it is unknown whether infant flora have the capacity to inactivate this drug. The pharmacokinetics of digoxin have been studied in 11 neonates who received digoxin transplacentally (Cahn et al., 1978). The half-life of placentally transferred digoxin ranged from 19.5 to 76.0 hr which is considerably longer than that of the adult (approximately 4 hr). The digoxin concentration of milk samples taken from both breasts of the mothers of these neonates postpartum was approximately 59% of maternal serum concentration.

H. Diuretics

Diuretics used in the puerperal period for the treatment of edema and hypertension may be transported into human milk. Chlorothiazide is a thiazide diuretic whose use has been associated with numerous side effects, including hypokalemia, hyponatremia, hyperbilirubinemia, and thrombocytopenia. To avoid exposure of the infant, it is generally recommended that nursing be discontinued if thiazide therapy must be maintained. In a study of 11 lactating women who ingested 500 mg of chlorothiazide (Werthman and Krees, 1972), all maternal serum and milk samples collected at 1, 2, and 3 hr after drug ingestion contained less than 0.1 mg per 100 ml chlorothizide, indicating that the sensitivity of the method employed was not adequate to measure quantitatively the fraction of the drug transferred to the milk after a single dose. Based on these findings, the investigators concluded that the risk of the infant acquiring harmful amounts of this drug from human milk was slight. However, the effects of cumulative thiazide use during lactation have not been assessed and until such information is available, it is not possible to make a reasonable recommendation to mothers who wish to nurse their infants and not discontinue drug therapy.

Chlorthalidone is a diuretic whose double-ring structure distinguishes it from the thiazide diuretics and is known to be long acting and low in toxicity. Its presence in milk has been demonstrated in nine women receiving 50 mg per day of chlorthalidone continuously during pregnancy and for 3 days postpartum for treatment of toxemia of pregnancy (Mulley et al., 1978). Milk concentrations ranged from none detected to 0.86 μg/ml, while maternal plasma concentrations ranged from 4.10 to 9.75 μg/ml. From cord blood chlorthalidone concentrations obtained at birth, it was calculated that a 3.5-kg newborn would have 250 μg of chlorthalidone in its circulation at birth and would receive an additional 180 μg per day if breast-fed. Although the half-life of chlorthalidone in the adult is relatively long (60 hr), chlorthalidone kinetics in the neonate have not been studied, so the effects of seemingly insignificant amounts of this diuretic in the neonate are unknown.

Moderate restriction of fluid in combination with furosemide therapy has been reported to be effective in suppressing lactation (Cominos et al., 1976) in a study of 120 women. This study has been criticized, however (Friedman, 1976), since restriction of fluid and tightly binding of breasts alone could suppress lactation without adjuvant diuretic therapy.

I. Ergot Derivatives

Ergot derivatives are frequently used in the stimulation of uterine involution to avoid hemorrhage and infection during the puerperium. Administration of 0.6 mg/day of ergonovine maleate has been demonstrated to decrease maternal serum prolactin levels compared to control levels, and to suppress the prolactin rise normally induced by the suckling of the infant (Canales et al., 1976). Clinical observations in this study revealed that of the 10 women in the drug treatment group, lactation was progressively inhibited in three mothers and painful engorgement with spontaneous milk ejection episodes were experienced by seven mothers.

In a study of eight women taking a single dose of 0.250 mg of methylergometrine after a 5-day therapy regime consisting of 0.125 mg, three times daily, drug concentrations in maternal plasma and milk were determined at 1 and 8 hr after drug administration (Erkkola et al., 1980). After 1 hr, concentration in maternal plasma ranged from 0.6 to 4.4 ng/ml, and after 8 hr the maternal plasma concentration either bordered or was below the detection limit of 0.5 ng/ml in all eight cases. Milk concentrations after 1 hr ranged from 0.6 to 1.3 ng/ml in half of the cases, and were less than 0.5 ng/ml in the other half. After 8 hr, measurable milk levels (1.2 ng/ml) of methylergometrine were detected in only one subject. The human milk fed infants ingesting approximately

800 ml of milk per day would receive approximately 1 μg of methylergometrine, which is merely a fraction of a percentage of the 0.375-mg
daily oral adult dose.

J. Hormones

Since natural hormones such as thyroxine, triiodothyronine (Bode et
al. , 1978), and prolactin (Gala and Van de Walle, 1977) are present in
human milk and may serve in the normal physiologic functioning of the
infant, it is not surprising to discover that exogenous hormones administered to the mother may also be excreted in the milk. Whether these
exogenous hormones alter the hormone balance of the infant and have
any untoward long-term effects is unknown. In the rat, maternal cortisone administration has been shown to have noxious effects on the pup
(Mercier-Parot, 1955). The long-term effects of hormone antagonists
such as carbamizole and propylthiouracil, which are antithyroid drugs,
are also unknown. Measurements of these two agents in human milk
samples revealed that only 0.47% of a radioactive dose of [^{35}S]carbami-
zole was excreted in human milk, while 0.077% of a [^{35}S]propylthioura-
cil dose was excreted in the milk samples after 24 hr (Low et al. , 1979).
These results led the authors to suggest that of the two drugs, propylthiouracil would be the preferred antithyroid drug for use in the
nursing mother and that infant circulating levels of thyroid hormones
must be carefully monitored when such agents are prescribed.

Tolbutamide stimulates synthesis and release of endogenous insulin,
and in a study of two women, concentrations reported in human milk
and maternal serum averaged 0.3 and 3.5 mg per 100 ml, respectively,
at 4 hr after a 500-mg oral dose (Moiel and Ryan, 1967). Although the
infants were not studied in this investigation, it would be interesting
to monitor the glucose response to feeding of these infants.

Prednisolone is used in patients requiring corticosteroid therapy, and
its excretion into human milk has been quantitated in seven nursing
women (McKenzie et al., 1975). After a 5-mg dose of prednisolone containing 10 μCi of [^{3}H]prednisolone, milk samples were expressed at
varying intervals for 48 hr, and it was found that the mean total recovery in milk ranged from 3.5 to 11.5 μg/liter. In urine collected
from two women, approximately 30—32% of the radioactive dose was excreted in 48 hr. At 2 hr after a single 10-mg oral dose of prednisone,
milk prednisone levels were 2.67 μg/liter, and those of prednisolone
were 0.16 μg/liter (Katz and Duncan, 1975). The authors suggested
that these amounts of steroids were unlikely to have a deleterious effect
on the infant.

The effects of oral contraceptive agents on lactation have been summarized (Vorherr, 1974), and in general it appears that these steroids
suppress the maintenance and not the establishment of lactation (Rosa,
1976). The appearance of oral contraceptive agents in human milk has

been reported (Nilsson et al., 1978;1977; Koetsawang, 1977; Pincus et al., 1966). Since long-term side effects of neonatal exposure to steroid hormones via human milk are unknown, it has been recommended that use of these agents not coincide with nursing of the infant (Szefler and Shen, 1981). Gynecomastia in a human milk-fed male infant which subsided upon cessation of nursing has been attributed to maternal use of norethynodrel and ethynylestradiol 3-methyl ether (Curtis, 1964). A relatively high incidence of jaundice among human milk-fed infants whose mothers had taken oral contraceptives prior to pregnancy has also been reported (Wong and Wood, 1971). Pregnane-3d,20β-diol has been isolated from the milk of mothers of seven jaundiced infants (Arias and Gartner, 1964), and milk samples from these women who were not taking oral contraceptives consistently inhibited glucuronyl transferase activity in vitro. Oral administration of pregnane-3d,20β-diol in amounts equivalent to those consumed by those jaundiced infants to two normal infants resulted in symptoms of hyperbilirubinemia. Since information presently available is fragmentary, it seems that the relationship between maternal use of steroids and jaundice in the infant needs to be investigated.

It is known that nutrient requirements for vitamin B_6 are increased in women taking oral contraceptives. Whether nutrient content of human milk may be altered by oral contraceptive use has been studied to a limited extent, and available data indicate that in apparently healthy women, the lactose and fat content (Toaff et al., 1969), as well as the normal variation of nonprotein nitrogen, α-lactalbumin, and serum albumin (Lönnerdal et al., 1980), are not altered by their use, and that total protein content may be increased (Toaff et al., 1969). On the other hand, results of a study of women who used oral contraceptives prior to pregnancy revealed lowered colostrum manganese concentrations (Kirksey et al., 1979) and decreased maternal serum copper concentrations. Three cases of vitamin B_6 deficiency have been reported in nursing infants of mothers who had been long-term users of oral contraceptives prior to pregnancy (Kirksey and Roepke, 1981). Available evidence implicates steroids as agents with long-term effects on both the lactating mother and her infant.

K. Laxatives

In a study of 175 women who were treated for constipation, gastrointestinal stimulants corrected the problem on a higher percentage of patients than did bulk-forming agents, but there were greater side effects of diarrhea, abdominal pain, and nausea in both the mother and infants of women administered the gastrointestinal stimulants (Greenhalf and Leonard, 1973). Phenolphthalein, a compound that stimulates the motor activity of the lower gastrointestinal tract, was undetected in milk of nursing women administered varying drug doses, but the conjugated variety of the drug was present in all specimens of milk analyzed (Fantus and Dyniewicz, 1936). It has been suggested that bulk-forming agents such as bran, plantago ovata coating, and psyllium hydrophyllic mucilloid may be the laxatives of choice for the nursing mother (Wilson et al., 1980).

L. Psychotherapeutic Agents

Chlorpromazine and its metabolites have been qualitatively determined in human milk when the daily maternal dose exceeded 200 mg (Uhlíř and Rýznar, 1973). Concentrations of chlorpromazine in maternal plasma and milk were reported for a woman who ingested 1200 mg/day of the drug (Blacker et al., 1962). Although barely detectable, milk levels of chlorpromazine paralleled those of maternal plasma and peak milk concentration was achieved at 120 min after the drug was administered. The therapeutic pediatric dose of chlorpromazine (250 µg/kg every 4-6 hr) is considerably more than the dose of 10 µg in 124 ml of milk received by the nursing infant in this case report. Levels of chlorpromazine have been reported to be higher in milk than in maternal plasma for some individuals, and symptoms of drowsiness and lethargy have been observed for one nursing infant when maternal serum chlorpromazine concentration was 92 ng/ml (Wiles et al., 1978). Extrapyramidal symptoms have also been reported in a newborn infant who received chlorpromazine transplacentally (Levy and Wisniewski, 1974).

Lithium, a widely used antidepressant, has been recently reported to decrease brain sodium-potassium ATPase activity (Guerri et al., 1981). Serum lithium levels of human milk-fed infants have been measured and found to be one-third to one-half of maternal serum values (Schou and Amdisen, 1973). In this study, milk concentrations averaged 0.35 mmol/liter. It appears that lithium, with its low molecular weight, readily passes into human milk. Moreover, its toxic effects of cyanosis and hypotonicity in a newborn have been described (Tunnessen and Hertz, 1972). These observations suggest that lithium therapy is contraindicated for the lactating woman.

Tricyclic antidepressants are often prescribed for postpartum depression. Imipramine and its demethylated metabolite have been detected in the plasma and milk of a woman who received a daily dose of 200 mg (Sovner and Orsulak, 1979). Milk concentrations of these compounds were similar to those of plasma (20-40 ng/ml) and since both are highly lipophilic compounds, it is likely that they are passively transported into milk. Two additional tricyclic antidepressants, amitriptyline and nortriptyline, were quantitated in maternal and infant serum (Erickson et al., 1979), and although the maternal serum concentrations of these drugs were 90 and 146 ng/ml, respectively, they were undetected in infant sera. A possible explanation for these findings is rapid transport of amitriptyline and nortriptyline to extravascular tissues in both humans and rat (Eschenhof and Rieder, 1969). These investigators have reported tissue concentrations of 3−70 times those of blood.

Human milk content of the antidepressant, dothiepin, was reported to be one-third of maternal serum concentration in a single case report (Rees et al., 1976). Levels of a relatively new antidepressant, amoxapine, and its active metabolite, 8-OH-amoxapine, were measured in milk and maternal serum of one user (Gelenberg, 1979). Amoxapine levels in the milk (< 20 ng/ml) were less than those of maternal plasma (97 ng/ml), as were the levels of 8-OH-amoxapine in milk (168 ng/ml) compared to those of maternal plasma (375 ng/ml). Although these antidepressants are known to be transferred to human milk, the consequence of such milk ingestion by the nursing infant has not been assessed.

M. Radiopharmaceuticals

Radiopharmaceuticals are commonly used in nuclear scanning procedures of the thyroid gland, kidney, brain, and bone. The utmost care must be taken to avoid exposure of the infant to these compounds. Accidental exposure of ^{99m}T via human milk has been reported in a 10-week-old infant whose mother was administered 15 mCi of ^{99m}T (Rumble et al., 1978). In a single feeding, 4 hr after the maternal dose, the infant ingested 82.5 μCi of this radioisotope as determined by total-body gamma ray measurement. These authors recommended a 48-hr abstinence from breast-feeding after a dose of 15 mCi of technetium. This recommendation is supported by the findings of Pittard et al. (1979). These investigators found that after 48 hr, the level of ^{99m}T in milk from a woman who received 20 mCi was slightly above background. There is an interesting case report of an unusual concentration of ^{67}G citrate in the milk of a lactating woman (Larson and Schall, 1971), which rendered the use of nuclear scanning procedures for the diagnosis of malignant breast disease in this nursing mother impossible. The half-life of ^{67}Ga in human milk was 9 days in another case report (Tobin and Schneider, 1976). A selective concentration of ^{131}I has also been observed in human milk (Miller and Weetch, 1955), and in saliva and gastric juice (Myant et al,, 1950). In a study of six nursing mothers (Weaver et al., 1960), milk samples were obtained at intervals of 2, 6, 24, and 48 hr after doses of 10 and 30 μCi ^{131}I. At 48 hr after the ^{131}I dosage, maternal plasma concentrations were approximately 1% of the dose. The suggestion that iodine is transferred to the milk by passive diffusion (Miller and Swanson, 1963) is supported by the observation of an increase in total amount of ^{131}I excreted as the volume of milk produced is increased. The maximum ^{131}I concentration of milk from women receiving 10- and 6-μCi dosages was 0.7 and 0.15 μCi/liter, respectively (Bland et al., 1969). Based on these milk concentrations of ^{131}I and assuming that infants ingest only 300 ml of milk per day, these investigators calculated that infants' exposures would be 0.5—0.6 μCi every 8 days. However, most infants consume more than 300 ml/day of human milk and thus these investigators have underestimated infant exposure by at least 50% (Picciano and Deering, 1977). In a study of ^{125}I excretion in human milk after maternal administration of 100 μCi as radiolabeled fibrinogen for investigations of postpartum deep leg vein thrombosis, the effective half-life of this radioisotope in milk was 80 hr, roughly the same as the half-life in maternal plasma (Palmer, 1979). Radioactive sodium appeared in human milk within 20 min after ingestion and maximum concentration occurred at 2 hr (Pommerenke and Hahn, 1943). The use of ^{131}I- and ^{99m}T-labeled macroaggregates of serum albumin and ferrous hydroxide in lactating women is also associated with detectable radioactivity in their milk (Wyburn, 1973) and should be avoided.

N. Sedative-Hypnotics

In general, sedative and hypnotic drugs are excreted in human milk and since their effects on the infant are unknown, careful observation of the nursing infant should be undertaken. Although certain anticonvulsants such as diphenylhydantoin may be classified in the sedative-hypnotic category, they have been referred to in a separate section.

Diazepam is a widely used tranquilizer and has been associated with drowsiness and altered encephalogram readings in the nursing neonate (Patrick et al., 1972). In a study of nine lactating mothers administered diazepam (doses not stated), milk to maternal plasma ratios were variable (0.21 to 2.78) and averaged approximately 0.5 (Cole and Hailey, 1975). Although analytical values were not given, these investigators reported that there were "appreciable" amounts of the active metabolite (desmethyldiazepam) in the serum of one infant 10 days after a single maternal dose during labor, indicating reduced drug metabolism of the neonate. No adverse clinical symptoms except mild jaundice in three infants were noted. Both diazepam and desmethyldiazepam concentrations tend to be higher in evening milk than morning milk (Brandt, 1976). This report is especially interesting considering that diazepam is a highly protein-bound drug, and that protein concentrations in human milk exhibit this same diurnal variation pattern (Janas and Picciano, 1981).

Several other sedative-hypnotic drugs have been reported in human milk. In an early study, Tyson et al. (1938b) quantitatively reported bromides in 97% of samples analyzed from mothers administered 5.8 g of sodium bromide per day. One-half-ounce milk samples were collected at each feeding in a 24-hr period. In all mothers and infants, a marked decrease in irritability was noted. In a nursing mother administered 1125 mg of pentothal sodium as anesthetic agent 12 days postpartum, a

20-min blood sample, 25-min milk sample from the left breast, and 30-min urine sample were analyzed and found to contain 0.45, 0.75, and 1.00 mg per 100 ml of barbiturate, respectively (Mayo and Schticke, 1942). In a milk sample taken from the right breast 14 min after injection of the drug was discontinued, the milk concentration was 2 mg per 100 ml. Since pentothal sodium exhibits a cyclic appearance and disappearance in the general circulation (Mayo and Schticke, 1942), an investigation of its elimination via human milk must take its blood variance pattern into consideration; otherwise, results will be misleading. Another anesthetic agent, halothane, has been measured in fore-milk samples of a lactating anesthetist after 1.5, 4.0, and 5.0 hr in the operating room (Coté et al., 1976). Milk concentrations were equivalent to environmental (air) concentrations (2 ppm) in the operating room, where air was replaced about five times per hour. Although halothane is the only volatile anesthetic agent reported in human milk thus far, it is probable that others may similarly be transported into the milk.

O. Social and Recreational Drugs

1. Alcohol

Ethanol inhibits oxytocin release from the neurohypophysis in humans (Fuchs and Wagner, 1963). Ethanol administration of 1--2 g/kg to lactating women has been shown to result in a dose-dependent inhibition of the milk-ejecting response (Cobo, 1973). It seems that the concentrations of nonionized substances such as ethanol and urea are comparable in maternal plasma and milk (Rasmussen, 1966). In a study of ethanol and acetaldehyde levels in human milk of 12 nursing mothers after an oral dose of 0.6 g of ethanol per kilogram of body weight, a dose corresponding to moderate social drinking, milk and maternal blood samples were obtained at 30-min intervals (Kesaniemi, 1974). Analyses revealed no detection of acetaldehyde in milk samples at mean maternal blood levels of 44.4 nmol/ml observed at 30 min, indicating an exclusion of acetaldehyde from the milk. Ethanol levels in milk samples (15.8 ± 5.4 μmol/ml) were comparable to those of maternal blood (19.1 ± 6.5 μmol/ml). Although only rarely, symptoms of intoxication of the infant, attributed to excessive maternal alcohol ingestion, have been reported (Bisdom, 1937). Increased blood cortisol levels and symptoms of Cushing's syndrome in an infant whose mother consumed excessive quantities of alcohol have been attributed to alcohol ingestion via human milk (Binkiewicz et al., 1978). Since a 4-month-old infant has approximately one-fourth of adult levels of alcohol dehydrogenase activity (Pikkarainen and Raiha, 1967), moderation in alcohol consumption is wise advice for the nursing mother. It is not until a child is 5 years of age that activity of this enzyme approaches adult levels.

2. Caffeine, Theophylline, Theobromine

The methylxanthines, caffeine, theophylline, and theobromine, are widely consumed in coffee, tea, soft drinks, and chocolate products, as well as in certain nonprescription medications. Although their effects on the infant are unknown, it has been suggested that these compounds might have a deleterious effect on the developing human brain (Allan and Volpe, 1978). Exposure of C-6 glial cells in vitro to 1×10^{-3} M concentrations of caffeine, theophylline, and aminophylline for 24 hr resulted in decreased cholesterol synthesis and reduction in activity of the rate-limiting enzyme of cholesterol synthesis, hydroxymethylglutaryl coenzyme A reductase. The pharmacokinetics of both caffeine and theophylline in low-birth-weight infants treated for apnea have been evaluated (Aranda et al., 1979a,1977,1976). In full-term neonates, the reported half-life for transplacentally acquired caffeine was 80 ± 26 hr (Parsons et al., 1976), which is considerably longer than in the adult (3.5 hr). The infant has been observed to achieve adult values for plasma half-life of caffeine at 4−6 months of age (Aranda et al., 1979b).

The transport of caffeine into human milk has been studied in five nursing mothers after 150 mg of caffeine sodium benzoate was administered orally (Tyrala and Dodson 1979). Milk and maternal serum were analyzed at 0, 30, 60, and 120 min, and peak milk and serum concentrations of 1.4−2.4 and 2.39−4.05 g/ml, respectively, were observed at 60 min. Doubling the dose of caffeine to one woman resulted in a corresponding elevation in serum caffeine concentration and the milk/maternal serum ratio (0.52) was not altered. In order to determine whether accumulation of caffeine may occur in the young nursing infant, further studies, including assessment of infant absorption, metabolism, and excretion, are needed.

Due to its use as a maintenance drug in treatment of asthma, theophylline levels in milk of five nursing women were quantitated to estimate transport of this compound into human milk. Three women received a single 4.25-mg/kg dose (Yurchak and Jusko, 1976), while two others received 200-mg doses four times daily together with 15−20 mg of prednisone. Milk and maternal saliva and serum were analyzed by high-pressure liquid chromatography. Peak serum theophylline levels were observed at 30 min, and the serum half-life was approximately 4 hr. Saliva and milk theophylline concentrations declined in parallel with serum concentrations. Peak milk levels of 4.0 mg/liter were observed at 1−3 hr, and the milk/maternal serum ratio and saliva/serum ratios were 0.73 and 0.58, respectively. The estimated maximum intake of the human milk fed infant was 8 mg/day, and it was suggested that the drug be taken after nursing to avoid peak milk concentrations at the time of feeding. Following this advice may not always achieve its intended purpose since, in early infancy, the interval between nursing is often only 2 hr. However, it would be prudent to advise the lactating woman using theophylline medication to reduce her dietary intake of methylxanthines, as this is easily accomplished with the elimination of a few foods and beverages. The average half-life of theophylline in infants and children, ages 3 months to 6 years, has been reported to be 4.92 ± 1.88 hr in a study of 54 subjects, where no relationship between half-life and age was found (Kadlec et al., 1978). These results indicate that as is the case for caffeine, theophylline metabolism is relatively well established at approximately 3 months of age, so it is only the very young infant who may be at risk from theophylline exposure.

Milk, plasma, and saliva levels of theombromine were measured in six lactating women after ingestion of 240 mg of theobromine contained in 113 g of chocolate (Resman et al., 1977). Peak levels of 3.7--8.2 mg/ liter were observed at 2–3 hr after chocolate ingestion in all three fluids, and the half-life of theobromine averaged approximately 7 hr. The milk/plasma and saliva/plasma ratios were 0.82 and 0.92, respectively. No adverse effects were noted in any of the nursing infants. It was estimated that a woman ingesting a 4-oz chocolate bar every 6 hr could deliver approximately 10 mg per day of theobromine to her infant. It is probable that the half-life of theobromine is prolonged in the first few months of life, as are the half-lives of theophylline and caffeine, so that the neonate might be more vulnerable to effects of theobromine than the older infant.

In a study of 10 nursing mothers ingesting 60 mg of theobromine and 6 mg of caffeine in a single chocolate bar, milk and saliva samples were obtained at 1, 2, 3, 5, 8, 12, and 15 hr (Berlin and Daniel, 1981). Peak milk (1.5– 3.67 µg/ml) and saliva levels (1.76– 3.55 µg/ml) were achieved by 3 hr. Milk and saliva half-lives were 14.7 ± 8.6 and 9.8 ± 8.65 hr, respectively. Neither theobromine nor caffeine were detected in the infant urine samples, indicating minimal or negligible absorption, and no adverse effects on the infant were noted. While there exists a lot of anecdotal testimony that maternal chocolate ingestion and coffee and tea consumption produce behavioral and bowel disturbances in the nursing infant, controlled clinical studies have been unable to confirm such allegations. It may be a methylxanthine dose-related phenomenon, and available information indicates only that moderate consumption of methylxanthine-containing foods is without consequence on the nursing infant.

Although we are unaware of any measurements of pyrrolizadine alkaloids in human milk, these compounds are present in herbal teas and are likely to be transported into human milk. Some of the problems with their use, such as toxicity and potential mutagenicity and carcinogenicity, have been reviewed (Huxtable, 1980). Herbal teas are frequently sold in health food stores to consumers who lack cultural knowledge of the use of these herbs and, consequently, they may be misused quite easily. Needless to say, the human milk fed infant should be protected from exposure to pyrrolizadine alkaloids.

3. Nicotine

Nicotine is excreted in milk of women who smoke, and although there are case reports of toxic symptoms in the infant attributed to nicotine in the milk (Bisdom, 1937; Perraudin and Sorin, 1978), which include vomiting, diarrhea, elevated pulse levels, and apnea, there are much greater numbers of nursing infants of smoking mothers who demonstrate no observable symptoms whatsoever. In an early study of Perlman et al. (1942), a correlation between the number of cigarettes smoked by 55 lactating women and the quantity of nicotine in their milk and urine was found. The average concentrations of nicotine in morning defatted samples were 0.116 mg/liter in occasional smokers (1−4 cigarettes/day), 0.225 mg/liter in moderate smokers (5−10 cigarettes/day), and 0.445 mg/liter in heavy smokers (11−20 cigarettes/day). A diurnal variation was observed with highest nicotine values observed in afternoon milk and urine samples. No increased failure of lactation in smoking mothers compared to nonsmoking mothers as suggested by Meyer (1979) was observed. In a study of milk samples from 15 mothers (Ferguson et al., 1976), nicotine levels ranged from 0.020 to 0.512 mg/liter. In this study, however, concentration of nicotine did not display a diurnal variation, and there was no correlation between milk nicotine level and number of cigarettes smoked. These investigators commented that the concentrations of nicotine observed in human milk are not hazardous to the infant and that lactation is not contraindicated for the smoking mother. Although the adult responds to nicotine use with induction of liver microsomal enzyme activity, as demonstrated by the increased body clearance of both caffeine and theophylline in the smoker compared to the nonsmoker (Parsons and Neims, 1978; Powell et al., 1977), maternal smoking does not appear to enhance ability to eliminate caffeine in term infants (Parsons et al., 1976).

4. Marihuana

We are unaware of any measurements of the psychoactive tetrahydrocannabinol compounds in human milk; however, after a single maternal intravenous injection of [^{14}C]tetrahydrocannabinol, radioactivity was detected in the feces and urine of suckling lambs reflecting transport of the drug and its metabolites through the milk (Jakubovič et al., 1974). A reduction in the number of ribosomes attached to the nuclear membrane in brain tissue of the suckled rat pup has also been observed (Jakubovič et al., 1973). Results of the studies of the metabolism of intravenously administered tetrahydrocannabinol indicated that most of a radioactive dose was excreted in the feces, and that the drug and its metabolites are involved in enterohepatic circulation (Klausner and Dingell, 1971). An extensive review of the physiological and pharmacological implications of marihuana use has been published (Vijay and Manocha, 1976). Nursing mothers should be aware that use of marihuana is likely to result in exposure of the infant to tetrahydrocannabinol compounds.

5. Environmental

The passage of environmental contaminants to the infant via human milk is an important concern; unfortunately, it is an emotional issue. The risks associated with these contaminants in human milk are unknown. For this reason it is important that nursing mothers be aware of the risks and benefits associated with human milk feeding so that they may make a decision whether to nurse their infants without the anxiety that they may be poisoning them. Although exposure to some environmental contaminants may be avoided, certain contaminants are widely distributed throughout the food chain and ecosystem and consequently impossible to avoid. The exposure of the infant to these contaminants in utero may be much greater than the exposure associated with human milk feeding (Nutrition Reviews, 1977). For example, DDT content of adipose tissue of fresh stillborn infants has been reported to be one-third of the adult (Abbott et al., 1968). Since the DDT concentration in adult adipose tissue is about 30 times greater than that in breast-milk (Egan et al., 1965), it is likely that the infant acquires more insecticide transplacentally than via human milk.

The literature is filled with reports of human milk excretion of environmental contaminants, and excellent review articles exist (Olszyna-Marzys, 1978; Sinaiko, 1981; West, 1964). Unfortunately, available data are difficult to evaluate due to differences in methodologies. Systematic studies are necessary which consider variations in the lipid composition of human milk with respect to maternal energy balance, stage of lactation, time of day, and time of sample collection during a single nursing period, since these factors influence the quality and quantity of human milk lipids. The amount of fat in a milk sample has a great bearing on contaminant concentration, as most are lipid soluble. Within a single nursing period, the fat content increases from the beginning to the end, and lipid-soluble contaminant concentrations will also increase. Samples taken at the end of the nursing period may then overestimate, while those taken at the beginning of the nursing period may underestimate levels ingested by the infant. Lactating women in negative energy balance will mobilize bodily fat- and lipid-soluble contaminants and influence milk concentrations accordingly. It is therefore not surprising that great variation is reported for contaminant levels in milk from a single mother on different days (World Health Organization, 1969). Until results from well-designed studies are available, it is difficult to assess the amounts of environmental contaminants which are passed to the nursing infant. Studies must also focus on the metabolism of such contaminants in the infant.

IV. CLINICAL CONSIDERATIONS

The nursing mother should be aware that virtually every drug appearing in the maternal circulation will also appear in the milk. Although milk content of most drugs may only be a small fraction of the maternal dose, short-term side effects in the infant have been reported after maternal drug use, and long-term effects of seemingly minute levels of drug are unknown. It is therefore prudent to suggest alternative therapy practices wherever possible and advise nursing mothers to curtail certain social and recreational practices which result in infant drug exposure. In cases where drug therapy must be continued, mothers taking drugs contraindicated during lactation must discontinue nursing their infants. In situations where drug therapy is not necessarily contraindicated, a dosage regime may be scheduled so that the mother can avoid nursing her infant at times when milk levels of drug are highest. Use of a supplemental bottle of either previously expressed human milk or formula may facilitate the nursing mother's scheduling of drug therapy, as peak milk levels of drug may not be avoided in infants who nurse either quite frequently or at irregular intervals.

V. FUTURE RESEARCH NEEDS

From the foregoing discussion, it is obvious that there is a dearth of information regarding the excretion of drugs in human milk and resulting exposures to the infant. Much available information stems from studies in which random milk samples from only one or several lactating women have been analyzed. Individual variability in drug metabolism is great and, consequently, recommendations for the entire population on the basis of such spurious data may be misleading.

Since protein binding and lipid solubility of drugs are important determinants of drug pharmacodynamics, the importance of well-planned sample collection procedures which consider the pharmacokinetics of the drug in question is evident. The half-life of the drug will help to define the sampling intervals after maternal drug administration, and only in light of such information will milk concentrations of drugs have any meaning. Use of typical dosage patterns, whether single or chronic, and of therapeutic dosage levels in studies of drug transport into human milk are important. Although the infant receives only a small fraction of the maternal dose in most cases, the long-term consequences of this type of exposure are unknown, and short-term effects are not readily discerned unless the infant expresses outward symptoms. Fortunately, recent developments in technology have improved analytic methods so that nanogram and picogram levels of drugs and their metabolites may be quantified. Use of microtechniques allows analyses of smaller sample aliquots than were required in the past. Although few studies have investigated infant urine, saliva, or blood to estimate drug exposure via human milk feeding, it is extremely important that pharmacokinetics and pharmacodynamics of drugs to which infants are exposed be evaluated in the infant.

At present, the majority of pharmacological agents used in pediatric therapy have not been proven safe and effective for this population (Mirkin, 1980). Consequently, reasonable recommendations for their use in therapy of the infant or nursing mother cannot be made. Research aimed at assessing the drugs used in this population, as well as those to which the infant may be inadvertently exposed to via human milk, is desperately needed. In learning more about basic pharmacokinetics of drugs in the infant, their transport into human milk, levels of drugs absorbed by the infant, and side effects, potential risks to the infant associated with our present state of ignorance might be averted.

REFERENCES

Abbott, D. C., Goulding, R., and Tatton, J. O. (1968). Organochlorine pesticide residues in human fat in Great Britain. *Br. Med. J.* 3:146-149.

Allan, W. C., and Volpe, J. J. (1978). Methylxanthines cause a marked reduction in cholesterol synthesis in cultured glial cells. *Pediatr. Res.* 12:401.

Allgén, L. G., Holmberg, G., Persson, B., and Sörbo, B. (1979). Biological fate of methenamine in man. Absorption, renal excretion and passage to the umbilical cord, amniotic fluid and breast milk. *Acta Obstet. Gynecol. Scand.* 58(3):287-293.

Amato, D., and Niblett, J. S. (1977). Neutropenia from cyclophosphamide in breast milk. *Med. J. Aust.* 1:383-384.

American Academy of Pediatrics Committee on Drugs (1979). Anticonvulsants and pregnancy. *Pediatrics* 63(2):331-333.

Ananth, J. (1978). Side effects in the neonate from psychotropic agents excreted through breast-feeding. *Am. J. Psychiatry* 135:801-805.

Aranda, J. V., Macleod, S. M., Renton, K. W., Eeade, N. R., and Phil, D. (1974). Hepatic microsomal drug oxidation and electron transport in newborn infants. *J. Pediatr.* 85(4):534-542.

Aranda, J. V., Sitar, D. S., Parsons, W. D., Loughnan, P. M., and Neims, A. H. (1976). Pharmacokinetic aspects of theophylline in premature newborns. *N. Engl. J. Med.* 295(8):413-416.

Aranda, J. V., Gorman, W., Bergsteinsson, H., and Gunn, T. (1977). Efficacy of caffeine in treatment of apnea in the low-birth-weight infant. *J. Pediatr.* 90(3):467-472.

Aranda, J. V., Cook, C. E., Gorman, W., Collinge, J. M., Loughnan, P. M., Outerbridge, E. W., Aldrige, A., and Neims, A. H.
(1979a). Pharmacokinetic profile of caffeine in the premature newborn infant with apnea. *J. Pediatr. 94*(4):663-668.

Aranda, J. V., Collinge, J. M., Zinman, R., and Watters, G.
(1979b). Maturation of caffeine elimination in infancy. *Arch.
Dis. Child. 54*(12):946-949.

Arias, I. M., and Gartner, L. M. (1964). Production of unconjugated
hyperbilirubinemia in full-term new-born infants following administration of pregnane-3(alpha), 20-(beta)-diol. *Nature 203*:1292-
1293.

Atkinson, S. A., Anderson, G. H., and Bryan, M. H. (1980). Human milk: comparison of the nitrogen composition in milk from
mothers of premature and full-term infants. *Am. J. Clin. Nutr.
33*:811-815.

Barsivala, V. M., and Virkar, K. D. (1973). The effect of oral contraceptives on concentrations of various components of human
milk. *Contraception 7*:307-312.

Bauer, J. H., Pape, B., Zajicek, J., and Groshong, T. (1979).
Propranolol in human plasma and breast milk. *Am. J. Cardiol.
43*:860-862.

Berger, H. (1941). Excretion of mandelic acid in breast milk. *Am.
J. Dis. Child. 61*:256-261.

Berlin, C. M. (1980). The excretion of drugs and chemicals in human milk. In *Pediatric Pharmacology. Therapeutic Principles in
Practice*, S. J. Yaffe, Ed., Grune & Stratton, New York, pp.
137-147.

Berlin, C. M., and Daniel, C. H. (1981). Excretion of theobromine
in human milk and saliva. *12th Int. Congr. Nutr.*, Abstr. 897,
p. 156.

Berlin, C. M., and Lee, C. (1979). Isoniazid and acetyl isoniazid
disposition in human milk, saliva and plasma. *Fed. Proc. 38*:
426.

Berlin, C. M., Yaffee, S. J., and Ragni, N. (1980). Disposition of
acetaminophen in milk, saliva, and plasma of lactating women.
Pediatr. Pharmacol. 1:135-141.

Binkiewicz, A., Robinson, M. J., and Senior, B. (1978). Pseudo-
Cushing syndrome caused by alcohol in breast milk. *J. Pediatr.
93*(6):965-967.

Bisdom, C. J. W. (1937). Alcohol and nicotine poisoning in nurs-
lings. *Maandsch. Kindergeneesk. 6*:332-341.

Blacker, K. H., Weinstein, B. J., and Ellman, G. L. (1962).
Mother's milk and chlorpromazine. *Am. J. Psychiatry 119*:178-
179.

Bland, E. P., Crawford, J. S., Decker, M. E., and Farr, R. F. (1969). Radioactive iodine uptake by thyroid of breast-fed infants after maternal blood-volume measurements. *Lancet.* 2:1039-1041.

Bode, H. H., Vanjonack, W. J., and Crawford, J. D. (1978). Mitigation of cretinism by breast-feeding. *Pediatrics* 62(1):13-16.

Borderon, J. C., Bernard, J. C., Vergnaud, R., Gold, F., Soutoul, J. H., and Laugier, J. (1980). Effect de l'antibiothérapie de la mère sur la colonisation du noveau-né par enterobactéries. *Arch. Fr. Pediatr.* 37:371-376.

Brambel, C. E., and Hunter, R. E. (1950). Effect of dicoumarol on the nursing infant. *Am. J. Obstet. Gynecol.* 59:1153-1159.

Brandt, R. (1976). Passage of diazepam and desmethyldiazepam into breast milk. *Arzneim. Forsch.* 26(3):454-457.

Braunlich, H. (1976). Kidney development: drug elimination mechanisms. In *Drug Disposition During Development*, P. L. Morselli, Ed., Spectrum Publications, Jamaica, N. Y., pp. 89-100.

Brown, T. C. K. (1973). Pediatric pharmacology. *Anaesthesiol. Intensive Care* 1:473-479.

Brown, A. K., and Cevik, N. (1965). Hemolysis and jaundice in the newborn following maternal treatment with sulfamethoxypyridazine (Kynex). *Pediatrics* 36(5):742-744.

Buchanan, R. A., Eaton, C. J., Koeff, S. T., and Kinkel, A. W. (1968). The breast milk excretion of mefenamic acid. *Curr. Ther. Res.* 10(11):592-596.

Buchanan, R. A., Eaton, C. J., Koeff, S. T., and Kinkel, A. W. (1969). The breast milk excretion of flufenamic acid. *Curr. Ther. Res.* 11(8):533-538.

Buimovici-Klein, E., Hite, R. L., Byrne, T., and Cooper, L. Z. (1977). Isolation of rubella virus in milk after postpartum immunization. *J. Pediatr.* 91(6):939-941.

Canales, E. S., Garrido, J. T., Zárate, A., Mason, M., and Soria, J. (1976). Effect of ergonovine on prolactin secretion and milk let down. *Obstet. Gynecol.* 48(2):228-229.

Casey, C. E. (1976). Concentrations of some trace elements in human and cow's milk. *Proc. Univ. Otago Med. Sch.* 54:7-8.

Chan, V., Tse, T. F., and Wong, V. (1978). Transfer of digoxin across the placenta and into breast milk. *Br. J. Obstet. Gynaecol.* 85:605-609.

Clark, J. H., and Wilson, W. G. (1981). A 16-day-old breast-fed infant with metabolic acidosis caused by salicylate. *Clin. Pediatr.* 20(1):53-54.

Clayman, C. B. (1977). Evaluation of cimetidine (Tagamet). An antagonist of hydrochloric acid secretion. *JAMA* 238(12):1289-1290.

Clyde, D. F. (1960). Prolonged malaria prophylaxis through pyrimethamine in mother's milk. *East. Afr. Med. J.* 37(10):659-660.

Clyde, D. F., and Shute, G. T. (1956). Transfer of pyrimethamine in human milk. *J. Trop. Med. Hyg.* 59:277-284.

Cobo, E. (1973). Effect of different doses of ethanol on the milk-ejecting reflex in lactating women. *Am. J. Obstet. Gynecol.* 115(6):817-821.

Cole, A. P., and Hailey, D. M. (1975). Diazepam and active metabolite in breast milk and their transfer to the neonate. *Arch. Dis. Child.* 50:741-742.

Cominos, D. C., Van der Walt, A., and Van Rooyen, A. J. L. (1976). Suppression of post-partum lactation with furosemide. *S. Afr. Med. J.* 50(8):251-252.

Coryell, M. N., Harris, M. E., Miller, S., Williams, H. H., and Macy, I. G. (1945). Human milk studies. XXII. Nicotinic acid, pantothenic acid, and biotin contents of colostrum and mature human milk. *Am. J. Dis. Child.* 70:150-161.

Coté, C. J., Kenepp, N. B., Reed, S. B., and Strobel, G. E. (1976). Trace concentrations of halothane in human breast milk. *J. Anaesth.* 48:541-543.

Criep, L. H., Arbesman, C. E., Sheldon, J. M., Siegel, B. B., and Weinstein, H. I. (1959-1960). The present status and problems involved in human sensitization to antiobiotics. *Antibiot. Annu.* 7:979-1000.

Curtis, E. M. (1964). Oral contraceptive feminization of a normal male infant. Report of a case. *Obstet. Gynecol.* 23:295-296.

DeForest, A., Parker, P. B., DiLiberti, J. H., Yates, H. T., Sibinga, M. S., and Smith, D. S. (1973). The effect of breast-feeding on the antibody response of infants to trivalent oral poliovirus vaccine. *J. Pediatr.* 83(1):93-95.

Deodhar, A. D., Rajalakshmi, R., and Ramakreshan, C. V. (1964). Studies on human lactation: 3. Effect of dietary vitamin supplementation on vitamin contents of breast milk. *Acta Paediatr. Scand.* 53:42-48.

Department of Health and Social Security (1977). *The Composition of Mature Human Milk*, H. M. Stationery Office, London.

Eckstein, H. B., and Jack, B. (1970). Breast feeding and anticoagulant therapy. *Lancet* 1:672-673.

Ecobichon, D. J., and Stephens, D. S. (1973). Perinatal development of human blood esterases. *Clin. Pharmacol. Ther.* 14:11-17.

Edelman, C. M., and Spitzer, A. (1976). The kidney. In *The Physiology of the New born Infant*, 4th ed., C. A. Smith and N. M. Nelson, Eds., Charles C. Thomas, Springfield, Ill., pp. 416-458.

Eeg-Olofsson, O., Malmros, I., Elwin, C. E., and Steen, B. (1978). Convulsions in a breast-fed infant after maternal indomethacin. *Lancet 2*:215.

Egan, H., Goulding, R., Roburn, J., and Tatton, J. O. (1965). Organochlorine pesticide residues in human fat and human milk. *Br. Med. J. 2*:66-69.

Erickson, S. H., and Oppenheim, G. L. (1979). Aspirin in breast milk. *J. Fam. Pract. 8*:189-190.

Erickson, S. H., Oppenheim, G. L., and Smith, G. H. (1981). Metronidazole in breast milk. *Obstet. Gynecol. 57*(1):48-50.

Erkkola, R., Kanto, J., Allonen, H., Kleimola, T., and Mäntylä, R. (1980). Excretion of methylergometrine (methylergonovine) into the human breast milk. *Int. J. Clin. Pharmacol. Biopharm. 16*(12):579-580.

Eschenhof, E., and Rieder, J. (1969). Untersuchungen über das Schicksal des Antidepressivums Amitriptylin in Organismus der Ratte und des Menschen. *Arzneim. Forsch. 19*:957-966.

Fantus, B., and Dyniewicz, J. M. (1936). Phenolphthalein administration to nursing women. *Am. J. Dig. Dis. 3*:184-185.

Farquhar, J. D. (1972). Follow-up on rubella vaccinations and experiences with subclinical reinfection. *J. Pediatr. 81*(3):460-465.

Fell, B. F., Smith, K. A., and Campbell, R. M. (1963). Hypertrophic and hyperplastic changes in the alimentary canal of the lactating rat. *J. Pathol. Bacteriol. 85*:179-188.

Ferguson, B. B., Wilson, D. J., and Schaffner, W. (1976). Determination of nicotine concentrations in human milk. *Am. J. Dis. Child. 130*:837-839.

Finch, E., and Lorber, J. (1954). Methemoglobinaemia in the newborn probably due to phenytoin excreted in human milk. *J. Obstet. Gynaecol. Br. Emp. 61*:833-834.

Finley, J. P., Waxman, M. B., Wong, P. Y., and Lickrish, G. M. (1979). Digoxin excretion in human milk. *J. Pediatr. 94*:339-340.

Friedman, B. A. (1976). Suppression of postpartum lactation with furosemide. *S. Afr. Med. J. 50*(10):651.

Fuchs, A. R., and Wagner, G. (1963). Effect of alcohol on release of oxytocin. *Nature 198*:92-94.

Gala, R. R., and Van de Walle, C. (1977). Prolactin heterogeneity in the serum and milk during lactation. *Life Sci. 21*:99-104.

Garrett, E. R. (1971). The physiochemical and pharmacokinetic bases for the biopharmaceutical evaluation of drug biological availability in pharmaceutical formulations. *Acta Pharmacol. Toxicol. 29*(Suppl. 3):1-29.

Gelenberg, A. J. (1979). Amoxapine, a new antidepressant, appears in human milk. *J. Nerv. Ment. Dis. 167*(10):635-636.

Glass, R. L., Troolin, H. A., and Jenness, R. (1967). Comparative biochemical studies of milks. IV. Constituent fatty acids of milk fats. *Comp. Biochem. Physiol.* 22:415-425.

Glazer, J. P., Danish, M. A., Plotkin, S. A., and Yaffee, S. J. (1980). Disposition of chloramphenicol in low birth weight infants. *Pediatrics* 66(4):573-577.

Gostof, Homolka, and Zelenka (1952). Les substances dérivées du tromexane dans le lait maternel et leurs actions paradoxales sur la prothrombine. *Schweiz. Med. Wochenschr.* 30:764-765.

Green, H. J., Burkhart, B., and Hobby, G. L. (1946). Excretion of penicillin in human milk following parturition. *Am. J. Obstet. Gynecol.* 51:732-733.

Greenhalf, J. O., and Leonard, H. S. D. (1973). Laxatives in the treatment of constipation in pregnant and breast-feeding mothers. *Practitioner* 210:259-263.

Guerri, C., Ribelles, M., and Grisolia, S. (1981). Effects of lithium and lithium and alcohol administration on (Na + K)-ATPase. *Biochem. Pharmacol.* 30:25-30.

Gugler, R., Shoeman, D. W., and Azarroff, D. L. (1974). Effect of in vivo elevation of free fatty acids on protein binding of drugs. *Pharmacology.* 12:160-165.

Gunther, M., and Stancier, J. E. (1949). Diurnal variation in the fat content of breast milk. *Lancet* 1:235-237.

Gunther, M., Hawkins, D. E., and Whyley, G. A. (1965). Some observations on the sodium and potassium content of human milk. *J. Obstet. Gynaecol. Br. Commonw.* 72:69-74.

Guthrie, H. A., Picciano, M. F., and Sheehe, D. (1977). Fatty acid patterns of human milk. *J. Pediatr.* 90:39-41.

Hall, B. (1975). Changing composition of human milk and early development of an appetite control. *Lancet* 1:779-781.

Hanwell, A., and Linzell, J. L. (1973a). The time course of cardiovascular changes in lactation in the rat. *J. Physiol. 233:* 93-109.

Hanwell, A., and Linzell, J. L. (1973b). The effects of engorgement with milk and of suckling on mammary gland blood flow in the rat. *J. Physiol.* 233:111-125.

Harley, J. D., and Robin, H. (1966). "Late" neonatal jaundice following maternal treatment with sulfamethoxypyridazine. *Pediatrics* 37:855-856.

Havelka, J., Hejzlar, M., Popov, V., Viktorinová, D., and Procházka, J. (1968). Excretion of chloramphenicol in human milk. *Chemotherapy.* 13:204-211.

Higginbottom, M. D., Sweetman, L., and Nyhan, W. L. (1978). A syndrome of methylmalonic aciduria, homocystinura, megaloblastic anemia and neurological abnormalities in a vitamin B-12 deficient breast-fed infant of a strict vegetarian. *N. Engl. J. Med. 299*: 377-323.

Hosbach, R. E., and Foster, R. B. (1967). Absence of nitrofurantoin from human milk. *JAMA 202*:1057.

Huxtable, R. J. (1980). Herbal teas and toxins: novel aspects of pyrrolizidine poisoning in the United States. *Perspect. Biol. Med. 24*(1):1-14.

Hytten, F. E. (1954a). Clinical and chemical studies in human lactation. II. Variation in major constituents during a feeding. *Br. Med. J. 1*:176-179.

Hytten, F. E. (1954b). Clinical and chemical studies in human lactation. III. Diurnal variation in major constituents of milk. *Br. Med. J. 1*:179-182.

Insull, W., and Ahrens, E. H. (1959). The fatty acids of human milk from mothers on diets taken ad libitum. *Biochem. J. 72*:27-33.

Insull, W., Hirsch, J., James, T., and Ahrens, E. H. (1959). The fatty acids of manipulation of caloric balance and exchange of dietary fats. *J. Clin. Invest. 38*:443-450.

Jadhay, M., Webb, J. K. G., Vaishnava, S., and Baker, S. J. (1962). Vitamin B-12 deficiency in Indian infants: a new syndrome. *Lancet 2*:903-907.

Jakubovič, A., Hattori, T., and McGeer, P. L. (1973). Radioactivity in suckled rats after giving ^{14}C-tetrahydrocannabinol to the mother. *Eur. J. Pharmacol. 22*:221-223.

Jakubovič, A., Tait, R. M., and McGeer, P. L. (1974). Excretion of THC and its metabolites in ewes' milk. *Toxicol. Appl. Pharmacol. 28*:38-43.

Janas, L. M., and Picciano, M. F. (1981). A profile of the nucleotide content of human milk. *Fed. Proc. 40*(3):876.

Jensen, R. L., Thomas, L. N., Bergman, K. E., Filer, L. J., and Fomon, S. J. (1972). *Composition of Milk of Iowa City Women*, Unpublished data. Cited by Fomon, S. J. (1974). *Infant Nutrition*. W. B. Saunders. Philadelphia, pp. 361, 364-365.

John, T. J., Devarajan, L. V., Luther, L., and Vijayarathnam, P. (1976). Effect of breast-feeding on sero-response of infants to oral poliovirus vaccination. *Pediatrics 57*:47-53.

Johns, D. G., Rutherford, L. D., Leighton, P. C., and Vogel, C. L. (1972). Secretion of methotrexate into human milk. *Am. J. Obstet. Gynecol. 112*:978.

Juul, S. (1969). Barbituate poisoning via breast milk. *Ugeskr. Laeg. 131*:2257-2258.

Kadlec, G. J., Ha, L. T., Jarboe, C. H., Richards, D. R., and Karibo, J. M. (1978). Theophylline half-life in infants and young children. *Ann. Allergy 40*(5):303-310.

Kafetzis, D. H., Lazarides, C. V., Siafas, C. A., Georgakopoulos, P. A., and Papadatos, C. J. (1980). Transfer of cefotaxime in human milk and from mother to fetus. *J. Antimicrob. Chemother.* *6*(Suppl. A): 135-141.

Kaneko, S., Sato, T., and Suzuki, K. (1979). The levels of anticonvulsants in breast milk. *Br. J. Clin. Pharmacol.* *7*(6):624-627.

Karlberg, B., Lundberg, D., and Aberg, H. (1974). Excretion of propranolol in human breast milk. *Acta Pharmacol. Toxicol.* *34*: 222-223.

Katz, F. H., and Duncan, B. R. (1975). Entry of prednisone into human milk. *N. Engl. J. Med.* *293*:1154.

Kautz, H. D. (1959). Penicillin and other antibiotics in milk. *JAMA* *171*(1):135-137.

Kermack, W. O., and Miller, R. A. (1951). Electrical conductivity and chloride content of women's milk. 2. The effect of factors relating to lactation. *Arch. Dis. Child.* *26*:320-324.

Kesaniemi, Y. A. (1974). Ethanol and acetaldehyde in the milk and peripheral blood of lactating women after ethanol administration. *J. Obstet. Gynaecol. Br. Commonwealth* *81*:84-86.

Khan, A. K. A., and Truelove, S. C. (1979). Placental and mammary transfer of sulphasalazine. *Br. Med. J.* *15*:2(6204):1553.

Kirskey, A., and Roepke, J. L. B. (1981). Vitamin B_6 nutriture of mothers of three breast-fed neonates with central nervous system disorders. *Fed. Proc.* *40*(3):864.

Kirskey, A., Ernst, J. A., Roepke, J. L., and Tsai, T.-L. (1979). Influence of mineral intake and use of oral contraceptives before pregnancy on the mineral content of human colostrum and of more mature milk. *Am. J. Clin. Nutr.* *32*:30-39.

Klausner, H. A., and Dingell, J. V. (1971). The metabolism and excretion of Δ^9-tetrahydrocannabinol in the rat. *Life Sci.* *10*(1): 49-59.

Koetsawang, S. (1977). Injected long-acting medroxyprogesterone acetate. Effect on human lactation and concentrations in milk. *J. Med. Assoc. Thai.* *60*(2):57-60.

Larson, S. M., and Schall, G. L. (1971). Gallium 67 concentrations in human breast milk. *JAMA* *218*:257.

Leck, J. B., and Park, B. K. (1981). A comparative study of the effects of warfarin and brodifacoum on the relationship between vitamin K_1 metabolism and clotting factor activity in warfarin-susceptible and warfarin-resistant rats. *Biochem. Pharmacol.* *30*:123-128.

Levy, W., and Wisniewski, K. (1974). Chlorpromazine causing extra pyramidal dysfunction in newborn infant of psychotic mother. *N. Y. St. J. Med.* *74*:684-685.

Levy, G., Khanna, N. N., Soda, D. M., Tsuzuki, O., and Stern, L. (1975). Pharmacokinetics of acetaminophen in the human neonate: formation of acetaminophen glucuronide and sulfate in relation to plasma bilirubin concentration and d-glucaric acid excretion. *Pediatrics* 55(6):818-825.

Lindblad, B. S., and Rahimtoola, R. J. (1974). A pilot study of the quality of human milk in a lower socio-economic group in Karachi, Pakistan. *Acta Paediatr. Scand.* 63:125-128.

Lindenbaum, J., Rund, D. G., Butler, V. P., Tse-Eng, D., and Saha, J. R. (1981). Inactivation of digoxin by the gut flora: reversal by antibiotic therapy. *N. Engl. J. Med.* 305(14):789-794.

Lönnerdal, B., Forsum, E., Gebre-Medhin, M., and Hambraeus, L. (1976). Breast milk composition in Ethiopian and Swedish mothers. II. Lactose, nitrogen and protein contents. *Am. J. Clin. Nutr.* 29:1134-1141.

Lönnerdal, B., Forsum, E., and Hambraeus, L. (1980). Effect of oral contraceptives on composition and volume of breast milk. *Am. J. Clin. Nutr.* 33:816-824.

Loughnan, P. M. (1978). Digoxin in human breast milk. *J. Pediatr.* 92:1019-1020.

Low, L. C. K., Lang, J., and Alexander, W. D. (1979). Excretion of carbamizole and propylthiouracil in breast milk. *Lancet* 2:1011.

Macy, I. G., Nims, B., Brown, M., and Huncher, H. A. (1931). Human milk studies. VII. Chemical analysis of milk representative of the entire first and last halves of the nursing period. *Am. J. Dis. Child* 42:569-589.

Macy, I. G., Kelly, H. J., and Sloan, R. E. (1953). The composition of milks. *NAS-NRC Res. Counc. Publ. 254.*

Mayo, C. C., and Schticke, C. P. (1942). Appearance of a barbiturate in human milk. *Proc. Staff Meetings Mayo Clin.* 17:87-88.

McClelland, D. B. L., McGrath, J., and Samson, R. R. (1978). Antimicrobial factors in human milk: studies of concentration and transfer to the infant during the early stages of lactation. *Acta Paediatr. Scand. Suppl.* 271:1-20.

McKenzie, S. A., Selley, J. A., and Agnew, J. E. (1975). Secretion of prednisolone into breast milk. *Arch. Dis. Child.* 50:894-896.

Meffin, P., Long, G. I., and Thomas, J. (1973). Clearance and metabolism of mepivacaine in the human neonate. *Clin. Pharmacol. Ther.* 14:218-225.

Mercier-Parot, L. (1955). Disturbances in post natal development in rats after maternal administration of cortisone during pregnancy or lactation. *Compt. Rend.* 240:2259-2261.

Meyer, M. B. (1979). Breast-feeding and smoking. *Lancet* 1:975-976.

Miller, R. A., and Jackson, I. I. A. (1951). Electrical conductivity and chloride content of human milk. 4. Results and their relationship to milk yield and to duration of lactation. *Arch. Dis. Child* 26:329-332.

Miller, J. K., and Swanson, E. W. (1963). Some factors affecting iodine secretion in milk. *J. Dairy Sci.* 46:927-932.

Miller, H., and Weetch, R. S. (1955). The excretion of radioactive iodine in human milk. *Lancet* 2:1013.

Mills, J. N. (1966). Human circadian rhythms. *Physiol. Rev.* 46: 128-171.

Mirkin, B. L. (1971). Diphenylhydantoin: placental transport, fetal localization neonatal metabolism, and possible teratogenic effects. *J. Pediatr.* 78(2):329-337.

Mirkin, J. N. (1980). Evaluation of drugs in children and pregnant women: an ineluctable conundrum. *Trends Pharmacol. Sci.*, Nov., pp. 1-4.

Mischler, T. W., Corson, S. L., Larranaga, A., Bolognese, R. J., Neiss, E. S., and Vukovich, R. A. (1978). Cephradine and epicillin in body fluids of lactating and pregnant women. *J. Reprod. Med.* 21(3):130-136.

Moiel, R. H., and Ryan, J. R. (1967). Tolbutamide orinase in human breast milk. *Clin. Pediatr.* 6(8):480.

Morganti, G., Ceccarelli, G., and Ciaffi, G. (1968). Comparative concentrations of a tetracycline antibiotic in serum and maternal milk. *Antibiotica* 6:216-223.

Morselli, P. C. (1976). Clinical pharmacokinetics in neonates. *Clin. Pharmacokinet.* 1:81-98.

Morselli, P. L., Ed. (1977). *Drug Disposition During Development*, Spectrum Publications, Jamaica, N. Y., pp. 51-69.

Mortimer, E. A. (1977). Drug toxicity from breast milk? *Pediatrics* 60(5):780-781.

Mulley, B. A., Parr, G. D., Pau, W. K., Rye, R. M., Mould, J. J., and Siddle, N. C. (1978). Placental transfer of chlorthalidone and its elimination in maternal milk. *Eur. J. Clin. Pharmacol.* 13(2):129-131.

Murphy, G. M., and Singer, E. (1974). Bile acid metabolism in infants and children. *Gut* 15:151-163.

Myant, N. B., Corbett, B. D., Honour, A. J., and Pochin, E. E. (1950). Distribution of radio iodine in man. *Clin. Sci.* 9:405-419.

New Scientist (1981). A cure for schistosomiasis. *New Sci.* 89(1236): 130.

Niebyl, J. R., Blake, D. A., Freeman, J. M., and Luff, R. D. (1979). Carbamazepine levels in pregnancy and lactation. *Obstet. Gynecol.* 53(1):139-140.

Nilsson, S., Nygren, K. G., and Johansson, E. D. B. (1977). D-Norgestrel concentrations in maternal plasma, milk, and child plasma during administration of oral contraceptives to nursing women. *Am. J. Obstet. Gynecol.* 129:178-184.

Nilsson, S., Nygren, K. G., and Johansson, E. D. B. (1978).

Transfer of estradiol to human milk. *Am. J. Obstet. Gynecol.* *132*(6):653-657.

Nutrition Reviews (1977). Insecticides in breast milk. *Nutr. Rev.* *35*(4):72-73.

O'Brien, J. R., Finch, W., and Clark, E. (1970). A comparison of an effect of different anti-inflammatory drugs on human platelets. *J. Clin. Pathol.* *23*:522-525.

Odell, G. B. (1973). Influence of binding on the toxicity of bilirubin. *Ann. N. Y. Acad. Sci.* *226*:225-237.

Olszyna-Marzys, A. E. (1978). Contaminants in human milk. *Acta Paediatr. Scand.* *67*:571-576.

Orme, M. L., Lewis, P. J., de Swiet, M., Serlin, M. J., Sibcon, R., Baty, J. D., and Breckenridge, A. M. (1977). May mothers given warfarin breast-feed their infants? *Br. Med. J.* *1*:1564-1565.

Painter, M. J., Pippenger, C., MacDonald, H., and Pitlick, W. (1978). Phenobarbital and diphenylhydantoin levels in neonates with seizures. *J. Pediatr.* *92*:315-319.

Palmer, K. E.(1979). Excretion of ^{125}I in breast milk following administration of labelled fibrinogen. *Br. J. Radiol.* *52*:672-673.

Parsons, W. D., and Neims, A. H. (1978). Effect of smoking on caffeine clearance. *Clin. Pharmacol.* *24*(1):40-45.

Parsons, W. B., Aranda, J. V., and Neims, A. H. (1976). Elimination of transplacentally acquired caffein in full-term neonates. *Pediatr. Res.* *10*:333.

Patrick, M. J., Tilstone, W. J., and Reavey, P. (1972). Diazepam and breast-feeding. *Lancet* *1*:542-543.

Peaker, M. (1976). Lactation: some cardiovascular and metabolic consequences, and the mechanisms of lactose and iron secretion into milk. *Ciba Found. Symp.* *45*:87-101.

Perlman, H. H., Dannenberg, A. M., and Sokofoff, N. (1942). The excretion of nicotine in breast milk and urine from cigarette smoking. *JAMA* *120*(13):1003-1009.

Perraudin, M. L., and Sorin, M. (1978). Intoxication probable d'un nouveau-né par la nicotine présente dans le lait de sa mère. *Ann. Pediatr.* *25*(1):41-44.

Picciano, M. F. (1978). Mineral content of human milk during a single nursing. *Nutr. Rep. Int.* *18*:5-10.

Picciano, M. F., and Deering, R. H. (1977). Milk, copper, iron, and zinc intakes of totally breast-fed infants. *Fed. Proc. Fed. Am. Soc. Exp. Biol.* *36*:1175.

Picciano, M. F., and Guthrie, H. A. (1976). Copper, iron and zinc contents of mature human milk. *Am. J. Clin. Nutr.* *29*: 242-254.

Picciano, M. F., Guthrie, H. A., and Sheehe, D. M. (1978). The cholesterol content of human milk. A variable constituent among

cholesterol content of hyman milk. A variable constituent among women and within the same woman. *Clin. Pediatr. 17*:359-362.

Pikkarainen, P. H., and Raiha, N. C. R. (1967). Development of alcohol dehydrogenase activity in the human liver. *Pediatr. Res. 1*:165-168.

Pincus, G., Bialy, G., Layne, D. S., Paniagua, M., and Williams, K. I. H. (1966). Radioactivity in the milk of subjects receiving radioactive 19-norsteroids. *Nature 212*:924.

Pittard, W. B., Bill, K., and Fletcher, B.D. (1979). Excretion of technetium in human milk. *J. Pediatr. 94*(4):605-607.

Plotkin, S. A., Katz, M., Brown, R. E., and Pagano, J. S. (1966). Oral poliovirus vaccination in newborn African infants. The inhibitory effect of breast feeding. *Am. J. Dis. Child 111*:27-30.

Pommerenke, W. T., and Hahn, P. F. (1943). Secretion of radioactive sodium in human milk. *Proc. Soc. Exp. Biol. Med. 52*: 223-224.

Posner, A. C., Konicoff, N. G., and Prigot, A. (1956). Tetracycline in obstetric infections. *Antibiot. Annu. 1955—1956*:345-348.

Potter, J. M., and Nestel, P. (1976). The effects of dietary fatty acids and cholesterol on the milk lipids of lactating women and the plasma cholesterol of breast-fed infants. *Am. J. Clin. Nutr. 29*:54-60.

Powell, J. R., Thiercelin, J. F., Vozeh, S., Sansom, L., and Riegelman, S. (1977). The influence of cigarette smoking and sex on theophylline disposition. *Ann. Rev. Respir. Dis. 116*: 17-23.

Pütter, J., and Held, F. (1979). Quantitative studies on the occurrence of praziquantel in milk and plasma of lactating women. *Eur. J. Drug. Metab. Pharmacokinet. 4*(4):193-198.

Pynnönen, S., and Sillanpää, M. (1975). Carbamazepine and mother's milk. *Lancet 2*:563.

Rane, A. (1974). Urinary excretion of diphenylhydantoin metabolites in newborn infants. *J. Pediatr. 85*(4):543-545.

Rasmussen, F. (1959). Mammary excretion of benzylpenicillin, erythromycin and penethamate hydroiodide. *Acta. Pharmacol. Toxicol. 16*:194-200.

Rasmussen, F. (1966). *Studies on the mammary excretion and absorption of drugs.* Mortensen, Copenhagen. pp. 9-83.

Read, W. W. C., Lutz, P. G., and Tashjian, A. (1965). Human milk lipids. II. The influence of dietary carbohydrates and fat on the fatty acids of mature milk. A study in four ethnic groups. *Am. J. Clin. Nutr. 17*:180-183.

Reed, P. I., Haines, K., Smith, P. L. R., House, F. R., and Walters, C. L. (1981). Gastric juice N-nitrosamines in health and gastroduodenal disease. *Lancet 2*:550-552.

Rees, J. A., Glass, R. C., and Sporne, G. H. (1976). Serum and breast milk concentrations of dothiepin. *Practitioner* 217:686.

Resman, B. H., Blumenthal, H. P., and Jusko, W. J. (1977). Breast milk distribution of theobromine from chocolate. *J. Pediatr.* 91:477-480.

Rosa, F. W. (1976). Resolving the "public health dilemma" of steroid contraception and its effects on lactation. *Am. J. Public Health* 66(8):791-792.

Rozansky, R., and Brzezinsky, A. (1969). The excretion of penicillin in human milk. *J. Lab. Clin. Med.* 34:497-500.

Rumble, W. F., Aamodt, R. L., Jones, A. E., Henkin, R. I., and Johnston, G. S. (1978). Accidental ingestion of Tc-99m in breast milk by a 10-week-old child. *J. Nucl. Med.* 19(8):913-915.

Sack, C. M., Koup, J. R., and Smith, A. L. (1980). Chloramphenicol pharmacokinetics in infants and young children. *Pediatrics* 66(4):579-584.

Schou, M., and Amdisen, A. (1973). Lithium and pregnancy-III, lithium ingestion by children breast-fed by women on lithium treatment. *Br. Med. J.* 2:138.

Sereni, F., Mandelli, M., Principi, N., Tognoni, G., Pardi, G., and Morselli, P. L. (1973). Induction of drug metabolizing enzymes activities in the human fetus and in the newborn infant. *Enzyme* 15:318-329.

Shirkey, H. C. (1980). Pediatric clinical pharmacology and therapeutics. In *Drug Treatment: Principles and Practice of Clinical Pharmacology and Therapeutics*, 2nd ed., G. S. Avery, Ed., Adis Press, New York, pp. 95-157.

Sinaiko, A. R. (1981). Environmental contaminants in human breast milk: potential effect on infant development. In *Textbook of Gastroenterology and Nutrition in Infancy*, E. Lebenthal, Ed., Raven Press, New York, pp. 339-346.

Smith, C. A. (1976). Physiology of the digestive tract. In *The Physiology of the Newborn Infant*, C. A. Smith and N. M. Nelson, Eds., Charles C Thomas, Springfield, Ill., pp. 459-479.

Smith, J. A., Morgan, J. R., Rachlis, A. R., and Papsin, F. R. (1975). Clindamycin in human breast milk. *Can. Med. Assoc. J.* 112:806.

Somogyi, A., and Gugler, R. (1979). Cimetidine excretion into breast milk. *Br. J. Clin. Pharmacol.* 7:627-629.

Sovner, R., and Orsulak, P. J. (1979). Excretion of imipramine and desipramine in human breast milk. *Am. J. Psychiatr.* 136(4A):451-452.

Sparr, R. A., and Pritchard, J. A. (1958). Maternal and newborn distribution of sulfamethoxypyridazine (Kynex). *Obstet. Gynecol.* 12:131-134.

Spector, A. A., Santos, E. C., Ashbrook, J. D., and Fletcher, J. E. (1973). Influence of free fatty acid concentration on drug binding to plasma albumin. _Ann. N. Y. Acad. Sci._ 226:247-258.

Stanbury, S. W., and Thomson, A. E. (1951). Diurnal variation in electrolyte excretion. _Clin. Sci._ 10:268-293.

Stern, L., Khanna, N. N., Levy, G., and Yaffe, S. (1970). Effect of phenobarbital on hyperbilirubinemia and glucuronide formation in newborns. _Am. J. Dis. Child._ 120:26-31.

Szefler, S. J., and Shen, D. D. (1981). Drug excretion in breast milk. In _Textbook of Gastroenterology and Nutrition in Infancy_, E. Lebenthal, Ed., Raven Press, New York.

Toaff, R., Ashkenazi, H., Schwartz, A., and Herzberg, M. (1969). Effects of oestrogen and progestagen on the composition of human milk. _J. Reprod. Fertil._ 19:475-482.

Tobin, R. E., and Schneider, P. B. (1976). Uptake of ^{67}Ga in the lactating breast and its persistence in milk. _J. Nucl. Med._ 17: 1055-1056.

Tunnessen, W. W., and Hertz, C. G. (1972). Toxic effects of lithium in newborn infants: a commentary. _Pediatr. Pharmacol. Ther._ 81(4):804-807.

Tyrala, E. E., and Dodson, W. E. (1979). Caffeine secretion into breast milk. _Arch. Dis. Child_ 54:787-800.

Tyson, R. M., Shrader, E. A., and Perlman, H. H. (1938a). Drugs transmitted through breast milk. II. Barbiturates. _J. Pediatr._ 13:86-90.

Tyson, R. M., Shrader, E. A., and Perlman, H. H. (1938b). Drugs transmitted through breast milk. III. Bromides. _J. Pediatr._ 13: 91-93.

Uhlíř, F., and Rýznar, J. (1973). Appearance of chlorpromazine in the mother's milk. _Act. Nerv. Super._ 15(2):106.

Varsano, I., Fischl, J., and Shochet, S. B. (1973). The excretion of orally ingested nitrofurantoin in human milk. _J. Pediatr._ 82(5):886-887.

Vest, M. F. (1965). The development of conjugation mechanisms and drug toxicity in the newborn. _Biol. Neonate_ 8:258-266.

Vijay, K. K., and Manocha, S. L. (1976). Pharmaco-physiological implications of marihuana use. _Baroda J. Nutr._ 3:197-216.

Vorherr, H. (1974). Excretion of drugs into milk—potential hazards to the breast-fed infant. In _The Breast: Morphology, Physiology, and Lactation_, Academic Press, New York, pp. 107-124.

Warren, R. J., Lepow, M. L., Bartsch, G. E., and Robbins, F. C. (1964). The relationship of maternal antibody, breast feeding, and age to the susceptibility of newborn infants to infection with attenuated polioviruses. _Pediatrics_ 34:4-13.

Watkins, J. B., Ingall, D., Szczepanik, P., Klein, P. D., and

Lester, R. (1973). Bile salt metabolism in the newborn. Measurement of pool size and synthesis by stable isotope technique. *N. Engl. J. Med.* *288*:431-434.

Weaver, J. C., Kamm, M. L., and Dobson, R. L. (1960). Excretion of radioiodine in human milk. *JAMA* *173*:872-875.

Werthman, M. W., and Krees, S. V. (1972). Excretion of chlorthiazine in human breast milk. *J. Pediatr.* *81*:781-783.

West, I. (1964). Pesticides as contaminants. *Arch. Environ. Health* *9*(5):626-633.

West, K. D., and Kirksey, A. (1976). Influence of vitamin B-6 intake on the content of the vitamin in human milk. *Am. J. Clin. Nutr.* *29*:961-969.

Wiernik, P. H., and Duncan, J. H. (1971). Cyclophosphamide in human milk. *Lancet* *1*:912.

Wiles, D. H., Orr, M. W., and Kolakowska, T. (1978). Chlorpromazine levels in plasma and milk of nursing mothers. *Br. Med. Clin. Pharmacol.* *5*:272-273.

Wilson, J. T., Brown, R. D., Cherek, D. R., Dailey, J. W., Hilman, B., Jobe, P. C., Manno, B. R., Manno, J. E., Redetzki, H. M., and Stewart, J. J. (1980). Drug excretion in human breast milk: principles, pharmacokinetics and projected consequences. *Clin. Pharmacokinet.* *5*(1):1-66.

Windorfer, A., Jr., Kvenzer, W., and Urbanek, R. (1974). The influence of age on the activity of acetylsalicyclic acid-enterase and protein salicylate binding. *Eur. J. Clin. Pharmacol.* *7*:227-231.

Wong, Y. K., and Wood, B. S. (1971). Breast-milk jaundice and oral contraceptives. *Br. Med. J.* *4*:403-404.

World Health Organization (1969). *WHO Technical Report Series 417*, Geneva.

Wurtman, J. J., and Fernstrom, J. D. (1979). Free amino acid, protein, and fat contents of breast milk from Guatemalan mothers consuming a corn-based diet. *Early Hum. Dev.* *3*:67-77.

Wyburn, J. R. (1973). Human breast milk excretion of radionuclides following administration of radiopharmaceuticals. *J. Nucl. Med.* *14*:115-117.

Yoshioka, H., Cho, K., Takimoto, M., Maruyama, S., and Shimizu, T. (1979). Transfer of cefazolin into human milk. *J. Pediatr.* *94*(1):151-152.

Yurchak, A. M., and Jusko, W. J. (1976). Theophylline secretion into breast milk. *Pediatrics* *57*:518-520.

10
Drugs, Appetite, and Body Weight

David A. Levitsky
Cornell University, Ithaca, New York

I. INTRODUCTION

Nearly 75% of the ingested drugs that are currently cited in the *Physician's Desk Reference* (PDR) list nausea, change in appetite, or body weight as an adverse symptom. For most of these drugs the nausea and loss of appetite is a general reaction to a pharmacological insult to the body. In some cases the loss of appetite and body weight caused by drug therapy is sufficiently serious, such as drug chemotherapy for cancer, that the other medication must be taken to enhance appetite. In other cases, slow and subtle changes in body weight and appetite were first noted in people chronically taking certain medications. These observations can now be combined with a large body of information on the biochemistry of appetite and weight regulation. As this information accumulates, a clear understanding is emerging of the fundamental processes underlying the control of appetite and the regulation of body weight. This allows us not only to understand why certain drugs cause changes in body weight, but also will help us predict what drugs will affect appetite and body weight in humans.

The intent of this chapter is to review the literature on the effect of drugs on appetite and body weight, explain the possible mechanism through which they are believed to operate, and suggest a conceptual framework to account for the myriad of drugs that affect appetite and body weight.

II. APPETITE AND BODY WEIGHT REGULATION

Before beginning this review it is necessary to discuss the relationship
between appetite and body weight and to realize the limitations on our
ability to establish a clear relationship between them. There are few
contradictions to the fact that drugs that depress appetite and food intake depress body weight. Similarly, most drugs that increase appetite also increase body weight. These relationships however do not
prove that the mechanism of drug-induced weight change is through
changes in appetite. In many cases the change in body weight and
the change in food intake merely represent the expression of similar
changes in energy balance (Levitsky and Strupp, 1981), not a causal
link between them.

A major difficulty in trying to link changes in body weight to changes
in food intake is that it is quite difficult to detect small changes in food
intake in humans because our present methods of monitoring for food
intake are simply too insensitive to detect changes smaller than 10%. It
is very possible that many drugs do cause such subtle changes in food
intake. It is because of these problems that one is compelled to look for
consistency between the human and the animal literature before drawing
conclusions concerning the acceptance of a relativity between drugs and
appetite and the mechanisms of action. There are few exceptions to the
rule that drugs that affect appetite and body weight in humans affect
monogastric mammals in a similar way. Therefore, the emphasis of this
review is on these major classes of drugs in which we have a substantial
amount of empirical information on both human and animal subjects.

III. APPETITE DEPRESSANTS

The first drug that was specifically used as an appetite suppressant is
amphetamine (Nathanson, 1937). Its anorectic effect was discovered
accidentally as a side effect of its use as an antinarcoleptic. It is interesting to note that although the weight-reducing effects of amphetamine are well accepted today, a controversy remained for several
years over whether the major mechanism of its action was due to its
anorexia or to the increased motor activity it produces. The argument seemed to be settled by a declaration that the amphetamine's
effect on weight loss occurred through its anorectic characteristics
(Stowe and Miller, 1957).

Although there exists little doubt as to the effectiveness of amphetamine and amphetamine-like drugs in promoting weight loss (Sullivan and
Comai, 1978), the continual use of these kinds of drugs has severe limitations as an ideal therapeutic technique for treatment of the overweight. Many patients taking amphetamines for weight loss complain
of excessive central nervous system stimulation—they have difficulty

sleeping, feel nervous and tense, and sometimes undergo personality changes. Moreover, tolerance develops quite quickly to the weight-reducing effects of the drug, but not to the general stimulating effects. As a consequence, patients come to rely on the drug to maintain alertness. Finally, the drug has a fairly high abuse potential.

As a result of these problems with amphetamines, the pharmaceutical industry has been actively searching for a more specific appetite suppressant than amphetamine and has led to the marketing of a large number of drugs listed in Table 1. Most of the drugs currently being used as appetite suppressants are structurally very similar to the amphetamines, being basically a phenylethylamine. Although small modifications of the basic phenylethylamine structure result in different degrees of central nervous system (CNS) stimulation and anorexia, most of these drugs act to inhibit appetite in a manner almost identical to amphetamines. There are two major exceptions, however: fenfluramine and mazindole.

A. Mode of Action of Major Anorectics

It is generally agreed that the mechanism through which amphetamines and the other amphetamine-like anorectics act is through modulation of the activity of catecholamine-containing neurons in the brain (Baez, 1974). Although amphetamine is structurally quite similar to norepinephrine and dopamine, the major brain catecholamines, it does not seem to directly stimulate postsynaptic catecholamine receptors. Instead, it seems to facilitate the release of catecholamines from the presynaptic ending and prevent reuptake of the neurotransmitters back into the presynaptic nerve ending. The effect of these two actions of amphetamine is to potentiate the natural role of the catecholamines in the brain. One almost invariant function of enhanced brain catecholamine output is an increase in central nervous system general arousal, increase in motor activity (Kelly, 1977), and a depression in appetite (Hoebel, 1977). Efforts began very early in the history of anorectic research to find a way to suppress appetite without causing an increase in CNS arousal. The first attempt was to add CNS depressants to amphetamines (Dexamyl, Eskatrol). Other efforts went into finding a completely new drug.

In 1971, it was believed that such a drug was found. That drug was fenfluramine. Although fenfluramine is structurally similar to amphetamine and is an effective anorectic in both animals and humans, its mechanism of action was found to be quite different from amphetamine. Rather than stimulating the central nervous system, fenfluramine seems to act as a mild CNS depressant. At doses that cause significant anorexia, fenfluramine causes a depression in motor activity in the animal, as indicative of CNS depression. Amphetamine and other amphetamine-like drugs, on the other hand, almost always cause an increase in motor activity. Moreover, one of the most common complaints of patients

Table 1 Anorectic Drugs

Generic name	Commercial name
Amphetamine	Benzedrine
	Dexedrine
	Obetral
Benzphetamine	Didrex
Chlorphentiramine	Pre-Sate
Chortermine	Voranil
Diethylpropion	Tenuate
	Tepanil
Fenfluramine	Pondimin
Mazindole	Sanorex
Methamphetamine	Desoxyn
Phendimetrazine	Bacarate
	Bontril
	Melfiat
	Phenazine
	Plegine
	Prelu-2
	SPRX-105
	Statobex
	Trimstat-Trimtab, Wehless-35
Phenmetrazine	Preludin
Phentermine	Adipex
	Fastin
	Ionamin
	Phentermine
	T-Diet
	Teramine
Phenylpropanolamine	Control
Phenylpropanolamine and caffeine	Anorexin
	Appedrine
	Cenadex
	Dexatrim
	Prolamine

taking fenfluramine for the treatment of obesity is that it causes mild depression and a loss of alertness (Sullivan and Comai, 1978) rather than insomnia and nervousness, the most common complaint of the amphetamine-like drugs.

The reason for these differences in CNS arousal is that unlike the amphetamine-type drugs, fenfluramine appears to cause its anorectic effect by facilitating the release of serotonin from serotonin-containing neurons in the central nervous system and blocking its reuptake (Fristrom et al., 1977). Drugs such as methylsergide which block serotonin receptors, block the anorexia produced by fenfluramine, but have no effect in blocking the anorexia produced by amphetamine. On the other hand, drugs that block catecholamine receptors block amphetamine-induced anorexia but have no effect on anorexia produced by fenfluramine (Clineschmidt et al., 1978).

In addition to this pharmacological difference between fenfluramine and amphetamine, the kind of anorexia they produce is different. Blundell et al. (1976) observed that amphetamine depresses food intake by delaying the onset of eating, interpreted as delaying hunger. In contrast, fenfluramine has little effect on delaying the onset of a meal, but once the meal is begun, it is terminated more rapidly, suggesting that fenfluramine enhances the satiety value of the food. This behavior difference between the two drugs observed in rats by Blundell has also been seen in humans (Wooley et al., 1977). The investigations of the mode of actions of these two drugs have suggested that two major neurotransmitter systems exist in the brain which are involved in the different aspects of the control of appetite: a catecholamine hunger system which, when activated, delays the onset of meals, and a serotonergic satiety system which potentiates the satiety value of food.

Recently, a structurally different anorectic drug has been introduced, mazindole. Although mazindole produces anorexia by potentiating the catecholamine system, it appears to be more selective in specifically blocking the presynaptic reuptake pump than the amphetamine-type anorectics (Carrube et al., 1977). As a consequence of this difference and other subtle pharmacological differences between mazindole and the amphetamines, mazindole inhibits appetite at doses far lower than necessary to produce increases in motor behavior (Gogerty et al., 1968), a sign of general CNS arousal. At higher doses, however, the anorexia is accompanied by excessive motor movement.

The only over-the-counter (OTC) anorectic drug sold in the United States is phenylpropylethylamine. When used as an appetite suppressant the drug is usually mixed with a large amount of caffeine. Phenylpropylethylamine is structurally similar to amphetamine and seems to share its mode of action in curbing appetite (Hoebel et al., 1975a), although the anorectic effect and the subsequent weight loss seems quite small (Hoebel et al., 1975b; Gruboff et al., 1975) compared to the other commercially available drugs.

B. Development of "Tolerance" to Anorectic Drugs

Perhaps one of the major drawbacks to the use of anorectic drugs for the treatment of obesity is the development of tolerance. With chronic use, the effectiveness of all the commercially available anorectic drugs in suppressing appetite decreases. As a result, the rate of weight loss decreases. Increasing the dose of the drug reestablishes the anorectic properties of the drug and further loss in weight ensues, but this effect is only temporary.

Recent research into the nature of the development of tolerance to the anorectic properties of drugs has revealed some unusual findings which suggest that what appears as tolerance may not be tolerance in the strict pharmacological sense of the term. One of the unusual features of the tolerance to anorectic drugs is that tolerance seems to develop only to the anorectic properties of the drug (Gotestam and Lewander, 1975). Very little tolerance seems to develop to most of the CNS excitation effects of these drugs, such as the increased motor activity or the antinarcoleptic effect (Lewander, 1971; Magour et al., 1974). Moreover, appetite suppression by these drugs is more closely related to body weight loss than to chronic drug administration (Levitsky et al., 1981). If the body weights of animals are reduced before they are administered anorectic drugs, the anorectic effect of the drugs can be completely blocked. Furthermore, the anorectic effect of these drugs can be reestablished in drug-tolerant animals by artifically raising body weight.

Perhaps the most interesting point of all is the fact that the depression in body weight in the "drug-tolerant" animal is maintained even though food intake returns to normal. The latter observation strongly suggests that increasing energy expenditure may be one of the major effects of the anorectic drugs. Unfortunately for the patient, body weight returns to predrug levels as soon as the drug use is discontinued.

C. Special Problems with the Use of Stimulants with Children

The use of central nervous system stimulants has not been restricted to weight control. Central nervous system stimulants have been effectively used to treat children suffering from various kinds of attentional disorders for almost 50 years. The fact that CNS stimulants were also appetite depressants was noted in the very first report describing the use of these amphetamines in children (Bradley, 1937). Since then other stimulants, considerably more mild than amphetamine, have been used for the treatment of childhood attentional disorders, of which the most popular is methylphenidate. Other CNS stimulants, such as imipramine (Gross, 1976; Waizer et al., 1974), pemoline (Dickerson et al.,

1979; Freidman et al., 1981), and hydroxyzine (Greenberg et al., 1972); have also been used effectively.

Safer et al. (1972,1975) noted that others, particularly Knight and Horton (1969), had observed a depression in appetite in children taking CNS medication for attentional disorders, and examined the effects of those drugs on their growth. They observed that the chronic use of CNS stimulants in children resulted in a significant reduction in body weight and linear growth. This observation was confirmed in children taking methylphenidate (Gross, 1976; Knights and Horton, 1969; Millichap and Millichap, 1975; Quinn and Rapoport, 1975; Weiss et al., 1975), pemoline (Dickinson et al., 1979; Friedman et al., 1981), imipramine (Quinn and Rapoport, 1975; Greenberg et al., 1972; Waizer et al., 1974), and amphetamine (Goss, 1976; Rayner and Conit, 1974).

Part of this suppression in growth is due to the direct suppression in appetite (Conners and Eisenberg, 1963) as observed in both humans and animals (Barone et al., 1979a,b; Greeley and Kizer, 1980). The reduction in appetite, however, is not the entire explanation for the growth retardation. Greeley and Kizer (1980) have shown that young growing rats receiving methylphenidate daily have impaired growth even when compared to pair-fed controls. Moreover, the reduction in appetite is seen primarily at the onset of drug treatment, but as seen in adults, disappears with continual usage. The growth-suppressing effects of these drugs continue but may depend on the particular drug (Greenhill et al., 1980). Fortunately, the growth-suppressing effects of stimulants in children appear to be totally reversible with discontinuation of treatment when major rebounds in growth occur (Safer et al., 1975). No evidence exists to suggest a permanent depression in growth or body weight to result from the use of CNS stimulants in childhood (Roche et al., 1979).

D. Final Comments About Anorectic Drugs

The theory behind the use of appetite suppressants as a treatment for obesity is that the drugs depress certain appetite pathways in the brain, helping an individual to maintain a calorically restricted diet, and thus aiding the patient to return to a "normal" body weight. It seems clear by now that this notion is both theoretically unsound and therapeutically ineffective in the long-term treatment of obesity. There are a number of reasons for this.

First, brain research conducted in the last 10 years has demonstrated repeatedly that the neural systems that influence feeding behaviors, such as the norepinephrine, dopamine, and serotonin pathways, are involved in many different kinds of behavior, not just the control of food intake, a concept suggested by Valenstein et al. in 1970). Second, even if there were a specific feeding or appetite system that could be activated or inactivated by direct application of specific chemicals to specific areas in the brain, it is highly unlikely that a drug will be discovered that will have that degree of specificity. More likely, if a drug is a specific receptor blocker, it will block all those receptors throughout the brain, not just those receptors located in an area most closely related to feeding behavior (if such a system exists). This may explain why almost none of the currently used anorectic drugs have specific anorectic activity, and why they produce other, usually unacceptable, behavorial changes as well.

The final fallacy in the underlying philosophy of using anorectic drugs in the treatment of obesity is the idea that reducing a patient to a "normal" body weight is sufficient for the alleviation of the problem of obesity. Any dieter knows that this is not true. There are hundreds of ways to lose weight (Berland, 1976), but the most important aspect of an effective treatment for obesity is the maintenance of the lowered body weight. Anorectic drugs are currently used only to help an individual lose weight, not maintain it. In most cases, when the drug is discontinued, body weight returns to its pretreatment values. Perhaps, in the light of the continued weight-suppressing effect of anorectic drugs, other drugs will be developed that are more directed to the continued weight maintenance characteristics, rather than to their appetite-suppressing effects.

In summary, many drugs are currently available which effectively depress appetite for short intervals of time and promote weight loss in humans. Most act by enhancing the catecholamine pathways in the brain. Some enhance serotonergic pathways. The activation of these neurochemical systems affects many behaviors, of which feeding behavior is only one, thereby causing many untoward effects. Finally, although anorectic drugs have been found to be effective in the short run as an aid to weight loss, there is no evidence that they are any more effective for maintaining the weight loss following discontinuance of the drug than merely restricting calories. Perhaps, continuing research into the mechanisms involved in the long-term maintenance of body weight will give us the "magic pill"; so far, we do nor have it.

IV. DRUGS THAT STIMULATE APPETITE

Just as almost all CNS stimulants depress appetite and cause a loss in weight, CNS depressants increase appetite and are associated with an increase in body weight. The appetite and weight-enhancing effect of depressants were mostly discovered by accident, as side effects. Of these drugs, cyproheptadine has received the most attention.

A. Cyproheptadine

The appetite-stimulating effects of cyproheptadine were discovered inadvertently in a study of the antiasthmatic effectiveness of cyproheptadine and chlorphenteramine in asthmatic children by Lavenstein et al. (1962). They observed a clear facilitation of the growth in the children treated with cyproheptadine, but not with chlorphenteramine. The increased growth appeared normal with proportional increases in height as well as weight. Moreover, the distribution of body fat appeared normal, unlike the morphological disfiguration commonly seen following chronic corticoid therapy. The fact that the growth effect was related to the drug was clearly demonstrated by the fact that the enhanced growth ceased on the termination of the use of the drug.

Since the publication of the original report by Lavenstein et al. (1962), many papers have appeared in the literature attesting to the appetite-stimulating effect of cyproheptadine. The appetite-stimulating effects have been observed in adults (Noble, 1969) as well as children (Bergen, 1964) and laboratory animals (Ghosh and Parvathy, 1973; Oomwa et al., 1973). What is important from a medical perspective is that the drug seems to be effective in stimulating growth in growth-retarded children (Sanzgiri et al., 1970) and in treating patients with anorexia nervosa (Mainguet, 1972; Pawlowski, 1975; Goldberg et al., 1979).

Although the appetite-stimulating effects of cyproheptadine are well founded (Silverstone and Schuyler, 1975), its mode of action is not. Cyproheptadine has both potent antiserotonergic and antihistaminergic properties. Blocking either one of these neurotransmitter pathways will lead to an increase in eating. As discussed above, fenfluramine causes an increase in serotonin at the postsynaptic receptor and produces satiety. Similarly, a systemic injection of 5-hydroxytryptophan, the immediate precursor of serotonin, causes an increase in brain serotonin and a decrease in food intake. It is also known that depleting the brain of serotonin by injecting animals intracerebrally with p-chlorophenylalanine will cause rats to overeat and gain weight (Breisch et al., 1976). Thus it seems reasonable that blocking a serotonergic receptor should also cause an increase in food intake.

However, the serotonergic blocking property of cyproheptadine is not the total explanation for the drug's appetite-stimulating characteristics. Other drugs, many times more specific as a serotonin blocker than cyproheptadine, such as methylsergide, do not stimulate feeding behavior by themselves, although they do block the anorectic effects of fenfluramine (Blundell and Leshem, 1973; Blundell et al., 1973). Moreover, the depletion of brain serotonin systems usually results in hyperactivity (Harvey et al., 1963), whereas one of the major complaints of patients taking cyproheptadine is drowsiness.

The other receptor system that cyproheptadine blocks is histamine. Although the role of histamine in the brain has not been studied as ex-

tensively as that of the catecholamines and serotonin, it is fairly well
accepted as a central neurotransmitter in the central nervous system
(Garbarg et al., 1974). There is some evidence to suggest that increased brain histamine levels suppress appetite in animals (Clineschmidt and Lotti, 1973) and in humans (Henkin et al., 1972). If increasing brain histamine inhibits appetite, it is reasonable to expect
that blocking histamine receptors should increase appetite. However,
like serotonin, blocking histamine may not be the whole story because
other antihistaminic drugs, such as chlorphenteramine, do not seem to
cause great increases in appetite. It seems that a depression of both
histamine and serotonin receptors may be responsible for the appetite-
stimulating effects of cyprohistadine.

It should also be pointed out that part of the weight gain seen in human patients recovering from anorexia nervosa may be due to the decrease in motor activity. Stiel et al. (1970) examined the weight gain
in volunteers who were limited to their normal food intake while taking
cyproheptadine and observed that although weight gain was less than
in subjects that had free access to food, it was significantly higher than
nondrug controls. Further analysis of the weight gain suggested that
the effect was not caused by a change in water balance brought about
by a differential sodium loss. Since the drug was found to cause drowsiness and sleep, the authors speculated that the patients may have
spent more time in low-energy-expenditure behaviors than was spent
by the controls, and this may have contributed to their weight gain.

B. Lithium

In 1949, Cade published the first study on the remarkable ameliorating
effect of lithium ingestion on manics. Since then, its use as a major
therapeutic tool has grown until today it is one of the drugs of choice
for treating not only manics, but also cyclic depressives (Johnson,
1975). Twenty years later Freidrich (1969) noted that his patients taking lithium seemed to gain weight at an unusually fast rate. This observation was soon verified by Kerry et al. (1970) and others (Schou
et al., 1970; O'Connell, 1971).

The mechanism through which lithium produces the increase in body
weight is still not well understood. There is evidence that at least part
of the increase in body weight is due to an increase in appetite.
Vendsborg et al. (1976) observed that about one-third of the patients
who gain weight on lithium show marked increased in appetite. Increased food intake in animals following small doses of lithium have also been reported (Opitz and Schafer, 1976), although higher doses
cause nausea and food aversion (Marini et al., 1978). Moreover, small
amounts of lithium also cause rats to ingest not only food, but also non-
foods such as pure cellulose (Kratz and Levitsky, 1978). Unfortunately, there are no published data demonstrating that lithium causes a

clear increase in food eaten by human subjects.

One reason why no clear data exist on the relationship between lithium usage and appetite may lie in our crude methods of measuring food
intake in humans. There exist huge variations in daily energy con-
sumptions both between human subjects, even of the same body weight
(Widdowson, 1962), and within the same subject from day to day (Edholm et al., 1955). Garrow (1955) has estimated that our techniques
for measuring food intake in nonconfined humans cannot detect a difference of less than about 10%. If lithium caused an increase in food
consumption of only about 250 cal per day, we could not measure it, but
we would see the effects of this small increment in caloric intake as an
increase of about 2 lb of body weight a month. Considering the fact
that patients usually remain on these medications for many months, it
is no wonder that slow insidious effects of a small positive energy balance become evident in patients before changes in appetite are recognized.

The earliest explanation for the weight gain of patients taking lithium
was offered by Kerry et al. (1970). They suggest that what appears
as a rapid weight gain in patients taking lithium for either mania or depression is actually a return of their body weight to their pre-illness
value. A decrease in appetite and a loss in body weight is a symptom
of both depression and mania. Thus increased appetite may be taken
as a sign that the patient is recovering from the illness.

Others, however, argue that the weight gain observed during lithium
therapy is too large to be considered as a return to "normal" weight.
Vendsborg et al. (1976) considered the weight gain with lithium a true
increase in body weight above normal levels. They support this idea
by demonstrating that only those patients who have a propensity for
obesity show the weight gain due to lithium. These individuals are
usually overweight before therapy and gain the most weight during
therapy. Moreover, those who gained the most weight with lithium had
significantly greater numbers of fat cells. It is known that individuals
with a greater number of fat cells have a greater tendency to gain
weight and are more likely to have a history of being overweight than
those who have fewer fat cells (Sjostom, 1980). It should also be recalled that chronic lithium administration to animals stimulates overfeeding and excessive weight gain (Opitz and Schafer, 1976).

Another mechanism proposed to explain how lithium ingestion might
produce an increase in food intake and body weight is related to one of
the most persistent symptoms reported by patients: increased thirst.
This explanation suggests that the excessive weight gain may be due to
an increased consumption of calories in the form of beverages such as
soda or fruit juices. This theory would explain why Vendsborg et al.
(1976) observed a higher correlation between weight gain and patients'
ratings of their thirst than their ratings of hunger.

Another novel explanation for the weight-gaining effects of lithium
was proposed by Mellerup et al. (1972). They observed an increase in

serum insulin levels in patients undergoing lithium therapy. They suggested that the increased insulin promotes the increased glucose uptake
and glycogen synthesis and is responsible for the excessive weight
gain. Unfortunately, they observed no differences in serum insulin
levels between those patients who gained weight and those who did not
during the lithium therapy.

Another physiological effect of lithium that might lead to an increase
in body weight is its inhibition of thyroxine. Ohlin and Soderberg
(1970) noted the appearance of goiter in several patients taking lithium
medication. Decreases in thyroid production leads to a decrease in
metabolic rate which may then lead to an increased accumulation of body
fat. Therefore, it is not unreasonable to propose that the decrease in
thyroxine release by lithium may contribute to weight gain of patients
chronically recovering lithium.

The appetite-stimulating effects of lithium are consistent with what
we know about the effect of lithium on CNS neurotransmitters and their
role in the control of food intake. One of the major effects of lithium
is to increase to reuptake of the catecholamines into the presynaptic
nerve ending (Byck, 1975). We have already seen that increased
synaptic receptors by the major tranquilizers also increases appetite.
Therefore, the decrease of postsynaptic catecholamines may be one of
the causes of the increase in appetite and weight gain.

C. Minor Tranquilizers

In 1960, Randall reported in a classic drug study many of the behavorial effects of minor tranquilizers on behavior, including an increase in
food intake. Since then, the administration of minor tranquilizers has
been observed to cause an increase in food intake and body weight of
rats (Fletcher et al., 1980; Wise and Dawson, 1974; Poschel, 1971; Randall, 1961; Soper and Wise, 1971), cats (Fratta, 1976; Rosenberg, 1980;
Mereu et al., 1976), dogs (Randall, 1960; 1961), horses (Brown et al.,
1976; Della Fera et al., 1978), pigs (McLaughlin et al., 1976), sheep
(Baile and McLaughlin, 1977;1978) cattle (Baile and McLaughlin, 1978),
and chicks (McLaughlin et al., 1976).

The brain mechanism responsible for the enhanced appetite seems to
involve the neurotransmitter, γ-aminobutyric acid (GABA). There
exist specific receptors in the brain for an endogenous benzodiazepine-
like substance. When these benzodiazepine receptors are activated by
the minor tranquilizers, they facilitate the release of GABA (Fuxe et
al., 1975). The effectiveness of the minor tranquilizers in stimulating
appetite depends on the integrity of GABAnergic neurons. The administration of the drug picrotoxin, a powerful GABA antagonist, inhibits
benzodiazepine-induced eating (Fletcher et al., 1980). Moreover, the
administration of a GABA agonist, muscumol, directly into the central
hypothalamic areas stimulates feeding (Kelly and Grossman, 1979).

Finally, when the amount of GABA in the brain is raised by treating an animal with the drug ethanolamine-O-sulfate, an irreversible inhibitor of GABA transaminase, feeding behavior is increased (Fletcher et al., 1980), although the site in the brain where GABA is altered determines whether an increase or a decrease in feeding behavior will occur (Cooper et al., 1980; Kelly et al., 1977,1979).

It is important to point out that although the appetite-stimulating effects are well documented in animals, there is little evidence of excessive eating or weight gain due to the use of minor tranquilizers in humans. The reason for the discrepancy is that unlike lithium, minor tranquilizers are not usually taken chronically. Since minor tranquilizers are not usually used chronically, changes in body weight are not as evident as with lithium as the major tranquilizer.

D. Major Tranquilizers

There is little question of the significant effect the major tranquilizers have on appetite and excessive weight gain. Large increase in body weight were first observed in patients chronically taking the major tranquilizers, chlorpromazine and reserpine (Hollister, 1971). Since then significant weight gains have been observed in patients taking thiothixine, fluphenazine, haloperidol, thioridazine (Doss, 1979), and clozapine (Norris and Israelstam, 1975). The weight gain appears just as readily when the tranquilizers are given as depot neuroleptics (Johnson and Breen, 1979; Korsgaard and Skausig, 1979). In fact, the only major tranquilizer that has been reported not to cause a weight gain is loxapine, which appears to produce a weight loss (Doss, 1979).

Although the effects of the major tranquilizers on appetite in humans are not well documented, their hyperphagic effect in animals is clear. Administration of moderate doses of the major tranquilizers to animals causes a clear hyperphagia and subsequent increase in body weight (Reynolds and Carlisle, 1961; Stolerman, 1970; Robinson et al., 1975; Antelman et al., 1977). Moreover, the pharmacological action of the drug on central neurotransmitters is consistent with our understanding of the biochemistry of appetite. The major effect of these drugs appears to be to block many postsynaptic receptors, including the catecholamines serotonin and histamine (Jarvick, 1970). Indeed, as we have already reviewed, a depression in these neurotransmitter systems seems to correlate with increases in appetite. Thus blocking these two neurotransmitter pathways may be one of the mechanisms through which these drugs may cause an increased appetite.

Even though the weight gain observed in patients chronically taking the major tranquilizer is thought to result from an increase in food intake, two other mechanisms must be considered. The first was suggested by Shah et al. (1973). They observed significant elevation in plasma antidiuretic hormone levels in patients ingesting chlorpromazine

daily for 18 days. This suggests that perhaps part of the increased
weight gain may be due to increased fluid retention.

The other contributing factor to the weight gain may be due to the
significant depression in motor activity commonly observed to result
from the administration of the major tranquilizers (Stolerman, 1970).
It is becoming increasingly clear that a depression in motor activity
may be a major contributor to an increase in body fat (Levitsky and
Strupp, 1981).

Regardless of the mechanism through which the major tranquilizers
induced increases in body weight, there is evidence that the use of
such drugs in the treatment of anorexia nervosa may be quite helpful
(Dally and Sargant, 1966; Dally, 1967).

E. Cannabis

Although cannabis is used primarily for nonmedical reasons, there are
at least two recognized potential medical applications: treatment of
glaucoma (Cohen, 1980) and as an antiemetic for patients undergoing
treatment for cancer (Sallan et al,, 1975; Lemberger, 1980). Both
chemotherapy and radiotherapy often cause nausea and a loss of appetite. This depression in appetite can aggrevate a cachexic condition
caused by the cancer and results in further deterioration of the patient. Cannabis has been observed not only to work as an effective
antiemetic for these patients (Chang et al., 1979; Ekert et al., 1979),
but also appears to stimulate appetite.

The observation of the appetite-stimulating effects of cannabis, commonly known as the "munchies", is not new. Reports by physicians of
patients claiming that cannabis stimulates appetite have been documented for over 100 years (O'Shaughnessy, 1938). Many appeared during
the early part of this century, when this country experienced much
concern over the popular use of marijuana (Siler et al., 1933; Adams,
1941-42; Allentuck and Bowman, 1942; Williams et al., 1946; Stockings,
1977; Ames, 1958). These studies were mostly case reports of patients.
There exist, however, only two experimental studies of the effects of
cannabis on appetite (Abel, 1971; Hollister, 1971). Both of these studies confirmed the earlier observations that cannabis does not increase
food intake in humans.

Unfortunately, the data on the effects of cannabis on the appetite of
animals are not only unclear, but seem contradictory to the human literature [see Abel (1975) for a comprehensive discussion]. For the most
part, when animals are treated with cannabis extracts of pure tetrahydrocannabinol (THC, active psychogen in cannabis) they show a decrease in food intake. This anorectic action of THC has been demonstrated in cats (Marshall, 1898; Chopra and Chopra, 1939), chicks
(Abel et al., 1972;1974), dogs (Dewey et al., 1972; Thompson et al.,
1973a,b), hamsters (Geber and Schramm, 1969), monkeys (Scheckel

et al., 1968; Grunfeld and Edery, 1969; Thompson et al., 1973a,b),
pigeons (McMillan et al., 1970); rabbits (Gerber and Schramm, 1969),
and rats (Abel and Schiff, 1969; Borgen et al., 1971; Fernandez et al.,
1971; Manning et al., 1971; Wetle and Singstake, 1971; Gonzales et al.,
1972; Rating et al., 1972; Graham and Li, 1973; Jarbe and Henriksson,
1973; Nahas et al., 1973; Siemans, 1973; Wayner et al., 1973; Sofia
and Barry, 1974). On the other hand, several investigators have observed increases in feeding behavior to result from cannabis administration in dogs (Huy et al., 1974) and rats (Carlini and Kramer, 1965;
Glick and Milloy, 1972; Thompson et al., 1973a,b; Gluck and Ferraro,
1974; Rosenkrantz and Braude, 1974).

The cause of the conflicting data is unclear. It is possible that subhuman mammals are quite different from humans in their biochemical
response and particularly their appetite response to cannabis. This
possibility, however, seems doubtful in light of the overwhelming consistency in the biochemical effects and in the feeding responses in all
mammals studied, particularly in response to drugs that alter appetite.

A more likely explanation for the discrepancy is that the drug does
not directly affect the biochemical system underlying appetite, but
rather affects feeding behavior indirectly. Unlike the other drugs discussed above which seem to stimulate appetite, cannabis is a social
drug. Eating is a behavior that occurs at social occasions in both humans and animals. It is possible that it is not the drug that stimulates
eating, but rather the social occasion that is responsible for the increased appetite (Hollister, 1971).

This explanation is not restricted to humans. It is fairly well known
that most social animals eat more food in groups than when they eat
alone (Harlow, 1932; James, 1953; Ross and Ross, 1949a,b; Yerkes,
1934). Of the five studies that observed an increase in food intake in
rats in response to the administration of cannabis, two tested their animals in groups (Thompson et al., 1973a,b; Rosenkrantz and Braude,
1974), while none of the studies that found a depression in food intake
tested their animals in a group feeding situation.

A second indirect effect of cannabis that may account for the apparent increase in appetite in humans is its hallucinogenic effect. The
most noticeable physological effect of any hallucinogen is the increase
in sensitivity and awareness of almost all sensory stimuli, including
taste. Thus subjects, particularly novice users, become aware of the
sensory dimension of ordinary foods of which they are normally not
aware. This sensory-enhancing characteristic may facilitate consumption.

Finally, the antiemetic effects may be the major reason why cannabis
is effective in stimulating the appetite of patients recovering from chemotherapy for treatment of cancer. It is well known that nausea-pro-
ducing chemicals or radiation produces significant depression in food
intake (Garcia and Ervin, 1968; Donaldson et al., 1975). It is interest-

ing to note that cannabis was suggested as an appetite stimulant for
patients recovering from morphine addiction in which nausea is a common symptom (Mayor's Committee on Marihuana, 1944).

Indeed, these interpretations of the indirect appetite-stimulating effect may explain why obesity is never mentioned as an effect of chronic
cannabis users. On the contrary, loss of appetite and body wasting
have been cited as areas of concern (Bouquet, 1951).

F. Antidepressants

Unlike the other classes of drugs cited in this section, the relationship
between antidepressant on appetite and body weight is inconsistent and
unclear. In 1973, Paykel et al. observed abnormally rapid weight gain
in patients receiving the tricyclic antidepressant drug, amitriptyline.
They reported a study of two groups of depressed patients. One group
was taken off the drug at the end of 3 months, the other was taken off
at the end of 9 months. Both groups gained weight in response to the
drug administration. However, the group that remained on the drug
continued to gain weight, whereas the group in which the drug was discontinued did not gain any further weight. When the drug was finally
withdrawn from the latter group, the group lost weight. Interestingly,
while on the drug, this group expressed a specific craving for carbohydrates.

Since the publication of this important paper, weight gain in patients
receiving antidepressant medication has frequently been reported (Harris and Harper, 1980; Jobson et al., 1978). Aware of the weight-gaining effect of the antidepressants, several researchers have used it to
treat anorexia nervosa with some success (Mills, 1976; Moore, 1977;
Needleman and Waber, 1976).

There exists a considerable problem in understanding the weight-
enhancing effect of the antidepressants. At the neurotransmitter level,
the antidepressants are believed to act by decreasing the presynaptic
catecholamine reuptake pump, thereby allowing more of the transmitter
to activate the postsynaptic receptor (Ciaranello and Patrick, 1977).
Recently, evidence has been presented which indicate that the tricyclic
antidepressants may act postsynaptically (Nagayama et al., 1981) to
sensitize the postsynaptive membrane to receptor activation. In either
case, an increase in brain catecholamines or an increase in catecholamine receptor sensitivity would be expected to produce a depression in
appetite.

There are areas in the brain in which an increased catecholamine level stimulates eating. The injection of the antidepressant desimpramine
into these areas causes increased food intake (Leibowitz and Brown,
1980). This observation, however, cannot be taken as evidence that
peripherally administered antidepressants cause overeating. In fact,

there is evidence to suggest that peripherally administered desimpramin produces a clear suppression in food intake and a loss in body weight in animals (Lupoli, 1977).

The simplest explanation of the apparent increase in body weight in patients taking antidepressants is to consider the weight gain as a return to their normal body weight. It is well known that one of the classic symptoms of endogenous depression is a loss of appetite and subsequent loss in body weight (Spitzer et al., 1978). It is possible, therefore, as has been argued for the weight-enhancing effect of lithium, that the increase in body weight following the administration of antidepressant medication to depressed patients is a reflection of the return of a stable "psychological" state.

The major argument against this interpretation is that ratings of the depression of patients taking antidepressants do not correlate with the amount of weight gained (Kupfer et al., 1979). There are two reasons, however, that could explain this lack of correlation. First, the rating scales may not be sufficiently sensitive to reflect the physiological and biochemical return of the patients to normalcy. Second, since nothing is known of the predepression body weight, it is not known how much weight was lost during the illness and therefore there is no indication of how much weight is recovered. Until accurate body weight measurements are observed before and following an episode of depression, or accurate measurements of food intake and body weight are made in normal subjects, we must be cautious in accepting the weight gain induced by antidepressants as anything more than a return to "normal" weight values.

The reason for accepting to "return to pre-illness weight" hypothesis with the antidepressant, while rejecting it with lithium, rests with the consistency of the chemical and brain neurotransmitter effects. Only under very unusual situations such as in "tail-pinch-induced eating (Antelman et al., 1977) does a rise in catecholamines activation cause eating behavior. In all other situations increasing catecholamine activities produces a depression in food intake and a loss in body weight. Moreover, the animal work is consistent with this view, in that lithium causes an increase in food consumed, while administration of antidepressants cause a decrease in food intake and a loss in body weight.

V. OTHER COMMONLY USED DRUGS AND THEIR EFFECTS ON APPETITE

A. Caffeine

Caffeine is one of the most commonly used psychoactive drugs. It is consumed primarily in drinks such as coffee, tea, and various carbonated soft drinks. There is no evidence that caffeine causes either a change in food intake or affects body weight in humans, other than the obvious depression in food intake caused by the nausea that results from high consumption of caffeine and other methylxanthines. However, there exists a considerable amount of indirect evidence which strongly suggests that caffeine might act as a mild anorectic.

The first clue that caffeine may act as an anorectic comes from the animal literature. Several studies have shown that caffeine suppresses food intake in the non-food-deprived rat (Dobrzanski and Doggett, 1976; Fajardo et al., 1974; Merkel et al., 1981; Peters and Boyd, 1967). The use of nondeprived rats is important, since no effect of caffeine on food intake was observed in deprived rats (Barone et al., 1979a,b; Dobrzanski and Doggett, 1976). Other methylxanthines have also been shown to reduce food intake and suppress body weight in rats. Theophylline, the major methylxanthine in tea, has been shown to depress food intake (Sakata et al., 1973; Fajardo et al., 1974), and similar decreases in food intake and reductions in body weight were observed in animals chronically treated with theobromine, the major methylxanthine in chocolate (Tarka et al., 1979; Fajardo et al., 1974).

Further evidence of the appetite-depressing effect of caffeine can be derived from the fact that caffeine acts very similar to amphetamine: that both drugs potentiate eating elicited by the drug 2-deoxyglucose. Moreover, like the anorectic drugs, there appears to be a tolerance to the appetite-suppressing effects of chronic treatment (Sakata et al., 1973) but not to weight-suppressing effects of the drug (Wurzner et al., 1977).

But perhaps one of the most intriguing aspects of the possible anorectic effects of caffeine is its possible mode of action. Three mechanisms are possible. First, it is well known that caffeine increase metabolic rate (Haldi et al., 1941; Miller et al., 1974; Acheson et al., 1980). Increase in heat production is known to inhibit appetite (Brobeck, 1960; Hamilton, 1963). The second mechanism through which caffeine may suppress food intake is through its ability to block the activation of benzodiazepine receptors (Skolnick et al., 1980). It should be recalled that the activation of benzodiazepine receptors by the minor tranquilizers clearly causes an increase in food intake of animals. Finally, recent studies have suggested that caffeine has a very high affinity for adenosine receptors in the brain (Synder et al., 1981). Capogrossi et al. (1979) found that the administration of adenosine or its metabolite, inosine, suppresses food intake in nondeprived rats. Thus all indication from the animal research strongly suggests that caffeine consumption should produce a mild anorectic effect in humans and support a mildly depressed body weight.

B. Nicotine

The relationship between nicotine and body weight was first noticed by people who stopped smoking and found themselves gaining weight (Brozek and Keys, 1957). Indeed, the scientific validity of this relationship is well documented (Blitzer et al., 1977; Comstock and Stone, 1972; Erikssen and Enger, 1978; Eysenck, 1964; Gordon et al., 1975; Hjermann et al, 1976; Howell, 1971; Jacobs and Gottenborg, 1981; Noppa and Bengtsson, 1980; Trahair, 1967; Wynder et al., 1967). It is important to point out that the weight gain observed following the cessation of cigarette smoking is greater than the normal increase in body weight which, unfortunately, accompanies an increase in age (Clark et al., 1967; Comstock and Stone, 1972; Jacobs and Gottenborg, 1981). The only study in which a gain in weight did not occur following the cessation of smoking was reported by Hickey and Mulcahy (1973). However, the population studied by these researchers consisted of patients who had experienced a myocardial infarction and were instructed not to gain weight.

Further support for the weight-suppressing effect of nicotine on body weight can be derived from the frequently made observation that people who smoke are lighter than nonsmokers (Noppa and Bengtsson, 1980; Noppa et al., 1978; Kittel et al., 1978; Khosla and Lowe, 1971; Hjermann et al., 1976; Blackburn et al., 1960; Erikssen and Enger, 1978; Damon, 1961), although the relationship between the number of cigarettes per day and body weight is not linear. Light smokers (more than 5 cigarettes per day) weigh less than nonsmokers, but heavy smokers (more than 20-30 cigarettes per day) do not show a body weight significantly different from nonsmokers (Jacobs and Gottenborg, 1981; Noppa and Bengtsson, 1980). Such a curvilinear relationship between number of cigarettes smoked and body weight may be related to the biphasic effects of nicotine: in low doses nicotine acts as a ganglionic stimulant and in high doses it is a ganglionic blocker (Volle and Koelle, 1971).

The mechanism of action through which cigarette smoking causes a suppression in body weight is far from clear. The most obvious mechanism is a direct anorectic effect of nicotine. Indeed, several studies show that nicotine administration does cause a depression in appetite (Munster and Battig, 1975; Baettig et al., 1980) in animals. However, there also exist several investigations which demonstrate a loss in body weight following the administration of nicotine, but without a decrease in food intake (Elson and Passey, 1963; Schechter and Cook, 1976). It is interesting to note that Damon (1961), working with humans, could not find any difference in food intake between smokers and nonsmokers, although smokers were significantly lighter than the nonsmokers. When chronic smokers give up smoking, however, a significant increase in appetite ensues (Glauser et al., 1970), especially for sweet-tasting foods (Eysenck, 1964).

Another mechanism contributing to the difference in body weight between smokers and nonsmokers is the enhanced metabolic rate caused by nicotine. Increase in resting metabolism has been observed to result from nicotine administration in both humans (Glauser et al., 1970) and animals (Burse et al., 1975; Ilebekk et al., 1975). Unfortunately, the data are unclear as to the effect on metabolic rate when chronic smokers cease smoking. Glauser et al. (1970) observed a significant decrease in metabolic rate, but Burse et al. (1975) were unable to confirm the effect. The latter research, however, also did not find the usual increase in body weight that occurs following the cessation of smoking, although they did increase in appetite among their ex-smokers.

VI. GENERALIZATIONS AND CONCLUSIONS

One generalization that can be made concerning the effects of various drugs, particularly psychoactive drugs, on appetite is that drugs that cause an increase in central nervous system arousal depress appetite and cause a loss in weight; while drugs that depress CNS arousal increase appetite and cause a gain in body weight. The two apparent exceptions to this generalization are fenfluramine, a CNS-depressing anorectic, and the tricyclic antidepressants. However, fenfluramine, while affecting appetite through the serotonergic system rather than the catecholamine system like the amphetamine, still has many of the same physiological effects of amphetamine, particularly in the peripheral sympathomemetic properties (Le Donarec and Neven, 1970), and a question still remains as to whether the weight-gaining effect of the tricyclics represents a real weight gain or a return to "normal" weight following an illness. However, despite these possible exceptions, observations of the overwhelming number of drug effects seem to support the generalization that CNS stimulants depress appetite and CNS depressants increase them. Thus any drug that affects the level of CNS arousal would be expected to affect appetite and body weight.

It is clear that a considerable amount of research still needs to be done on the long-term effects of drugs on appetite and body weight regulation. We are not only confronted with increasing pressure by the public to create a chemical cure for obesity, but are faced with the serious problem of weight loss due to anorexia nervosa and cancer. As we collect and compile more information on effects of drugs on appetite, a clearer understanding of the basic mechanisms underlying appetite and weight control will emerge, and perhaps one day we will be able to find effective and safe medication for treatment of appetite and weight disorders.

ACKNOWLEDGMENTS

The author is particularly grateful to Mr. James Schuster for his unselfish help in preparing the references, to Ms. Eva Obarzanek for her careful reading of the manuscript, and to Ms. Beverly Hastings for her careful typing.

REFERENCES

Abel, E. L. (1971). Effects of marihuana on the solution of anagrams, memory, and appetite. *Nature 231*:260.

Abel, E. L. (1975). Cannabis: effects on hunger and thirst. *Behav. Biol. 15*:255-281.

Abel, E. L., and Schiff, B. B. (1969). The effects of the marihuana homologue, pyrahexyl, on food and water intake and curiosity in the rat. *Psychon. Sci. 16*:38.

Abel, E. L., McMillan, D. E., and Harris, L. S. (1972). Tolerance to the behavioral and hypothermic effects of 1-Δ^9-tetrahydrocannabinol in neonatal chicks. *Experientia 28*:1188.

Abel, E. L., Cooper, C. W., and Harris, L. S. (1974). Effects of delta-9-tetrahydrocannabinol on body weight and brain electrolytes in the chicken. *Psychopharmacologia 35*(4):335-339.

Acheson, K. J. B., Zahorska-Morkiewic, Y., Pittel, P., Anantharaman, K., and Jequier, E. (1980). Caffeine and coffee: their influence on metabolic rate and substrate utilization in normal weight and obese individuals. *Am. J. Clin. Nutr. 33*:989-997.

Adams, R. (1941-1942). Marihuana. *Harvard Lect. 37*:169-195.

Allentuck, S., and Bowman, K. (1942). Psychiatric aspects of marihuana intoxication. *Am. J. Psychiatry 99*:248-251.

Ames, F. (1958). A clinical and metabolic study of acute intoxication with *Cannabis sativa* and its role in the model psychosis. *J. Ment. Sci. 104*:972-999.

Antelman, S. M., Black, C. A., and Rowland, N. E. (1977). Clozapine induces hyperphagia in undeprived rats. *Life Sci. 21*(12):1747-1749.

Baettig, K., Martin, J. R., and Classen, W. (1980). Nicotine and amphetamine; differential tolerance and no cross-tolerance for ingestive effects. *Pharmacol. Biochem. Behav. 12*:107-111.

Baez, D. A. (1974). The role of catecholamines in the anorectic effects of amphetamine in rats. *Psychopharmacologia 35*(2):91-98.

Baile, C. A., and McLaughlin, C. L. (1977). Feeding behavior of sheep following intravenous injections of imidazo benzodiazepines. *Fed. Proc. 36*:460.

Baile, C. A., and McLaughlin, C. L. (1978). Chemically stimulated feed intake in ruminants. *Cereal Foods Worlds 23*:291-294,323-328.

Barone, R. C., Wayner, M. J. and Kleinrock, S. (1979a). Effects of caffein on FT-1 min schedule induced drinking at different body weights. *Pharmacol. Biochem. Behav. 11*:347-350.

Barone, F. C., Wayner, M. J., Lee, H. K., Tsai, W. H., Dehaven, D. L., and Woodson, W., Jr. (1979b). Effects of methylphenidate on food and water consumption at different body weights. *Pharmacol. Biol. Behav. 10*(4):591-595.

Bergen, S. S. (1964). Appetite stimulating properties of cyproheptadine. *Am. J. Dis. Child. 108*:270-273.

Berland, T. (1976). Rating the Diets. *Consumer Guide*. Publ. Intern. Ltd., Skokie, Ill.

Blackburn, H., Brozek, J., and Taylor, H. L. (1960). Common circulatory measurements in smokers and nonsmokers. *Circulation 22*:1112-1124.

Blitzer, P. H., Rimm, A. A., and Giefer, E. E. (1977). The effect of cessation of smoking on body weight in 57,032 women: cross sectional and longitudinal analysis. *J. Chronic Dis. 30*:415-429.

Blundell, J. E., and Leshem, M. M. (1973). Dissociation of the anorectic effects of fenfluramine and amphetamine following intrahypothalamic injection. *Br. J. Pharmacol. 47*:183-185.

Blundell, J. E., Latham, C. J., and Leshem, M. B. (1973). Biphasic action of a 5-hydroxytryptamine inhibitor on fenfluramine induced anorexia. *J. Pharm. Pharmacol. 25*(6):492-494.

Blundell, J. E., Latham, C. J., and Leshem, M. B. (1976). Differences between the anorexic actions of emphetamine and fenfluramine—possible effects on hunger and satiety. *J. Pharm. Pharmacol. 28*:471-477.

Borgen, L. A., Davis, W. M., and Pace, H. B. (1971). Effects of synthetic delta-9-tetrahydrocannabinol on pregnancy and offspring in the rat. *Toxicol. Appl. Pharmacol. 20*:480-486.

Bouquet, J. Cannabis. (1951). *Bull. Narc. 3*:22-45.

Bradley, C. (1937). The behavior of children receiving benzadrine. *Am. J. Psychiatry 94*:577-585.

Breisch, S. T., Zemlan, F. P., and Hoebel, B. G. (1976). Hyperphagia and obesity following serotonin depletion with intraventricular parachlorophenylalanine. *Science 192*:382-385.

Brobeck, J. R. (1960). Food and temperature. In *Recent Progress in Hormone Research*, Vol. 16, G. Pincus, Ed., Academic Press, New York.

Brown, R. F., Houpt, K. A., and Schryver, H. F. (1976). Stimulation of food intake in horses by diazepam and promazine. *Pharmacol. Biochem. Behav. 5*:495-497.

Brozek, J., and Keys, A. (1957). Changes in body weight in normal men who stop smoking cigarettes. *Science 125*:1203.

Burse, R. L., Bynum, G. D., Pandolf, K. B., Goldman, B. F., Sims, E. A. H., and Danforth, E. R. (1975). Increased appetite and unchanged metabolism upon cessation of smoking with diet held constant. *Physiologist 18*:157.

Byck, R. (1975). Drugs and the treatment of psychiatric disorders. In *The Pharmacological Basis of Therapeutics*, 5th ed., L. S. Goodman and A. Gilman, Eds., Macmillan, New York, pp. 152-200.

Cade, J. F. J. (1949). Lithium salts in the treatment of psychotic excitement. *Med. J. Aust.* 2:349.

Capogrossi, M. C., Francendese, A., and DiGirolamo, M. (1979). Suppression of food intake by adenosine and inosine. *Am. J. Clin. Nutr.* 32:1762-1768.

Carlini, E. A., and Kramer, C. (1965). Effects of *Cannabis sativa* (marihuana) on maze performance of the rat. *Psychopharmacology* 7:175-181.

Carruba, M. P., Picotti, G. B., Zambotti, F., and Mantegazzo, P. (1977). Blockade of mazindol of brain 5-HT depletion induced by p-chloromethamphetamine. *J. Pharm. Pharmacol.* 29(4):242-243.

Chang, A. E., Shiling, D. J., Stillman, R. C., Goldberg, N. H., Seipp, C. A., Barofsky, I., Simon, R. M., and Rosenburg, S. A. (1979). Delta-9-THC as an antiemetic in cancer patients receiving high dose methotrexate. *Ann. Intern. Med.* 91:819-824.

Chopra, R. N., and Chopra, G. S. (1939). The present position of hemp-drug addiction in India. *Ind. Med. Res. Mem.* 31:1-119.

Ciaranello, R. D., and Patrick, R. L. (1977). Catecholamine neuroregulators. In *Psychopharmacology: From Theory to Practice*, J. D. Barchas, P. A. Bergen, R. D. Ciaranello, and G. R. Elliott, Eds., Oxford University Press, New York.

Clark, D. A., Allen, M. G., and Wilson, F. H. (1967). Longitudinal study of serum lipids: 12-year report. *Am. J. Clin. Nutr.* 20:743.

Clineschmidt, B. V., and Lotti, V. J. (1973). Histamine: intraventricular injection suppresses ingestion behavior in the cat. *Arch. Int. Pharmacodyn. Ther.* 206:288-298.

Clineschmidt, B. V., McGuffin, J. C., Pflueger, A. B., and Totaro, J. A. (1978). A 5-hydroxytryptamine-like mode of anorectic action for 6-chloro-2-1-piperazinyl-pyrazine (MK-212). *Br. J. Pharmacol.* 62(4):579-589.

Cohen, S. (1980). Marijuana research findings: therapeutic aspects. *Natl. Inst. Drug. Abuse Res. Monogr. Ser.* 31:199-221.

Comstock, G. W., and Stone, R. W. (1972). Changes in body weight and subcutaneous fatness related to smoking habits. *Arch. Environ. Health* 24:271-276.

Conners, C. K., and Eisenberg, L. (1963). The effects of methylphenidate on symptomatology and learning in disturbed children. *Am. J. Psychiatry* 120:458-464.

Cooper, B. R., Howard, J. L., White, H. L., Soroko, F., Ingold, K., and Maxwell, R. A. (1980). Anorexic effects of ethanolamine-0-sulfate and muscimol in the rat: evidence that GABA inhibits ingestive behavior. *Life Sci.* *26*(23):1997-2002.

Dally, P. J. (1967). Anorexia nervosa: long term follow-up and effects of treatment. *J. Psychosom. Res.* *11*:151-155.

Dally, P. J., and Sargant, W. (1966). Treatment and outcome in anorexia nervosa. *Br. Med. J.* *2*:793-795.

Damon, A. (1961). Constitution and smoking. *Science* *134*:339-341.

Della Fera, M. A., Naylor, J. N., and Baille, C. A. (1978). Benzodiazepines stimulate feeding in clinically debilitated animals. *Fed. Proc.* *37*:401.

Della Fera, M. A., Baile, C. A., and McLaughlin, C. L. (1980). Feeding elicited by benzodiazepine-like chemicals in puppies and cats—structure-activity relationships. *Pharmacol. Biochem. Behav.* *12*(2):195-200.

Dewey, W. L., Jenkins, J., O'Rourke, T., and Harris, L. S. (1972). The effects of chronic administration of trans-delta-9-tetrahydrocannabinol on behavior and the cardiovascular systems of dogs. *Arch. Int. Pharmacodyn. Ther.* *198*:118-131.

Dickinson, L. C., Lee, J., Ringdahl, J. C., Schedewie, H. K., Kilgore, B. S., and Elders, I. C. (1979). Impaired growth in hyperkinetic children receiving pemoline. *J. Pediatry* *94*:538-541.

Dobrzanski, S., and Doggett, N. S. (1976). The effects of (D)-amphetamine and fenfluramine on feeding in starved and satiated mice. *Psychopharmacology* *48*:283-286.

Donaldson, S. S., Jundt, S., Ricour, C., Sarrazin, D., Lemberle, J., and Schwersguth, O. (1975). Radiation enteritis in children. A retrospectus review, clinicopathologic correlations, and dietary management. *Cancer* *35*:1167-1178.

Doss, F. W. (1979). The effect of antipsychotic drugs on body weight: a retrospective review. *J. Clin. Psychiatry* *40*(12):528-530.

Edholm, O. G., Fletcher, J. G., Widdowson, E. M., and McCance, R. A. (1965). The energy expenditure and food intake of individual men. *Br. J. Nutr.* *9*:286-300.

Ekert, H., Waters, K. D., Jurk, I. H., Mobilia, J., and Loughnan, P. (1979). Amelioration of cancer chemotherapy-induced nausea and vomiting by delta-9-tetrahydrocannabinol. *Med. J. Aust.* *2*(12):657-659.

Elson, L. A., and Passey, R. D. (1963). Biochemical effects of tobacco smoke and nicotine inhalation. *Acta Unio. Int. Cancer* *19*:715.

Erikssen, J., and Enger, S. C. (1978). The effect of smoking on selected coronary heart disease risk factors in middle-aged men. *Acta. Med. Scand.* *203*:27-30.

Eysenck, H. J. (1964). Personality and cigarette smoking. *Life Sci.* 3:777-792.

Fajardo, M., Vidal, C., and Carela, G. (1974). Influence of zanthine and some of its methyl derivatives on the nutritive value of a diet. *Minerva Dietol.* 13:54-55.

Fernandez, M., Rating, D., and Klume, S. (1971). The influence of subchronic tetrahydrocannabinol and cannabis treatment of food and water intake, body weight, and body temperature of rats. *Acta Pharmacol. Toxicol.* 29:89.

Fletcher, A., Green, S. E., and Hodges, H. M. (1980). Evidence for a role for GABA in benzodiazepine effects on feeding in rats. *Br. J. Pharmacol.* 69(2):274-275.

Fratta, W. (1976). Benzodiazepine-induced voraciousness in cats and inhibition of amphetamine-anorexia. *Life Sci.* 18(10):1157-1166.

Friedman, N., Thomas, J., Carr, R., Elders, J., Ringdahl, I., and Roche, A. (1981). Effect on growth in pemoline-treated children with attendant deficit disorder. *Am. J. Dis. Child.* 155:429-432.

Friedrich, P. (1969). In: Lithium in Psychiatry. *Acta Psychiatr. Scand. Suppl.* 207.

Fristrom, S., Airaksinen, M. M., and Halmekoski, J. (1977). Release of platelet 5-hydroxytryptamine by some anorexic and other sympathomimetics and their acetyl derivatives. *Acta Pharmacol. Toxicol.* 41(3):281-224.

Fuxe, K., Agnati, L. F., Bolme, P., Hokfelt, T., Ledbrink, P., Ljungdahl, A., Perez de la Mora, M., and Ogren, S. O. (1975). The possible involvement of GABA mechanisms in the action of benzodiazepine on central catecholamine neurons. *Acta Biochem. Psychopharm.* 14:45-61.

Garbarg, M., Barbin, G., Feger, J., and Schwartz, J. (1974). Histaminergic pathway in rat brain evidenced by lesions of the medial forebrain bundle. *Science* 186:833-835.

Garcia, J., and Ervin, F. R. (1968). Appetites, aversions, and addiction: a model for visceral memory. *Rec. Adv. Biol. Psychiatry* 10:284-293.

Garrow, J. S. (1974). *Energy Balance and Obesity in Man*, North-Holland, Amsterdam.

Geber, W. F., and Schramm, L. C. (1969). Effect in marihuana extract on fetal hamsters and rabbits. *Toxicol. Appl. Pharmacol.* 14:276-282.

Ghosh, M. N., and Parvathy, S. (1973). The effect of cyproheptadine on water and food intake and on body weight in the fasted adult and weanling rats. *Br. J. Pharmacol.* 48(2):328-329.

Glauser, S. C., Glauser, E. M., Reidenberg, M. M., Rusy, B. F., and Tallarid, R. J. (1970). Metabolic changes associated with the cessation of cigarette smoking. *Arch. Environ. Health 20*:277-381.

Glick, S. D., and Milloy, S. (1972). Increased and decreased eating following THC administration. *Psychon. Sci. 29*:6.

Gluck, J. P., and Ferraro, D. P. (1974). Effects of delta-9-THC on food and water intake of deprivation experienced rats. *Behav. Biol. 11*:395-401.

Gogerty, J. H., Houlihan, W., Galen, M., Eden, P., and Penberthy, C. (1968). Neuropharmacological studies on an imidazo-isoindole derivative. *Fed. Proc. 27*:501.

Goldberg, S. C., Halmi, K. A., Eckert, E. D., Casper, R. C., and Davis, J. M. (1979). Cyproheptadine in anorexia nervosa. *Br. J. Psychiatry 134*:67-70.

Gonzales, S. C., Karniol, I. G., and Carlini, E. A. (1972). Effects of *Cannabis sativa* on conditioned fear. *Behav. Biol. 7*:83-94.

Gordon, T., Kannel, W. B., Dawber, T. R., and McGee, D. (1975). Changes associated with quitting cigarette smoking: the Framingham Study. *Am. Heart. J. 90*:322-328.

Gross, M. D. (1976). Growth of hyperkinetic children taking methylphenidate, dextroamphetamine, or imipramine/desipramine. *Pediatrics 58*:423-461.

Gotestam, K. G., and Lewander, T. (1975). The duration of tolerance to the anorexigenic effect of amphetamine in rats. *Psychopharmacologia 42*(1):41-45.

Graham, J. D. P., and Li, D. M. F. (1973). Cardiovascular and respiratory effects of cannabis in cat and rat. *Br. J. Pharmacol. 49*:1-10.

Greeley, G. H., and Kizer, J. S. (1980). The effects of chronic methylphenidate treatment on growth and endocrine function in the developing rat. *J. Pharmacol. Exp. Ther. 215*:545-551.

Greenberg, L. M., Deem, M. A., and McMahon, S. (1972). Effects of dextroamphetamines, chlorpromazine, and hydroxyzine on behavior and performance in hyperactive children. *Am. J. Psychiatry 129*:532-539.

Greenhill, L. L., Ping-Antich, J., Halpern, F., Sacher, E. J., Dubinstein, B., Chambers, W., Fiscina, B., and Florea, J. (1980). Growth disturbances in hyperkinetic children. *Pediatrics 66*:152-153.

Gruboff, S. I., Berman, R., and Silverman, H. I. (1975). A double-blind clinical evaluation of a phenylpropanolamine caffeine-vitamin combination and a placebo in the treatment of exogenous obesity. *Curr. Ther. Res. 17*(6):535-543.

Grunfeld, Y., and Edery, H. (1969). Psychopharmacologic activity of the active constituents of hashish and some related cannabinols. *Psychopharmacology 14*:200-210.

Haldi, J., Bachmann, G., Ensor, C., and Wynn, W. (1941). The effect of various amounts of caffeine on the gaseous exchange and the respiratory quotient in man. *J. Nutr.* 21:307-320.

Hamilton, C. L. (1963). Interaction on food intake and temperature regulation in the rat. *J. Comp. Physiol. Psychiol.* 56:476-488.

Harlow, H. F. (1932). Social facilitation of feeding in the albino rat. *J. Genet. Psychol.* 41:211-221.

Harris, B., and Harper, M. (1980). Unusual appetites in patients on mianserin. *Lancet* 1:8168,590.

Harvey, J. A., Heller, A., and Moore, R. Y. (1963). The effect of unilateral and bilateral medial bundle lesions on brain serotonin. *J. Pharmacol. Exp. Ther.* 140:103-110.

Henkin, R. I., Keiser, H. R., and Bronzert, D. (1972). Histidine-dependent zinc loss, hypogeusia, anorexia, and hyposomia. *J. Clin. Invest.* 51:44A.

Hickey, N., and Mulcahy, R. (1973). Effect of cessation of smoking on body weight after myocardial infarction. *Am. J. Clin. Nutr.* 26:385-386.

Hjermann, I., Helgeland, A., Holme, I., Lund-Larsen, P. G., and Leren, P. (1976). The intercorrelation of serum cholesterol, cigarette smoking and body weight—Oslo study. *Acta Med. Scand.* 200:479.

Hoebel, B. C. (1977). The pharmacology of feeding. In *Handbook of Psychopharmacology*, Vol. 8, L. L. Iversen, S. D. Iversen, and S. H. Synder, Eds., Plenum Press, New York.

Hoebel, B. G., Hernandez, L., and Thompson, R. D. (1975a). Phenylpropanolamine inhibits feeding, but not drinking, induced by hypothalamic stimulation. *J. Comp. Physiol. Psychol.* 89:1046-1052.

Hoebel, B. G., Krauss, I. K., Cooper, J., and Willard, D. (1975b). Body weight decreased in humans by phenylpropanolamine taken before meals. *Obesity Bariatr. Med.* 4:200-206.

Hollister, L. E. (1971). Hunger and appetite after single doses of marijuana, alcohol and dextroamphetamine. *Clin. Pharmacol. Ther.* 12:44.

Howell, R. W. (1971). Obesity and smoking habits. *Br. Med. J.* 4:625.

Huy, N. D., Gailes, L., and Roy, P. E. (1974). Effets après trois mois de l'inhalation de marihuana et de tabac chez le chien. *Union Med. Can.* 103:65-71.

Ilebekk, A., Miller, N. E., and Mjos, O. D. (1975). Effects of nicotine and inhalation of cigarette smoke on total body oxygen consumption in dogs. *Scand. J. Clin. Lab. Invest.* 35:67-72.

Jacobs, D. R., and Gottenberg, S. (1981). Smoking and weight: the Minnesota Lipid Research Clinic. *Am. J. Public Health* 71:391-396.

James, W. T. (1953). Social facilitation of eating behavior in puppies after satiation. *J. Comp. Physiol. Psychol.* 46:427-428.

Jarbe, T. V. C., and Henriksson, B. G. (1973). Influence of tetrahydrocannabinols (Δ^8-THC and Δ^9-THC) on body weight, food, and water intake in rats. *Pharmacol. Biochem. Behav.* 1:395-399.

Jarvick, M. E. (1970). Drugs used in the treatment of psychiatric disorders. In *The Pharmacological Basis of Therapeutics,* L. S. Goodman and A. Gilman, Eds., Macmillan, London.

Jobson, K., Burnett, G., and Linnoila, M. (1978). Weight loss and a concommitant change in plasma tricyclic levels. *Am. J. Psychiatry* 135(1):237-238.

Johnson, F. N. (1975). *Lithium Research and Therapy,* Academic Press, New York.

Johnson, D. A., and Breen, M. (1979). Weight changes with depot neuroleptic maintenance therapy. *Acta Psychiatr. Scand.* 59(5):525-528.

Kelly, P. H. (1977). Drug-induced motor behavior. In *Handbook of Psychopharmacology,* Vol. 8, L. L. Iversen, S. D. Iversen, and S. H. Synder, Eds., Plenum Press, New York.

Kelly, J., and Grossman, S. P. (1979). GABA and hypothalamic feeding systems. II. A comparison of glycine and acetylcholine and their antagonists. *Pharmacol. Biochem. Behav.* 11(6):647-652.

Kelly, J., Alheid, G. F., Newberg, A., and Grossman, S. P. (1977). GABA stimulation and blockade in the hypothalamus and midbrain: effects of feeding and locomotor activity. *Pharmacol. Biochem. Behav.* 7:537-541.

Kelly, J., Rothstein, J., and Grossman, S. P. (1979). GABA and hypothalamic feeding systems. I. Topographic analysis of the effects of microinjections of muscimol. *Physiol. Behav.* 23(6):1123-1134.

Kerry, R. J., Liebling, L. I., and Owen, G. (1970). Weight changes in lithium responders. *Acta Psychiatr. Scand.* 46:238-243.

Khosla, T., and Lowe, C. R. (1971). Obesity and smoking habits. *Br. Med. J.* 4:10-13.

Kittel, F., Rustin, R. M., Dramaix, M., de Backer, G., and Kornitzer, M. (1978). Psycho-socio-biological correlates of moderate overweight in an industrial population. *J. Psychosom. Res.* 22:145-158.

Knights, R. M., and Horton, G. G. (1969). The effects of methylphenidate (Ritalin) on the motor skills and behavior of children with learning problems. *J. Nerv. Ment. Dis.* 148:643-653.

Korsgaard, S., and Skausig, O. B. (1979). Increase in weight after treatment with depot neuroleptics. *Acta Psychiatr. Scand.* 59(2):139-144.

Kratz, C. M., and Levitsky, D. A. (1978). Post-ingestive effects of quinine on intake of nutritive and non-nutritive substances. *Physiol. Behav.* 21:851-854.

Kupfer, D. J., Coble, P. A., and Rubinstein, D. (1979). Changes in weight during treatment for depression. *Psychosom. Med.* 41:535-543.

Lavenstein, A. F., Dacaney, E. P., Lasagna, L., and Van Metre, T. E. (1962). Effects of cyproheptadine on asthamatic children. *JAMA* 180:912-916.

Le Donarec, J. C., and Neven, C. (1970). Pharmacology and biochemistry of fenfluramine. In *Amphetamines and Related Compounds*, E. Costa and S. Garattini, Eds., Raven Press, New York.

Leibowitz, S. F., and Brown, L. L. (1980). Histochemical and pharmacological analysis of noradrenergic projections to the paraventricular hypothalamus in relation to feeding stimulation. *Brain Res.* 201:289-314.

Lemberger, L. (1980). Potential therapeutic usefulness of marijuana. *Annu. Rev. Pharmacol. Toxicol.* 20:151-172.

Levitsky, D. A., and Strupp, B. J. (1981). Behavorial control of energy expenditure. In *Body Weight Regulatory Systems: Normal and Disturbed Mechanisms*, L. A. Cioffi, W. P. T. James, and T. B. Van Itallie, Eds., Raven Press, New York.

Levitsky, D. A., Strupp, B. J., and Lupoli, J. (1981). Tolerance to anorectic drugs: pharmacological or artifactual. *Pharmacol. Biochem. Behav.* 14(5):661-667.

Lewander, T. (1971). A mechanism for the development of tolerance to amphetamines in rats. *Psychopharmacologia* 21:17-31.

Lupoli, J. C. (1977). The effects of desipramine hydrochloride and amphetamine sulfate on food intake and body weight in the rat. M. S. thesis, Cornell University, Ithaca, N. Y.

Magour, S., Coper, H., and Fahndrich, C. (1974). The effects of chronic treatment with d-amphetamine on food intake, body weight, locomotor activity and subcellular distribution of the drug in rat brain. *Psychopharmacologia* 34(1):45-54.

Mainguet, P. (1972). Effect of cyproheptadine on anorexia and loss of weight in adults. *Practitioner* 208:797-800.

Manning, F. J., McDonough, J. H., Elsmore, T. F., Saller, C., and Sodetz, F. J. (1971). Inhibition of normal growth by chronic administration of Δ^9-tetrahydrocannabinol. *Science* 174:424-427.

Marini, J. L., Williams, S. P., and Sheard, M. H. (1978). Repeated sustained-release lithium carbonate administration to cats. *Toxicol. Appl. Pharmacol.* 43:559-567.

Marshall, C. R. (1898). A contribution to the pharmacology of *Cannabis indica*. *Am. Med. J.* 31:882-891.

Mayor's Committee on Marihuana. (1944). *The Marihuana Problem in the City of New York,* Jaques Cattrell, Lancaster, Pa.

McLaughlin, C. L., Kraybill, L. F., Scott, G. C., and Baille, C. A. (1976). Chemical stimulants of animals. *Fed. Proc. 35:*579.

McMillan, D. E., Harris, L. S., Frankenheim, J. M., and Kennedy, J. S. (1970). $1-\Delta^9$-trans-tetrahydrocannabinol in pigeons: tolerance to the behavorial effects. *Science 169:*501-503.

Mellerup, E. T., Thomson, H. G., Bjorum, N., and Rafaelsen, O. J. (1972). Lithium, weight gain, and serum insulin in manic-depressive patients. *Acta Psychiatr. Scand. 48:*332-336.

Mereu, G. P., Fratta, W., Chessa, P., and Gessa, G. L. (1976). Voraciousness induced in cats by benzodiazepines. *Psychopharmacology 47:*101-103.

Merkel, A. D., Wayner, M. J., Jolicoeur, F. B., and Mintz, R. (1981). Effects of caffeine administration on food and water consumption under various experimental conditions. *Pharmacol. Biochem. Behav. 14:*235-240.

Miller, D. S., Stock, M. J., and Stuart, J. A. (1974). The effects of caffeine and carnitine on the oxygen consumption of fed and fasted subjects. *Proc. Nutr. Soc. 33:*28A-29A.

Millichap, J. C., and Millichap, M. (1975). Growth of hyperkinetic children. *N. Engl. J. Med. 292:*1300.

Mills, I. H. (1976). Amitriptyline therapy in anorexia nervosa. *Lancet 2:*687.

Moore, D. C. (1977). Amitriptyline therapy in anorexia nervosa. *Am. J. Psychiatry 134*(11):1303-1304.

Munster, G., and Battig, K. (1975). Nicotine-induced hypophagia and hypodipsia in deprived and in hypothalamically stimulated rats. *Psychopharmacologia 41*(3):211-217.

Nagayama, H., Hingtgen, J. N., and Aprison, M. H. (1981). Postsynaptic action by four antidepressive drugs in an animal model of depression. *Pharmacol. Biochem. Behav. 15:*125-130.

Nahas, G. G., Schwartz, I. W., Adamec, J., and Manger, W. M. (1973). Tolerance to delta-9-tetrahydrocannibinol in the spontaneously hypertensive rat. *Proc. Soc. Exp. Biol. Med. 14L:* 58-60.

Nathanson, M. H. (1937). The central action of beta-aminopropylbenzene (Benzadrine): Clinical observations. *JAMA 108:*528-531.

Needleman, H. L., and Waber, D. (1976). Amitriptyline therapy in patients with anorexia nervosa. *Lancet 2:*580.

Noble, R. E. (1969). Effect of cyproheptadine on appetite and weight gain in adults. *JAMA 209:*2054-2055.

Noppa, H. and Bengtsson, C. (1980). Obesity in relation to smoking: a population study of women in Goteborg, Sweden. *Prev. Med. 9:*534-543.

Noppa, H., Bengtsson, C., Bjorntorp, P., Smith, U., and Tibblin, E. (1978). Overweight in woman—metabolic aspects. *Acta Med.*

Scand. 203:135-141.

Norris, D. L., and Isrealstam, K. (1975). Letter: Clozapine (Leponex) overdosage. *S. Afr. Med. J. 49*(11):388.

O'Connel, R. A. (1971). Lithium's site of action: clues from side effects. *Comp. Psychiatry 12*:224-229.

Ohlin, G., and Soderberg, U. (1970). Inhibition of peripheral utilization of thyroid hormones induced by lithium. *Acta Physiol. Scand 79*:24A-25A.

Oomwa, Y., Ono, T., Sugimori, M., and Nakamura, T. (1973). Effects of cyproheptidine on the feeding and satiety center in the rat. *Pharmacol. Biochem. Behav. 1*:449-459.

Opitz, K., and Schafer, G. (1976). Effect of lithium on food intake in rats. *Int. Pharmacopsychiatry 11*(4):197-205.

O'Shaughnessy, W. B. (1938). On the preparation of the Indian hemp or gunjah. *Trans. Med. Physiol. Soc. Beng.*, 421-461.

Pawlowski, G. J. (1975). Cyproheptadine: weight-gain and appetite stimulation in essential anorexic adults. *Curr. Ther. Res. 18*(5): 673-678.

Paykel, E. S., Mueller, P. S., and DeLaVergue, P. M. (1973). Amitriptyline, weight gain and carbohydrate craving: a side effect. *Br. J. Psychiatry 123*(576):501-507.

Peters, J. M., and Boyd, E. M. (1967). The influence of sex and age in albino rat given a daily oral dose of caffeine at a high dose level. *Can. J. Physiol. Toxicol. 45*:305.

Poschel, B. P. H. (1971). A simple and specific screen for benzodiazepine-like drugs. *Psychopharmacology 19*:193-198.

Quinn, P. O., and Rapoport, J. L. (1975). One year follow-up of hyperactive boys treated with imipramine or methylphenidate. *Am. J. Psychiatry 132*:241-245.

Randall, L. O. (1960). Pharmacology of methaminodiazepoxide. *Dis. Nerv. Syst. 22*:7-15.

Randall, L. O. (1961). Pharmacology of chlordiazepoxide. *Dis. Nerv. Syst. 22*:7-15.

Rating, D., Broermann, I., Horecker, H., Klume, S., and Coper, H. (1972). Effect of subchronic treatment with $(-)\Delta^8$-transtetrahydrocannabinol (Δ^8THC) on food intake, body temperature, hexobarbital sleeping time and hexobarbital elimination rate. *Psychopharmacology 27*:349-357.

Rayner, P. H. W., and Conit, J. M. (1974). Effect of dietary restriction and anorectic drugs on linear growth in childhood obesity. *Arch. Dis. Child. 49*:822-823.

Reynolds, R. W., and Carlisle, H. J. (1961). The effect of chlorpromazine on food intake in the albino rat. *J. Comp. Physiol. Psychol. 54*:354-356.

Robinson, R. G., McHugh, P. R., and Bloom, F. E. (1975). Chlorpromazine induced hyperphagia in the rat. *Psychopharmacol. Commun. 1*(1):37-50.

Roche, A. F., Lipman, R. S., Overall, J. E., and Hunsz, W. (1979).
The effect of stimulant medication on the growth of hyperkinetic
children. *Pediatrics* 63:847-850.

Rosekrantz, H., and Braude, M. C. (1974). Acute, subacute and
23 day chronic marihuana inhalation toxicities in the rat. *Toxicol.
Appl. Pharmacol.* 28:428-441.

Rosenberg, H. C. (1980). Central excitatory actions of flurazepan.
Pharmacol. Biochem. Behav. 13:415-420.

Ross, S., and Ross. J. G. (1949a). Social facilitation of feeding behavior in dogs. I. Group and solitary feeding. *J. Genet. Psychol.*
74:97-108.

Ross, S., and Ross, J. G. (1949b). Social facilitation of feeding behavior in dogs. II. Feeding after satiation. *J. Genet. Psychol.*
74:293-304.

Safer, D., Allen, R., and Barr, F. (1972). Depression of growth
in hyperactive children on stimulant drugs. *N. Engl. J. Med.*
287:217.

Safer, D. J., Allen, R. P., and Barr, E. (1975). Growth rebound
after termination of stimulant drugs. *J. Pediatr.* 86(1):113-116.

Sakata, T., Kodama, J., and Fukushima, M. (1973). Feeding patterns of theophyllinized rats and effects of dextrose on their
food intake. *Physiol. Behav.* 17:797-802.

Sallan, S. E., Zinberg, N. E., and Frei, D. (1975). Antiemetic effect of delta-9-tetrahydrocannabinol in patients receiving cancer
chemotherapy. *N. Engl. J. Med.* 293:795-797.

Sanzgiri, R. R., Mohamad, H. A., and Raja, Z. (1970). Appetite
stimulation and weight gain with cyproheptadine, a double-blind
study in underweight children. *J. Postgrad. Med. Bombay 16*:
12-17.

Schechter, M. D., and Cook, P. G. (1976). Nicotine induced weight
loss without an effect on appetite. *Eur. J. Pharmacol.* 38:63-
69.

Scheckel, C. L., Buff, E., Dahlen, P., and Smart, T. (1968).
Behavorial effects in monkeys of racemates of two biologically
active marihuana constituents. *Science* 160:1467-1469.

Schou, M., Baastrup, P. C., Grof, P., Weis, P., and Angst, J.
(1970). Pharmacological and clinical problems of lithium prophylaxis. *Br. J. Psychiatry 116*:615-619.

Seltzer, C. (1963). Morphological constituents and smoking. *JAMA
183*:639-645.

Shah, D. K., Wig, N. N., and Chaudhury, R. R. (1973). Antidiuretic hormone levels in patients with weight gain after clor-
promazine therapy. *Indian J. Med. Res.* 61(5):771-776.

Siemens, A. J. (1973). Acute and chronic metabolic interaction of
Δ^1-tetrahydrocannabinol and other drugs. Ph. D. thesis,
University of Toronto, Toronto.

Siler, J. F., Sheep, W. L., Bates, L. B., Clark, G. F., Cook, G. W., and Smith, W. H. (1933). Marihuana smoking in Panama. *Mil. Surg.* 73:269-280.

Silverstone, T., and Schuyler, D. (1975). The effect of cyproheptadine on hunger, food intake and body weight in man. *Psychopharmacologia* 40(4):335-340.

Sjostom, L. (1980). Fat cells and body weight. *In Obesity,* A. J. Stunkard, Ed., W. B. Saunders, Philadelphia.

Skolnick, P., Paul, S. M., and Marangos, P. J. (1980). Purines as endogenous ligands of the benzodiazepine receptor. *Fed. Proc., Fed. Am. Soc. Exp. Biol.* 39:3050-3055.

Synder, S. H., Katims, J. J., Anna, Z., Burns, R. F., and Daly, J. W. (1981). Adenosine receptors and behavorial actions of methylxanthines. *Proc. Natl. Acad. Sci. USA* 78:3260-3264.

Sofia, R. D., and Barry, H. D. (1974). Acute and chronic effects of delta-9-tetrahydrocannabinol on food intake by rats. *Psychopharmacologia* 39(3):213-222.

Soper, W. Y., and Wise, R. A. (1971). Hypothalamically induced eating: eating from "noneater" with diazepam. *Life Sci.* 1:79-84.

Spitzer, R. L., Endicott, J., and Robins, E. (1978). Research diagnostic criteria. *Arch. Gen. Psychiatry* 35:773-783.

Stiel, J. N., Liddle, G. W., and Lacy, W. W. (1970). Studies of mechanism of cyproheptadine-induced weight gain in human subjects. *Metabolism* 19:192-200.

Stockings, G. T. (1977). A new euphoriant for depressive mental stress. *Br. Med. J.* 1:918-922.

Stolerman, I. P. (1970). Eating, drinking and spontaneous activity in rats after the administration of chlorpromazine. *Neuropharmacology* 9:405-417.

Stowe, F. R., and Miller, A. T. (1957). The effect of amphetamine on food intake in rats with hypothiamin hyperphagia. *Experientia* 13:114-115.

Sullivan, A. C., and Comai, K. (1978). Pharmacological treatment of obesity. *Int. J. Obesity* 2:167-189.

Tarka, S. M., Jr., Zoumas, B. L., and Gans, J. H. (1979). Short term effects of graded levels of theobromine in laboratory rodents. *Toxicol. Appl. Pharmacol.* 49(1):127-149.

Thompson, G. R., Rosekrantz, H., Schaeppi, V. H., and Braude, M. C. (1973a). Comparison of acute oral toxicity of cannabinoids in rats, dogs, and monkeys. *Toxicol. Appl. Pharmacol.* 25:363-372.

Thompson, G. R., Mason, M. M., Rosekrantz, H., and Braude, M. C. (1973b). Chronic oral toxicity of cannabinoids in rats. *Toxicol. Appl. Pharmacol.* 25:373-390.

Trahair, R. C. S. (1967). Giving up cigarettes: 222 case studies. *Med. J. Aust.* 1:929-932.

Valenstein, E. S., Cox, V. C., and Kakolewski, J. K. (1970). Re-examination of the role of the hypothalamus in motivation. *Psychol. Rev.* 77:16-31.

Vendsborg, P. B., Bech, P., and Rafaelsen, O. J. (1976). Lithium treatment and weight gain. *Acta Psychiatr. Scand.* 53:139-147.

Volle, R. L., and Koelle, G. B. (1971). Ganglionic stimulating and blocking agents. In *The Pharmacological Basis of Therapeutics,* 4th Ed., L. S. Goodman and A. Gilman, Eds., Macmillan, New York, Chap. 27.

Waizer, J., Hoffman, S. P., and Polizos, P. (1974). Outpatient treatment of hyperactive school children with imipramine. *Am. J. Psychiatry* 131:587-591.

Wayner, M. J., Greenberg, I., Fraley, S., and Fisher, S. (1973). Effects of Δ^9-tetrahydrocannabinol and ethyl alcohol on adjunctive behavior and the lateral hypothalamus. *Physiol. Behav.* 10:109-132.

Weiss, G., Kruger, E., and Danielson, V. (1975). Effect of long-term treatment of hyperkinetic children with methylphenidate. *Can. Med. Assoc. J.* 112:159-165.

Wetle, T., and Singstake, C. B. (1971). The effects of tetrahydrocannibinol on eating behavior of rats. Paper presented at Western Psychological Association, San Francisco.

Widdowson, E. M. (1962). Nutritional individuality. *Proc. Nutr. Soc.* 21:121-128.

Williams, E. G., Himmelsbach, C. K., Wikler, A., Ruble, P. C., and Lloyd, B. J. (1946). Studies on marihuana and pyrahexyl compound. *Public Health Rep.* 61:1059-1070.

Wise, R. A., and Dawson, V. (1974). Diazepam-induced eating and lever pressing for food in sated rats. *J. Comp. Physiol. Psychol.* 86:930-941.

Wooley, O. W., Wooley, S. C., Williams, B. S., and Nurre, C. (1977). Differential effects of amphetamine and fenfluramine on appetite for palatable food in humans. *Int. J. Obesity* 1:293-300.

Wurzner, H. P., Lindstrom, E., Vuataz, L., and Luginbuhl, H. (1977). A 2-year feeding study of instant coffees in rats. I. Body weight, food consumption, haematological parameters and plasma chemistry. *Food. Cosmet. Toxicol.* 15:7-16.

Wynder, E. L., Kaufman, P. L., and Lesser, R. L. (1967). A short-term follow up study on ex-cigarette smokers with special emphasis on persistent cough and weight gain. *Am. Rev. Respir. Dis.* 96:645-655.

Yerkes, R. M. (1934). Suggestibility in chimpanzees. *J. Abnorm. Soc. Psychol.* 5:271-282.

11
Anticonvulsant-Drug-Induced Mineral Disorders

Theodore J. Hahn
University of California at Los Angeles, and The Wadsworth Medical Center, Los Angeles, California

Louis V. Avioli
The Jewish Hospital at Washington University, St. Louis, Missouri

I. INTRODUCTION

In recent years, it has become apparent that chronic treatment with anticonvulsant drugs can result in a variety of disorders of vitamin D, mineral, and bone metabolism. Among the most commonly observed clinical abnormalities are hypocalcemia, increased serum alkaline phosphatase concentration, reduced serum of 25-hydroxyvitamin D (25OHD) levels, mild increase in serum immunoreactive parathyroid hormone (iPTH) concentration, radiological evidence of decreased bone mass, increased incidence of bone fractures, and histologic evidence of osteomalacia. Drug-induced alterations in the hepatic and renal metabolism of vitamin D, and direct inhibitory effects of certain drugs on transmembrane mineral transport mechanisms, appear to be the basis of most of these clinical manifestations. This group of drug-induced mineral disorders is frequently referred to as "anticonvulsant osteomalacia."

II. CLINICAL FEATURES

The earliest descriptions of anticonvulsant osteomalacia appeared primarily in the European literature, presumably a reflection of the somewhat lower levels of vitamin D intake and sunlight exposure which prevail in many European populations. In 1968, Kruse reported a 15% incidence of hypocalcemia and radiological evidence of rickets in a German pediatric epileptic population (Kruse, 1968). Subsequently, English investigators reported the occurrence of hypocalcemia in 23–30%

of institutionalized adult and pediatric epileptic patients treated chronically with anticonvulsant drugs (Richens and Rowe, 1970; Hunter et al., 1971). More recently, this disorder has been detected in epileptic populations throughout the world, with the reported incidence varying from 4 to 70% depending on the population studied and the sensitivity of the techniques employed (Hahn et al., 1972b; 1975; Rodbro et al., 1974; Tolman et al., 1975).

The rather delayed general awareness of the existence of anticonvulsant osteomalacia may be a function of the broad clinical spectrum of this disorder. Rarely, a patient may exhibit the full clinical presentation: repeated bone fractures, severe hypocalcemia and hypophosphatemia, marked muscle weakness, and routine radiographic evidence of osteopenia with signs of rickets (in children) or pseudofractures (in adults). Upon occasion, a patient may experience a paradoxical increase in seizure frequency following an increase in anticonvulsant drug dose, presumably due to increased neuromuscular instability resulting from progressive drug-induced hypocalcemia (Glynne et al., 1972). In addition, a myopathy of variable severity is frequently observed in patients with other apparent manifestations of anticonvulsant osteomalacia (Dent et al., 1970; Marsden et al., 1973; Lindgren et al., 1979). Finally, in severe cases bone histology exhibits a marked degree of osteomalacia with increased number and width of osteoid seams in addition to increased bone osteoclastic resorptive activity, the latter presumably reflecting a degree of secondary hyperparathyroidism (Dent et al., 1970; Melsen and Mosekilde, 1976; Mosekilde et al., 1977). In one large series, an increase in unmineralized osteoid was demonstrated in 53% of patients, while an increase in osteoclastic resorption surfaces occurred in 69% (Mosekilde and Melsen, 1976).

In contrast to this array of severe manifestations, the usual patient generally has a much more subtle clinical presentation. Bone symtoms are usually minimal or absent, while serum calcium, phosphate, and alkaline phosphatase concentrations may be within the normal range, and routine x-ray techniques may not reveal a clear-cut deficiency in bone mass. In most large series, the average reduction in serum calcium concentration in patients receiving chronic anticonvulsant drug therapy ranges between 0.3 and 0.8 mg per 100 ml relative to matched control subjects, while the incidence of frank hypocalcemia varies from 4 to 30% and the incidence of significant elevations in serum alkaline phosphatase levels ranges from 24 to 40%. Mean fasting serum phosphate levels are occasionally reduced but often lie within the noral range.

However, the use of recently developed more sensitive means of assessing vitamin D and bone mineral status now permits the demonstration of mild but significant derangements in mineral metabolism even in the group of patients lacking clear-cut routine biochemical or radiologic abnormalities. For example, serum 25OHD concentrations in anticonvulsant-treated patients are reduced an average of 40 to 70% relative to matched controls (Hahn et al., 1972b,1975b; Stamp et al., 1972; Bouillon et al., 1975). Moreover, mild elevations in serum iPTH concentrations occur in a significant proportion of patients, and the degree of iPTH elevation correlates inversely with serum calcium and 25OHD levels (Bouillon et al., 1975; Mosekilde et al., 1977; Hahn and Halstead, 1979).

The increased application of photon absorption bone mass measurement techniques in these patients has also led to a greatly increased rate of detection of abnormalities in mineral metabolism. Although routine radiographic techniques are not capable of reliably detecting a less than 30 to 50% loss of bone mass, the photon absorption technique has an accuracy of 4% in the estimation of bone loss (Hahn et al., 1974a). Using this technique it has been demonstrated that mean bone mass in various epileptic populations is usually reduced by 10−30% from age-normal values (Christiansen et al., 1973;1975; Hahn et al., 1975b; Hahn and Halstead, 1979).

The statistics above represent mean values obtained from large population studies. However, within any group of anticonvulsant-treated patients there is a surprisingly wide range in the severity of clinical manifestations. In recent years it has become apparent that a number of specific risk factors affect this severity of anticonvulsant-induced mineral disorders.

Numerous studies have demonstrated that the *dose and duration of drug therapy* are extremely important factors in determining the incidence of clinical abnormalities. Multiple-drug regimens produce more severe reductions in serum calcium, serum 25OHD, and bone mass than do single-drug regimens. Moreover, the larger the total daily dose of drug received, the more severe are the derangements in mineral metabolism (Richens and Rowe, 1970; Hahn et al., 1972b,1975b). In addition, the incidence of these abnormalities increases with duration of therapy, although significant changes in mineral parameters have been reported after as little as 6 months of treatment (Lifshitz and Maclaren, 1973; Rodbro et al., 1974; Tolman et al., 1975).

It is generally felt that the various anticonvulsant drugs exhibit significant differences in their ability to disorder vitamin D and mineral metabolism (Richens and Rowe, 1970). This has yet to be specifically confirmed. However, considering the varying potency of drugs with regard to their ability to induce hepatic microsomal enzyme activity and the additional variability in direct effects of drugs on cell membrane mineral transport, it is quite likely that the various agents do differ in their clinical effects on mineral metabolism.

In both normal individuals and in patients on anticonvulsant drug therapy, serum 25OHD levels show a positive correlation with quantitative estimates of customary *vitamin D intake*. However, at any given level of vitamin D intake, mean serum 25OHD levels in patients receiving anticonvulsant drugs are lower than those in matched control subjects

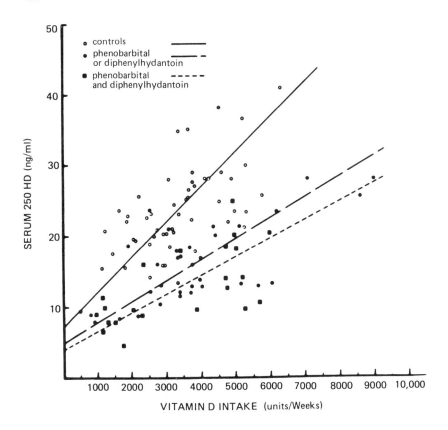

Figure 1 Correlation of serum 25OHD concentrations versus customary
vitamin D intake in normal individuals and patients treated chronically
with single or combined anticonvulsant drug therapy. (Reproduced
from Hahn et al., 1975b, with permission of the Editor of the New England Journal of Medicine.)

(Figure 1), with the degree of reduction related directly to total daily
drug dosage (Hahn et al., 1972b; Hahn et al., 1975b; Mosekilde et al.,
1977). Moreover, at any given drug dose, the lower the average daily
vitamin D intake, the more likely is the patient to develop clinical manifestations of vitamin D deficiency. Based on regression analysis of
the relationship between vitamin D intake and serum 25OHD levels in
epileptic patients and normals, it appears that multiple-drug regimens
increase the intake of vitamin D required to maintain normal 25OHD levels by roughly 400—1000 IU/day (Hahn et al., 1972b,1975b). These
estimates are supported by evidence that maintenance of positive calcium

balance in anticonvulsant-treated subjects requires an increase in vitamin D intake of approximately 600 IU/day relative to control subjects (Peterson et al., 1976).

The other major source of vitamin D activity in humans, in addition to dietary intake, is *sunlight exposure*, which accelerates the conversion of cutaneous 7-dehydrocholesterol stores to vitamin D_3 (DeLuca, 1976). In situations where sunlight exposure is reduced, the incidence of significant vitamin D deficiency is increased. Thus, not unexpectedly, biochemical and radiological abnormalities occur much more frequently in instutionalized epileptic patients who are largely confined indoors (Richens and Rowe, 1970; Lifshitz and Maclaren, 1973). Even among outpatients where the incidence of detectable abnormalities is usually lower, individuals with limited sunlight exposure have significantly lower serum calcium and 25OHD levels than do those who spend much of their time out-of-doors (Hahn et al., 1972b). An additional consideration is the seasonal effect on serum 25OHD concentrations. Levels of 25OHD are highest in the summer when sunlight exposure is maximum and fall by 30−50% in late winter (Haddad and Hahn, 1973). This seasonal variation correlates with the increased incidence of nutritional rickets in the winter months. Similarly, in patients receiving anticonvulsant drug therapy, the period of lowest 25OHD concentration and greatest risk of deranged mineral metabolism is during the winter months.

In adults, a very potent stimulus for bone formation is *physical activity*, which appears to mediate its effect by stimulating production of piezoelectric forces in bone, resulting in increases osteoblastic bone-forming activity. Hence any significant degree of immobilization results in a marked decrease in the rate of bone mass. Moreover, even relatively minor degrees of immobilization, such as the limitation in activity that accompanies advanced rheumatoid arthritis, produce significant decreases in bone mass readily detectable by photon absorption densitometry measurement techniques (Hahn and Hahn, 1976). Thus it is not surprising that radiological evidence of osteopenia in anticonvulsant-treated patients is most marked in nonambulatory individuals (Lifshitz and Maclaren, 1973). Indeed, a major portion of the osteopenia seen in certain patients with seizure disorders may be the result of decreased levels of physical activity resulting from the sedative effects of anticonvulsant drugs, in combination with the physical limitations imposed by associated neurological disorders (Murchison et al., 1975).

In severe or atypical cases of epilepsy, various forms of *adjuvant therapy* are often employed which may in themselves aggravate the already disordered state of mineral metabolism. Acetazolamide, which is frequently added to conventional drug regimens in poorly controlled patients, has been reported to accelerate markedly the course of drug-induced osteomalacia (Mallette, 1977). The adverse effects of this agent have been attributed to its phosphaturic action (Beck and Goldberg, 1973) and to the production of a systemic acidosis which may directly accelerate bone mineral loss and in addition may impair renal conversion of 25OHD to $1,25(OH)_2D$ (Lee et al., 1977). Similarly, the greater degree of bone loss seen in epileptic patients treated with ketogenic diet therapy in addition to anticonvulsant drugs may be attributable to the systemic acidosis produced by this regimen (Hahn et al., 1979).

III. PATHOGENESIS OF DRUG-INDUCED MINERAL DISORDERS

The majority of the clinical manifestations of anticonvulsant osteomalacia appear to be the end result of two processes: (1) drug-induced derangements in vitamin D metabolism, and (2) drug inhibition of cellular ion transport and metabolism.

A. Disordered Vitamin D Metabolism

It is commonly recognized that many drugs, including virtually all of the common anticonvulsants, induce increased hepatic microsomal mixed-function oxidase enzyme activity. A major physiological consequence of this increased enzymatic activity is that degradative metabolism of steroid hormones proceeds at an accelerated pace. As a result, there is increased hepatic formation of polar, hydroxylated, biologically inactive steroid metabolites which are eliminated in the bile and urine (Conney, 1967). This phenomenon has been particularly well demonstrated in the case of estrogens, progesterone, and corticosteroids. Clinical deficiencies of these hormones are not commonly observed as a result of anticonvulsant drug treatment, since in individuals with intact hypothalmic-pituitary function, normal feedback control mechanisms can increase endogenous steroid hormone production rates up to 10-fold, so that normal levels of biologically active hormones are maintained despite increased catabolism. On the other hand, it has been shown that the biological effects of *exogenously* administered steroid hormones are significantly reduced following chronic treatment with hepatic microsomal inducing agents such as phenobarbital and phenytoin (Levin et al., 1967; Jubiz et al., 1970).

In humans, body stores of vitamin D are normally derived from two sources: (1) through cutaneous conversion of 7-dehydrocholesterol to vitamin D_3 (cholecalciferol) in a process accelerated by solar ultraviolet (UV) irradiation; and (2) through ingestion of vitamin D_3 derived from animal food sources and vitamin D_2 (ergocalciferol) from multivitamin supplements and vitamin D-supplemented foods. Vitamin D_2 and D_3 as well as their subsequent metabolites appear to be equipotent in normal humans. Customary vitamin D intake varies widely, but mean intake levels in the United States range from approximately 200–400 units/day in normal adults to several-fold higher values in children, the higher values in the latter being due to their increased use of vitamin supplements and increased intake of vitamin D-supplemented foods such as milk and cereals (Hahn et al., 1972b,1975b). The absolute minimum vitamin D requirement in normal adults appears to be on the order of 80 IU/day. In temperate zones, the relative contributions of intake and sunlight exposure to total vitamin D nutritional status vary with the season (Haddad and Hahn, 1973).

After ingestion or cutaneous production vitamin D (herein used to indicate both vitamin D_2 and vitamin D_3), which is essentially a prohormone, is stored in adipose tissue and muscle, from whence it is delivered in an apparently unregulated process to the liver for subsequent metabolism. In the liver, two distinct vitamin D-25-hydroxylase enzyme systems effect the conversion to 25OH vitamin D (25OHD): a partially product-feedback-regulated high-affinity microsomal system (DeLuca, 1976) and a non-product-regulated lower-affinity mitochondrial system (Bjorkhem and Holmberg, 1978). It is uncertain at present which system plays the quantitatively dominant role in normal vitamin D metabolism. Once produced, 25OHD is delivered to the circulation where it is transported, as are vitamin D and its other metabolites, on vitamin D metabolite binding protein (DBP) (Haddad and Walgate, 1976). 25OHD is the quantitatively major circulating vitamin D metabolite, being present in normal serum at concentrations from 10 to 60 ng/ml (Hahn et al., 1972b,1975b). Subsequent conversion to other metabolites of biologic significance occurs in the proximal renal tubular cell, where separate mitochondrial enzyme systems catalyze conversion to either $24,25(OH)_2D$ or $1,25(OH)_2D$. Activity of the 1-hydroxylase system is stimulated by increased circulating levels of PTH, decreased serum calcium concentration, and possibly also by decreased serum phosphate concentrations. The opposite conditions favor the activity of the 24-hydroxylase system (DeLuca, 1976). In normal humans $24,25(OH)_2D$ circulates at a concentration of approximately 0.5–3.0 ng/ml, while the normal serum concentration of $1,25(OH)_2D$ is 20–60 pg/ml (Hahn et al., 1981a). $1,25(OH)_2D$ is currently accepted to be the major biologically active metabolite of vitamin D, being at least 1000 times more potent than 25OHD in stimulating intestinal calcium transport and 1000-5000 times more potent in directly stimulating release of calcium from bone (DeLuca, 1976; Haussler and McCain, 1977). The biological role of $24,25(OH)_2D$ is uncertain. However, the metabolite has been suggested to have unique effects on the maintenance of normal bone formation processes (Bordier et al., 1978; Ornoy et al., 1978). Vitamin D, 25OHD $24,25(OH)_2D$, and $1,25(OH)_2D$ have all been demonstrated to undergo enterohepatic recirculation (Silver et al., 1974; Arnaud et al., 1975; Kumar et al., 1980a,b). with the parent metabolites and their hepatic products excreted in the bile and reabsorbed in the proximal intestine.

Vitamin D and its active metabolites bear certain structural similarities to the steroid hormones. Thus it has been suggested that the vitamin D sterols may undergo increased hepatic microsomal metabolism in
anticonvulsant-drug-treated patients in a manner similar to the steroid
hormones. Although the hepatic vitamin D-25-hydroxylase system is
subject to a degree of product feedback regulation (DeLuca, 1976),
this feedback control is incomplete. Hence alterations in vitamin D input and vitamin D metabolite elimination can significantly alter serum
and tissue vitamin D metabolite levels. Moreover, total vitamin D input
is limited by the individual's extent of dietary vitamin D intake and
sunlight exposure. Thus drug-induced accelerated hepatic catabolism
of the vitamin D sterols could quite readily lead to the degree of reduction in serum 25OHD concentration which is observed in patients
with anticonvulsant osteomalacia. The serum 25OHD levels in these individuals (in the range 2–12 ng/ml) are comparable to those achieved
in other clinical states of vitamin D deficiency such as severe deficiency
of vitamin D intake and intestinal fat malabsorption syndromes (Arnaud
et al., 1976; Teitelbaum et al., 1977; Krawitt and Chastenay, 1980).
Morever, anticonvulsant-drug administration does not alter either the
intestinal absorption of vitamin D (Hahn and Halstead, 1979) or the
binding of 25OHD by serum DBP (Hahn et al., 1972b); hence it is clear
that drug-induced reductions in serum 25OHD concentration must be due
to alterations in the metabolism of vitamin D *subsequent* to its absorption.

Chronic administration of anticonvulsant drugs in humans and animal
results in a marked acceleration of the serum disappearance of vitamin
D and 25OHD, with an associated increase in the rate of appearance of
polar products other than the known biologically active metabolites
(Hahn et al., 1972a; Silver et al., 1974). Additionally, administration
of phenobarbital in animals results in increased in vivo hepatic microsomal accumulation and metabolism of vitamin D (Hahn et al., 1974b),
enhanced biliary excretion of vitamin D metabolites (Silver et al.,
1974), and accelerated in vitro liver microsomal conversion of vitamin
D and 25OHD to polar inactive products (Hahn et al., 1972a). In con-
cert with this evidence for a drug-stimulated increase in the rate of
degradative metabolism of vitamin D, it has been shown that treatment
with anticonvulsant drugs reduces the biological effectiveness of exogenously administered vitamin D (Gascon-Barre and Cote, 1978; Norman et al., 1975), and that chronic administration of phenytoin produces classic biochemical and histological changes of vitamin D-deficien-
cy osteomalacia in animals (Villareale et al., 1974,1978; Harris et al.,
1978).

The precise molecular mechanisms whereby drugs alter hepatic vitamin D metabolism are currently under investigation. It has been shown
that vitamin D and 25OHD are tightly bound by the hepatic microsomal
P-450 system and appear to compete with aminopyrine for metabolism in

this system (Cinti et al., 1976), thus suggesting a common hepatic pathway for degradative processing of drugs and vitamin D sterols. On the other hand, it has been reported that phenobarbital stimulates the activity of the hepatic mitochondrial vitamin D 25-hydroxylase system (Bjorkhem and Holmberg, 1978), a finding which correlates with the observation that administration of high doses of phenobarbital in the rat results in an initial rise in serum 25OHD concentration followed by a subsequent decline to subnormal levels (Hahn et al., 1975a), and an increased rate of conversion of vitamin D_3 to $25OHD_3$ by the perfused rat liver (Baran et al., 1979).

The effects of anticonvulsant drugs on dihydroxyvitamin D metabolite turnover are less well defined. Serum $1,25(OH)_2D$ levels have frequently been reported to be significantly elevated to anticonvulsant-drug-treated patients (Jubiz et al., 1977; Bell et al., 1979; Hahn et al., 1981b). In contrast, serum $24,25(OH)_2D$ concentrations are markedly reduced, showing a direct correlation with serum 25OHD concentration (Hahn et al., 1980). Although this increase in serum 1, $1,25(OH)_2D$ concentration could be considered to represent a normal physiologic response to reduced serum calcium and increased serum PTH levels, short-term supplementation with large doses of vitamin D results in a paradoxical further *increase* in serum $1,25(OH)_2D$ concentration in the face of a rise in serum calcium and a fall in serum PTH concentration (Hahn et al., 1981b). This paradoxical response suggests that renal metabolism of 25OHD may be directly altered by anticonvulsant drugs. Possible mechanisms include (1) drug inhibition of renal cell membrane transport of calcium ion, analogous to that seen in other tissues (Ferendelli and Kinscherf, 1977), with consequent decreased calcium feedback inhibition of 25OHD-1-hydroxylase activity; or (2) drug induction of renal mitochondrial 25OHD-1-hydroxylase activity analogous to recently demonstrated drug induction of hepatic mitochondrial vitamin D-25-hydroxylase (Bjorkhem and Holmberg, 1978). The latter possibility is supported by the observation that in vivo administration of both phenobarbital and phenytoin enhance in vitro renal 25OHD-1-hydroxylase activity in severely vitamin D-deficient chicks (Levinson et al., 1977).

The fact that clinical measures of vitamin D biologic activity in this disorder change in parallel with serum 25OHD [and $24,25(OH)_2D$] concentration has a rather profound implication. Since it appears that in the presence of a reduced circulating concentration of 25OHD even elevated levels of $1,25(OH)_2D$ are incapable of maintaining a normal serum calcium concentration, it must be surmised that 25OHD, or a metabolite of vitamin D other than $1,25(OH)_2D$, may play a more important direct role in the maintenance of normal calcium homeostasis than has therefore been suspected. In addition, it could be theorized that elevated $1,25(OH)_2D$ levels in the presence of reduced levels of 25OHD and $24,25(OH)_2D$ might lead to an increased tendency for net bone resorption (Bordier et al., 1978); however, at present this must remain an interesting but unproved hypothesis.

B. Direct Effects on Cellular Metabolism

There is considerable evidence indicating that the anticonvulsant drugs have direct effects on mineral metabolism independent of their effects on vitamin D. This is particularly true in the case of phenytoin, which showed well-documented inhibitory effects on cation transport in a variety of tissues (Ferendelli and Kinscherf, 1977). For example, it has been demonstrated in the rat that doses of phenytoin which do not appear to alter vitamin D metabolism significantly inhibit intestinal calcium transport, while comparable doses of phenobarbitone do not (Koch et al., 1972). In addition, short-term combined phenobarbital-phenytoin treatment in the rat results in decreased vitamin D and 25OHD-stimulated in vitro intestinal calcium transport, an effect that appears to be due to a specific inhibition of energy-dependent calcium transport processes (Harrison and Harrison, 1976). Moreover, there is evidence that supranormal circulating levels of vitamin D metabolites are required to produce normal intestinal calcium absorption in patients receiving combined drug anticonvulsant therapy (Hahn and Halstead, 1979).

Recent in vitro studies have demonstrated that both phenobarbital and phenytoin are capable of inhibiting the bone resorptive response to PTH and vitamin D metabolites (Jenkins et al., 1974; Hahn et al., 1978;1980). However, phenytoin is several-fold more potent than phenobarbital in this regard (Figure 2), and appears to have a somewhat different mechanism of action, since phenytoin, but not phenobarbital, is capable of suppressing PTH-stimulated cyclic AMP production and interacting synergistically with calcitonin (Hahn et al., 1978). Phenytoin has also been shown to have a potent direct inhibitory effect on collagen synthesis (Dietrich and Duffield, 1980) and lysosomal enzyme release (Lerner and Hanstrom, 1980) in cultured bone, indicating inhibition of both osteoblast and osteoclast activity. This contrast of in vitro evidence of direct drug inhibition of bone cell function with the frequent in vivo histological evidence of variable degrees of increased osteoclastic activity in anticonvulsant-treated patients (Mosekilde et al., 1977) indicates that the final effects of anticonvulsant drugs on bone metabolism involve an interaction of vitamin D- and PTH-related actions and direct inhibitory metabolic effects. In this regard, it is of interest that a paradoxical thickening of the calvarium has been reported in children treated chronically with phenytoin (Kattan, 1970). Moreover, phenytoin has been reported to accelerate fracture healing in animals (Frymoyer, 1976). Thus it appears that phenytoin has somewhat variable direct effects on bone formation and resorption processes.

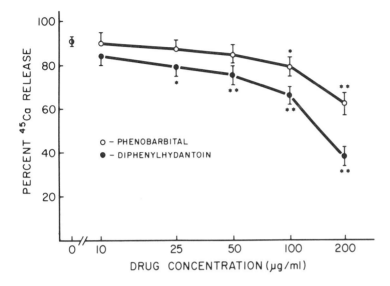

Figure 2 Inhibition by phenobarbital and diphenylhydantoin of PTH-stimulated ^{45}Ca release in 5-day cultures of fetal *rat* forelimb rudiments. PTH was present at a concentration of 50 ng/ml. Significant inhibition of ^{45}Ca release is produced by diphenylhydantoin at a concentration of 25 µg/ml, which phenobarbital produced significant inhibition only at concentrations of 100 µg/ml or greater.*, Significantly different from control at P < 0.02; **, Significantly different from control at P < 0.01.

IV. DIAGNOSTIC PROCEDURES

Probably the most sensitive and reliable means of rapidly establishing the diagnosis of drug-induced osteomalacia is by measurement of serum 25OHD concentration and determination of bone mass by photon absorption densitometry. However, more conventional diagnostic techniques may also suffice. If the mean of several determinations of fasting serum calcium and phosphate concentrations lies at or below the lower limits of normal, a significant derangement of mineral metabolism is probable. Elevation of the serum alkaline phosphatase concentration per se does not unequivocally indicate osteomalacia, since liver alkaline phosphatase levels are generally increased soon after initiation of anticonvulsant therapy at a time when serum bone alkaline phosphatase concentration is normal (Hahn et al., 1972b). However, at the very least, an elevated serum alkaline phosphatase level suggests hepatic enzyme

induction and thus warrants intensive investigation of the patient's
mineral status.

In addition, the assessment of 24-h urinary calcium excretion can be
a very useful diagnostic aid, since urinary calcium excretion reflects
the mean serum ionized calcium concentration as well as the effects of
parathyroid hormone on the renal tubule. The reduction of urinary
calcium excretion to less than 80 mg/day in an adult with normal calcium
intake and normal renal function is good presumptive evidence of decreased intestinal calcium absorption.

In patients in whom there is reason to suspect significant osteomalacia, an extensive radiologic examination for radiological evidence of
bone disease should be performed. The presence of rachitic changes

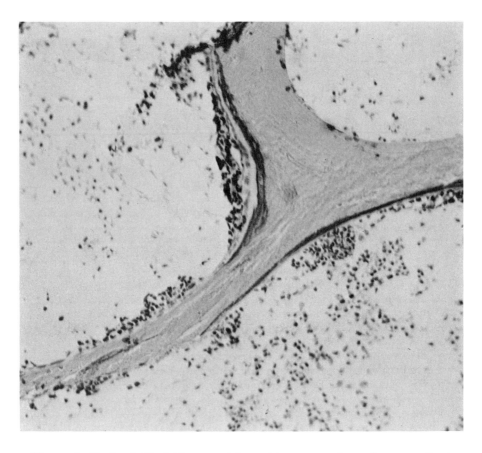

Figure 3 Undecalcified iliac crest bone biopsy specimen from a patient
with anticonvulsant-drug-induced bone disease. Note increased osteoclastic resorptive activity.

in children or pseudofractures in adults would be strong presumptive evidence for this diagnosis. However, in the usual case of anticonvulsant osteomalacia, a degree of generalized demineralization is all that is observed. When the diagnosis is in doubt, one may employ needle bone biopsy of the iliac crest, with examination of undecalcified sections to confirm the presence of increased osteoid tissue and elevated osteoclastic activity (Figure 3). However, in most cases of relatively severe disease, the diagnosis can be established by the above-mentioned clinical criteria.

V. TREATMENT

A variety of treatment regimens have been employed in patients with clinically overt drug-induced osteomalacia bone disease. Christiansen and co-workers have shown that treatment with vitamin D 2000—4000 units/day for 3 months produces a 3—5% increase in bone mass in various groups of pediatric and adult patients (Christiansen et al., 1973, 1975). Similarly, we have recently reported that administration of vitamin D_3 4000 units/day for 4 months produces significant improvement in intestinal calcium absorption, serum mineral and iPTH levels, urinary calcium and hydroxyproline excretion, and bone mass (Hahn and Halstead, 1979). Moreover, a reduced incidence of osteopenia has been reported in anticonvulsant-treated patients receiving a routine daily multivitamin supplement (Barden et al., 1980). On the other hand, other investigators have reported that in certain cases as much as 15,000 units of vitamin D per day may be required to produce significant healing of radiologic lesions (Maclaren and Lifshitz, 1973). In addition, it has been suggested that 25OHD in relatively small doses (100—2000 units/day) may be more rapidly effective than vitamin D (Stamp et al., 1972; Maclaren and Lifshitz, 1973). This suggestion has some theoretical merit since 25OHD administration would bypass the requirement for hepatic accumulation and metabolism of vitamin D.

In patients with clinically or radiologically apparent bone disease and/ or definite hypocalcemia, we recommend initial treatment with vitamin D 4000 units per square meter of body area, or $25OHD_3$ 20 $\mu g/m^2$ body area, plus 500 mg of supplemental calcium per day, generally for a period of 3—6 months. When the appropriate biochemical parameters (serum 25OHD, serum and urine calcium, and urinary hydroxyproline) are normalized, patients are placed on chronic maintenance therapy with approximately 800 units of vitamin D, or 5 μg of $25OHD_3$ per day. It is extremely important to maintain careful patient monitoring so that the dose of vitamin D and calcium supplements can be adjusted to meet individual requirements and thereby inadvertent vitamin D overdosage can be avoided.

There is considerable controversy over the question of whether routine vitamin D metabolite supplementation should necessarily be given to all patients who are receiving chronic anticonvulsant drug therapy, even those in whom standard routine parameters of mineral metabolism are normal. The objections to this approach are based on the economic burden imposed by chronic vitamin D therapy and the risk of inadvertent vitamin D overdosage. On the other hand, it has been observed that the single most costly aspect of medical management in institutionalized epileptic patients may be the treatment of pathological bone fractures resulting from demineralized bone (Tolman et al., 1975). Furthermore, moderate levels of vitamin D supplementation have been shown to decrease the incidence of significant bone loss (Barden et al., 1980) and sharply reduce the incidence of fractures in epileptic populations (Sherk et al., 1977). A theoretical factor of equal importance is that it seems likely that a chronic mild reduction in bone mass due to anticonvulsant drug therapy, when combined with the normal decrease in bone mass occurring with age, should lead to a significant increase in the incidence of clinically significant osteopenia in older patients who have been maintained on anticonvulsant drugs throughout life.

If it is accepted that prophylactic treatment with vitamin D is indicated, the question arises as to when therapy should be started. This is not a trivial question since it has been shown that significant reductions in bone mass can be demonstrated in patients who have received anticonvulsant therapy for less than 1 year (Christiansen et al., 1973). However, it has been our experience that significant decreases in serum 25OHD and elevations in bone alkaline phosphatase usually occur only after 6 months or more of therapy. In addition, there are animal data suggesting that a transient paradoxical *rise* in serum 25OHD. concentration and evidence of vitamin D biologic activity occurs immediately after initiation of drug therapy, presumably due to a temporary competitive block of catabolic pathways (Hahn et al., 1975a). Therefore, it is our current feeling that prophylactic vitamin D treatment should instituted only in patients who have been on therapy for 6 months or longer and who exhibit reduced serum concentrations of 25OHD.

REFERENCES

Arnaud, S. B., Goldsmith, R. S., Lambert, P. W., and Go, V. L. W. (1975). 25-Hydroxyvitamin D_3: evidence of an enterohepatic circulation in man. *Proc. Soc. Exp. Biol. Med.* *149*:570-572.

Arnaud, S. B., Stickler, G. B., and Haworth, J. C. (1976). Serum 25-hydroxyvitamin D in infantile rickets. *Pediatrics* 57:221-225.

Baran, D. T., Fausto, A. C., Roberts, M. L., Karl, I., and Avioli, L. V. (1979). Phenobarbital-induced alterations in the metabolism of (^{3}H) vitamin D_3 by the perfused rachitic rat liver in vitro. *J. Clin. Invest.* *64*:1112-1117.

Barden, H. S., Mazess, R. B., Rose, P. G., and McAweeney, W. (1980). Bone mineral status measured by direct photon absorptiometry in institutionalized adults receiving long-term anticonvulsant therapy and multivitamin supplementation. *Calcif. Tissue. Int.* 31:117-121.

Beck, L. H., and Goldberg, M. (1973). Effects of acetazolamide and parathyroidectomy on renal transport of sodium, calcium and phosphate. *Am. J. Physiol.* 224:1136-1142.

Bell, R. D., Pak, C. Y. C., Zerwekh, J., Barilla, D. E., and Vasko, M. (1979). Effect of phenytoin on bone and vitamin D metabolism. *Ann. Neurol.* 5:374-378.

Bjorkhem, I., and Holmberg, I. (1978). Assay and properties of a mitochondrial 25-hydroxylase activity on vitamin D. *J. Biol. Chem.* 253:842-849.

Bordier, P., Rasmussen, H., Marie, P., Miravet, L., Gueris, J., and Ryckwaert, A. (1978). Vitamin D metabolites and bone mineralization in man. *J. Clin. Endocrinol. Metab.* 46:284-294.

Bouillon, R., Reynaert, J., Claes, J. H., Lissens, W., and DeMoor, P. (1975). The effect of anticonvulsant therapy on serum levels of 25-hydroxyvitamin D, calcium, and parathyroid hormone. *J. Clin. Endocrinol. Metab.* 41:1130-1135.

Christiansen, C., Rodbro, P., and Lund, P. (1973). Incidence of anticonvulsant osteomalacia and effect of vitamin D: controlled therapeutic trial. *Br. Med. J.* 4:695-701.

Christiansen, C., Rodbro, P., and Nielsen, C. T. (1975). Iatrogenic osteomalacia in epileptic children. A controlled therapeutic trial. *Acta Paediatr. Scand.* 64:219-224.

Cinti, D. L., Glorieux, F. H., Delvin, E. E., Bolub, E. E., and Bronner, F. (1976). 25-Hydroxycholecalciferol: high affinity substrate for hepatic cytochrome P-450. *Biochem. Biophys. Res. Commun.* 72:546-553.

Conney, A. H. (1967). Pharmacologic implications of microsomal enzyme induction. *Pharmacol. Rev.* 19:317-366.

DeLuca, H. F. (1976). Recent advances in our understanding of the vitamin D endocrine system. *J. Lab. Clin. Med.* 87:7-26.

Dent, C. E., Richens, A., Rowe, D. J. F., and Stamp, T. C. B. (1970). Osteomalacia with long-term anticonvulsant therapy in epilepsy. *Br. Med. J.* 4:69-72.

Dietrich, J. W., and Duffield, R. (1980). Effects of diphenylhydantoin on synthesis of collagen and noncollagen protein in tissue culture. *Endocrinology* 106:606-610.

Ferrendelli, J. A., and Kinscherf, D. A. (1977). Phenytoin: effects on calcium flux and cyclic nucleotides. *Epilepsia* 18:331-336.

Frymoyer, J. W. (1976). Fracture healing in rats treated with diphenylhydantoin. *J. Trauma* 16:368-370.

Gascon-Barre, M., and Cote, M. G. (1978). Effects of phenobarbital and diphenylhydantoin on acute vitamin D toxicity in the
rat. *Toxicol. Appl. Pharmacol. 43*:125-135.

Glynne, A., Hunter, I. P., and Thomson, J. A. (1972). Pseudohy-
poparathyroidism with paradoxical increase in hypocalcemic seizures due to long-term anticonvulsant therapy. *Postgrad. Med.
J. 48*:632-636.

Haddad, J. G., Jr., and Hahn, T. J. (1973). Natural and synthetic
sources of circulating 25-hydroxyvitamin D in man. *Nature
244*:515-518.

Haddad, J. G., Jr., and Walgate, J. (1976). 25-Hydroxyvitamin D
transport in human plasma: isolation and partial characterization
of calcifidiol-binding protein. *J. Biol. Chem. 251*:4803-4809.

Hahn, T. J., and Hahn, B. H. (1976). Osteopenia in patients with
rheumatic diseases: principles of diagnosis and therapy. *Sem.
Arthritis Rheum. 6*:165-186.

Hahn, T. J., and Halstead, L. R. (1979). Anticonvulsant drug-
induced osteomalacia: alterations in mineral metabolism and response to vitamin D_3 administration. *Calcif. Tissue Int. 27*:13-
18.

Hahn, T. J., Birge, S. J., Scharp, C. R., and Avioli, L. V.
(1972a). Phenobarbital induced alterations in vitamin D metabolism. *J. Clin. Invest. 51*:741-748.

Hahn, T. J., Hendin, B. A., Scharp, C. R., and Haddad, J. G.,
Jr. (1972b). Effect of chronic anticonvulsant therapy on serum
25-hydroxycholecalciferol levels in adults. *N. Engl. J. Med.
287*:900-904.

Hahn, T. J., Boisseau, V. C., and Avioli, L. V. (1974a). Effect
of chronic corticosteroid administration on diaphyseal and meta-
physeal bone mass. *J. Clin. Endocrinol. Metab. 39*:274-282.

Hahn, T. J., Scharp, C. R., and Avioli, L. V. (1974b). Effect
of phenobarbital administration on the subcellular distribution of
vitamin D_3-^3H in rat liver. *Endocrinology 94*:1489-1495.

Hahn, T. J., Halstead, L. R., Scharp, C. R., and Haddad, J. G.,
Jr. (1975a). Enhanced biotransformation and biologic efficacy
of vitamin D following phenobarbital administration in the rat.
Clin. Res. 23:111A.

Hahn, T. J., Hendin, B. A., Scharp, C. R., Boisseau, V. C., and
Haddad, J. G., Jr. (1975b). Serum 25-hydroxycalciferol levels
and bone mass in children on chronic anticonvulsant therapy.
N. Engl. J. Med. 292:550-554.

Hahn, T. J., Scharp, C. R., Richardson, C. A., Halstead, L. R.,
Kahn, A. J., and Teitelbaum, S. L. (1978). Interaction of
diphenylhydantoin (phenytoin) and phenobarbital with hormonal
mediation of fetal rat bone resorption in vitro. *J. Clin. Invest.
62*:406-414.

Hahn, T. J., Halstead, L. R., and DeVivo, D. C. (1979). Disordered mineral metabolism produced by ketogenic diet therapy. *Calcif. Tissue Int. 28*:17-22.

Hahn, T. J., DeBartolo, T. F., and Halstead, L. R. (1980). Ouabain effects on hormonally-stimulated bone resorption and cyclic AMP content in cultured fetal rat bones. *Endocr. Res. Commun. 7*:189-200.

Hahn, T. J., Halstead, L. R., and Baran, D. T. (1981a). Effects of short-term glucocorticoid administration on intestinal calcium absorption and circulating vitamin D metabolite concentrations in man. *J. Clin. Endocrinol. Metab. 52*:111-115.

Hahn, T. J., Shires, R. A., and Halstead, L. R. (1981b). Serum vitamin D metabolite concentrations in anticonvulsant drug-treated patients. *Clin. Res. 29*:407A.

Harris, M., Rowe, D. J. F., and Darby, A. J. (1978). Anticonvulsant osteomalacia induced in the rat by diphenylhydantoin. *Calcif. Tissue Res. 25*:13-17.

Harrison, H. C., and Harrison, H. E. (1976). Inhibition of vitamin D-stimulated active transport of calcium of rat intestine by diphenylhydantoin-phenobarbital treatment. *Proc. Soc. Exp. Biol. Med. 153*:220-224.

Haussler, M. R., and McCain, T. A. (1977). Basic and clinical concepts related to vitamin D metabolism and action. *N. Engl. J. Med. 297*:974-983,1041-1050.

Hunter, J., Maxwell, J. D., Stewart, D. A., Parsons, V., and Williams, R. (1971). Altered calcium metabolim in epileptic children on anticonvulsants. *Br. Med. J. 2*:202-204.

Jenkins, M. V., Harris, M., and Wills, M. R. (1974). The effect of phenytoin on parathyroid extract and 25-hydroxycholecalciferol-induced bone resorption: adenosine 3',5'-cyclic monophosphate production. *Calcif. Tissue Res. 16*:163-167.

Jubiz, W., Meikle, A. W., and Levinson, R. A. (1970). Effect of diphenylhydantoin on the metabolism of dexamethasone: mechanism of the abnormal dexamethasone suppression in humans. *N. Engl. J. Med. 283*:11-14.

Jubiz, W., Haussler, M. R., McCain, T. A., and Tolman, K. G. (1977). Plasma 1,25-dihydroxyvitamin D levels in patients receiving anticonvulsant drugs. *J. Clin. Endocrinol. Med. 44*: 617-621.

Kattan, K. R. (1970). Calvarial thickening after dilantin medication. *Invest. Radiol. 110*:102-105.

Koch, H. C., Kraft, D., and von Herrath, D. (1972). Influence of diphenylhydantoin and phenobarbital on intestinal calcium transport in the rat. *Epilepsia 13*:829-841.

Krawitt, E. L., and Chastenay, B. F. (1980). 25-Hydroxyvitamin D absorption test in patients with gastrointestinal disorders. *Calcif. Tissue Int. 32*:183-187.

Kruse, R. (1968). Osteopathien bei antiepilptischer Langzeit-therapie (vorlaufige Mitteilung). *Monatchri. Kinderheilkd. 116*:378-380.

Kumar, R., Nagubandi, S., Mattox, V. R., and Londowski, J. M. (1980a). Enterohepatic physiology of 1,25-dihydroxyvitamin D₃. *J. Clin. Invest. 65*:277-284.

Kumar, R., Nagubandi, S., and Londowski, J. M. (1980b). The enterohepatic physiology of 24,25-dihydroxyvitamin D₃. *J. Lab. Clin. Med. 96*:278-284.

Lee, S. W., Russell, J., and Avioli, L. V. (1977). 25-Hydroxycholecalciferol to 1,25-dihydroxycholecalciferol: conversion impaired by systemic metabolic acidosis. *Science 195*:994-996.

Lerner, U., and Hanstrom, L. (1980). Influence of diphenylhydantoin on lysosomal enzyme release during bone resorption in vitro. *Acta Pharmacol. 47*:144-150.

Levin, W., Welch, R. M., and Conney, A. H. (1967). Effect of chronic phenobarbital treatment on the liver microsomal metabolism and uterotrophic action of 17β estradiol. *Endocrinology 80*:135-140.

Levinson, J. C., Kent, G. N., Worth, G. K., and Retallack, R. W. (1977). Anticonvulsant induced increase in 25-hydroxyvitamin D₃-1α hydroxylase. *Endocrinology 101*:1898-1901.

Lifshitz, F., and Maclaren, N. K. (1973). Vitamin D-dependent rickets in institutionalized mentally retarded children receiving long-term anticonvulsant therapy. I. A survey of 288 patients. *J. Pediatr. 83*:612-620.

Lindgren, L., Nilsson, B. E., and Walloe, A. (1979). Bone mineral content in epileptics. *Calcif. Tissue Int. 28*:99-102.

Maclaren, N. K., and Lifshitz, F. (1973). Vitamin D dependency rickets in institutionalized, mentally retarded children on long-term anticonvulsant therapy. II. The response to 25-hydroxycholecalciferol and vitamin D. *Pediatr. Res. 7*:914-923.

Mallette, L. E. (1977). Acetazolamide-accelerated anticonvulsant osteomalacia. *Arch. Int. Med. 137*:1013-1017.

Marsden, C. D., Reynolds, E. H., Parson, V., Harris, R., and Duchan, L. (1973). Myopathy associated with anticonvulsant osteomalacia. *Br. Med. J. 4*:526-527.

Melsen, F., and Mosekilde, L. (1976). *Proc. 11th Eur. Symp. Calcified Tissues*, FADL's, Forlag, Copenhagen, p. 247.

Mosekilde, L., and Melsen, F. (1976). Anticonvulsant osteomalacia determined by quantitative analysis of bone changes. *Acta Med. Scand. 199*:349-355.

Mosekilde, L., Christensen, M. S., Lund, B., Sorensen, O. H., and Melsen, F. (1977). The interrelationships between serum 25-hydroxycholecalciferol, serum parathyroid hormone and bone changes in anticonvulsant osteomalacia. *Acta Endocrinol. 84*:559-565.

Murchison, L. E., Bewsher, P. D., Chesters, M., Gilbert, J., Catto, G., Law, E., McKay, E., and Ross, H. S. (1975). Effects of anticonvulsants and inactivity on bone disease in epileptics. *Postgrad. Med. J. 51*:18-21.

Norman, A. W., Bayless, J. D., and Tsai, H. C. (1975). Biologic effects of short-term phenobarbital treatment on the response to vitamin D and its metabolites in the chick. *Biochem. Pharmacol. 25*:161-168.

Ornoy, A., Goodwin, D., Noff, D., and Edelstein, S. (1978). 24, 25-Dihydroxyvitamin D is a metabolite of vitamin D essential for bone formation. *Nature 276*:517-519.

Peterson, P., Gray, P., and Tolman, K. G. (1976). Calcium balance in drug-induced osteomalacia: response to vitamin D. *Clin. Pharmacol. Ther. 19*:63-67.

Richens, A., and Rowe, D. J. F. (1970). Disturbance of calcium metabolism by anticonvulsant drugs. *Br. Med. J. 3*:73-76.

Rodbro, P., Christiansen, C., and Lund, M. (1974). Development of anticonvulsant osteomalacia in epileptic patients on phenytoin treatment. *Acta Neurol. Scand. 50*:527-532.

Sherk, H. H., Cruz, M., and Stamburgh, J. (1977). Vitamin D prophylaxis and the lowered incidence of fractures in anticonvulsant rickets and osteomalacia. *Clin. Orthop. Relat. Res. 129*:251-257.

Silver, J., Neale, G., and Thompson, G. R. (1974). Effect of phenobarbitone treatment on vitamin D metabolism in mammals. *Clin. Sci. Mol. Med. 46*:433-448.

Stamp, T. C. B., Round, J. M., Rowe, D. J. F., and Haddad, J. G. (1972). Plasma levels and therapeutic effect of 25-hydroxycholecalciferol in epileptic patients taking anticonvulsant drugs. *Br. Med. J. 4*:9-12.

Teitelbaum, S. L., Halverson, J. D., Bates, M., Wise, L., and Haddad, J. G., Jr. (1977). Abnormalities of circulating 25-OH vitamin D after jejunal-ileal bypass for obesity: evidence of an adaptive response. *Ann. Intern. Med. 86*:289-293.

Tolman, K. G., Jubiz, W., Sannella, J. J., and Madsen, J. A. (1975). Osteomalacia associated with anticonvulsant drug therapy in mentally retarded children. *Pediatrics 56*:45-51.

Villareale, M., Gould, L. V., Wasserman, R. H., Garr, A., Chiroff, R. T., and Bergstrom, W. H. (1974). Diphenylhydantoin: effects on calcium metabolism in the chick. *Science 183*:671-673.

Villareale, M. E., Chiroff, R. T., Bergstrom, W. H., Gould, L. V., Wasserman, R H., and Romano, F. A. (1978). Bone changes induced by diphenylhydantoin in checks on a controlled vitamin D intake. *J. Bone Joint Surg. 60*:911-916.

12

Vitamin K and Vitamin K Antagonists

Thorir D. Bjornsson
Duke University Medical Center, Durham, North Carolina

I. INTRODUCTION

Vitamin K was discovered by Henrik Dam in 1929 in studies of sterol metabolism in chicks fed fat-free diets (1). The antihemorrhagic fat-soluble agent was called vitamin K, K being short for "Koagulation" (the German word for coagulation). Since then there have been two major eras of extensive research on this vitamin. The first era was in the 1930s and it culminated in 1939 with the characterization and synthesis of vitamin K_1 (phylloquinone) and a year later of "vitamin K_2" (menaquinone-7). The chemical structures of the different vitamins K are shown in Figure 1. During this period it was shown that the hemorrhagic disease associated with vitamin K deficiency was due to the absence of prothrombin activity in plasma, and shortly thereafter, it was demonstrated that a combination therapy with vitamin K and bile salts was effective in the treatment of hemorrhagic tendency in patients with obstructive jaundice and diseases of the liver. Thus the relationship between vitamin K, liver function, and blood coagulation became established. The second era of extensive research on vitamin K has focused on its function. It started in the late 1960s and it culminated, at least temporarily, in the mid-1970s, when the product of post-translational vitamin K-dependent carboxylation, γ-carboxyglutamic acid (Gla), was identified (2-4). It was demonstrated that this modified amino acid gave the vitamin K-dependent clotting factors the calcium binding properties which are necessary for their normal function in blood coagulation. In the years between these two eras, several vitamin K antagonists, such as dicumarol, warfarin, phenpro-

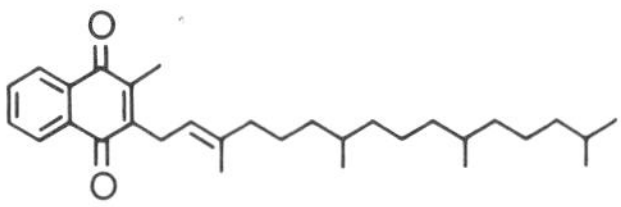

PHYLLOQUINONE (VITAMIN K$_1$)

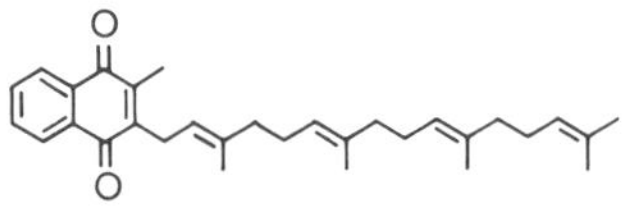

MENAQUINONE - 4 (VITAMIN K$_2$)

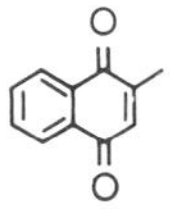

MENADIONE (VITAMIN K$_3$)

Figure 1 Chemical structures of phylloquinone (vitamin K$_1$), mena-quinone (vitamin K$_2$), and menadione (vitamin K$_3$). The particular form of menaquinone shown has four prenyl units, hence menaquinone-4. A menaquinone with six prenyl units would be called menaquinone-6.

coumon, and phenidione, were identified and their place in therapeutics was established (i.e., in the prevention of thrombosis).

Several reviews are available on the different aspects of vitamin K. The early history of the vitamin (5—8) and its absorption and metabolism (9) have been reviewed, and several excellent reviews are available on the biochemistry of vitamin K function and on theories of the mode of action of vitamin K antagonists (7,8,10—12). This chapter will review the available data on the physiological disposition of vitamin K, including absorption, distribution, and metabolism, and on the biochemistry and pharmacology of vitamin K-dependent carboxylation, emphasizing current understanding of the roles of the different enzymes involved. It will also review how drugs and other factors can affect both its physiological disposition and function.

II. DISPOSITION OF VITAMIN K

A. Absorption

Absorption of compounds with vitamin K activity from the intestine varies with their solubility characteristics and other factors. Absorption of the naturally occurring vitamin K compounds, phylloquinone and menaquinones, which takes place in the small intestine by way of the lymph, requires the presence of both bile and pancreatic juices to allow adequate or maximum absorption (7,9).

1. Extent, Site, and Mechanism of Absorption

The rate and extent of absorption of phylloquinone has been studied in normal subjects following the oral administration of [^{3}H]phylloquinone (9,13). The rate of absorption is relatively rapid, with peak concentrations occurring at 2−4 hr after administration. Absorption of phylloquinone from food, however, would be expected to be somewhat slower since it has to be preceded by digestion. Net absorption of the vitamin in normal subjects, based on recovery of radioactivity in the feces over 5 days, has been estimated to be about 80% (9,13). The radioactivity recovered in the feces over 5 days, however, was 52−56% of the administered dose, with 15−22% of the dose as unchanged phylloquinone. The difference consists of radioactivity excreted via the bile. Studies in patients with cannulated thoracic ducts showed that 19−62% of the administered radioactive dose was recovered in the thoracic duct lymph over 24 hr following the administration of [^{3}H]phylloquinone in a formula meal (14). Appearance of radioactivity in the lymph occurred mainly 2−8 hr after administration. In a patient with biliary tract obstruction, less than 3% of the administered dose was recovered in the lymph (14). Treatment of patients with chronic pancreatitis with Cotazyme (a preparation containing pancreatic enzymes) resulted in a marked increase in the absorption of [^{3}H]phylloquinone (9).

The location in the intestinal tract and the mechanism of absorption of compounds with vitamin K activity has been studied extensively in rats. Studies on the intestinal absorption of phylloquinone in rats, both in vitro using everted intestinal sacs and in vivo using perfused intestinal segments, have demonstrated that the vitamin is absorbed by an energy-requiring saturable transport process (15,16). The in vivo studies showed no differences in absorption rates of the vitamin by the proximal or distal small intestine, but previous in vitro studies had shown that the absorption was more rapid by the proximal intestine. These studies also showed that alkalinization of the perfusate and the addition of the unsaturated fatty acids, oleic and linoleic acids, to the perfusate decreased the rate of phylloquinone absorption, while the addition of medium- and long-chain saturated fatty acids, a menaquinone, or menadione to the perfusate, or increasing the concentration of taurocholate, had no effects on the absorption rate of the vitamin (16,17). The addition of butyric acid, however, to the perfusate increased the total absorption of phylloquinone (16,17). Because of these interactions of fatty acids with the rate of absorption of phylloquinone, it has been suggested that an intestinal fatty acid binding protein (18) may be involved in the absorption of phylloquinone (16).

Using the same in vivo perfused intestinal segment system, a circadian rhythm was demonstrated in the rate of absorption of phylloquinone, with most rapid absorption occurring during the evening and at midnight, but slowest absorption occurring in early morning and at noon (19). It was concluded that this circadian rhythm was related to synchronization of digestive and absorptive functions in relation to the time of feeding (19).

Studies on the intestinal absorption of menaquinone-9 in rats, both in vitro using everted intestinal sacs and in vivo using perfused intestinal segments, have shown that the menaquinone is absorbed by a passive diffusion by both the ileum and colon (20—23). However, absorption of the menaquinone was found to be dependent on the presence of bile salts for micellar solubilization. The rate of absorption was faster in the proximal than in the distal small intestine. Studies on the effects of different saturated and unsaturated fatty acids on the rate of absorption of menaquinone-9 showed different effects in the in vitro and in vivo systems, but in general, the fatty acids decreased its absorption in the in vivo system. As with phylloquinone, absorption of menaquinones is though to be primarily by way of the lymph.

Menadione, which is lipid-soluble like phylloquinine and menaquinones, and its water-soluble derivatives, may be absorbed in the absence of bile, unlike the other forms of the vitamin (9). Studies using in vitro everted perfused rat small intestine and colonic segments have shown that menadione is absorbed by passive diffusion in both proximal and distal portions of the small intestine and in the colon (23, 24). The absorption was more rapid by the distal small bowel than the proximal small bowel (23). Under physiological conditions, however, the proximal bowel comes first in contact with the ingested lipids and is likely to absorb most of the menadione. Menadione and its derivatives are thought to enter the portal system (9).

2. Factors Affecting Absorption

Compounds that interfere with the micelle formation involving the bile salts and phylloquinone or menaquinones will prevent absorption of the vitamin. The addition of mineral oil to vitamin K-deficient diets has been shown to enhance markedly the hypoprothrombinemic effect of the diets in rats (25,26); this effect was more pronounced in male than in female rats (25). Similarly, the oral administration of phylloquinone in a neutral oil solution to warfarin-treated rats did not affect the anticoagulant effect, while the oral administration of the same dose of phylloquinone solubilized in a nonionic surfactant [polyoxyethylene (20) glyceryloleate] reverted the coagulation times to control values (27). The addition of squalene and oxidized squalene to vitamin K-deficient diet had an effect similar to that of mineral oil in male rats, but was ineffective in female rats, while the addition of castor oil to the diet was without an effect in both sexes (25,28). The relative resistance of female rats to vitamin K deficiency may be due to the effects of female sex hormones on phylloquinone absorption, since estrogen treatment in rats has been shown to increase absorption of the vitamin (29). It is not known, however, whether this occurs in humans. Abuse of laxatives and cathartics in patients has been reported to result in hypoprothrombinemia; specific agents involved have been mineral oil and bisacodyl (30–32). Long-term administration of the nonabsorbable anion exchange resin cholestyramine, which binds bile acids and thereby prevents solubilization of vitamin K, may result in reduced absorption of the vitamin and subsequently in hypoprothrombinemia (9,33–35).

Other compounds that have been implicated in causing reduced absorption of vitamin K are the other fat-soluble vitamins (i.e., vitamins A, D, and E). Of these it appears that only vitamin A interferes with vitamin K absorption. Rats and chicks given an excess of vitamin A develop hypoprothrombinemia which can be reversed by vitamin K administration (28,36,37). The antivitamin K effect of vitamin A appears to be an inhibition of intestinal absorption, since parenteral administration of neither retinyl acetate nor retinoic acid was associated with hypoprothrombinemia (28). Vitamin E has been shown to have an antivitamin K effect in rats which can be prevented by the administration of a menaquinone (38), and to potentiate the anticoagulant effect of warfarin and dicumarol in rats and in humans (39,40). Both the quinone and hydroquinone forms of vitamin E have antivitamin K activity, and it has been suggested that its antivitamin K effect is pharmacodynamic; possibly that d-α-tocopheryl hydroquinone acts as a competitive inhibitor of vitamin K (39,41). The effects of excess doses of vitamin D on the absorption of vitamin K are unclear, although studies in rats have shown an antivitamin K effect (40).

Numerous diseases can be associated with diminished absorption of vitamin K (42,43). Diseases resulting in diminished secretion of bile and pancreatic juices into the gastrointestinal tract are the most common causes of insufficient absorption of the vitamin. This includes biliary tract obstruction, caused by gallstones, strictures or tumors, liver diseases, and chronic pancreatitis. Other diseases involving the intestinal tract resulting in malabsorption (e.g., celiac disease and sprue) can also result in insufficient absorption of vitamin K.

In summary, phylloquinone requires bile salts for absorption and is absorbed by an energy-requiring saturable transport process in the small intestine. Menaquinones, which also require bile salts for absorption, and menadione, whose absorption is not dependent on bile salts, are apparently absorbed by passive diffusion. Although the synthetic menadione and its derivatives are effective in preventing hypoprothrombinemia in malabsorption states and other causes of vitamin K deficiency, it is ineffective in the treatment of overdoses of warfarin and other vitamin K antagonists (44,45). Most of phylloquinone absorption probably takes place in the proximal part of the small intestine. The role of the bacterially produced menaquinones as a source of vitamin K in humans remains unsettled since the terminal ileum is the primary site of bile salt active absorption and most of menaquinone production takes place in the large intestine. It is therefore presently unclear how much of menaquinones can be solubilized and absorbed.

B. Transport, Distribution, and Disposition Kinetics

Following absorption phylloquinone is first taken up by the lymphatic vessels, and subsequently delivered into the systemic circulation. In the circulation, it is apparently associated with chylomicrons and lipoproteins. It distributes into the different tissues of the body and appears to have rapid turnover in humans. Very limited data are available on menaquinones.

1. Transport

Phylloquinone is primarily taken up into the lymph after absorption from the intestinal tract. After oral administration of [^{3}H]phylloquinone to patients with cannulated thoracic ducts, about 70—80% of the lymph radioactivity was found in the chylomicron fraction (14). In another study, after oral administration of [^{3}H]phylloquinone and at the time of peak serum radioactivity, more than 97% of the total serum radioactivity was in the lipid phase (13). Following ultracentrifugation, 65% of the radioactivity was found in the surface pellicle, presumably containing chylomicrons and lipoproteins. Using gel filtration, the major radioactivity was eluted in a peak thought to contain α- and β-lipoproteins (13).

Abetalipoproteinemia, a genetic disease characterized by the absence of β-lipoproteins, may be associated with symptoms of vitamin K deficiency, and a case has been reported that presented as severe vitamin K deficiency (46). Attempts to measure the plasma binding of phylloquinone in human plasma samples obtained 5 min after the intravenous injection of [^{3}H]phylloquinone and using equilibrium dialysis against a physiological buffer revealed that essentially all the radioactivity was bound in plasma (47). No specific plasma binding protein has been identified, such as exist for the fat-soluble vitamins A and D.

2. Distribution

Phylloquinone is taken up by the liver and a number of extrahepatic tissues. The vitamin and its metabolites accumulate much more in the liver than in other organs, although it is also found in the spleen, bones, kidneys and lungs (7,48—50). It had been suggested that vitamin K might have a function in tissues, where it accumulates, and indeed, vitamin K-dependent carboxylation has been demonstrated in all of these tissues (50). Vitamin K epoxidase activity is also found in most of these organs (51). Menaquinone-4 appeared to have somewhat similar tissue distribution as phylloquinone (52), but menadione and its water-soluble derivatives distribute differently within the body than phylloquinone; specifically, they do not accumulate in the liver and distribute more into kidneys and skeletal muscle (7,53). Within the rat liver cells, most of phylloquinone is located in the mitochondria and in the endoplasmic reticulum (49,54,55), probably reflecting preferential localization of the vitamin in the various cellular membranes due to its lipid solubility characteristics (7).

3. *Disposition and Turnover Kinetics*

Present knowledge about the disposition and turnover kinetics of phylloquinone is limited to data obtained by the use of a radiolabel. Studies in normal subjects on the disposition and turnover of phylloquinone, using tracer doses of [^{3}H]phylloquinone, showed that phylloquinone concentrations decline biexponentially after intravenous administration, with $t_{\frac{1}{2}\alpha}$ of 26 ± 8 min (56,57) or 20−24 min (58), and $t_{\frac{1}{2}\beta}$ of 2.8 ± 0.2 hr (56,57) or 121−150 min (58). Pharmacokinetic analysis revealed total clearance, Cl, of 115 ± 26 ml/min, apparent volume of distribution Vd, of 17.6 ± 3.9 l, and turnover time, t_t, calculated as

$$t_t = \frac{Vd}{Cl}$$

of 153 ± 12 min, suggesting very low plasma concentrations and a small body pool size of the vitamin in humans (56,57). Warfarin administration to normal subjects did not change the disposition and turnover parameters of phylloquinone, in spite of a marked accumulation of phylloquinone-2,3-epoxide, in plasma (56). Neither did clofibrate administration, a hypolipidemic agent, change the disposition and turnover kinetics of phylloquinone (56). The body pool size, P, can be calculated only if the true turnover time and rate of intake, R, are known, using the expression

$$P = R \times t_t$$

Intake of about 10 times the minimum daily requirement would therefore be expected to result in a body pool size of about 100 µg. This estimate is of interest since it has been shown that the human liver contains about 100 µg of phylloquinone (59), and since a substantial portion (about one-half) of phylloquinone in animals is found in the liver (7,48,52). In spite of the apparent short turnover time and small body pool size of phylloquinone, the acute development of vitamin K deficiency is apparently avoided by the presence of higher-molecular-weight storage forms of the vitamin in humans or by the bacterially produced menaquinones (60). It should be emphasized, however, that

these values for turnover time and pool size are only estimates. They
are based on the observed biexponential decline of phylloquinone in
plasma. It is possible that a final elimination phase was not identified,
in which case total clearance will be overestimated and volume of distribution and turnover time underestimated. These questions of relative turnover, pool sizes, and roles of phylloquinone and menaquinones
will only be solved when reliable chemical assays become available.

C. Metabolism

Phylloquinone is metabolized by the liver and subsequently eliminated
by renal and biliary excretion. Its metabolism is affected by warfarin
and other vitamin K antagonists, and it is thought that the changed
phylloquinone metabolism is involved in the mechanism of action of the
oral anticoagulants. Essentially no data are available on the metabolism
of menaquinones.

1. Routes of Elimination

Phylloquinone is rapidly metabolized in humans to more polar metabolites
which are eliminated by renal and biliary excretion (13,58). The biliary route of elimination is apparently of greater importance quantitatively in all species studied. After intravenous administration of 45
$\mu g-1$ mg of [^{3}H]phylloquinone to normal subjects, 8−26% of the administered dose was recovered in the urine over a period of 3 days,
while 34−51% of the dose was recovered in the feces over a period of
5 days (9,58,61). Excretion in bile appears to be the only mechanism
by which phylloquinone metabolites enter the intestinal lumen (58).
Studies in humans using oral doses of [^{3}H]phylloquinone have recovered 8−19% of the administered dose in the urine and 52−56% of the dose
in the feces (13). The apparent differences in the relative recoveries
of the administered dose in urine and feces, depending on route of administration, are due to incomplete absorption of the vitamin after oral
administration, as was mentioned earlier. In patients with a T-tube
drain in the bile duct, 5−25% of the administered dose was recovered in
the bile (58,62). Biliary excretion also appears to be the main route
of elimination of phylloquinone metabolites in other animal species. In
rats only about 5% of a dose of [^{3}H]phylloquinone was excreted in the
urine over 3 days (48), and about 25% of a dose of [^{14}C]phylloquinone
was excreted in the urine over 4 days; in hepatectomized rats, however, only 0.5% of the dose was recovered in the urine over the first
day compared with 10% in the control rats (63), suggesting that phylloquinone has to be metabolized first by the liver to more-water-soluble
metabolites before it can be excreted in the urine.

Studies in rats on the metabolism of menadione and menadiol diphosphate suggest that its metabolites are eliminated primarily by urinary

excretion (53,63,64), but no studies are available on the metabolism of menaquinones.

2. Identity of Metabolites

The major urinary metabolites of phylloquinone have been identified in humans (65,66) and rabbits (67) as being conjugates of acidic metabolites. The two major urinary aglycones in humans have been isolated and identified as 2-methyl-3-(5'-carboxy-3'-methyl-2'-pentenyl)-1,4-naphthoquinone (metabolite I) and 2-methyl-3-(3'-carboxy-3'-methyl-propyl)-1,4-naphthoquinone (metabolite II), based on comparisons of chromatographic and spectral data with model synthetic compounds (65,66). A third minor aglycone in humans has been isolated and tentatively identified as 2-methyl-3-(7'-carboxy-3',7'-dimethyl-2'-heptenyl)-1,4-naphthoquinone (metabolite III) (66). A phylloquinone metabolite previously identified in rats, a γ-lactone of metabolite I (48), was shown to be an artifact (65,66). In humans, approximately 80–90% of the urinary metabolites of phylloquinone appear to be excreted in the urine as glucuronide conjugates, since they can be hydrolyzed by treatment with bovine liver β-glucuronidase (65,66). The possibility that sulfate or other conjugates of phylloquinone metabolites are formed in humans has not been investigated, but sulfate conjugates have been reported for metabolites of menadione in rats (68,69) and ubiquinone in rabbits (70). Although there is no direct evidence, it has been postulated that the conjugation of the urinary metabolites of phylloquinone with glucuronic acid occurs at one or both of the 1,4-hydroxyl groups formed by reduction of the quinone to the hydroquinone by a vitamin K reductase (DT-diaphorase) present in the liver (66). This is supported by the identification by mass spectroscopy of a monoglucuronide conjugate of reduced menadione in rat bile (71). It was not possible, however, to determine to which hydroxyl group (1- or 4-) the glucuronic acid moiety is attached. The sulfate conjugate of reduced menadione, however, was shown to be a 1-sulfate conjugate (72).

A metabolism scheme has been proposed for the urinary metabolites of phylloquinone, involving first ω oxidation of phylloquinone to a 15'-carboxyl metabolite [2-methyl-3-(15'-carboxy-3',7',11',15'-tetramethyl-2'-pentadecenyl)-1,4-naphthoquinone], followed by successive removal of C_2 units from the phytyl side chain of phylloquinone by the β-oxidation pathway in mitochondria (66). This scheme is identical to that proposed for the side chain of ubiquinone (70). The relative amounts of metabolites I, II, and III in the urine appear to be phylloquinone dose dependent; at physiological doses, the vitamin is largely metabolized to the terminal metabolite II, whereas at higher doses, there is an increasing proportion of urinary metabolites with less extensively metabolized aglycones (i.e., with longer side chains) (66). Figure 2 summarizes the metabolism scheme of the urinary metabolites of phylloquinone in humans.

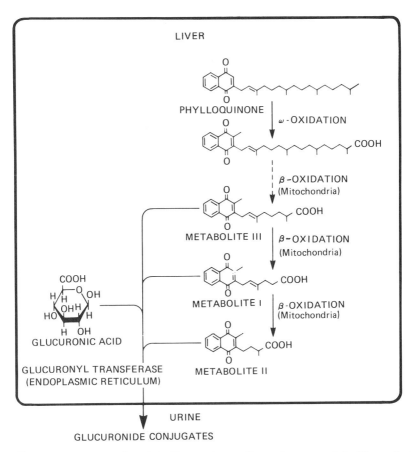

Figure 2 Proposed metabolism scheme for urinary metabolites of phylloquinone. (Modified from Refs. 10 and 11.)

The major biliary and fecal metabolites of phylloquinone in humans have not been identified. After intravenous administration of [3H]-phylloquinone to patients in whom duodenal contents or bile was collected, most of the radioactivity (85–95% in bile and 70–90% in duodenal contents) was found as water-soluble metabolites (58). In feces, however, the radioactivity is largely (94–99%) found as lipid-soluble metabolites (58). Most of the radioactivity in the bile can be rendered lipid soluble by treatment with β-glucuronidase, suggesting that the explanation for the difference in solubility characteristics of the radioactive material recovered in bile and feces is that in bile the phylloquinone metabolites are as glucuronide conjugates which are subsequently deconjugated by β-glucuronidases derived from bacterial flora and/or intestinal cells (9,58). A small portion of the biliary aglycones has solubility and chromatographic characteristics compatible with metabolites I and II (9). A major portion of the biliary aglycones exhibits lipid-solubility characteristics between that of phylloquinone and the γ-lactone compound. It is much less polar than the aglycones I and II. In feces, this metabolite(s) accounts for essentially all the radioactivity, and only traces are compatible with aglycones I and II (9,58).

3. Factors Affecting Metabolism

Warfarin administration has significant effects on the metabolism of phylloquinone. The major effect is the accumulation of phylloquinone-2,3-epoxide, and this will be discussed later. In humans, treatment with therapeutic doses of warfarin results in approximately a twofold increase in the 3-day urinary excretion of radioactivity after an intravenous administration of 45μg–1 mg doses of [^{3}H] phylloquinone (61, 73,74). These urinary metabolites are 80–96% water-soluble compared with 96–99% in control subjects (73,74). Another difference is that after warfarin only 50–55% of ether-extracted urinary metabolites are rendered lipid soluble by treatment with bovine liver β-glucuronide, compared with 85–90% in control subjects, suggesting a relative decrease in glucuronide conjugates (61,73,74). A considerable fraction of the warfarin-induced urinary metabolites of phylloquinone appears to be sulfate conjugates, since simple solvolysis renders 20–40% of the ether-extracted radioactivity lipid soluble (73,74). A third difference is an absolute reduction in urinary excretion of metabolites I and II; after warfarin these metabolites account only for about 10% of ether-extracted material treated with β-glucuronidase compared with about 60% in control subjects (9,73,74). Indeed, there appears to be a warfarin-dose-dependent decline in the urinary excretion of metabolites I and II which is associated with an increase in the warfarin-induced urinary metabolites of phylloquinone (73). The remainder consists of several (at least three) warfarin-induced metabolites of phylloquinone whose identity and metabolic pathways are not known. The major warfarin-induced aglycones, however, are organic acids which have greater polarity than aglycones I and II and they apparently contain hydroxyl group(s), since they react with silyl ethers, and they have an ultraviolet absorption spectra similar to that of phylloquinone-2,3-epoxide and one of them has a molecular weight of 326 (74). It has been suggested that the warfarin-induced metabolites may be 2,3-dihydrodiol metabolites, formed by the microsomal epoxide hydratase (74). Studies in rats have shown that warfarin and phenindione treatment results in a marked increase in polar metabolites of phylloquinone in the liver (75,76). In addition to both quantitative and qualitative changes in urinary excretion of phylloquinone metabolites, warfarin also decreases biliary excretion of phylloquinone metabolites in humans (9). Studies in rats showed that treatment with the 2-chloro analog of phylloquinone

(chloro-K) resulted in a two- to threefold increase in the percentage
of administered phylloquinone dose found in the liver, primarily in the
mitochondria, and it was suggested that chloro-K inhibited phylloquinone metabolism (49). The cytochrome P-450 inhibitor SKF-525A decreased elimination of phylloquinone in rats, although the amounts of
polar metabolites in the liver appeared unchanged (75). These studies
suggest that cytochrome P-450 may be involved in the metabolism of
phylloquinone.

In summary, phylloquinone metabolites are eliminated by biliary and
urinary excretion as water-soluble metabolites, primarily glucuronide
conjugates. Presently, only the identity of the major urinary aglycones
is known. Warfarin treatment has major effects on the metabolite pattern of phylloquinone in humans; the effects of other vitamin K antagonists have not been investigated. It should be noted that all studies
on the metabolites of phylloquinone have used a mixture of varying
ratios of the cis and trans isomers of phylloquinone. Only the trans
isomer is found naturally and the cis isomer has essentially no biological activity (55,77—79). Since differential metabolism of isomers is not
uncommonly observed for drugs and endogenous compounds, the available data on phylloquinone may not correctly reflect the metabolism and
disposition of the biologically active isomer of the vitamin.

D. Daily Requirement and Deficiency

1. Daily Requirement

The daily intake requirement of phylloquinone in humans is not accurately known, but it appears to be very small. It is though that the
minimum daily requirement is lower than 1.5 $\mu g/kg$ of body weight,
probably in the range 0.5—1.0 $\mu g/kg$ (7). In the infant, 10 $\mu g/kg$ of
body weight of phylloquinone is thought to be sufficient to prevent
hypoprothrombinemia. The recommendations of the Food and Nutrition
Board, National Research Council, for safe and adequate daily dietary
intake of vitamin K in the various age groups are shown in Table 1.

Dietary needs are generally satisfied by the average diet, where
vitamin K is provided primarily by the various vegetables. Certain
vegetables, such as lettuce, cabbage, broccoli, spinach, and kale, have
a high content (> 100 μg per 100 g) of vitamin K_1 (80). Vitamin K_1
content of infant formula products varies considerably and cow's milk,
which contains more vitamin K_1 than mother's milk, shows seasonal and
regional variation in its vitamin K_1 content (80).

2. Vitamin K Deficiency

Vitamin K deficiency may be more common than is presently recognized
due to our inability so far to diagnose it chemically. The more obvious
causes of vitamin K deficiency are diminished absorption of the vitamin

Table 1 Estimated Safe and Adequate Daily Dietary Intake of Vitamin K at Various Ages (Years)

	Infants		Children				Adults
	0−0.5	0.5−1	1−3	4−6	7−10	11+	
Vitamin K (μg)	12	10-20	15-30	20-40	30-60	50-100	70-140

Source: Modified from Food and Nutrition Board, National Research Council, 1979.

due to diseases associated with diminished secretion of bile and pancreatic juices into the gastrointestinal tract (e.g., biliary tract obstruction and primary liver diseases) and malabsorption syndromes (e.g., celiac disease and sprue). Another less well recognized and probably a far more common cause is dietary deficiency. This is not infrequently seen in hospitalized patients, particularly those receiving prolonged intensive care, postoperative patients, and in cancer and renal failure patients (81−84), in the elderly (85), and in the newborn (86,87).

To date, vitamin K deficiency has been diagnosed by prolonged coagulation test times which are normalized after administration of the vitamin. It is possible that such methods are not sensitive enough for diagnosing low degrees of vitamin K deficiency. Chemical assays for measuring plasma concentrations of phylloquinone have to be able to measure the predicted few ng/ml concentrations in normals and lower than ng/ml concentrations in patients with vitamin K deficiency (57). The availability of chemical assays for determining plasma concentrations of phylloquinone and the menaquinones will help define the clinical significance of vitamin K deficiency. One such method has been reported for phylloquinone (88), but none for the different menaquinones.

III. FUNCTION OF VITAMIN K

A. Vitamin K Epoxide and Hydroquinone

Vitamin K epoxide and vitamin K hydroquinone (Figure 3) are the two metabolites of vitamin K, which are thought to be involved in the biological function of the vitamin (i.e., carboxylation of glutamyl residues of precursor protein molecules). Vitamin K epoxide was isolated and identified in 1970 (89), and vitamin K hydroquinone was shown to be involved in vitamin K-dependent carboxylation in 1975 (90) and identified in microsomal preparations in 1980 (91).

1. *Vitamin K Epoxide*

Phylloquinone-2,3-epoxide (vitamin K_1 epoxide) is the major known metabolite of phylloquinone. It is seen primarily when vitamin K antagonists are present. It was first isolated and identified as a metabolite of phylloquinone from rat livers in studies where [^{14}C]phylloquinone was administered to rats that had previously received warfarin (89). Subsequently, warfarin-induced phylloquinone epoxide accumulation in rat livers has been extensively studied, and this metabolite has been thought to play a central role in both the mechanism of action of vitamin K and vitamin K antagonists. Phylloquinone epoxide has also been shown to accumulate in human plasma after the administration of [^{3}H]-phylloquinone to normal volunteers who had been administered warfarin (9,56,61,73). Indeed, the accumulation of phylloquinone epoxide in human plasma has been shown to be warfarin dose dependent (73). The epoxide has also been detected in the livers of rats not receiving warfarin (89), and in human plasma after administration of [^{3}H]phylloquinone in the absence of warfarin (47), although in very low quantities in both cases. Thus vitamin K_1 epoxide is a natural metabolite of vitamin K_1, which accumulates in the presence of warfarin and several other vitamin K antagonists. In humans, vitamin K_1 epoxide accumulation has been studied only after warfarin. In rats, it has been shown to occur after numerous vitamin K antagonists, although to different degrees: for example, after the coumarin derivatives warfarin, phenprocoumon, coumatetralyl, dicumarol, 4-hydroxycoumarin, and 3-phenyl-4-hydroxycoumarin, and indandione and its derivatives phenindione and diphenadione, and to a very small degree after the 2-chloro analog of vitamin K_1 and tetrachloro-4-pyridinol (92,93).

Vitamin K_1 epoxide appears to have the same biological activity as vitamin K_1 in stimulating prothrombin synthesis when given to vitamin K-deficient rats and chicks (94,95). It is thought that vitamin K_1 epoxide acts only after being converted to vitamin K_1. This is supported by studies using radiolabeled compounds showing that vitamin K epoxide is converted to vitamin K_1, a conversion that is inhibited by warfarin (95,96). Vitamin K_1 epoxide was essentially ineffective in counteracting a warfarin-induced anticoagulant effect unless it was administered 15 min before warfarin (95), and it was much less effective than vitamin K_1 in overcoming inhibition of prothrombin synthesis by phenindione (92), and did not counteract the anticoagulant effect of phenprocoumon and 3-(phenylbenzyl)-4-hydroxycoumarin (76). However, vitamin K_1 epoxide is as effective as vitamin K_1 in reversing the anticoagulant effect of chloro-K and tetrachloropyridinol (92), and vitamin K_1 epoxide has been reported to be effective in antagonizing the anticoagulant effect of dicumarol in humans and rats, although less effectively than vitamin K_1 (97–99). Vitamin K_1 epoxide is also effective against 3-phenyl-4-hydroxycoumarin (76). In general, these data sug-

VITAMIN K EPOXIDE   VITAMIN K HYDROQUINONE

Figure 3   Chemical structures of vitamin K epoxide and vitamin K hydroquinone.

gest that vitamin K_1 epoxide is only effective in reversing the inhibition of vitamin K-dependent carboxylation caused by compounds that do not cause or cause only a minor accumulation of the epoxide, such as chloro-K, tetrachloropyridinol, and 3-phenyl-4-hydroxycoumarin, but is not effective against the inhibition by compounds causing accumulation of the epoxide, such as warfarin, phenprocoumon, and phenindione.

Soon after vitamin K_1 epoxide was identified, it was postulated that it was a competitive inhibitor of vitamin K, and that warfarin exerted its anticoagulant effect by causing accumulation of the epoxide (95, 100). When rats pretreated with warfarin were given varying doses and ratios of vitamin K_1 and vitamin K_1 epoxide, high doses of vitamin K_1 epoxide appeared to inhibit the effectiveness of lower doses of vitamin K_1 (100). Subsequent studies in normal rats and warfarin-resistant rats, however, did not reveal any direct inhibiting effects of vitamin K_1 epoxide (101). It was later proposed that warfarin and other coumarin and indandione vitamin K antagonists worked by inhibiting the enzyme converting vitamin K epoxide back to vitamin K (i.e., vitamin K epoxide reductase), thus resulting in accumulation of vitamin K epoxide and lower concentration of vitamin K itself (100,102). Several studies in animals tried to establish specific ratios of vitamin K epoxide/vitamin K that would be associated with anticoagulant effect (75,76,92,96,102). However, results were inconsistent, both with respect to specific ratios and with respect to different drugs, and the precise role of phylloquinone epoxide in vitamin K function and metabolism remains unknown.

2. *Vitamin K Hydroquinone*

Vitamin K_1 hydroquinone, the reduced form of vitamin K_1, is thought to be the active form of the vitamin. This was first demonstrated when it was shown that the hydroquinone could replace the quinone form of the vitamin and NADH in driving the carboxylation reaction (90). Subsequently, most investigators have used the vitamin K_1 hydroquinone for initiating the vitamin K-dependent carboxylation in in vitro studies. Recently, vitamin K_1 hydroquinone was identified in a microsomal preparation, and it was shown that it could be formed from both vitamin K_1 and vitamin K_1 epoxide (91). In addition, it has been demonstrated that vitamin K_1 hydroquinone is the immediate substrate for vitamin K epoxides (103). It was also mentioned earlier that it has been assumed that the reduced forms of phylloquinone metabolites are the substrates for glucuronyl transferase (66). This suggests that vitamin K_1 hydroquinone, and possibly also hydroquinones of its metabolites, play a central role in the regulation of vitamin K function and metabolism.

B. Vitamin K Oxidoreductase

Vitamin K oxidoreductase [DT-diaphorase, NAD(P)H dehydrogenase, vitamin K reductase] has been thought to play an important role in the metabolism or function of vitamin K for more than 20 years. It appears safe to assume that vitamin K oxidoreductase is the same enzyme as DT-diaphorase. The major features of this enzyme are its ability to react with vitamins K and other quinones to form hydroquinones and its sensitivity to inhibition by coumarin and indandione vitamin K antagonists (104–108).

1. Distribution and Localization

DT-diaphorase is found in greatest quantities in the liver, but it is also found in several other organs, including the kidneys, brain, and Ehrlich ascites tumor cells (105,108). In the liver, it is found primarily in the soluble fraction of the cytoplasm, which contains about 90% of the cell enzyme activity, but it is also found in the endoplasmic reticulum and mitochondria (104,109). The cytoplasmic DT-diaphorase catalyzes the oxidation of NADH and NADPH at equal rates (hence its name, DT-diaphorase, from DPNH and TPNH, i.e., the old terminology for NADH and NADPH, respectively), but both the microsomal and mitochondrial enzymes exhibit greater activities with respect to NADH than NADPH (110). DT-diaphorase has been found in several animal species, including rats, cows, pigs, dogs, and rabbits (108). Considerable strain differences have been found in liver DT-diaphorase activity in rats, but the enzyme activity is apparently normal in warfarin-resistant rats (111–113), indicating that both the abnormally high vitamin K requirements and resistance to warfarin's effects in these rats is not due to abnormalities in vitamin K hydroquinone generation.

2. Requirements and Characteristics

This enzyme is a flavoprotein containing one molecule of FAD as a prosthetic group per molecule of enzyme, has a molecular weight of about

55,000, and is apparently comprised of two nonidentical subunits (108, 114,115). In its purified form, DT-diaphorase is activated by serum albumin, polyvinylpyrrolidone, certain nonionic detergents, such as Tween-20 and Triton X-100, and by neutral phospholipids, such as phosphatidylcholine, phosphatidylethanolamine, lysophosphatidylcholine, and lysophosphatidylethanolamine (104,110,116). Treatment with Tween 20, Triton X-100, and lysophosphatidylethanolamine is associated with diminished sensitivity to inhibition by dicumarol and warfarin and an apparent increased activity with respect to NAD(P)H, whereas treatment with phosphatidylcholine had the opposite effect (116,117), suggesting that the immediate phospholipid environment may have modulating effects on its activity. Various com， unds will accept electrons from DT-diaphorase, but the best electron acceptors are certain benzo- and naphthoquinones. Among the quinones, those without a side chain in the 3-position are the most active [e.g., 1,4-naphthoquinone, 1,2-naphthoquinone, 2-methyl-1,4-naphthoquinone (menadione), 2-ethyl-1,4-naphthoquinone, p-benzoquinone, and certain derivatives of benzoquinone] (104,105,108). The activity appears to decrease with increasing length of the side chain in the 3-position; for example, 2,3-dimethyl-1,4-naphthoquinone is less active than 2-methyl-1,4-naphthoquinone and 2-methyl-3-phytyl-1,4-napthoquinone (phylloquinone) has little activity (104,105,108). It is not known if the DT-diaphorase exhibits isomer-specific activity, for example, with respect to cis and trans phylloquinone. Substitution of a methyl group in the 2-position has little influence on the efficiency as electron acceptors. However, substitution of a hydroxy group in the 2- or 3-position renders quinones inactive as electron acceptors for DT-diaphorase (e.g., 2-hydroxy-1,4-naphthoquinone and 2-methyl-3-hydroxy-1,4-naphthoquinone are inactive) (105,110). Certain quinones are able to mediate electron transfer from DT-diaphorase to cytochrome c or coenzyme Q_{10}. In both cases, 2-methyl-1,4-naphthoquinone and 1,4-naphthoquinone are the best mediators (110). A different quinone, 2,6-dichlorophenolindophenol, is a potent electron acceptor and is indeed used in assays of the DT-diaphorase activity (105,110). Both 2,6-dichlorophenolindophenol and various quinones can inhibit DT-diaphorase activity when used in high concentrations (105). No reaction takes place when reduced menadione is used as a substrate and the oxidized pyridine nucleotides as electron acceptors, indicating that the equilibrium of the reaction is shifted strongly in favor of the reduced quinone (110).

DT-diaphorase can be induced by phenobarbital, 3-methylcholanthrene, and butylated hydroxytoluene (117,118). Treatment of rats with 3-methylcholanthrene causes a four- to five-fold increase in liver DT-diaphorase activity (118); this increase occurs both in the cytosolic and microsomal fractions of the enzyme. However, treatment with phenobarbital resulted in an increase of only 1.5- to 2-fold in activities of both the cytosolic and microsomal DT-diaphorase (118).

3. Role and Inhibitors

The precise role of DT-diaphorase in the metabolism and function of vitamin K has not been elucidated. As was mentioned earlier, it is currently thought that the reduced form of vitamin K_1, vitamin K_1 hydroquinone, is the active form of the vitamin, since the hydroquinone can replace the quinone form of the vitamin and NAD(P)H in driving the carboxylation reaction in in vitro rat liver microsomal preparations (90, 119—121). This suggests that a NAD(P)H-dependent enzymatic reduction of vitamin K_1 quinone to vitamin K_1 hydroquinone is a prerequisite for vitamin K-dependent carboxylation reactions. Indeed, recent studies using DT-diaphorase purified from rat liver by affinity chromatography have shown that it will restore carboxylation, when vitamin K_1 quinone and NADH are added, in a solubilized rat liver microsomal carboxylation system from which the DT-diaphorase has been selectively removed by the affinity chromatography method (115,121). Thus there remains little doubt that the DT-diaphorase is necessary for the activation and reduction of vitamin K_1 quinone, presumably to vitamin K_1 hydroquinone. It has also been proposed that vitamin K semiquinone is the active form of the vitamin and that it is formed by the DT-diaphorase (122). DT-diaphorase may also have other roles in the metabolism of vitamin K, since a functional relationship has been suggested between DT-diaphorase and the aryl hydrocarbon hydroxylase system (118).

DT-diaphorase is highly sensitive to inhibition by various vitamin K antagonists, particularly dicumarol, and numerous other compounds. These compounds can be divided into four groups, vitamin K antagonists (coumarin and indandione derivatives), sulfhydryl inhibitors, thyroid hormones and analogs, and others. These various inhibitors are listed in Table 2, which gives concentrations associated with 50% inhibition of DT-diaphorase activity (104,105,108,113,115,117). Most of the vitamin K antagonists are effective inhibitors at $10^{-5}-10^{-7}$ M concentrations. Compounds that have been shown not to inhibit DT-diaphorase activity include amobarbital, rotenone, antimycin A, EDTA, and Mg^{2+} and Mn^{2+} (105,110). The inhibition of DT-diaphorase activity, caused by the inhibitors listed in Table 2, is competitive with respect to the reduced pyridine nucleotides but noncompetitive with respect to menadione (110). It has been suggested that the different inhibitors of DT-diaphorase can be divided into two classes, acting on two different sites on the enzyme, in a synergetic fashion, one specific for the coumarin derivatives and another for the indandione derivatives (116). It remains to be established what role inhibition of DT-diaphorase activity plays in the mechanism of action of vitamin K antagonists.

C. Vitamin K Epoxidase

Vitamin K epoxidase catalyses the reaction of vitamin K to vitamin K epoxide. For the last 10 years, this enzyme or enzyme system has been thought to be intimately involved in the function of vitamin K. However, in spite of numerous similarities between epoxidation of vitamin K and vitamin K-dependent carboxylation of glutamyl residues, there is no definite proof that these reactions are functionally related.

1. Distribution and Localization

Vitamin K epoxidase is found in greatest quantities in the liver, where it shows increasing activity in fetal, newborn, to adult rat livers (51). It is also found in rat kidneys, placenta, spleen, and bone extracts, but it was not detected in lungs, heart, skeletal muscle, pancreas, brain, skin, and small intestine (51). In the rat liver, it is located primarily in the rough endoplasmic reticulum, which has been found to have two or four to five times greater epoxidase activity than the smooth endoplasmic reticulum (123–125), indicating that as much as 80% of the total enzyme activity may be present in the rough endoplasmic reticulum. It is primarily on the cisternal surface. Epoxidase activity is also found in significant amounts in the nuclear fraction (126).

2. Requirements and Characteristics

The vitamin K epoxidation reaction requires a microsomal fraction, which contains the enzyme activity, a soluble protein, a heat-stable soluble factor, and molecular oxygen (103,127). The soluble cytosolic components can be replaced by either NADH or NADPH, while NAD^+ and $NADP^+$ were inactive in the absence of cytosolic components (103). Epoxidation of vitamin K_1 is not supported by DTT. The requirement for a reduced pyridine nucleotide for vitamin K_1 epoxidation, as well as for vitamin K-dependent carboxylation, is eliminated if the vitamin is supplied as vitamin K_1 hydroquinone, and in the absence of NADH, vitamin K_1 epoxide is formed only from vitamin K_1 hydroquinone, not from the vitamin K quinone (103). This indicates that vitamin K hydroquinone is the substrate for the epoxidase and it has been suggested that the hydroquinone itself provides the reducing equivalents for the epoxidation (103,123). While the carboxylation reaction is dependent on HCO_3^- concentration, epoxidation of vitamin K_1 is not (103), indicating that epoxidation is independent of or precedes carboxylation.

The epoxidase is apparently geometric isomer specific, since the cis isomer of vitamin K_1 is poorly converted to vitamin K_1 epoxide, both in vivo and in vitro (128,129). Menaquinone-2 and menaquinone-3 were more readily epoxidazed than phylloquinone in rat liver microsomes, while menadione and 2-demethylphylloquinone are apparently not epoxidized (130). Menaquinone-2 and menaquinone-3 also were more active than phylloquinone in carboxylation (119,130). This suggests

Table 2 Concentrations of Several Inhibitors Associated with 50% Inhibition of Enzyme Activities Involved in Vitamin K-Dependent Carboxylation and Related Vitamin K Biotransformations

Inhibitors	Enzymes inhibited (IC-50[a], M)			
	DT-Diaphorase (104,105,108, 113,117b)	Epoxidase (103,113, 135,136b)	Epoxide reductase (113,138b)	Carboxylase (113,131,166,180, 183,192,201b)
Coumarin derivatives				
Coumarin	1×10^{-4}			
4-Hydroxycoumarin	2×10^{-6}	$> 5 \times 10^{-1}$		
Dicumarol[3,3-methylene-bis(4-hydroxycoumarin)]	$1 \times 10^{-7}-1 \times 10^{-9}$	9×10^{-4}		
3,3-Methylene-bis(4-methoxycoumarin)	5×10^{-7}			
3,3-Methylene-bis(4-chlorocoumarin)	1×10^{-6}			
3-Phenyl-4-hydroxycoumarin		8×10^{-4}		
Acenocoumarol	2×10^{-5}			
Phenprocoumon	1×10^{-5}	6×10^{-4}		
Ethyl biscoumacetate	$6 \times 10^{-5}-5 \times 10^{-6}$			
Warfarin	$9 \times 10^{-5}-2 \times 10^{-5}$	1×10^{-2}	$2 \times 10^{-6}-1 \times 10^{-6}$	$> 1 \times 10^{-4}-1 \times 10^{-6c}$
Coumatetralyl	2×10^{-6}	3×10^{-3}		

Indandione derivatives

Indandione		6 × 10^{-2}		
Phenindione (2-phenyl-1,3-indandione)	2 × 10^{-6}	7 × 10^{-4}		
2-Pivaloyl-1,3-indandione	3 × 10^{-5}			
2-(4'-chlorophenyl)-1,3-indandione	2 × 10^{-7}			
Others				
Tetrachloro-4-pyridinol	4 × 10^{-4}	3 × 10^{-5}—1 × 10^{-5}	7 × 10^{-4}	1 × 10^{-5}—1 × 10^{-6}
2-Chloro-3-phytyl-1,4-naphthoquinone		3 × 10^{-6}—5 × 10^{-7}		< 1 × 10^{-5}—1 × 10^{-6}
Chlorpromazine	2 × 10^{-3}—5 × 10^{-4}			
Quinacrine	2 × 10^{-3}			
1-Hydroxy-2-trifluoromethylimidazo-[4,5-b]-3-chloropyridine	1 × 10^{-3}	4 × 10^{-4}	2 × 10^{-3}	
Thyroid hormones/analogs				
Thyroxine	6 × 10^{-5}			
Triiodothyronine	6 × 10^{-5}			
Sulfhydryl inhibitors				
p-Chloromercuribenzoate	1 × 10^{-4}			< 1 × 10^{-3}
o-Iodosobenzoate	7 × 10^{-4}—4 × 10^{-4}			

aMost of the IC-50s are available in the literature, but some had to be calculated from tables or estimated from graphs.
bSome of the concentrations had to be calculated from the original publications.
cConsiderably higher concentrations in solubilized microsomal systems.

that an alkyl group has to be present in both the 2-position and the 3-position for vitamin K to be a substrate for epoxidase, that the specific side chain in the 3-position is important, and also that only those vitamins K which are converted to their respective epoxides will support carboxylation (130). However, neither group appears to be modified during either epoxidation or carboxylation (103).

Phylloquinone epoxidase activity increases when plasma prothrombin is lowered either after warfarin administration or by inducing vitamin K deficiency in rats (127). In warfarin-resistant rats, however, warfarin administration that caused a reduction in plasma prothrombin in normal rats but not in the warfarin-resistant rats did not change epoxidase activity (127). The activity of the enzyme returns rapidly to normal after vitamin K administration to hypoprothrombinemic rats (127). The cause for increased enzyme activity was found to reside in the microsomal fraction, not in the cytosolic fraction. The activity of the epoxidase was found to be directly related to the amount of prothrombin precursors in the liver (127). Phylloquinone epoxidase is induced by phenobarbital treatment in vitamin K-deficient rats (103). The epoxidase activity doubles after phenobarbital, which is almost as much an increase as in carboxylase activity after phenobarbital (103). A sex difference has been reported in epoxidase activity in rats, with normal male rats fed normal diet having higher epoxidase activity than female rats fed the same diet (127). It should be noted that vitamin K epoxidase activity is determined in the presence of warfarin, which is used to inhibit epoxidase reductase activity, allowing the accumulation of vitamin K epoxidase (103,124,127). Variable activity of the vitamin K epoxide reductase can therefore account for some differences in vitamin K epoxide accumulation.

3. Role and Inhibitors

The precise role of vitamin K epoxidase in vitamin K metabolism and function remains unclear. Ever since phylloquinone epoxide was identified, epoxide formation has been thought to be involved in vitamin K function, either directly or indirectly. Indeed, several similarities and relationships exist between the epoxidation of vitamin K and the vitamin K-dependent carboxylation of glutamyl residues (123). First, these two reactions have similar requirements, that is, require a microsomal fraction and cytosolic components, which can be replaced by reduced pyridine nucleotides or the hydroquinone form of the vitamin, and molecular oxygen (78,103,127,131). Second, both are primarily located on the rough endoplasmic reticulum (124–127). Third, there is a good relationship between the two enzyme activities; both are increased by vitamin K deficiency and warfarin administration (127,132). Fourth, both are induced by phenobarbital (103,123). Fifth, there is a direct relationship between both enzyme activities and the amount of prothrombin precursors present in the liver of hypoprothrombinemic rats (127,133), and immunospecific removal of prothrombin precursors from solubilized microsomes has been shown to lower vitamin K epoxidase activity (134). Sixth, there is an overall relationship in concentrations and order of compounds that inhibit epoxidase and carboxylase activities (e.g., chloro-K is a potent inhibitor and warfarin a weak inhibitor) (135). However, no definite proof exists that the epoxidation of vitamin K and vitamin K-dependent carboxylation of glutamyl residues are related at all. In spite of all the similarities, these two reactions might be coincidental. In fact, it has recently been shown that there is no strict coupling of vitamin K-dependent carboxylation and vitamin K epoxidation in solubilized rat liver microsomal fractions, although carboxylation was increased when epoxidase containing fraction was added (121). This has led to the speculation that these two reactions might have a common intermediate (e.g., the semiquinone form of vitamin K).

Phylloquinone epoxidase activity is inhibited by the noncoumarin vitamin K antagonists chloro-K and tetrachloropyridinol, both in vivo and in vitro (103,121,136). Chloro-K is about 30 times as potent an inhibitor as tetrachloropyridinol (136). Both of these compounds are active in warfarin-resistant rats (92). Several coumarin and indandione derivatives inhibit vitamin K epoxidation; 3-phenyl-4-hydroxycoumarin, dicumarol, phenprocoumon, and phenindione were much more potent inhibitors than warfarin, 4-hydroxycoumarin, coumatetralyl, and indandione (135). The various epoxidase inhibitors are listed in Table 2, which gives concentrations associated with 50% inhibition of epoxidase activity. Glutathione peroxidase inhibits both epoxidation of phylloquinone and carboxylation, while catalase was without effect (123). This suggests a role of a hydroperoxide form of vitamin K in these reactions. Vitamin K epoxidase activity is not inhibited by CO, KCN, or EDTA (127), and is not inhibited by metyrapone, aminoglutethimide, glutethimide, benzphetamine, or norbenzphetamine, which are known cytochrome P-450 inhibitors (103), or by menadione sodium bisulfate (121). Based on these data it has been concluded that epoxidation of vitamin K_1 is not accomplished by the cytochrome P-450-metabolizing enzyme system (103).

D. Vitamin K Epoxide Reductase

Vitamin K epoxide accumulation in the presence of warfarin and numerous other vitamin K antagonists is caused by inhibition of the enzyme that converts vitamin K epoxide back to vitamin K (i.e., vitamin K epoxide reductase). The different vitamin K antagonists, however, cause different degrees of vitamin K epoxide accumulation for any given degree of anticoagulant effect, as was mentioned earlier in relation to studies investigating the effects of these compounds on the ratios of vitamin K epoxide to vitamin K (75,76,92,96,102).

The vitamin K epoxide reductase activity appears to be located primarily in the microsomal fraction, with little or no activity in the cytosolic fraction and no activity in nuclei or mitochondria (125,137). Vitamin K epoxide reductase activity is found both in the rough and smooth endoplasmic reticulum, with more in the rough endoplasmic reticulum; it is primarily located on the cisternal surface of the membrane (125,126).

The enzyme activity requires the presence of sulfhydryl reagents (137,138). The vitamin K epoxide reductase activity is not supported by NADH or NADPH, but is supported by DTT (137−139). Lipoic acid can also serve as a reductant in the conversion of the epoxide to the quinone (139), but the biological reductant is unknown. Cis and trans vitamin K epoxide are reduced equally to vitamin K_1 quinone (137), indicating that there is no geometric isomer specificity with respect to the substrate. However, in vivo studies in rats showed that there was more vitamin K epoxide accumulation in plasma after S(−) phenprocoumon and S(−) warfarin, the more active enantiomorphs, than after R(+) phenprocoumon and R(+) warfarin, indicating a steroselective difference with respect to the inhibitors (140).

Older rats were more sensitive to the vitamin K antagonists phenprocoumon (141) and warfarin (142). In the case of the phenprocoumon, this was found to be associated with increased maximal accumulation of vitamin K epoxide in the older rats (141). Older patients require smaller doses of oral anticoagulants than did younger patients (143,144). This suggests that vitamin K epoxide reductase activity changes with age and thereby results in greater sensitivity to warfarin and other vitamin K antagonists. It is not known if vitamin K epoxide reductase is induced by phenobarbital or 3-methylcholanthrene.

Warfarin-resistant rats have diminished vitamin K epoxide reductase activity (113,145,146), and they need 10−30 times higher or up to 70 times higher warfarin concentrations to cause similar inhibition as in normal rats (102,113,139). This suggests that the genetic defect is an abnormality in this enzyme. This strain of rats has also been shown to have diminished binding of warfarin to a specific microsomal binding protein (147). This protein is found in both the smooth and rough endoplasmic reticulum and has a molecular weight of 32,000. It exhibits preferential binding toward S(−) warfarin and warfarin is displaced by phylloquinone (147). It is presently not clear if this protein is related to vitamin K epoxide reductase. The warfarin-resistant rats have increased requirements of vitamin K (148,149). The same is found in hereditary warfarin resistance in humans (150). In the warfarin-resistant rats, chloro-K and coumatetralyl are effective vitamin K antagonists (149,151,152).

Vitamin K epoxide reductase is inhibited by warfarin in low concentration (139,153), while chloro-K and tetrachloropyridinol have small effect on epoxide reductase activity (154). The concentrations of these inhibitors that are associated with 50% inhibition are given in Table 2. It is widely accepted that the mechanism of action of most vitamin K antagonists, including warfarin, is most likely by inhibition of vitamin K epoxide reductase, which would result in lower effective concentrations of the vitamin (10,155). This theory, however, has not been unequivocally proven.

E. Vitamin K-Dependent Carboxylase

Various systems have been used to investigate the vitamin K-dependent formation of prothrombin and other vitamin K-dependent clotting factors and the inhibition of their formation by vitamin K antagonists. These include isolated perfused rat livers (156,157), hepatoma cells (158,159), and three different cell-free systems: postmitochondrial supernatant suspension, washed unsolubilized microsomes, and microsomes solubilized with detergents (8,10). Significant differences exist between the different cell-free systems with respect to vitamin K requirements and sensitivity to vitamin K antagonists; vitamin K requirements increase in the microsomal systems and warfarin sensitivity decreases with solubilization of microsomes. These and other characteristics of the microsomal systems have often made comparisons between studies difficult, and it is not inconceivable that different enzymes involved in vitamin K function and metabolism may be rate limiting in different systems, thereby making interpretation difficult.

1. Distribution and Localization

Vitamin K-dependent carboxylase activity has been found in numerous tissues other than the liver, including the lung (160), kidney (161, 162), bone (163), placenta (164), and spleen (161), and a Gla-containing protein has been found in atherosclerotic plaques (165). The biological roles of these vitamin K-dependent proteins are presently unknown, although the vitamin K-dependent protein found in bones, osteocalcin, appears to be necessary for new bone development. The vitamin K-dependent carboxylase, like other enzymes involved in vitamin K function, is found primarily in the rough endoplasmic reticulum. The rough endoplasmic reticulum has been found to have about four to six times greater carboxylase activity than the smooth endoplasmic reticulum, indicating that about 80−90% of the total enzyme activity is present in the rough endoplasmic reticulum (125,126,166−168). The carboxylase is apparently tightly bound to the endoplasmic reticular membrane, and studies using trypsin and detergents have demonstrated that the enzyme is located on the cisternal surface of the endoplasmic reticulum, like the epoxidase and the epoxide reductase (125,126,166,167). The biological substrate for the vitamin K-dependent carboxylase, acarboxyprothrombin or prothrombin precursors in the case of prothrombin,

is found primarily within the rough endoplasmic reticulum where it is
apparently bound to the cisternal surface (123,127,166−170). Prothrombin, however, is primarily found in the smooth endoplasmic reticulum (167). After warfarin treatment, acarboxyprothrombin is found
both in the rough and smooth endoplasmic reticulum, and this is
though to be due to spilling of the precursor molecules into the non-
ribosomal-containing endoplasmic reticulum. Studies on vitamin K-dependent carboxylation have been aided by the development of solubilized microsomal carboxylase systems (171,172) and the use of artificial
peptide substrates containing glutamic acids (173−177), of which the
pentapeptides Phe-Leu-Glu-Glu-Val, Phe-Leu-Glu-Glu-Ile, and Phe-
Leu-Glu-Glu-Leu are the most common. It appears that it is primarily
the first glutamyl residue that is carboxylated (178,179).

2. Requirements and Characteristics

For carboxylation of its biological substrates or synthetic peptide substrates, the vitamin K-dependent carboxylase requires cytosolic components (180,181), which can be replaced by the reduced pyridine nucleotides NADH or NADPH (78,131). The use of NADH in microsomal
systems is associated with similar or slightly greater carboxylation than
is seen with NADPH. It is possible that this difference in rates of carboxylation, depending on whether NADH or NADPH is used, is related
to the greater activity of microsomal vitamin K oxidoreductase when
NADH is used than NADPH (110). The oxidized cofactors, NAD^+ and
$NADP^+$, are ineffective in stimulating carboxylation in the presence of
phylloquinone (131). Optimal carboxylation was found to take place in
the presence of 1.5 mM NADH (131,182). DTT stimulated carboxylation
effectively; in fact, it promotes carboxylation faster than NAD(P)H
(78), presumably by enzymatic or nonenzymatic reduction of vitamin
K_1 quinone to the hydroquinone or other active form. At low concentrations of the hydroquinone, the addition of NADH markedly stimulates
carboxylation of prothrombin precursors, but at higher concentrations
of hydroquinone, the addition of NADH has little effect (131). This
suggests that the hydroquinone undergoes biotransformation, perhaps
associated with carboxylation, but can be recycled to the hydroquinone in the presence of NADH. The hydroquinone is slightly more active
in the present of DTT (78,175), also suggesting a recycling of the vitamin by a DTT-medicated reaction. DTT stimulates protein and peptide
carboxylations more when the vitamin K_1 quinone and NADH are used
than when the hydroquinone is used alone (175).

  In addition to vitamin K and reducing equivalents, the carboxylase
requires bicarbonate and molecular oxygen (78,131,183). The optimum
pH is 7.6−7.9 (178). Incorporation of radiolabeled bicarbonate into
prothrombin has been demonstrated in rats both in vivo and in vitro
(180,184). In vitro, the carboxylation reaction is dependent on bicar-

bonate concentration (131). The active species of "CO_2" which becomes the carboxyl group has been shown to be CO_2 (185). The carboxylation is apparently not associated with any electrical or chemical transmembrane gradient, since it was not inhibited by carbonylcyanide-m-chlorophenylhydrazone (167). Neither ATP (or an ATP-generating system) nor biotin is required for the carboxylation reaction (131,183,185,186). Biotin is a known carboxyl group carrier. Pyridoxal phosphate, which is involved in decarboxylation reactions, was shown to stimulate carboxylation of a peptide substrate, but not of the endogenous substrates, and to be due to binding of vitamin B_6 to the enzyme, and is not thought to be of physiological significance (187,188). Neither biotin nor vitamin B_6-deficient rats exhibit hypoprothrombinemia or reduced vitamin K-dependent carboxylase activity, respectively (185,186, 188). The available evidence therefore suggests that vitamin K is not involved in CO_2 transfer (e.g., as a CO_2 carrier), but that the vitamin functions in labilizing the hydrogen on the γ-carbon of the glutamyl residue so that some form of CO_2 may attack (179,189). In this respect it is interesting to note that the γ-carbon-hydrogen bond cleavage can be dissociated from carboxylation (190,191). The reason for the requirement for molecular oxygen in the carboxylation reaction is not known. It has been demonstrated that neither singlet oxygen, hydroxyl radical, nor superoxide is involved in the reaction (189). However, it appears that some type of vitamin K hydroperoxide is involved in the carboxylation since glutathione peroxidase inhibits both carboxylation and epoxidation (123).

The naphthoquinone ring system in vitamin K is essential for carboxylation activity. This is illustrated by two quinones, phytylubiquinone and phytylplastoquinone, both of which lack the benzenoid ring of the naphthoquinone structure and have no activity (78). The carboxylase exhibits geometric isomer specificity since only the trans isomer of phylloquinone is active, while the cis isomer is inactive (78). The methyl group in the 2-position is important since 2-demethylphylloquinone is essentially inactive (78). Menadione in the presence of NADH or menadione hydroquinone has essentially no activity (78,131, 192). Saturation of the 2'-3' double bond in the phytyl side chain of phylloquinone has a negligible effect on activity. The menaquinones containing one, two, three, and four isoprenyl units on their 3-position side chain have been shown to have essentially the same activity as phylloquinone in postmitochondrial supernatant preparations (193). However, in a microsomal system, menaquinone-2 and menaquinone-3 were found to have much greater activity than phylloquinone, while menaquinone-1 was essentially inactive (78). A possible explanation for this discrepancy are different structure-activity relationships between the cytosolic DT-diaphorase, on the one hand, and the vitamin K-dependent carboxylase, on the other, with respect to vitamins K. The DT-diaphor-

ase shows greatest activity toward quinones without a side chain in the
3-position, while the opposite appears to be true for the carboxylase.
Studies in a solubilized microsomal system on a variety of thioethers of
menadione in the 3-position have illustrated that a polyprenyl side
chain in the 3-position is not essential for carboxylation, but that this
position does need to be filled by an uncharged, relatively hydrophobic
group (192).

The activity of rat liver microsomal vitamin K-dependent carboxylase
appears to be dependent on the amount of prothrombin precursors
present in the microsomes and therefore directly related to the degree
of hypoprothrombinemia of the animals (126,133). Warfarin treatment
increases markedly the apparent activity of the carboxylase, but pretreatment of vitamin K-deficient or warfarin-treated rats with phylloquinone 15 min before sacrifice markedly reduces protein carboxylase
activity, presumably because of reduction in prothrombin precursor
levels, but has little influence on the high activity of peptide carboxylation (126). This increase in carboxylase activity after vitamin K deficiency or warfarin treatment has been demonstrated in several animal
species other than the rat, including hamster, guinea pig, mouse, rabbit, pig, and calf (194). Available data indicate that the carboxylase
has a rapid turnover and that the observed increase in enzyme activity
is a true increase in amount of enzyme (195). Apparent carboxylase
activity can also be increased by the addition of prothrombin precursors
and partially decarboxylated prothrombin (196) and of peptide substrate (134). Carboxylase activity is also increased after phenobarbital
treatment, indicating enzyme induction (123). Steroid hormones affect
the formation of vitamin K-dependent clotting factors; estrogens, progesterone and pituitary hormones increase, but androgens inhibit their
formation (197–199). These changes appear to be due both to changes
in synthesis of precursor proteins and in carboxylase activity. It has
been concluded that the microsomal cytochrome P-450 system is not involved in the carboxylation reaction, since several cytochrome P-450 inhibitors, such as SKF-525A, aminoglutethimide, metyrapone, quina-
crine, and 7,8-benzoflavone, were ineffective as inhibitors of hydro-
quinone-initiated carboxylation (192). However, these studies did not
establish if cytochrome P-450 was active in this system. Several copper
complexes, such as copper penicillamine, copper aspirinate, and copper
tyrosine, inhibit carboxylase activity, and it has been suggested that
copper complexes are inhibiting superoxide anion formation (187,200).

3. Inhibitors

The vitamin K-dependent carboxylase is effectively inhibited by chloro-
K, both in unsolubilized and solubilized microsomal systems, while warfarin is a potent inhibitor of carboxylase activity in unsolubilized systems, but is a weak inhibitor of carboxylase activity in solubilized mi-

crosomal systems. When vitamin K_1 quinone is used, with NADH or in postmitochondrial supernatant, chloro-K inhibits carboxylation or prothrombin synthesis over 80% in concentrations of $10^{-5}-10^{-6}$ M (131,180, 183,201). The hydroquinone form of chloro-K appears to be equally effective as an inhibitor (131). Tetrachloropyridinol is also an effective carboxylase activity inhibitor, with IC-50 in the range $10^{-5}-10^{-6}$ M (113,175,201). Warfarin inhibits carboxylation effectively in unsolubilized microsomal systems at low vitamin K concentrations but is rather ineffective at high vitamin concentrations (131). It was equally effective as an inhibitor when vitamin K_1 quinone and NADH or vitamin K_1 hydroquinone were used, suggesting that warfarin action is not on the reduction of the vitamin to the hydroquinone (131). In the unsolubilized systems, warfarin exhibits 15-50% inhibition in concentrations of $10^{-4}-10^{-6}$ M (138,166,201). In solubilized microsomal systems, however, it requires concentrations in the low mM range for inhibition, but dicumarol is apparently slightly more effective (192). The concentrations of these and other carboxylase inhibitors associated with significant inhibition are listed in Table 2. Numerous vitamin K analogs are inhibitors of vitamin K-dependent carboxylation when initiated by vitamin K_1 hydroquinone, such as menadione, 1,4-naphthoquinone, 2,3-dichloro-1, 4-naphthoquinone, 2-methyl-5-hydroxyl-1, 4-naphthoquinone, 2-methoxy-1, 4-naphthoquinone, and duroquinone (192). The sulfhydryl inhibitor p-hydroxymercuribenzoate almost totally inhibits carboxylation at 10^{-3} M concentration, both in solubilized and unsolubilized systems, and both when the quinone and hydroquinone forms of the vitamin are used (78,166,175,182,192). This suggests that the carboxylase system contains an essential sulfhydryl.

In summary, the vitamin K-dependent carboxylase is located on the cisternal surface of the rough endoplasmic reticulum, as are two other enzymes thought to be involved in vitamin K function, vitamin K epoxidase and vitamin K epoxide reductase. The fourth enzyme involved in vitamin metabolism, vitamin K oxidoreductase (DT-diaphorase), it also located on endoplasmic reticulum, but is found primarily in the cytoplasm. Figure 4 schematically depicts these enzymes, their function, and the formation by ribosomes and subsequent carboxylation of a vitamin K-dependent clotting factor. As has been reviewed in this chapter, each enzyme activity can be inhibited by various vitamin K antagonists, and several theories have been offered to explain the mechanism of action of these inhibitors (8,10,60,155). At present, however, no one theory can be considered compatible with all the available data. Increased knowledge of the molecular events involved in this unique oxygen-dependent carboxylation and of the different vitamin K biotransformation steps, their relative rates and sensitivities to different inhibitors, should lead to a clearer understanding of their pharmacological action.

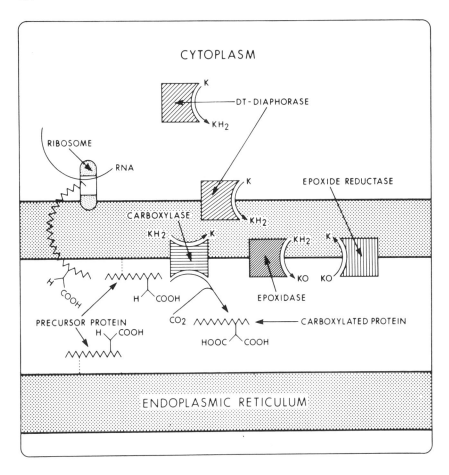

Figure 4 Schematic representation of enzymes involved in vitamin K-dependent carboxylation of clotting factors and related vitamin K biotransformations. K, vitamin K; KH_2 vitamin K hydroquinone; KO, vitamin K epoxide; RNA, ribonucleic acids. The precursor proteins, containing the glutamyl residues to be carboxylated, are sythesized by the ribosomes located on the outside of the rough endoplasmic reticulum. Each protein subsequently passes into the cisternal space of the endoplasmic reticulum, where it is tightly bound to the membrane. The three major enzymes involved in vitamin K function are all located on the cisternal surface of the endoplasmic reticular membrane. The respective functions of these enzymes—vitamin K-dependent carboxylation of several glutamyl residues on each protein and vitamin K biotransformations are indicated by arrows. It is assumed that vitamin K hydroquinone is transformed to some form of vitamin K during carboxylation.

ACKNOWLEDGMENTS

Supported in part by NIH Grants HL-24343 and NS-06233, Thorir D. Bjornsson is a recipient of a Pharmaceutical Manufacturers Association Foundation Development Award in Clinical Pharmacology.

REFERENCES

1. Dam, H. (1935). The antihaemorrhagic vitamin of the chick. *Biochem. J. 29*:1273-1285.
2. Stenflo, J., Fernlund, P., Egan, W., and Roepstorff, P. (1974). Vitamin K dependent modification of glutamic acid residues in prothrombin. *Proc. Natl. Acad. Sci. USA 71*:2730-2733.
3. Nelsestuen, G. L., Zytkovitz, T. H., and Howard, J. B. (1974). The mode of action of vitamin K. Identification of γ-carboxyglutamic acid as a component of prothrombin. *J. Biol. Chem. 249*:6347-6350.
4. Magnusson, S., Sottrup-Jensen, L., Petersen, T. E., Morris, H. R., and Dell, A. (1974). Primary structure of the vitamin K-dependent part of prothrombin. *FEBS Lett. 44*:189-193.
5. Almquist, H. J. (1975). The early history of vitamin K. *Am. J. Clin. Nutr. 28*:656-659.
6. van der Meer, J., Hemker, H. C., and Loeliger, E. A. (1968). I. The literature on vitamin K_1. *Thromb. Diath. Haemorrh. Suppl. 29*:1-11.
7. Suttie, J. W. (1978). Vitamin K. In *Handbook of Lipid Research. 2. The Fat-Soluble Vitamins*, H. F. DeLuca, Ed., Plenum Press, New York, pp. 211-277.
8. Olson, R. E., and Suttie, J. W. (1977). Vitamin K and γ-carboxyglutamate biosynthesis. In *Vitamins and Hormones. Advances in Research and Applications*, P. L. Munson, E. Diczfaluzy, J. Glover, and R. E. Olson, Eds., Academic Press, New York, pp. 59-108.
9. Shearer, M. J., McBurney, A., and Barkhan, P. (1974). Studies on the absorption and metabolism of phylloquinone (vitamin K_1) in man. *Vitam. Horm. 32*:513-542.
10. Suttie, J. W. (1980). Mechanism of action of vitamin K: synthesis of γ-carboxyglutamic acid. *CRC Crit. Rev. Biochem. 8*: 191-223.
11. Jackson, C. M., and Suttie, J. W. (1977). Recent developments in understanding the mechanism of vitamin K and vitamin K-antagonist drug action and the consequences of vitamin K action in blood coagulation. In *Progress in Hematology*, Vol. 10, E. B. Brown, Ed., Grune & Stratton, New York, pp. 333-359.

12. Stenflo, J. (1978). Vitamin K, prothrombin, and γ-carboxyglutamic acid. *Adv. Enzymol. Relat. Areas Mol. Biol.* 46:1-31.

13. Shearer, M. J., Barkhan, P., and Webster, G. R. (1970). Absorption and excretion of an oral dose of tritiated vitamin K_1 in man. *Br. J. Haematol.* 18:297-308.

14. Blomstrand, R., and Forsgren, L. (1968). Vitamin K_1-^{3}H in man. Its intestinal absorption and transport in the thoracic duct lymph. *Int. Z. Vitaminforsch.* 38:45-64.

15. Hollander, D. (1973). Vitamin K_1 absorption by everted intestinal sacs of the rat. *Am. J. Physiol.* 225:360-364.

16. Hollander, D., Rim, E., and Muralidhara, K. S. (1977). Vitamin K_1 intestinal absorption in vivo: influence of luminal contents or transport. *Am. J. Physiol.* 232:E69-E74.

17. Hollander, D., and Rim, E. (1978). Effect of luminal constituents on vitamin K_1 absorption into thoracic duct lymph. *Am. J. Physiol.* 234:E54-E59.

18. Ockner, R. K., and Manning, J. A. (1974). Fatty acid binding protein in small intestine. Identification, isolation, and evidence for its role in cellular fatty acid transport. *J. Clin. Invest.* 54:326-338.

19. Hollander, D., Kielb, M., and Rim, E. (1978). Diurnal rhythmicity of absorption of a lipid compound (vitamin K-1) in vivo in the rat. *Dig. Dis. Sci.* 23:1125-1128.

20. Hollander, D., Rim, E., and Ruble, P. E. (1977). Vitamin K_2 colonic and ileal in vivo absorption: bile, fatty acids, and pH effects on transport. *Am. J. Physiol.* 233:E124-E129.

21. Hollander, D., and Rim, E. (1976). Vitamin K_2 absorption by rat everted small intestinal sacs. *Am. J. Physiol.* 321:415-419.

22. Hollander, D., Muralidhara, K. S., and Rim, E. (1976). Colonic absorption of bacterially synthesized vitamin K_2 in the rat. *Am. J. Physiol.* 230:251-255.

23. Hollander, D., and Truscott, T. C. (1974). Mechanism and site of vitamin K-3 small intestinal transport. *Am. J. Physiol.* 226:1516-1522.

24. Hollander, D., and Truscott, T. C. (1974). Colonic absorption of vitamin K-3. *J. Lab. Clin. Med.* 83:648-656.

25. Matschiner, J. T., Hsia, S. L., and Doisy, E. A. (1967). Effect of indigestible oils on vitamin K deficiency in the rat. *J. Nutr.* 91:299-302.

26. Elliott, M. C., Isaacs, B., and Ivy, A. C. (1940). Production of prothrombin deficiency and response to vitamins A, D, and K. *Proc. Soc. Exp. Biol. Med.* 43:240-245.

27. Thoma, K., Pfaff, G., and Quiring, K. (1978). Biological effect of phytonadione administered orally as oily solution or solubilized with non-ionic surfactant in rats. *J. Pharm. Pharmacol.* 30:270-272.

28. Matschiner, J. T., Amelotti, J. M., and Doisy, E. A. (1967). Mechanism of the effect of retinoic acid and squalene on vitamin K deficiency in the rat. *J. Nutr. 91*:303-306.
29. Jolly, D. W., Craing, C., and Nelson, T. E. (1977). Estrogen and prothrombin synthesis: effect of estrogen on absorption of vitamin K_1. *Am. J. Physiol. 232*:H12-H17.
30. Javert, C. T., and Macri, C. (1941). Prothrombin concentration and mineral oil. *Am. J. Obstet. Gynecol. 42*:409-414.
31. Busse, K. (1968). Schwere Blutgerinnungsstörung bei Laxantienabusus. *Dtsch. Med. Wochenschr. 13*:653-655.
32. Fingl, E. (1980). Laxtives and cathartics. In *Goodman and Gilman's The Pharmacological Basis of Therapeutics*, 6th ed., A. G. Gilman, L. S. Goodman, and A. Gilman, Eds., Macmillan, New York, pp. 1002-1012.
33. Visintine, R. E., Michaelis, G. D., Fukayama, G., Conklin, J., and Kinsell, L. W. (1961). Xanthomatous biliary cirrhosis treated with cholestyramine. *Lancet 2*:341-343.
34. Scott, R. B., Lee, M., Mallinson, C. N., and Shearer, M. J. (1973). Failure to demonstrate a bile salt-independent pathway for absorption of vitamin K_1 in man. *Gut 14*:825.
35. West, J., and Lloyd, J. K. (1975). The effect of cholestyramine on intestinal absorption. *Gut 16*:93-98.
36. Poole, C. J. F. (1958). The effect of hypervitaminosis A on blood coagulation in the rat. *Q. J. Exp. Physiol. 43*:427-437.
37. Woodward, B., and March, B. E. (1974). Effects of vitamin A on blood coagulation and clot-lysis times. *Can. J. Physiol. Pharmacol. 52*:984-990.
38. Rao, G. H., and Mason, K. E. (1975). Antisterility and antivitamin K activity of d-α-tocopheryl hydroquinone in the vitamin E-deficient female rat. *J. Nutr. 105*:495-498.
39. Corrigan, J. J., and Marcus, F. I. (1974). Coagulopathy associated with vitamin E ingestion. *JAMA 230*:1300-1301.
40. Schrogie, J. J. (1975). Coagulopathy and fat soluble vitamins. *JAMA 232*:19.
41. Horwitt, M. K. (1976). Vitamin E: a reexamination. *Am. J. Clin. Nutr. 29*:569-578.
42. Beeson, P. B., McDermott, W., and Wyngaarden, J. B., Eds. (1979). *Cecil Loeb Textbook of Medicine*, W. B. Saunders, Philadelphia, Part XVI.
43. Mandel, H. G., and Cohn, V. H. (1980). Fat-soluble vitamins. Vitamins A, K, and E. In *Goodman and Gilman's The Pharmacological Basis of Therapeutics*, 6th ed., A. G. Gilman, L. S. Goodman, and A. Gilman, Eds., Macmillan, New York, pp. 1583-1601.
44. Udall, J. A. (1970). Don't use the wrong vitamin K. *Calif. Med. 112*:65-67.

45. Griminger, P. (1966). Biological activity of the various vitamin K forms. *Vitam. Horm.* 24:605-618.
46. Caballero, F. M., and Buchanan, G. R. (1980). Abetalipoproteinemia presenting as severe vitamin K deficiency. *Pediatrics* 65:161-163.
47. Bjornsson, T. D., Meffin, P. J., and Blaschke, T. F. (1976). Unpublished observations.
48. Wiss, O., and Gloor, H. (1966). Absorption, distribution, storage, and metabolites of vitamin K and related quinones. *Vitamin. Horm.* 24:575-586.
49. Thierry, M. J., and Suttie, J. W. (1971). Effect of warfarin and the chloro analog of vitamin K_1 on phylloquinone metabolism. *Arch. Biochem. Biophys.* 147:430-435.
50. Bell, R. A. (1980). Vitamin K dependent carboxylation in lung microsomes. In *Vitamin K Metabolism and Vitamin K-Dependent Proteins*, J. W. Suttie, Ed., University Park Press, Baltimore, Md., pp. 286-293.
51. Friedman, P. A., and Smith, M. W. (1977). A survey of rat tissues for phylloquinone epoxidase activity. *Biochem. Pharmacol.* 26:804-805.
52. Konishi, T., Baba, S., and Stone, H. (1973). Whole-body autoradiographic study of vitamin K distribution in rat. *Chem. Pharm. Bull.* 21:220-224.
53. Thierry, M. J., and Suttie, J. W. (1969). Distribution and metabolism of menadiol diphosphate in the rat. *J. Nutr.* 97: 512-516.
54. Nyquist, S. E., Matschiner, J. T., and Morre, D. J. D. (1971). Distribution of vitamin K among rat liver cell fractions. *Biochim. Biophys. Acta* 244:645-649.
55. Matschiner, J. T., and Bell, R. G. (1972). Metabolism and vitamin K activity of cis phylloquinone in rats. *J. Nutr.* 102: 625-630.
56. Bjornsson, T. D., Meffin, P. J., Swezey, S. E., and Blaschke, T. F. (1979). Effects of clofibrate and warfarin alone and in combination on the disposition of vitamin K_1. *J. Pharmacol. Exp. Ther.* 210:322-326.
57. Bjornsson, T. D., Meffin, P. J., Swezey, S. E., and Blaschke, T. F. (1980). Disposition and turnover of vitamin K_1 in man. In *Vitamin K Metabolism and Vitamin K-Dependent Proteins*, J. W. Suttie, Ed., University Park Press, Baltimore, Md., pp. 328-332.
58. Shearer, M. J., Mallinson, C. N., Webster, G. R., and Barkhan, P. (1972). Clearance from plasma and excretion in urine, faces, and bile of an intravenous dose of tritiated vitamin K_1 in man. *Br. J. Haematol.* 22:579-588.

59. Duello, T. J., and Matschiner, J. T. (1972). Characterization of vitamin K from human liver. *J. Nutr.* *102*:331-335.
60. O'Reilly, R. A. (1976). Vitamin K and the oral anticoagulant drugs. *Annu. Rev. Med.* *27*:245-261.
61. Shearer, M. J., McBurney, A., and Barkhan, P. (1973). Effect of warfarin anticoagulation on vitamin K_1 metabolism in man. *Br. J. Haematol.* *24*:471-479.
62. Forsgren, L. (1969). Studies on the intestinal absorption of labelled fat-soluble vitamins and fatty acids in the thoracic-duct in man. Clinical investigations with special reference to biliary obstruction. Dissertation, Kungl. Boktryckeriet, P. A. Norstedt and Söner, Stockholm.
63. Losito, R., Owen, C. A., and Flock, E. V. (1968). Metabolic studies of vitamin K_1-^{14}C and menadione-^{14}C in the normal and hepatectomized rats. *Thromb. Diath. Haemorrh.* *19*:383-388.
64. Taggart, W. V., and Matschiner, J. T. (1969). Metabolism of menadione-6,7-^3H in the rat. *Biochemistry* *8*:1141-1146.
65. Shearer, M. J., and Barkhan, P. (1973). Studies on the metabolites of phylloquinone (vitamin K_1) in the urine of man. *Biochim. Biophys. Acta* *297*:300-312.
66. McBurney, A., Shearer, M. J., and Barkhan, P. (1980). Preparative isolation and characterization of the urinary aglycones of vitamin K_1 (phylloquinone) in man. *Biochem. Med.* *24*:250-267.
67. Watanabe, M., Toyoda, M., Imada, I., and Morimoto, H. (1974). Ubiquinone and related compounds. XXVI. The urinary metabolites of phylloquinone and α-tocopherol. *Chem. Pharm. Bull.* *22*:176-182.
68. Hoskin, F. C. A., Spinks, J. W. T., and Jaques, L. B. (1954). Urinary excretion products of menadione (vitamin K_3). *Can. J. Biochem. Physiol.* *32*:240-250.
69. Losito, R., Owen, C. A., and Flock, E. V. (1967). Metabolism of ^{14}C-menadione. *Biochemistry* *6*:62-68.
70. Imada, I., Watanabe, M., Matsumoto, N., and Morimoto, H. (1970). Metabolism of ubiquinone-7. *Biochemistry* *9*:2870-2878.
71. Thompson, R. M., Gerber, N., Seibert, R. A., and Desiderio, M. (1972). Identification of 2-methyl-1,4-naphthohydroquinone monoglucuronide as a metabolite of 2-methyl-1,4-naphthoquinone (menadione) in rat bile. *Res. Commun. Chem. Pathol. Pharmacol.* *4*:543-552.
72. Richert, D. A. (1951). Studies on the detoxification of 2-methyl-1,4-naphthoquinone in rabbits. *J. Biol. Chem.* *189*:763-768.
73. Shearer, M. J., McBurney, A., Breckenridge, A. M., and Barkhan, P. (1977). Effect of warfarin on the metabolism of

phylloquinone (vitamin K$_1$): dose-response relationships in man. *Clin. Sci. Mol. Med.* 52:621-630.

74. McBurney, A., Shearer, M. J., and Barkhan, P. (1978). Changes in the urinary metabolites of phylloquinone (vitamin K$_1$) in man following therapeutic anticoagulation with warfarin. *Biochem. Pharmacol.* 27:273-278.

75. Caldwell, P. T., Ren, P., and Bell, R. G. (1974). Warfarin and metabolism of vitamin K$_1$. *Biochem. Pharmacol.* 23:3353-3362.

76. Sadowski, J. A., and Suttie, J. W. (1974). Mechanism of action of coumarins. Significance of vitamin K epoxide. *Biochemistry* 13:3696-3699.

77. Knauer, T. E., Siegfried, C., Willingham, A. K., and Matschiner, J. T. (1975). Metabolism and biological activity of cis and trans phylloquinone in the rat. *J. Nutr.* 105:1519-1524.

78. Friedman, P. A., and Shia, M. (1976). Some characteristics of a vitamin K-dependent carboxylating system from rat liver microsomes. *Biochem. Biophys. Res. Commun.* 70:647-654.

79. Lowenthal, J., and Rivera, G. M. V. (1979). Comparison of the activity of the cis and trans isomer of vitamin K$_1$ in vitamin K-deficient and coumarin anticoagulant-pretreated rats. *J. Pharmacol. Exp. Ther.* 209:330-333.

80. Shearer, M. J., Allan, V., Maroon, Y., and Barkhan, P. (1980). Nutritional aspects of vitamin K in the human. In *Vitamin K Metabolism and Vitamin K-Dependent Proteins*, J. W. Suttie, Ed., University Park Press, Baltimore, Md., pp. 317-327.

81. Pineo, G. F., Gallus, A. S., and Hirsh, J. (1973). Unexpected vitamin K deficiency in hospitalized patients. *Can. Med. Assoc. J.* 109:880-883.

82. Ham, J. M. (1971). Hypoprothrombinaemia in patients undergoing prolonged intensive care. *Med. J. Aust.* 22:716-718.

83. Colvin, B. T., and Lloyd, M. J. (1977). Severe coagulation defect due to a dietary deficiency of vitamin K. *J. Clin. Pathol.* 30:1147-1148.

84. Ansell, J. E., Kumar, R., and Deykin, D. (1977). The spectrum of vitamin K deficiency. *JAMA* 238:40-42.

85. Hazell, K., and Baloch, K. H. (1970). Vitamin K deficiency in the elderly. *Gerontol. Clin.* 12:10-17.

86. Editorial (1978). Vitamin K and the newborn. *Lancet* 1:755-757.

87. Fomon, S. J., and Strauss, R. G. (1978). Nutrient deficiencies in breast-fed infants. *N. Engl. J. Med.* 299:355-357.

88. Lefevere, M. F., DeLeenheer, A. P., and Claeys, A. E. (1979). High-performance liquid chromatographic assay of vitamin K in human serum. *J. Chromatogr.* 186:749-762.

89. Matschiner, J. T., Bell, R. G., Amelotti, J. M., and Knauer, T. E. (1970). Isolation and characterization of a new metabolite of phylloquinone in the rat. *Biochim. Biophys. Acta 201*:309-315.

90. Esmon, C., Sadowski, J., and Suttie, J. (1975). A new carboxylation reaction. The vitamin K-dependent incorporation of $H^{14}CO_3^-$ into prothrombin. *J. Biol. Chem. 250*:4744-4748.

91. Fasco, M. J., and Principe, L. M. (1980). Vitamin K hydroquinone formation catalyzed by a microsomal reductase system. *Biochem. Biophys. Res. Commun. 97*:1487-1492.

92. Ren, P., Laliberte, R. E., and Bell, R. G. (1974). Effect of warfarin, phenylindanedione and tetrachloropyridinol, and chloro-vitamin K_1 on prothrombin synthesis and vitamin K metabolism in normal and warfarin-resistant rats. *Mol. Pharmacol. 10*:373-380.

93. Ren, P., Stark, P. Y., Johnson, R. L., and Bell, R. G. (1977). Mechanism of action of anticoagulants: correlation between the inhibition of prothrombin synthesis and the regeneration of vitamin K_1 from vitamin K_1 epoxide. *J. Pharmacol. Exp. Ther. 201*:541-546.

94. Fieser, L. F., Tishler, M., and Sampson, W. L. (1941). Vitamin K activity and structure. *J. Biol. Chem. 137*:659-692.

95. Bell, R. G., and Matschiner, J. T. (1970). Vitamin K activity of phylloquinone oxide. *Arch. Biochem. Biophys. 141*:473-476.

96. Bell, R. G., Sadowski, J. A., and Matschiner, J. T. (1972). Mechanism of action of warfarin. Warfarin and metabolism of vitamin K_1. *Biochemistry 11*:1959-1961.

97. Davidson, C. S., Freed, J. H., and MacDonald, H. (1945). The effect of vitamin K_1 oxide upon the anticoagulant properties of dicumarol. *Am. J. Med. Sci. 210*:634-637.

98. James, D. F., Bennett, I. L., Scheinberg, P., and Butler, J. J. (1949). Clinical studies on dicumarol hypoprothrombinemia and vitamin K preparations. *Arch. Int. Med. 83*:632-652.

99. Miller, R., Harvey, W. P., and Finch, C. A. (1950). Antagonism of dicumarol by vitamin K preparations. *N. Engl. J. Med. 242*:211-215.

100. Bell, R. G., and Matschiner, J. T. (1972). Warfarin and the inhibition of vitamin K activity by an oxide metabolite. *Nature 237*:32-33.

101. Goodman, S. R., Houser, R. M., and Olson, R. E. (1974). Ineffectiveness of phylloquinone epoxide as an inhibitor of prothrombin synthesis in the rat. *Biochem. Biophys. Res. Commun. 61*:250-257.

102. Matschiner, J. T., Zimmerman, A., and Bell, R. G. (1974). The influence of warfarin on vitamin K epoxide reductase. *Thromb. Diath. Haemorrh. Suppl. 57*:45-52.

103. Sadowski, J. A., Schnoes, H. K., and Suttie, J. W. (1977). Vitamin K epoxidase: properties and relationship to prothombin synthesis. *Biochemistry* 16:3856-3863.
104. Ernster, L., Ljunggren, M., and Danielson, L. (1960). Purification and some properties of a highly dicumarol-sensitive liver diaphorase. *Biochem. Biophys. Res. Commun.* 2:88-92.
105. Ernster, L. (1967). DT diaphorase. *Methods Enzymol.* 10: 309-317.
106. Ernster, L., and Navazio, F. (1958). Soluble diaphorase in animal tissues. *Acta Chem. Scand.* 12:595.
107. Martius, C., and Strufe, R. (1954). Phyllochinonreduktase. Vorläufige Mitteilung. *Biochem. Z.* 326:24-25.
108. Märki, F., and Martius, C. (1960). Vitamin K-reduktase, Darstellung und Eigenschaften. *Biochem. Z.* 333:111-135.
109. Märki, F., and Martius, C. (1961). Vitamin K-reduktasen aus Rinds und Rattenleber. *Biochem. Z.* 334:293-303.
110. Ernster, L., Danielson, L., and Ljunggren, M. (1962). DT diaphorase. I. Purification from the soluble fraction of rat-liver cytoplasm, and properties. *Biochim. Biophys. Acta* 58:171-188.
111. Ernster, L., Lind, C., and Rase, B. (1972). A study of the DT-diaphorase activity of warfarin-resistant rats. *Eur. J. Biochem.* 25:198-206.
112. Lind, C., Rase, B., Ernster, L., Townsend, M. G., and Martin, A. D. (1973). Strain differences in liver DT diaphorase activities. *FEBS Lett.* 37:147-149.
113. Friedman, P. A., and Griep, A. E. (1980). In vitro inhibition of vitamin K dependent carboxylation by tetrachloropyridinol and the imidazopyridines. *Biochemistry* 19:3381-3386.
114. Rase, B., Bartfai, T., and Ernster, L. (1976). Purification of DT-diaphorase by affinity chromatography. Occurrence of two subunits and nonlinear Dixon and Scatchard plots of the inhibition by anticoagulants. *Arch. Biochem. Biophys.* 172:380-386.
115. Wallin, R., Gebhardt, O., and Prydz, H. (1978). NAD(P)H dehydrogenase and its role in the vitamin K_1 (2-methyl-3-phytyl-1,4-naphthoquinone)-dependent carboxylation reaction. *Biochem. J.* 169:95-101.
116. Hollander, P. M., and Ernster, L. (1975). Studies on the reaction mechanism of DT diaphorase. Action of dead-end inhibitors and effects of phospholipids. *Arch. Biochem. Biophys.* 169:560-567.
117. Hall, J. M., Lind, C., Golvano, M. P., Rase, B., and Ernster, L. (1972). DT-diaphorase-reaction mechanism and metabolic function. In *Structure and Function of Oxidation Reduction Enzymes*, A. Akeson and A. Ehrenberg, Eds., Pergamon Press, Oxford, pp. 433-443.

118. Lind, C., and Ernster, L. (1974). A possible relationship between DT diaphorase and the aryl hydrocarbon hydrolase system. *Biochem. Biophys. Res. Commun.* *56*:392-400.
119. Friedman, P., and Shia, M. (1976). Some characteristics of a vitamin K-dependent carboxylating system from rat liver microsomes. *Biochem. Biophys. Res. Commun.* *70*:647-654.
120. Sadowski, J. A., Esmon, C. T., and Suttie, J. W. (1976). Vitamin K-dependent carboxylase. Requirements of the rat liver microsomal enzyme system. *J. Biol. Chem.* *251*:2770-2776.
121. Wallin, R. (1979). No strict coupling of vitamin K_1 (2-methyl-3-phytyl-1,4-naphthoquinone)-dependent carboxylation and vitamin K_1 epoxidation in detergent-solubilized microsomal fractions from rat liver. *Biochem. J.* *178*:513-519.
122. Girardot, J. M., Mack, D. O., Floyd, R. A., and Johnson, B. C. (1976). Evidence for vitamin K semiquinone as the functional form of vitamin K in the liver vitamin K-dependent protein carboxylation reaction. *Biochem. Biophys. Res. Commun.* *70*:655-662.
123. Suttie, J. W., Larson, A. E., Canfield, L. M., and Carlisle, T. L. (1978). Relationship between vitamin K-dependent carboxylation and vitamin K epoxidation. *Fed. Proc.* *37*:2605-2609.
124. Egeberg, K., and Helgeland, L. (1980). Vitamin K epoxidase activity of rough and smooth microsomes from rat liver. *Biochim. Biophys. Acta* *627*:225-229.
125. Carlisle, T. L., and Suttie, J. W. (1980). Vitamin K dependent carboxylase: subcellular location of the carboxylase and enzymes involved in vitamin K metabolism in rat liver. *Biochemistry* *19*:1161-1167.
126. Carlisle, T. L., Shah, D. V., and Suttie, J. W. (1980). Species variation, induction, and subcellular localization of the liver vitamin K-dependent carboxylase. In *Vitamin K Metabolism and Vitamin K-Dependent Proteins*, J. W. Suttie, Ed., University Park Press, Baltimore, Md., pp. 443-449.
127. Willingham, A. K., and Matschiner, J. T. (1974). Changes in phylloquinone epoxidase activity related to prothrombin synthesis and microsomal clotting activity in the rat. *Biochem. J.* *140*:435-441.
128. Knauer, T. E., Willingham, A. K., and Matschiner, J. T. (1974). Biological activity and metabolism of cis and trans phylloquinone in the rat. *Fed. Proc.* *33*:1314.
129. Knauer, T., Siegfried, C., Willingham, A., and Matschiner, J. (1975). Metabolism and biological activity of cis and trans phylloquinone in the rat. *J. Nutr.* *105*:1519-1524.
130. Friedman, P. A., and Smith, M. W. (1979). Epoxidation of several vitamins K by rat liver microsomes. *Biochem. Pharmacol.* *28*:937-938.

131. Sadowski, J. A., Esmon, C. T., and Suttie, J. W. (1979). Vitamin K-dependent carboxylase. Requirements of the rat liver microsomal enzyme system. *J. Biol. Chem.* 251:2770-2776.

132. Grant, G. A., and Suttie, J. W. (1976). Rat liver prothrombin precursors: purification of a second, more basic form. *Biochemistry* 15:5387-5393.

133. Esmon, C. T., Sadowski, J. A., and Suttie, J. W. (1975). A new carboxylation reaction. The vitamin K-dependent incorporation of $H^{14}CO_3^-$ into prothrombin. *J. Biol. Chem.* 250:4744-4748.

134. Suttie, J. W., Geweke, L. O., Martin, S. L., and Willingham, A. K. (1980). Vitamin K epoxidase: dependence of epoxidase activity on substrates of the vitamin K-dependent carboxylation reaction. *FEBS Lett.* 109:267-270.

135. Bell, R. G., and Stark, P. (1976). Inhibition of prothrombin synthesis and epoxidation of vitamin K_1 by anticoagulants in vitro. *Biochem. Biophys. Res. Commun.* 72:619-625.

136. Willingham, A. K., Laliberte, R. E., Bell, R. G., and Matschiner, J. T. (1976). Inhibition of vitamin K epoxidase by two non-coumarin anticoagulants. *Biochem. Pharmacol.* 25: 1063-1066.

137. Elliott, G. R., Townsend, M. G., and Odam, E. M. (1980). Assay procedure for the vitamin K_1 2,3-epoxide-reducing system. *Methods Enzymol.* 67:160-165.

138. Siegfried, C. M. (1978). Solubilization of vitamin K epoxide reductase and vitamin K-dependent carboxylase from rat liver microsomes. *Biochem. Biophys. Res. Commun.* 83:1488-1495.

139. Whitlon, D. S., Sadowski, J. A., and Suttie, J. W. (1978). Mechanism of courmarin action: significance of vitamin K epoxide reductase inhibition. *Biochemistry* 17:1371-1377.

140. Schmidt, W., Beermann, D., Oesch, F., and Jähnchen, E. (1979). Differential effect of the enantiomers of phenprocoumon and warfarin on the vitamin K_1-epoxide/vitamin K_1 ratio in the rat plasma. *J. Pharm. Pharmacol.* 31:490-491.

141. Trenk, D., Beermann, D., Oesch, F., and Jähnchen, E. (1980). Age-dependent differences in the effect of phenprocoumon on the vitamin K_1-epoxide cycle in rats. *J. Pharm. Pharmacol.* 32:828-832.

142. Shepherd, A. M. M., Hewick, D. S., Moreland, T. A., and Stevenson, I. H. (1977). Age as a determinant of sensitivity to warfarin. *Br. J. Clin. Pharmacol.* 4:315-320.

143. Husted, S., and Andreasen, F. (1977). The influence of age on the response to anticoagulants. *Br. J. Clin. Pharmacol.* 4: 559-565.

144. Routledge, P. A., Chapman, P. H., Davies, D. M., and Rawlings, M. D. (1979). Factors affecting warfarin requirements.

A prospective population study. *Eur. J. Clin. Pharmacol. 15:* 319-322.

145. Bell, R. G., and Caldwell, P. T. (1973). Mechanism of warfarin resistance. Warfarin and the metabolism of vitamin K_1. *Biochemistry 12:*1759-1762.

146. Zimmerman, A., Matschiner, J. (1974). Biochemical basis of hereditary resistance to warfarin in the rat. *Biochem. Pharmacol. 23:*1033-1040.

147. Searcey, M. T., Graves, C. B., and Olson, R. E. (1977). Isolation of a warfarin binding protein from liver endoplasmic reticulum of Sprague-Dawley and warfarin-resistant rats. *J. Biol. Chem. 252:*6260-6267.

148. Hermodson, M. A., Suttie, J. W., and Link, K. P. (1969). Warfarin metabolism and vitamin K requirement in the warfarin-resistant rat. *Am. J. Physiol. 217:*1316-1319.

149. Shah, D. V., and Suttie, J. W. (1973). The chloro analog of vitamin K: antagonism of vitamin K action in normal and warfarin-resistant rats. *Proc. Soc. Exp. Biol. Med. 143:*775-779.

150. O'Reilly, R. A., Pool, J. G., and Aggeler, P. M. (1968). Hereditary resistance to coumarin anticoagulant drugs in man and rat. *Ann. N. Y. Acad. Sci. 151:*913-931.

151. Bell, R. G., Caldwell, P. T., and Holm, E. E. T. (1976). Coumarins and the vitamin K-K epoxide cycle. Lack of resistance to coumatetralyl in warfarin-resistant rats. *Biochem. Pharmacol. 25:*1067-1070.

152. Suttie, J. W. (1973). Anticoagulant-resistant rats: possible control by the use of the chloro analog of vitamin K_1. *Science 180:*741-743.

153. Matschiner, J. T., Zimmerman, A., and Bell, R. G. (1974). The influence of warfarin on vitamin K epoxide reductase. *Thromb. Diath. Haemorrh. Suppl. 57:*45-52.

154. Ren, P., Laliberte, R. E., and Bell, R. G. (1974). Effects of warfarin, phenylindanedione, tetrachloropyridinol, and chloro-vitamin K_1 on prothrombin synthesis and vitamin K metabolism in normal and warfarin-resistant rats. *Mol. Pharmacol. 10:*373-380.

155. Bell, R. G. (1978). Metabolism of vitamin K and prothrombin synthesis: anticoagulants and the vitamin K-epoxide cycle. *Fed. Proc. 37:*2599-2604.

156. Olsen, J. P., Miller, L. L., and Troup, S. B. (1966). Synthesis of clotting factors by the isolated perfused rat liver. *J. Clin. Invest. 45:*690-701.

157. Li, L. F., Kipfer, R. K., and Olson, R. E. (1970). Immunochemical measurement of vitamin K-induced biosynthesis of prothrombin by the isolated perfused rat liver. *Arch. Biochem. Biophys. 137:*494-499.

158. Rugstad, H. E., Prydz, H., and Johansson, B. (1972). Synthesis of coagulation factors by a clonal strain of rat hepatoma cells. *Exp. Cell Res.* 71:41-44.

159. Munns, T. W., Johnston, M. F. M., Liszewski, M. K., and Olson, R. E. (1976). Vitamin K-dependent synthesis and modification of precursor prothrombin in cultured H-35 hepatoma cells. *Proc. Natl. Acad. Sci. USA* 73:2803-2807.

160. Bell, R. G. (1980). Vitamin K dependent carboxylation in lung microsomes. In *Vitamin K Metabolism and Vitamin K-Dependent Proteins,* J. W. Suttie, Ed., University Park Press, Baltimore, Md., pp. 286-293.

161. Buchthal, S. D., and Bell, R. G. (1980). Vitamin K dependent carboxylation in spleen and kidney. In *Vitamin K Metabolism and Vitamin K-Dependent Proteins,* J. W. Suttie, Ed., University Park Press, Baltimore, Md., pp. 299-302.

162. Hauschka, P. V., Friedman, P. A., Traverso, H. P., and Gallop, P. M. (1976). Vitamin K-dependent γ-carboxyglutamic acid formation by kidney microsomes in vitro. *Biochem. Bio-Phys. Res. Commun.* 71:1207-1213.

163. Lian, J. B., and Friedman, P. A. (1978). The vitamin K-dependent synthesis of γ-carboxyglutamic acid by bone microsomes. *J. Biol. Chem.* 253:6623-6626.

164. Friedman, P. A., Hauschka, P. V., Shia, M. A., and Wallace, J. K. (1979). Characteristics of the vitamin K-dependent carboxylating system in human placenta. *Biochim. Biophys. Acta* 583:261-265.

165. Levy, R. J., Lian, J. B., and Gallop, P. M. (1980). γ-Carboxyglutamic acid and atherosclerotic plaque. In *Vitamin K Metabolism and Vitamin K-Dependent Proteins,* J. W. Suttie, Ed., University Park Press, Baltimore, Md., pp. 269-273.

166. Helgeland, L. (1977). The submicrosomal site for the conversion of prothrombin precursor to biologically active prothrombin in rat liver. *Biochim. Biophys. Acta* 499:181-193.

167. Wallin, R., and Prydz, H. (1979). Studies on a subcellular system for vitamin K-dependent carboxylation. *Thromb. Haemostasis* 41:529-536.

168. Helgeland, L. (1977). The submicrosomal site for the conversion of prothrombin precursor to biologically active prothrombin in rat liver. *Biochim. Biophys. Acta* 499:181-193.

169. Esmon, C. T., Grant, G. A., and Suttie, J. W. (1975). Purification of an apparent rat liver prothrombin precursor: characterization and comparison to normal rat prothrombin. *Biochemistry* 14:1595-1600.

170. Grant, G. A., and Suttie, J. W. (1976). Rat liver prothrombin precursors: purification of a second, more basic form. *Biochemistry* 15:5387-5393.

171. Johnson, B. C. (1980). Vitamin K-dependent carboxylation. *Methods Enzymol.* 67:165-180.
172. Suttie, J. W., Canfield, L. M., and Shah, D. V. (1980). Microsomal vitamin K-dependent carboxylation. *Methods Enzymol.* 67:180-185.
173. Suttie, J. W., Hageman, J. M., Lehrman, S. R., and Rich, D. H. (1976). Vitamin K-dependent carboxylase. Development of a peptide substrate. *J. Biol. Chem.* 251:5827-5830.
174. Houser, R. M., Carey, D. J., Dus, K. M., Marshall, G. R., and Olson, R. E. (1977). Partial sequence of rat prothrombin and the activity of two related pentapeptides as substrates for the vitamin K-dependent carboxylase system. *FEBS Lett.* 75: 226-230.
175. Suttie, J. W., Lehrman, S. R., Geweke, L. O., Hageman, J. M., and Rich, D. M. (1979). Vitamin K-dependent carboxylase: requirements for carboxylation of soluble peptide substrates and substrate specificity. *Biochem. Biophys. Res. Commun.* 86:500-507.
176. Rich, D. H., Lehrman, S. R., Kawai, M., Goodman, H. L., and Suttie, J. W. (1980). Rat liver vitamin K-dependent carboxylase: substrate specificity. In *Vitamin K Metabolism and Vitamin K-Dependent Proteins*, J. W. Suttie, Ed., University Park Press, Baltimore, Md., pp. 471-479.
177. Finnan, J. L., Goodman, H. L., and Suttie, J. W. (1980). Glutamic acid derivatives as substrates for the vitamin K-dependent carboxylase. In *Vitamin K Metabolism and Vitamin K-Dependent Proteins*, J. W. Suttie, Ed., University Park Press, Baltimore, Md., pp. 480-483.
178. Decottignies-Le Marechal, P., Rikong-Adie, H., Azerad, R., and Gaudry, M. (1979). Vitamin K-dependent carboxylation of synthetic substrates. Nature of the products. *Biochem. Biophys. Res. Commun.* 90:700-707.
179. Finnan, J. L., and Suttie, J. W. (1980). Carboxylation of low-molecular-weight substrates by the rat liver vitamin K-dependent carboxylase: characterization of products. In *Vitamin K Metabolism and Vitamin K-Dependent Proteins*, J. W. Suttie, Ed., University Park Press, Baltimore, Md., pp. 509-517.
180. Esmon, C. T., Sadowski, J. A., and Suttie, J. W. (1975). A new carboxylation reaction. The vitamin K-dependent incorporation of $H^{14}CO_3^-$ into prothrombin. *J. Biol. Chem* 250:4744-4748.
181. Lowenthal, J., and Jaeger, V. (1977). Synthesis of clotting factors by a cell-free system from rat liver in response to the addition of vitamin K_1 in vitro. *Biochem. Biophys. Res. Commun.* 74:25-32.
182. Mack, D. O., Suen, E. T., Girardot, J. M., Miller, J. A.,

Delaney, R., and Johnson, B. C. (1976). Soluble enzyme system for vitamin K-dependent carboxylation. *J. Biol. Chem.* 251:3269-3276.

183. Esmon, C. T., and Suttie, J. W. (1976). Vitamin K-dependent carboxylase. Solubilization and properties. *J. Biol. Chem.* 251: 6238-6243.

184. Girardot, J. M., Delaney, R., and Johnson, B. C. (1974). Carboxylation, the completion step in prothrombin biosynthesis. *Biochem. Biophys. Res. Commun.* 59:1197-1203.

185. Jones, J. P., Gardner, E. J., Cooper, T. G., and Olson, R. E. (1977). Vitamin K-dependent carboxylation of peptide-bound glutamate. The active species of "CO_2" utilized by the membrane-bound preprothrombin carboxylase. *J. Biol. Chem.* 252:7738-7742.

186. Friedman, P. A., and Shia, M. A. (1977). The apparent absence of involvement of biotin in the vitamin K-dependent carboxylation of glutamic acid residues of proteins. *Biochem. J.* 163:39-43.

187. Dubin, A., Suen, E. T., Delaney, R., Chiu, A., and Johnson, B. C. (1979). Stimulation of vitamin K-dependent carboxylation by pyridoxal-5-phosphate. *Biochem. Biophys. Res. Commun.* 88:1024-1029.

188. Suttie, J. W., Geweke, L. O., Finnan, J. L., Lehrman, S. R., and Suttie, J. W. (1980). Effect of pyridoxal phosphate on the vitamin K-dependent carboxylase. In *Vitamin K Metabolism and Vitamin K-dependent Proteins*, J. W. Suttie, Ed., University Park Press, Baltimore, Md., pp. 450-454.

189. Larson, A. E., Mctigue, J. J., and Suttie, J. W. (1980). Investigation of the role of oxygen in the vitamin K-dependent carboxylase reaction. In *Vitamin K Metabolism and Vitamin K-Dependent Proteins*, J. W. Suttie, Ed., University Park Press, Baltimore, Md., pp. 413-421.

190. Friedman, P. A., Shia, M. A., Gallop, P. M., and Griep, A. E. (1979). Vitamin K-dependent γ-carbon-hydrogen bond cleavage and nonmandatory concurrent carboxylation of peptide-bound glutamic acid residues. *Proc. Natl. Acad. Sci. USA* 76:3126-3129.

191. Friedman, P. A. (1980). Dissociation of vitamin K-dependent γ-carbon-hydrogen bond cleavage from carboxylation of peptide-bound glutamic acid residues. In *Vitamin K Metabolism and Vitamin K-Dependent Proteins*, J. W. Suttie, Ed., University Park Press, Baltimore, Md., pp. 401-407.

192. Johnson, B. C., Mack, D. O., Delaney, R., Wolfensberger, M. R., Esmon, C., Price, J. A., Suen, E., and Girardot, J. M. (1980). Vitamin K analogs in the study of vitamin K-dependent carboxylation. In *Vitamin K Metabolism and Vitamin*

K-Dependent Proteins, J. W. Suttie, Ed., University Park Press, Baltimore, Md., pp. 455-456.

193. Jones, J. P., Fausto, A., Houser, R. M., Gardner, E. J., and Olson, R. E. (1976). Effect of vitamin K homologues on the conversion of preprothrombin to prothrombin in rat liver microsomes. *Biochem. Biophys. Res. Commun.* 72:589-597.

194. Shah, D. V., and Suttie, J. W. (1979). Vitamin K-dependent carboxylase: liver activity in various species. *Proc. Soc. Exp. Biol. Med.* 161:498-501.

195. Shah, D. V., and Suttie, J. W. (1978). Vitamin K-dependent carboxylase: increased activity in a hypoprothrombinemia state. *Arch. Biochem. Biophys.* 191:571-577.

196. Dubin, A., Suen, E. T., Delaney, R., Chiu, A., and Johnson, B. C. (1980). Regulation of vitamin K-dependent carboxylation. *J. Biol. Chem.* 255:349-352.

197. Nishino, Y. (1979). Hormonal control of prothrombin synthesis in rat liver microsomes, with special reference to the role of estradiol, testosterone and prolactin. *Arch. Toxicol. Suppl.* 2:397-402.

198. Siegfried, C. M., Knauer, G. R., and Matschiner, J. T. (1979). Evidence for increased formation of preprothrombin and the noninvolvement of vitamin K-dependent reactions in sex-linked hyperprothrombinemia in rat. *Biochem. Biophys.* 194:486-495.

199. Jolly, D. W., McBride, R., Seibert, S., Kadis, B., and Nelson, T. E. (1980). Fetal/maternal vitamin K dependent reactions: some hormonal effects. In *Vitamin K Metabolism and Vitamin K-Dependent Proteins*, J. W., Suttie, Ed., University Park Press, Baltimore, Md., pp. 337-341.

200. Esnouf, M. P., Green, M. R., Hill, H. A. O., and Walters, S. J. (1979). Inhibition of the vitamin K-dependent carboxylation of glutamyl residues in prothrombin by some copper complexes. *FEBS Lett.* 107:146-150.

201. Shah, D. V., and Suttie, J. W. (1974). The vitamin K dependent, in vitro production of prothrombin. *Biochem. Biophys. Res. Commun.* 60:1397-1402.

13

Drug-Induced Maldigestion and Malabsorption

Philip G. Holtzapple and Sheldon E. Schwartz
Upstate Medical Center of the State University of New York, Syracuse, New York

I. INTRODUCTION

Drug-induced nutrient maldigestion and malabsorption occurs frequently, but the clinical manifestations of these drug-induced disorders—anemia, diarrhea and weight loss—are often attributed to the underlying disease. Therefore, the etiology may remain unrecognized by the physician. If one considers the complex and diverse intra- and extracellular events involved in the digestion and absorption of proteins, carbohydrates, and lipids, it is not surprising that many drug-related malabsorptive syndromes have been elucidated. There are many possible mechanisms by which drugs interfere with nutrient absorption. Most frequently, drugs alter the absorption of nutrients by disrupting the intestinal luminal or mucosal mechanisms of nutrient digestion and absorption. Drugs have little, if any, effect on the composition or flow of the hepatobiliary or pancreatic secretions.

II. NEOMYCIN

Neomycin, a poorly absorbed polybasic antibiotic, is used primarily to suppress colonic bacterial growth in preparation for bowel surgery or in the treatment of hepatic encephalopathy. Large doses of neomycin (3–10 g daily) reversibly depress absorption of lipids, nitrogen, carotene, iron, vitamin B_{12}, xylose, and glucose (1–8).
   In this classic model of drug-induced malabsorption, both mucosal and intraluminal absorptive functions are disrupted. In human volun-

teers, taking moderate doses of neomycin (6 g) daily for 8 days, morphologic alterations of small intestinal mucosa are observed. The histologic changes include shortening of mucosal villi, infiltration of the
lamina propria with inflammatory cells, an increased number of mitoses
in the mucosal crypts, and interstitial macrophages containing lyso-
somes. Ultrastructurally, villus tip epithelial cells appear normal,
while large numbers of crypt cells show evidence of injury, including
dilatation of endoplasmic reticulum, ballooning of mitochondria, and
clumping of nuclear chromatin (7,8). The metabolic consequences of
this change in morphology may account for the observed malabsorption
of carbohydrates as a result of inhibition of disaccharidase activity,
and alteration in the rate of glucose transport (9,10).

The malabsorption of lipid is attributed more to alterations in the
luminal phase of lipolysis rather than to a reduction in fatty acid transport. In vitro studies suggest that the strongly basic amino groups of
neomycin interact with the intraluminal dihydroxy bile acids, thus disrupting the micellar complex, causing its constituent components to
precipitate (11–14). Analysis of jejunal intraluminal contents in human
volunteers, who received a test meal to which 1 g of neomycin was added, confirmed this prediction (15). All micellar constituents had separated with cholesterol precipitation exceeding that of the fatty acids,
monoglycerides, and bile acids. Intraluminal lipolytic activity appar-
rently is unaltered by the administration of neomycin. Human lipase
activity measured by an in vitro micellar system consisting of triolein
and taurocholate is actually enhanced by the addition of neomycin (16).

A notable feature of this drug is the marked cholesterol-lowering effect, which is out of proportion to the severity of a malabsorptive disorder produced (3–5). Small doses of neomycin (2 g daily), which are
not sufficient to alter neutral lipid absorption, when prescribed for
long periods of time produces significant reductions in serum cholesterol levels. The explanation for this observation is that cholesterol
is absorbed only to a limited extent in the upper small intestine, while
fatty acid absorption occurs by diffusion and along the entire length
of small intestine, and bile acids are mainly absorbed by an active process in the ileum. By disrupting the micellar complex and inducing the
precipitation of cholesterol in the upper small intestine, neomycin apparently prevents cholesterol absorption to a greater degree than
either that of fatty acid or bile salts (17).

III. FOLATE ABSORPTION

Folates exist in nature as a mixture of pteroylpolyglutamic and pteroylmonoglutamic acid, with the polyglutamate forms predominating. About
65% of pteroylmonoglutamic acid is absorbed by the jejunum, while
pteroylheptaglutamic acid absorption is reduced to 70–90% of the efficiency of the monoglutamate form (18,19). There is now convincing

evidence that the intestinal mucosa is the source of the hydrolytic activity known as pteroylpoly-γ-carboxypeptidase (folate conjugase),
which splits off the glutamic acid groups (20−23). Incubation of radio-
active-labeled pteroylpolyglutamate with intestinal homogenates releases
the same product, pteroylmonoglutamate, found in the blood after ingestion of the polyglutamate forms (21,22). In human intestine,
pteroylpoly-γ-carboxypeptidase appears located in or near the brush
border membrane of the intestinal epithelial cell (20,23). As compared
to the activity in biliary, pancreatic, or intestinal secretions, folate
conjugase is concentrated several hundred-fold in jejunal mucosa (24),
has maximal activity at pH 6.5, and is capable of producing pteroylmonoglutamate from pteroylheptaglutamate by progressive hydrolysis
(20). Reports of a "pancreatic conjugase" have appeared, but "pancreatic conjugase" activity can be demonstrated only at a pH of 4.6,
a pH well below that generally encountered in pancreatic secretions
(24a).

Following uptake and mucosal hydrolysis, the pteroylmonoglutamate
is reduced and methylated by mucosal dihydrofolate reductase and
methylenetetrahydrofolate reductase (25,26). Reduced methylated folic
acid is not an obligatory form for intestinal transport, as inhibition of
metabolism by methotrexate does not effect intestinal transport (26-29),
and pteroylmonoglutamate appears in the portal blood (21). The most
critical factor in controlling intestinal absorption appears to be luminal
pH. Maximal folate absorption occurs at pH 6.0−6.2. Absorption
against a concentrate in gradient is eradicated at a luminal pH of 7.4
or higher (30).

IV. DRUGS AFFECTING FOLATE ABSORPTION: DIPHENYLHY-
DANTOIN

Folate deficiency and megaloblastic anemia have been observed in patients receiving diphenylhydantoin for seizure disorders (31−33). As
there is little to suggest that diphenylhydantoin affects the dietary intake or cellular metabolism of folic acid, clinical studies have focused
on alterations in intestinal absorption of folic acid (33).

There are still unresolved conflicting studies which suggest that
diphenylhydantoin either inhibits pteroylpoly-γ-carboxypeptidase activity (34,35) or has no effect at all on this enzyme system (36,37).
Fluctuations in intraluminal pH might be a more reasonable explanation
for the observed reduction in intestinal transport, since the pH of an
aqueous solution of diphenylhydantoin is 10. At this pH, intestinal
transport would be inhibited. However, in human volunteers when
the jejunum was perfused with diphenylhydantoin, 20 μg/ml buffered
at pH 6.8, folate absorption was reduced (38). Thus the mechanism
for impaired folate absorption with this drug remains to be elucidated.

V. DRUGS AFFECTING FOLATE ABSORPTION: SULFASALAZINE (SALICYLAZOSULFAPYRIDINE)

Sulfasalazine, a drug effective in the treatment of inflammatory bowel disease, consists of 5-aminosalicylate linked through an azo bond to sulfapyridine. Even though there are few structural similarities between sulfasalazine and folic acid (Figure 1), 60% of patients on long-term sulfasalazine therapy have low serum folate levels and 10% may demonstrate macrocytosis (39).

Folate absorption is impaired when either a standard oral folic acid tolerance test is performed or when tritiated pteroylmonoglutamic acid is given with sulfasalazine (39–41). In vivo kinetic studies suggest a competitive mode of transport inhibition (40,41). Only sulfasalazine itself is considered to inhibit folic acid transport, as the metabolites, 5-aminosalicylate or sulfapyridine, do not affect folate absorption in rat jejunal segments (39).

There potentially several additional mechanisms by which sulfasalazine may inhibit folic acid absorption, (40,41). Sulfasalazine competitively inhibits human jejunal pteroylpoly-γ-carboxypeptidase activity in vitro (42). In jejunal perfusion experiments in patients with ulcerative colitis, sulfasalazine inhibited both the hydrolysis of pteroylpolyglutamic acid folate and the disappearance of both polyglutamyl and monoglutamyl folates from the perfused segment (43). In liver, sulfasalazine inhibits folate dihydroreductase, methylene tetrahydrofolate

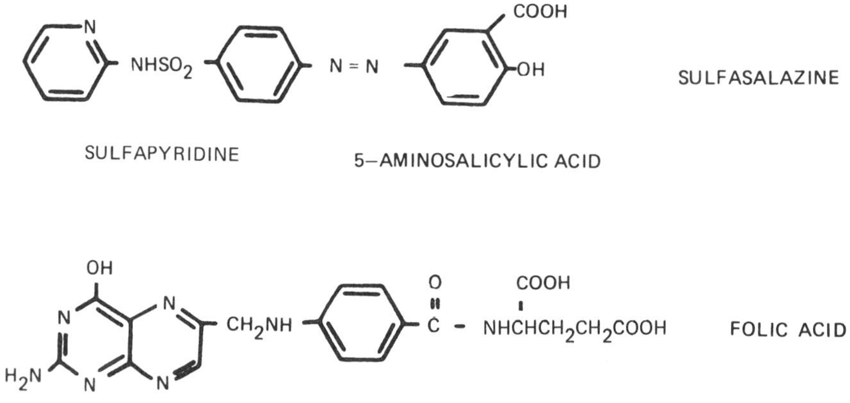

Figure 1   Chemical formulas of folic acid and sulfasalazine.

reductase, and transhydroxymethylase, all enzymes utilized in folate metabolism (44).

VI. ORAL CONTRACEPTIVES

Megaloblastic anemia, attributed to folate deficiency, has been reported in women on oral contraceptives. Low serum folate levels in these women have directed investigators to examine folate absorption during oral contraceptive usage.

In two clinical studies oral folic acid tolerance tests were performed in females using oral contraceptives (45,46). In each study, absorption of pteroylpolyglutamic acid was decreased compared to the absorption of the monoglutamate form. These studies suggest that oral contraceptives inhibit mucosal pteroylpoly-γ-carboxypeptidase activity, although there is no direct evidence for this. However, if tissue folate stores were repleted before performing the oral tolerance test, pteroylpolyglutamate absorption was not affected during long-term administration of oral contraceptives (47,48). Other observations suggest that the megaloblastic anemia associated with oral contraceptive use occurs only in women with a primary, unrelated, occult, malabsorptive syndrome (49,50).

VII. COLCHICINE

Colchicine, an agent used in patients with acute gouty arthritis and for the prevention of acute attacks of familial Mediterranean fever, causes diarrhea in essentially all patients and megaloblastic anemia or bone marrow suppression in an occasional patient (51,52). Cyanocobalamin is the only vitamin whose absorption is significantly altered by colchicine usage. In human volunteers colchicine reversibly reduced cyanocobalamin-intrinsic factor complex uptake and/or binding by the ileal mucosa. Gastric intrinsic factor secretion, activity, and B_{12} binding were not affected by colchicine administration (53).

In clinical practice colchicine is used only for brief limited periods of time. If taken chronically, colchicine would be associated with lipid malabsorption. Colchicine binds to tubulin, preventing helical polymerization of this protein and formation of microtubules. Microtubules, integrally involved in spindle formation during mitoses, are also important in cellular secretory processes. Chronic colchicine administration interferes with lipoprotein secretion in the intestinal epithelial cell and results in triglyceride and lipoprotein accumulation in the cytoplasm with markedly disorganized Golgi structures (54–56).

Diarrhea with colchicine usage occurs independently of nutrient uptake. Although colchicine alters epithelial cell generation and migration along the villus, and the rate and the activity of disaccharidases (57), other mechanisms must account for the diarrhea observed during the absence of nutrient intake. There is conflicting evidence of the effect of colchicine on water transport in the small intestine. Jejunal water absorption has been reported to be diminished by colchicine, with increases noted in mucosal PGE_2, cyclic AMP content, and adenylcyclase activity. Prostaglandins and cyclic AMP are potent effectors in stimulating intestinal secretion (58,59). In other studies, intestinal basal water transport was not effected by colchicine administration, and the expected secretory response to cholera toxin was blunted by colchicine administration (60,61). The relevance of these observations to clinical diarrhea remains to be determined.

VIII. PARA-AMINOSALICYLIC ACID

Para-aminosalicylic acid (PAS), effective in the treatment of tuberculosis, is associated with mild steatorrhea and vitamin B_{12} malabsorption. Mild steatorrhea developed in all volunteers taking large amounts of PAS daily (62). Jejunal biopsies remained normal in all. Addition of PAS to human bile or a model bile salt solution did not cause precipitation of bile acids as seen with neomycin (62,63). The intraluminal phase of fat absorption is reported to be normal (64). Therefore, the mechanism of the steatorrhea remains unknown.

In the absence of steatorrhea, PAS is associated with malabsorption of vitamin B_{12}. While depressed serum vitamin B_{12} levels vary directly with the duration of PAS therapy, abnormal Schilling tests occur within days to weeks of the initiation of PAS treatment (65–67). The abnormal Schilling tests are not corrected by intrinsic factor, pancreatic extract, intestinal juice, or tetracycline (68). In addition, there does not appear to be any defect in the production of intrinsic factor (64, 69) or in its binding of vitamin B_{12} (69,70).

The structural similarity of PAS and folic acid has led to the concept that folic acid is important for vitamin B_{12} absorption (71). Serum folate levels decrease during long-term PAS administration and correction of vitamin B_{12} malabsorption is noted in many patients when oral folic acid is administered concomitantly with PAS (69,71). In contrast, other patients do not normalize vitamin B_{12} absorption after taking folic acid (64,68). The mechanism for the impairment of vitamin B_{12} absorption remains to be elucidated.

REFERENCES

1. Jacobson, E. E., Chodos, R. B., and Falcon, W. W. (1960). An experimental malabsorption syndrome induced by neomycin. *Am. J. Med.* 28:524-533.

2. Faloon, W. W., Paes, I. C., Woolfolk, D., Nankin, H., Wallace, K., and Haro, E. N. (1966). Effect of neomycin and kanamycin upon intestinal absorption. *Ann. N. Y. Acad. Sci. 132*: 879-887.

3. Hvidt, S., and Kjeldsen, K. (1963). Malabsorption induced by small doses of neomycin sulphate. *Acta Med. Scand. 173*:699-705.

4. Eyssen, H., Evard, E., and Vanderhaegre, H. (1966). Cholesterol-lowering effects of N-methylated neomycin and basic antibiotics. *J. Lab. Clin. Med. 68*:753-768.

5. Samuel, P., and Meilman, E. (1967). Dietary lipids and reduction of serum cholesterol levels by neomycin in man. *J. Lab. Clin. Med. 70*:471-479.

6. Samuel, P. (1979). Treatment of hypercholesterolemia with neomycin. A time for reappraisal. *N. Engl. J. Med. 801*:595-597.

7. Dobbins, W. O., III, Herrero, B. A., and Mansbach, C. M. (1968). Morphologic alterations associated with neomycin-induced malabsorption. *Am. J. Med. Sci. 225*:63-77.

8. Jacobson, E. D., Prior, J. T., and Faloon, W. W. (1960). Malabsorptive syndrome induced by neomycin: morphologic alterations in the jejunal mucosa. *J. Lab. Clin. Med. 56*:245-250.

9. Paes, I. C., Searl, P., Rubert, M. W., and Faloon, W. W. (1967). Intestinal lactase deficiency and saccharide malabsorption during oral neomycin administration. *Gastroenterology 53*:49-58.

10. Cain, G. D., Reiner, E. B., and Patterson, M. (1968). Effects of neomycin on disaccharidase activity of the small bowel. *Arch. Intern. Med. 122*:314.

11. Van den Bosch, J. F., and Claes, D. J. (1967). Correlation between the bile salt-precipitating capacity of derivatives of basic antibiotics and their plasma cholesterol lowering effect in vivo. *Prog. Biochem. Pharmacol. 2*:97-104.

12. Thompson, G. R., MacMahon, M., and Claes, P. (1970). Precipitation by neomycin compounds of fatty acid and cholesterol from mixed micellular solution. *Eur. J. Clin. Invest. 1*:40-47.

13. DeSomer, P. H., Vanderhaeghe, H., and Eyssen, H. (1964). Influence of basic antibiotics on serum and liver cholesterol concentration in chicks. *Nature 204*:1306.

14. Miettinen, T. A. (1975). Mechanism of action of nonabsorbable lipid lowering drugs. *Proc. GI Int. Cong. Pharmacol*, Finnish Pharmacological Society, Vol. 11, pp. 149-158.

15. Thompson, G. R., Barrowman, J., Gutiennez, L., and Dowling, R. H. (1971). Action of neomycin on the intraluminal phase of lipid absorption. *J. Clin. Invest. 50*:319-323.

16. Rogers, A. L., and Bachouk, P. S. (1968). The effect of neomycin sulfate on pancreatic lipase activity. *Proc. Soc. Exp. Biol. Med. 127*:1236-1240.

17. Miettinen, T. A. (1979). Effects of neomycin alone and in combination with cholestyramine on serum cholesterol and fecal steroid in hypercholesterolemic subjects. *J. Clin. Invest. 64*: 1485-1493.

18. Godwin, H. A., and Rosenberg, I. H. (1975). Comparative studies of the intestinal absorption of ^{3}H-pteroylmonoglutamate and ^{3}H-pteroylheptaglutamate in man. *Gastroenterology 69*: 364-373.

19. Halsted, C. H., Baugh, C. M., and Butterworth, C. E., Jr. (1975). Jejunal perfusion of simple and conjugated folates in man. *Gastroenterology 68*:261-269.

20. Reisenauer, A. M., Krumdieck, C. L., and Halsted, C. H. (1977). Folate conjugase: two separate activities in human jejunum. *Science 198*:196-197.

21. Baugh, C. M., Krumdieck, C. L., Baker, J. H., and Butterworth, C. F., Jr. (1971). Studies on the absorption and metabolism of folic acid: folate absorption in the dog after exposure of isolated intestinal segments to synthetic pteroylpolyglutamates of various chain lengths. *J. Clin. Invest. 50*:2009-2021.

22. Rosenberg, I. H., and Neumann, H. (1974). Evidence for a multistep mechanism in the enzymatic hydrolysis of polyglutamyl folates by chicken intestine. *J. Biol. Chem. 249*:5126-5130.

23. Rosenberg, I. H., Sheiff, R. R., Godwin, H. A., and Castle, W. B. (1969). Absorption of polyglutamic folate: participation of deconjugating enzymes of intestinal mucosa. *N. Engl. J. Med. 280*:985-988.

24. Jagerstad, M., Lindstrand, K., and Westesson, A. K. (1972). Hydrolysis of conjugated folic acid by pancreatic conjugase. *Scand. J. Gastroenterol. 9*:639-643.

24a. Hoffbrand, A. V., and Peters, T. J. (1970). Recent advances in knowledge of clinical and biochemical aspects of folate. *Schweiz. Med. Wochenschr. 100*:1954-1960.

25. Whitehead, V. M., Pratt, R., Viallet, A., and Cooper, B. A. (1972). Intestinal conversion of folic acid to 5-methyltetrahydrofolate in man. *Br. J. Haematol. 22*:63-72.

26. Olinger, E. J., Bertino, J. R., and Binder, H. J. (1973). Intestinal folate absorption. II. Conversion and retention of pteroylmonoglutamate by jejunum. *J. Clin. Invest. 52*:2138-2145.

27. Baker, H., Frank, O., Feingold, S., Ziller, H., Gellene, R. A., Leavy, C. M., and Sobotka, H. (1965). The fate of orally and parenterally administered folates. *Am. J. Clin. Nutr. 17*:18-95.

28. Perry, J., and Chanarin, I. (1970). Intestinal absorption of reduced folate compounds in man. *Br. J. Haematol. 18*:329-339.
29. Selhub, J., Brin, H., and Grossowicz, N. (1973). Uptake and reduction of radioactive folate by everted sacs of rat small intestine. *Eur. J. Biochem. 33*:433-438.
30. Russel, R. M., Dhar, J. G., Dutta, S. K., and Rosenberg, I. H. (1979). Influence of intraluminal pH on folate absorption: studies in control subjects and in patients with pancreatic insufficiency. *J. Lab. Clin. Med. 93*:428-436.
31. Klipstein, F. A. (1964). Subnormal serum folate and macrocytosis associated with anticonvulsant drug therapy. *Blood 23*:68-86.
32. Meynall, M. J. (1966). Megaloblastic anemia in anticonvulsant therapy. *Lancet 1*:487.
33. Elsborg, L. (1974). Inhibition of intestinal absorption of folic acid by phenytoin. *Acta Haematol. 52*:24-28.
34. Rosenberg, I. H., Godwin, H. A., Streiff, R. R., and Castle, W. B. (1968). Impairment of intestinal deconjugation of dietary folate: a possible explanation of megaloblastic anemia associated with phenytoin therapy. *Lancet 2*:530-532.
35. Hoffbrand, A. V., and Necheles, R. F. (1968). Mechanism of folate deficiency in patients receiving phenytoin. *Lancet 2*:528-530.
36. Baugh, C. M., and Krumdieck, C. L. (1969). Effect of phenytoin on folic acid conjugases in man. *Lancet 2*:519-521.
37. Houlihan, M., Scott, J. M., Boyle, P. H., and Weir, D. B. (1972). The effect of phenytoin on the absorption of synthetic folic acid polyglutamate. *Gut 13*:189-190.
38. Gerson, C. D., Hepner, G. W., Brown, N., Cohen, H., Herbert, V., and Janowitz, H. D. (1972). Inhibition by diphenylhydantoin of folic acid absorption. *Gastroenterology 65*:246-251.
39. Franklin, J. L., and Rosenberg, I. H. (1973). Impaired folic acid absorption in inflammatory bowel disease: effects of salicylazosulfapyridine (Azulfidine). *Gastroenterology 64*:517-525.
40. Dhar, G. J., Selhub, J., and Rosenberg, I. (1976). Azulfidine inhibition of folic acid absorption: confirmation of a specific saturable transport mechanisn. *Gastroenterology 30*:898a.
41. Rosenberg, I. H. (1981). Intestinal Absorption of Folate. In *Physiology of the Gastrointestinal Tract*, Vol. 2, L. R. Johnson, Ed., Raven Press, New York. pp. 1221-1230.
42. Reisenauer, A. M., and Halsted, C. H. (1981). Human jejunal brush border folate conjugase. Characteristics and inhibition by salicylazosulfapyridine. *Biochim. Biophys. Acta 659*:62-69.

43. Halsted, C. H., Gandhi, G., and Tamura, T. (1981). Sulfasalazine inhibits the absorption of folate in ulcerative colitis. N. Engl. J. Med. 205:1513-1516.
44. Selhub, J., Dhar, G. J., and Rosenberg, I. H. (1978). Inhibition of folate enzymes by sulfasalazine. J. Clin. Invest. 61:221-224.
45. Streiff, R. (1970). Folate deficiency and oral contraceptives. JAMA 214:105-108.
46. Necheles, T. F., and Synder, L. M. (1970). Malabsorption of folate polyglutamates associated with oral contraceptive therapy. N. Engl. J. Med. 282:858-859.
47. Stephens, M. E. M., Craft, I., and Peters, J. (1972). Oral contraceptives and folate metabolism. Clin. Sci. 42:405-414.
48. Shojania, A. M., and Hornady, G. J. (1973). Oral contraceptives and folate absorption. J. Lab. Clin. Med. 82:869-875.
49. Toghill, F. J., and Smith, P. G. (1971). Folate deficiency and the pill. Br. Med. J. 1:608-609.
50. Wood, J. K., Goldstone, A. H., and Allan, N. C. (1972). Folic acid and the pill. Scand. J. Haematol. 9:539-544.
51. Hawkins, C. F., Ellis, H. A., and Rowson, A. (1965). Malignant gout with tophaceous small intestine and megaloblastic anemia. Ann. Rheum. Dis. 24:224-233.
52. Boruchow, I. B. (1966). Bone marrow depression associated with colchicine toxicity in presence of hepatic dysfunction. Cancer 19:541-543.
53. Webb, D. I., Chodos, R. B., Mahar, C. Q., and Faloon, W. W. (1970). Mechanism of B_{12} malabsorption in patients receiving colchicine. N. Engl. J. Med. 279:845-850.
54. Arreagza-Plaza, C. A., Bosch, V., and Otaysek, M. A. (1976). Lipid transport across the intestinal epithelial cell. Effect of colchicine. Biochim. Biophys. Acta 431:297-302.
55. Glickman, R. M., Perrotto, J. L., and Kirsch, K. (1976). Intestinal lipoprotein formation: effect of colchicine. Gastroenterology 70:347-352.
56. Race, T. F., Paes, I. C., and Faloon, W. W. (1970). Intestinal malabsorption induced by oral colchicine: comparison with neomycin and cathartic agents. Am. J. Med. Sci. 259:32-44.
57. Herbst, J. J., Hurwitz, R., Sunshine, P., and Kretchmer, N. (1970). Disaccharidases: correlation with biochemical aspects of cellular renewal. J. Clin. Invest. 49:530-536.
58. Rachmilewitz, D., Fogel, R., and Karmeli, F. (1978). Effect of colchicine and vinblastine on rat intestinal water transport and Na-K-ATPase activity. Gut 19:759-764.

59. Rachmilewitz, D., and Karmeli, F. (1980). Effect of colchicine on jejunal adenylate cyclase activity, PGE_2 and cAMP content. *Eur. J. Pharmacol.* 67:235-239.

60. Notis, W. M., Orellana, S. A., and Field, M. (1981). Inhibition of intestinal secretion in rats by colchicine and vinblastine. *Gastroenterology* 81:766-772.

61. Strombeck, D. R. (1973). Colchicine, cycloheximide, and serotonin inhibition of intestinal fluid production caused by vibrio cholera toxin. *Life Sci.* 12:211-218.

62. Levine, R. A. (1968). Steatorrhea induced by para-aminosalicylic acid. *Ann. Intern. Med.* 68:1265-1270.

63. Coltart, D. J. (1969). Malabsorption induced by para-aminosalicylate. *Br. Med. J.* 1:825-826.

64. Halsted, C. H., and McIntyne, T. A. (1972). Intestinal malabsorption caused by aminosalicylic acid therapy. *Arch. Intern. Med.* 150:935-939.

65. Heinivaara, O., and Palva, I. P. (1964). Malabsorption of vitamin B_{12} during treatment with para-aminosalicylic acid. Preliminary report. *Acta Med. Scand.* 175:469-471.

66. Heinivaara, O., and Palva, I. P. (1965). Malabsorption and deficiency of vitamin B_{12} caused by treatment with para-aminosalacylic acid. *Acta Med. Scand.* 17:337-341.

67. Paoby, P., and Norvin, E. (1966). The absorption of vitamin B_{12} during treatment with para-aminosalicylic acid. *Acta Med. Scand.* 180:561-564.

68. Toskes, P. P., and Deren, J. J. (1975). Selective inhibition of vitamin B_{12} absorption by para-aminosalicylic acid. *Gastroenterology* 62:1232-1237.

69. Thompson, J. B., Hess, D. R., Poley, J. R., Smalley, T. K., and Welsh, J. D. (1970). Intestinal malabsorption induced by para-aminosalicylic acid. *Gastroenterology* 58:1001a.

70. Palva, I. P., and Heinivaara, O. (1966). Drug-induced malabsorption of vitamin B_{12} in vitro using the dialysis technique. *Scand. J. Haematol.* 3:33-37.

71. Palva, I. P., Heinivaara, O., and Mattila, M. (1966). Drug-induced malabsorption of vitamin B_{12}. III. Interference of PAS and folic acid in the absorption of vitamin B_{12}. *Scand. J. Haematol.* 3:149-153.

14

Toxic Pancreatitis

R. J. Laugier and H. Sarles
Hôpital Sainte Marguerite, Marseilles, France

I. CHRONIC PANCREATITIS: ROLE OF ALCOHOL, TOXIC FOOD, AND ADDITIVES

A. Alcoholic Pancreatitis

Chronic alcohol consumption is generally considered as being a frequent cause of chronic pancreatitis (CP). In two international surveys (68,73), it has been shown that alcoholic chronic pancreatitis was particularly frequent in the rich countries when alcohol consumption was high (i.e., particularly in the Occidental world). As alcohol consumption is increasing tremendously, the frequency of alcoholic pancreatitis is also increasing (73). In the tropical countries of Africa and Asia but probably not of Latin America, CP is significantly associated with malnutrition in childhood (kwashiorkor), alcohol consumption being, nevertheless, the second cause of the disease (73).

1. Epidemiological Study

The relations and interrelations between alcohol consumption and diet, together with their effect on the risk of developing alcoholic chronic pancreatitis (ACP), have been studied (22). Daily alcohol consumption was recorded and patients were divided into groups at 20-g/day intervals with a separate group for no alcohol intake. There is a good correlation between the mean daily consumption of ethanol and the logarithm of the relative risk (risk related to the class of no alcohol consumption). However, the fit between observed and estimated risk can be improved by assuming that the risk is higher for the two first groups than for the others. This proves that there is no statistical threshold for the toxicity of alcohol on the pancreas but probably a continuous series of individual thresholds. The individual sensitivity of the pancreas to alcohol could be the result of different factors: acquired (associated diet, see below) and/or possibly hereditary (increased frequency of blood group O and other genetic markers) (45).

Neither the type of alcoholic beverage (wine, beer, whisky, saké, cachaça, etc.) nor the type of consumption (regular from one day to another or paroxysmal at the weekends) has an evident role (68). The duration of consumption plays a significant role (23): for the same group of mean daily alcohol consumption, the risk increases with the duration of consumption. This explains that the higher the consumption, the shorter the duration of consumption before the first symptoms appear (73). Nevertheless, mean daily consumption is a better statistical parameter of the risk than is total consumption. The risk of developing ACP is also linearly increased by a high intake of proteins but varies quadratically with fat intake, being the lowest for mean fat intake and higher for high than for low fat intakes. The effect of alcohol, fat, and protein are additive without potentiation. For instance, it can be calculated from our data (22) that a patient with a high-fat average-alcohol high-protein diet has a similar statistical risk than a patient with an average-fat high-alcohol low-protein diet. This explains that ACP is generally observed in alcoholic drinkers having a high-protein high-fat diet as, for instance, in France, Japan, Brazil (73), or Germany (29), but in some veterans' hospitals in the United States, ACP patients were found to have a low-protein low-fat diet (58, 73). Nevertheless, the U.S.A. veteran's patients presented with advanced lesions which could have modified secondarily their dietary habits, whereas the European patients selected for study were recent cases and had not modified their diet since the beginning of the disease, so that it was possible to calculate the diet before the beginning of the symptoms.

2. Pathological Anatomy

The lesions of ACP are similar to those of CP associated with hyperparathyroidism, tropical CP, hereditary CP, and idiopathic CP, and correspond to the pathological entity "chronic calcifying pancreatitis" (52,55): at the beginning of the disease, acinar and ductal cells are apparently normal at the electron microscopical level, but acinar cells present with signs of hyperfunction (82). The only pathological modification is the presence in the ducts of eosinophilic protein precipitates. In later stages ACP is characterized by (1) frequent dilatation of the lumen and atrophy of the epithelium of intra- and extralobular ducts; (2) a particular patchy distribution of the lesions, one lobule or group of lobules presenting with lesions of intensity different from the neighboring lobules (in contrast to the regular distribution of the lesions observed in CP distal to an obstruction on the main pancreatic duct); (3) frequent inflammatory lesions of the nerves; (4) intraductal protein plugs sometimes calcified, forming pancreatic stones or calculi.

Pancreatic stones have been redissolved (16,42). They are built up of different proportions of calcium carbonate in the form of calcite and a predominant or sole protein. This "stone protein" is found in normal pancreatic juice and has no known exzymatic action but inhibits both calcite crystal nucleation and growth (51a). Its molecular weight is 13,500. The intraductal protein precipitates contain the stone protein but also all the enzymatic proteins of pancreatic juice (77).

These findings are compatible with the assumption that the beginning of the disease is marked by the precipitation of all juice proteins and of calcium carbonate, when the capacity of the stone protein for preventing stone formation is overwhelmed or when the concentration of stone protein is too low (51b). As is true for stones from other secretory glands, pancreatic stones are responsible for the lesions: epithelial atrophy and stricture of the ducts, dilatation at the end of the ducts, atrophy or formation of cysts and retention extrapancreatic pseudocysts, or acute episodes of pancreatitis.

3. Clinical Evolution

The clinical evolution of ACP is not very different from the other forms of CP. Nevertheless, its evolution is more frequently marked by acute attacks than is tropical pancreatitis and probably less frequently than CP associated with hyperparathyroidism (35). The first symptoms are generally observed in 30- to 40-year-old men drinking for a mean of 17 years a mean of 150 g of alcohol per day. The disease is much more frequent in males than in females, the sex ratio varying from one country to another and probably being linked to drinking habits.

The evolution of the disease is characterized by recurrent attacks of acute pancreatitis on a background of progressive chronic lesions and a late onset of endocrine (diabetes) and exocrine (malabsorption) pancreatic insufficiency. In the first stages the lesions are so localized and spotty (see above) that pancreatic function tests may be normal, the only biological modification at some distance from the attacks being the secretion in the pancreatic juice of an abnormally high concentration of lactoferrin (51). The frequency of attacks is not predictable. Some attacks may follow within 12–24 hr after a high intake of alcohol (45). Alcohol withdrawal reduces the number of attacks, but frequently complete abstinence is unable to stop the course of the disease. Complications can modify the evolution: (1) formation of intrapancreatic cysts which are at the origin of extrapancreatic retention pseudocysts (exceptional necrotic pseudocysts); (2) stricture of neighboring organs by the peripancreatic fibrosis of by cysts: main bile duct (jaundice generally of the relapsing type), stomach and duodenum, colon, esophagus, arteries, portal and splenic veins (portal hypertension and digestive hemorrhages), and lymph vessels; (3) acute, generally recurrent episodes of fatty necrosis of the subcutaneous tissue (Weber-Christian syndrome), joints, and bones: and (4) serosal effusions (peritoneal, pleural, and pericardial), generally due to the communication of the serosal cavity with the cysts. Cancerization is rare. Finally, the course of the disease is not severe in patients who have stopped drinking, and death is more often due to another complication of alcoholism than to the pancreatic disease itself. Arteritis and respiratory cancers, probably due to dietary habits and to the frequent association of smoking with alcoholism, are frequently found (35).

4. Alcohol-Induced Modifications of Exocrine Pancreatic Secretion in Humans

In nonalcoholic humans, alcohol given intravenously inhibits pancreatic secretion induced by secretin and pancreozymin (12), but this effect is suppressed by anticholinergic drugs (48) and is not observed in chronic alcoholics (60). The pure pancreatic juice of alcoholics compared to normal abstinent controls has a higher protein concentration and a lower bicarbonate concentration. These modifications are probably greater and more significant when the juice collection is done the day following alcohol abuse than when done 1–3 weeks later (63,65,67). At the same time, frequent protein precipitates are observed, similar to the intraductal protein precipitates formed in the ducts of ACP. The data published (67) are compatible with the assumption that alcohol-induced modifications are due to the modifications of basal secretion and not of the response to hormones. Similar conclusions can be drawn from the study of the duodenal juice in basal conditions and after a meal in humans (60). These modifications of pancreatic function are seen at a time when no ultrastructural modifications can be observed with the exception of signs of hypersecretion by the acinar cell (82).

The increase in the protein/bicarbonate concentration ratio could play a part in the formation of precipitates. Calcium concentration is increased only when CP lesions are observed, and at this time it could favor the calcification of protein precipitates (77). The increase in serum protein content of pancreatic juice (14,51) is also probably a consequence and not the cause of the lesions. Lysosomal enzymes are increased (65). Trypsinogen is more easily activated than in controls. Therefore, the estimation of trypsin inhibitor by biochemical methods is of no value and the conclusion that the trypsinogen/trypsin inhibitor ratio is decreased remains to be verified (64). The decrease in the cationic/anionic trypsinogen ratio (66) is probably artifactual since we were unable to confirm it by more sophisticated methods of enzyme separation (77).

Finally, lactoferrin concentration is increased in duodenal (25) and pure pancreatic juice (28) of patients with alcoholic, idiopathic, and hereditary (51) pancreatitis and in a small percentage of normal controls. This increase is related neither to alcohol consumption nor to the intensity of the lesions. As it is not modified in tropical CP (unpublished results), it could be the marker of a defect (possibly congenital) which could express itself spontaneously (family and idiopathic cases) or be latent (controls) or be revealed by associated nutritional disorders (alcoholic pancreatitis).

5. *Alcohol-Induced Modifications of the Regulation of Pancreatic Secretion in Humans*

Chronic alcohol consumption in humans increases gastrin release in response to a meal (89), but does not modify secretin release in response to intraduodenal ethanol (27); cholecystokinin (CCK) release is increased when pancreatic insufficiency is observed and thus is a consequence and not the cause of the disease (32). On the contrary, pancreatic polypeptide (PP) release after a meal is no longer observed in CP patients (91). We have recently shown (76) that PP release was induced in humans by intravenous ethanol and that this release was no longer observed when intravenous ethanol was unable to inhibit pancreatic secretion. Therefore, PP could be the cause of the ethanol-induced inhibition of pancreatic secretion observed in nonalcoholics. Nevertheless, modifications of protein and bicarbonate secretion observed in chronically alcoholic humans are to date unexplained by modifications of the hormonal control of the exocrine pancreas. The fact that the secretion of Cl^- and Na^+ by the sweat is increased in ACP patients would be an argument for an increased release of acetylcholine at the level of the peripheral parasympathic ganglion cells, a modification which is better documented in dogs and which could explain the basal hypersecretion of protein.

6. *Animal Models (69)*

In the rat (79) chronic alcohol consumption (20% w/v for 12 weeks) did not stimulate NADPH oxidase or microsomal ethanol-oxidizing system in pancreatic cells. In contrast to what occurs in hepatic cells, no enzymatic induction by alcohol was found and since very little alcohol dehydrogenase (15,79) is present in the pancreas, it was considered that this organ is unable to metabolize ethanol. More recently, Estival provided evidence for the existence in the pancreas of three enzymatic activities, until now unknown, related or involved in ethanol oxidation (26). Nevertheless, unlike in the liver, a direct toxic action of alcohol on the pancreatic cells is almost ruled out by the fact that pancreatic stones and precipitates are observed before ultrastructural lesions (82).

Rats and dogs have been used for physiological studies. Rats develop lesions which are not very different from human CP; they are

observed spontaneously but are increased by alcohol consumption (78).
Results on secretory modifications observed in these animals are contradictory because the action of alcohol depends on the associated diet
(fat and protein) (70,71) and on the duration of alcohol consumption
(38). Furthermore, the secretory response of the normal rat pancreas
to alcohol differs from the response of the human gland (17). Therefore, the rat is not a suitable animal for research.

The response of the dog is much more like that of the human (69,72).
But in 2-year alcoholic dogs, the lesions are limited to intraductal protein precipitates (also found in the pancreatic juice of humans), peri-
ductal fibrosis, and duct reduplication in some animals (75). Like humans, nonalcoholic dogs respond to intravenous ethanol by an inhibition
of pancreatic secretion, mostly of protein (83), which is suppressed by
atropine, ganglion blockers and vagotomy (88). After 1 year of alcohol
consumption, this inhibition is not only suppressed as in humans, but
is reversed to an important increase of pancreatic secretion, mostly of
protein (85). This increase is suppressed by atropine (86) but no
longer by ganglion blockers or by the vagotomy (84). Therefore, at
this stage alcohol could act at the level of the intrapancreatic deuto-
neurones of the vagus nerve. At this time of alcohol consumption the
protein concentration is increased and the bicarbonate concentration is
decreased in basal secretion and protein precipitates are observed (53).
The response to a meal shows a decreased secretion of bicarbonate and
water with a hyperconcentration of proteins (87). After 2 years of alcohol consumption, the water and bicarbonate response to high doses
of secretin is increased (increased mass of ductal cells) (74); a similar
bicarbonate response had been found in the duodenal juice of alcoholic
human (19,35). But recent studies of pure human pancreatic juice did
not confirm this (see above). After 2 years the increased secretion in
response to a meal and the basal hypersecretion of proteins are no longer observed in the dog (unpublished results), a difference from what
is found in humans.

After 1 year of alcohol consumption secretin release is decreased
(7), CCK release is not modified (59), but gastrin release is increased
(90). A most interesting finding which could explain the increased
basal protein secretion is that in the intrapancreatic nerve endings,
acetylcholinesterase is decreased and choline-acetyltransferase increased, showing that acetylcholine release is increased in dog by chronic alcoholism (13,56).

The formation of protein precipitates in the ducts of humans and dogs
(and the formation of pancreatic stones in humans) is partly explained
by the above-mentioned findings. The modifications of the ionic environment of proteins (decreased ratio of protein to bicarbonate and
water) probably play an important role. A similar modification has been
found in the pancreatic juice of dogs treated with repeated injections
of calcium (54) and it is known that hypercalcemia following either hy-

perparathyroidism, vitamin D administration (39), calcium infusion test, or hemodialysis (33) is a cause of acute and chronic pancreatitis.

B. Tropical Pancreatitis

Tropical pancreatitis is generally associated with malnutrition in child-hood. But Pitchumoni is of the opinion that the toxicity of prussic acid from manioc, which is a common food in these countries, could be responsible (58).

II. ACUTE PANCREATITIS

A. Acute Alcoholic Pancreatitis

The frequency of acute pancreatitis in alcoholics is increasing in different countries. Acute alcoholic pancreatitis is generally observed in chronically alcoholic people and represents the beginning of an alcoholic chronic pancreatitis. There is no evidence that an isolated alcoholic bout can produce acute pancreatitis lesions (35,81). Therefore, it is reasonable to think that the mechanism of acute alcoholic lesions is due, like chronic pancreatitis, to a hypersecretion of protein (81). An argument in favor of this assumption is that scorpion venom (2), as well as an insecticide (20) able to produce acute pancreatitis, do so by increasing the secretion of the pancreatic gland. In the case of the insecticide 0,0-diethyl-0-(2-isopropyl-6-methyl-4-pyrimidyl)phosphozo-thioate, this is due to an inhibition of acetylcholinesterase and an increased release of acetylcholine, which focuses once more the importance of acetylcholine in chronic and acute pancreatitis. Other mechanisms could be responsible: spasms of the sphincter of Oddi observed in dogs (47) and in humans (11,57) or alcohol-induced hyperlipemia (10).

B. Role of Drugs

Many drugs have been implicated in pancreatic pathology. It seems reasonable now to separate them into three groups according to Mallory and Kern (43; see for complete literature).

1. Drugs That Seem to Cause Pancreatitis (Definite Association)

(a) *Estrogens* [originally described by Bank and Marks (1)]: Now-adays numerous evidences favor the existence of estrogen-induced acute pancreatitis (readministration of estrogens associated with attacks of pancreatitis and recovery observed after discontinuing the medication). Generally, pancreatic lesions are associated if not induced by hypertriglyceridemia (9). Whatever the reason for the estrogen therapy, pancreatic attacks may occur within 2–3 months of exposure to the hormone. The serum triglyceride level is generally high, with a possible relationship to the estrogen dosage.

(b) *Azathioprine*: Pancreatitis was reported in patients treated only with this drug, presenting with recurrent symptoms and associated laboratory findings after challenge with the drug. Usual doses were 50–150 mg/day. Symptoms of pancreatitis began within 2–3 weeks of exposure to the drug.

(c) *Tetracycline*: When abnormally high blood levels of tetracycline are attained, there is a risk of acute fatty degeneration of the liver, acute renal failure, and acute pancreatitis. Generally observed in the third trimester of pregnancy, these tetracycline-induced acute lesions may also be observed in nonpregnant women or in men. The role of the liver disease is still unclear—a cause rather than a consequence of the pancreatic disease. Acute pancreatitis is reported within 3 weeks of beginning tetracycline therapy, and is more commonly a severe hemorrhagic pancreatitis than a mild interstitial one.

(d) *Chlorothiazide*: This drug seems to induce acute pancreatitis only after a long treatment. Symptoms are reported to appear within 3–4 months and the severity of the attacks seems to be correlated with the duration of therapy.

(e) *Furosemide*: According to some similarities with the structure of chlorothiazide, furosemide has also been reported to be associated with acute pancreatitis. Furosemide was given orally (40–100 mg/day) and symptoms appeared within 3 weeks after beginning the therapy.

(f) *Sulfonamides*: These drugs were claimed to cause pancreatitis only 1–2 weeks after initiating therapy. Since fever, pruritis, and chills accompanied the pancreatic symptoms, a possible allergic mechanism can be suggested rather than a purely toxic effect.

2. Drugs That May Cause Pancreatitis (Probable Association)

(a) *L-Asparaginase*: This drug would be associated with acute pancreatitis in up to 25% of patients receiving the drug, but no challenge tests have been done. The onset of the symptoms was an average 6 days after beginning the therapy.

(b) *Corticosteroids*: These drugs have been claimed to be the cause of acute pancreatitis in numerous patients, but also in some experimental models pancreatic lesions may occur within the first week of therapy, although they usually do not begin until the end of the first year of exposure to corticosteroids. ACTH seems to act similarly. Moreover, chronic corticosteroid therapy can induce some pancreatic secretory changes resembling those observed in chronic pancreatitis (5,6).

(c) *Diuretics*: Among diuretics, chlorthalidone and ethacrynic acid have been claimed to be associated in one well-documented case, each with acute pancreatitis, but the evidence has not yet been confirmed; this is also the case for procainamide.

3. *Drugs That Are Unlikely to Cause Pancreatitis*

Drugs that are unlikely to cause pancreatitis include amphetamines, cholestyramine, diazoxide; propoxyphene; histamine; mercaptopurine; rifampicin, salicylates, and cimetidine. Opiates may act through a contraction of the sphincter of Oddi.

III. CANCER

Pancreatic cancers in humans originate most commonly from duct cells: exocrine adenocarcinomas (37). Their frequency is increasing rapidly, and both toxic and alimentary factors are now suspected.

A. Animal Models

For a long time it has been known that some chemical substances are able to promote pancreatic tumors in experimental animals; p-dimethyl-aminoazobenzene (34), 3-methylcholanthrene (31), methylnitrosourea, and methylnitrosourethane (21) are among them. More recently, in the hamster, 2,2'-dihydroxy-n-propylnitrosamine (62) and N-nitrosobis-(2-acetoxypropyl)amine (61) have been known to induce pancreatic adenocarcinomas that closely resemble those observed in humans.

The action of all these chemical carcinogens is not yet very well documented; nevertheless, it seems reasonable to assume that some of them are preferentially taken up by the pancreas and not metabolized (3). It must be pointed out that the tumorigenicity of the chemical carcinogens is increased by the stimulation of the pancreatic tissue to proliferate. For instance, in rats, azaserine, a well-known carcinogen, has a much more important carcinogenic effect (in terms of number and size of tumors) when associated with either ethionine diet or partial pancreatectomy (18). In the same manner, the carcinogenic effect of azaserine or of di(2-hydroxypropyl)nitrosamine was shown to be increased by raw soya flour-induced pancreatic hypertrophy (40,50). Even more interesting is the fact that chronic release of large amounts of digestive hormones by a long-term feeding with soya flour is able, alone, to induce pancreatic cancer in the rat (46).

Finally, some differentiation of acinar cells during tumor development has been shown in rats by using 7,12-dimethylbenz[a]anthracene (4) According to these authors, some apparently ductal tumors may well originate from acinar cells and be recognized erroneously as ductular cells, because of the loss of zymogen granules by the tumoral cells.

B. Epidemiological Data

In humans, the role played by chemical carcinogens can be evaluated only by surveys on the etiology of pancreatic diseases. For instance, some populations in contact with these substances have been shown to develop many more pancreatic tumors than control populations. This is the case for industrial workers exposed to betanaphthylamine or benzidine (44) and also for members of the American Chemical Society (41) compared to persons in other professions.

As in many other cancers, a high fat intake is observed (24,36,80, 93). A correlation with alcohol consumption has been found by certain authors (8,36), but not by others (49,93). Recently, this discrepancy has been explained (23): the frequency of pancreatic cancer is increased by beer consumption but decreased by the consumption of slight wines (alcohol concentration 12% v/v). The anticorrelation with wine could be due to the fact that ordinary wine consumers do not drink much beer. The toxicity of beer is very likely due to the high concentration of nitrosamine (as in whiskey but in contrast to wine and cognac) (30).

Various studies in the United States have found that pancreatic cancer is correlated with tobacco smoking (50,92,93). This is partially untrue in France (24), where dark tobacco (French type) is smoked, unlike the United States, where mild tobacco (American type) is preferentially smoked. Indeed, in this study a correlation was found only with mild tobacco, and not with dark tobacco.

REFERENCES

1. Bank, S., and Marks, I. N. (1970). Hyperlipaemic pancreatitis and the pill. *Postgrad. Med. J. 46*:576-588.
2. Bartholomew, C., Murphy, J. J., McGeeney, K. J., and Fitzgerald, O. (1977). Exocrine pancreatic response to the venom of the scorpion *Tityus. Gut 18*:623-625.
3. Black, O., and Webster, P. D. (1974). Uptake of methylcholanthrene in the rat pancreas. *Am. J. Dig. Dis. 19*:37-42.
4. Bockman, D. E., Black, O., Mills, L. R., and Webster, P. D. (1978). Origin of tubular complexes developing during induction of pancreatic adenocarcinoma by 7,12-dimethylbenz[a]-anthracene. *Am. J. Pathol. 90*:645-658.
5. Bourry, J., and Sarles, H. (1978). Influence de la corticothérapie prolongée sur la secrétion pancréatique externe de l'homme. *Gastroenterol. Clin. Biol. 2*:139-144.
6. Bourry, J., and Sarles, H. (1978). Secretory pattern and pathological study of the pancreas of steroid-treated rats. *Am. J. Dig. Dis. 23*:423-428.

7. Bretholz, A., Levesque, D., Voirol, M., Tiscornia, O. M., Bloom, S. R., and Sarles, H. (1978). Impaired secretin release in chronic alcoholic dogs. *Digestion* *17*:436-440.

8. Burch, G. E., and Ansari, A. (1968). Chronic alcoholism and carcinoma of the pancreas. *Arch. Intern. Med. 122*:273-275.

9. Cameron, J. L., Capuzzi, D. M., Zuidema, G. D., and Margolis, S. (1974). Acute pancreatitis with hyperlipemia: evidence for a persistent defect in lipid metabolism. *Am. J. Med. 56*: 482-487.

10. Cameron, J. L., Zuidema, G. D., and Margolis, S. (1975). A pathogenesis for alcohol pancreatitis. *Surgery 77*:755-763.

11. Capitaine, Y., and Sarles, H. (1971). Action de l'ethanol sur le tonus du sphincter d'Oddi chez l'homme. *Biol. Gastroenterol. 3*:231-236.

12. Capitaine, Y., Barros Mott, C., Gullo, L., and Sarles, H. (1971). Action de l'éthanol sur la secrétion pancréatique chez l'homme. *Biol. Gastroenterol. 3*:193-198.

13. Celener, D., Lechene de la Porte, P., Tiscornia, O. M., and Sarles, H. (1977). Histochemical study of cholinergic activities on exocrine pancreas of dogs. Modification related to chronic alcoholism. *Biomedicine 27*:161-165.

14. Clemente, F., Ribeiro, R., Figarella, C., and Sarles, H. (1971). Albumine IgG et IgA dans le suc pancréatique humain normal chez l'adulte. *Clin. Chim. Acta 33*:317-324.

15. Clemente, F., Durand, S., Laval, J., Thouvenot, J. P., and Ribet, A. (1977). Métabolisme de l'éthanol par le pancréas de rat. I. Recherche des éventuelles enzymes impliquées et de leur variation de niveau. *Gastroenterol. Clin. Biol. 1*:39-48.

16. De Caro, A., Lohse, J., and Sarles, H. (1979). Characterization of a protein isolated from pancreatic calculi of men suffering from chronic calcifying pancreatitis. *Biochem. Biophys. Res. Commun. 87*:1176-1182.

17. Demol, P., Andersen, B. N., and Sarles, H. (1980). Chronic ethanol consumption and exocrine pancreatic response to ethanol and acetaldehyde in the rat. *Digestion 20*:85-94.

18. Denda, A., Inui, A., Sunagawa, M., Takahashi, S., and Konishi, Y. (1978). Enhancing effect of partial pancreatectomy and ethionine-induced pancreatic regeneration on the tumorigenesis of azoserine in rats. *Gann 69*:633-639.

19. Dreiling, D. A., Greenstein, A., and Bordalo, O. (1973). The hypersecretory state of the pancreas. *Am. J. Gastroenterol. 59*:505-511.

20. Dressel, T. D., Goodale, R. L., Arneson, M. A., and Boorner, J. W. (1979). Pancreatitis as a complication of anticholinesterase insecticide intoxication. *Ann. Surg. 189*:199-204.

21. Druchrey, H., Ivankovic, S., Bucheler, J., Preussman, R.,

and Thomas, C. (1968). Production of stomach and pancreatic cancer. *Z. Krebsforsch. 71*:167-182.

22. Durbec, J. P., and Sarles, H. (1978). Multicenter survey on the etiology of pancreatic diseases. Relationship between the relative risk of developing chronic pancreatitis and alcohol, protein and lipid consumption. *Digestion 18*:337-350.

23. Durbec, J. P., Bidart, J. M., and Sarles, H. (1980). Inter-actions between alcohol and other foodstuffs. Epidemiological aspects. In *Alcohol and the Gastrointestinal Tract*, Colloques de l'INSERM 95.

24. Durbec, J. P., Bidart, J. M., Berthezene, P., and Sarles, H. (1980). Effects of diet and alcohol and tobacco consump-tions on the risk of cancer of pancreas. A case control study. In *Alcohol and Gastrointestinal Tract*, Colloques de l'INSERM 95.

25. Estevenon, J. P., Sarles, H., and Figarella, C. (1975). Lacto-ferrin in the duodenal juice of patients with chronic calcifying pancreatitis. *Scand. J. Gastroenterol. 10*:327-330.

26. Estival, A., Clemente, F., and Ribet, A. (1980). Ethanol metabolism by the rat pancreas. In *Alcohol and Gastrointestinal Tract*, Colloques de l'INSERM 95.

27. Fahrenkrug, A., and Schaffalitzky de Muckadell, O. B. (1977). Plasma secretin concentration in man: effect of intraduodenal glucose, fat, amino acid, ethanol, HCl and ingestion of a meal. *Eur. J. Clin. Invest. 7*:201-204.

28. Fedail, S. S., and Harvey, F. (1970). Radioimmunoassay of lactoferrin in pancreatic juice as a test for pancreatic diseases. *Lancet 1*:180-182.

29. Goebell, H., Hotz, J., and Hoffmeister, H. (1980). Hyper-caloric nutrition as aetiological factor in chronic pancreatitis. *Z. Gastroenterol. 18*:94-97.

30. Goff, E. U., and Fine, D. H. (1979). Analysis of volatile N-nitrosamines in alcoholic beverages. *Food Cosmet. Toxicol. 17*:569-573.

31. Gorski, T. (1959). Induction of experimental pancreas car-cinoma in mice. *Vopr. Onkol. 5*:413-415.

32. Harvey, R. F., Mathur, M. S., Dowsett, L., and Read, A. E. (1974). Measurement of cholecystokinin-pancreozymin levels in peripheral venous blood in man. *Gastroenterology 66*:707.

33. Hoch-Gelerent, E. L., and David, D. S. (1974). Acute pan-creatitis secondary to calcium infusion in a dialysis patient. *Arch. Surg. 108*:218-219.

34. Hoch-Ligeti, C. (1949). Primary pancreatic tumours in rat fed p-dimethylaminoazobenzene. *Br. J. Cancer 3*:285-288.

35. Howat, H. T., and Sarles, H. (1979). In *The Exocrine Pan-creas*, H. T. Howat and H. Sarles, Eds., W. B. Saunders, Philadelphia.

36. Ishii, K., Nakamura, K., Takeuchi, T., and Hirayama, T. (1973). Chronic calcifying pancreatitis and pancreatic carcinoma in Japan. *Digestion* 9:429-437.
37. Kircher, C. H., and Nielsen, S. W. (1976). Tumours of the pancreas. *Bull. WHO* 53:195-202.
38. Laugier, R., and Sarles, H. (1977). Effets de la consommation chronique d'alcool sur la secrétion pancréatique exocrine du rat. Variations en fonction de la durée de consommation. *Gastroenterol. Clin. Biol.* 1:767-774.
39. Leeson, P. M., and Fourman, P. (1966). Acute pancreatitis from vitamin D poisoning in a patient with parathyroid deficiency. *Lancet* 1:1185-1186.
40. Levison, D. A., Morgan, R. G. H., Brimacombe, J. S., Hopwood, D., Coghill, G., and Wormsley, K. G. (1979). Carcinogenic effect of di(2-hydroxypropyl)nitrosamine (DHPN) in male Wistar rats: promotion of pancreatic cancer by a raw soya flour diet. *Scand. J. Gastroenterol.* 14:217-224.
41. Li, F. P., Fraumeni, F. J., Mantel, N., and Miller, R. W. (1969). Cancer mortality among chemists. *J. Nat. Cancer Inst.* 43:1159-1163.
42. Lohse, J., Verine, H., and Sarles, H. (1980). Studies on pancreatic stones. I. In vitro dissolution. *Digestion* 21 (in press.
43. Mallory, A., and Kern, F. (1980). Drug-induced pancreatitis: a critical review. *Gastroenterology* 78:813-820.
44. Mancuso, T. F., and El-Attar, A. A. (1967). Cohort study of workers exposed to betanaphtylamine and benzidine. *J. Occup. Med.* 9:277-285.
45. Marks, I. N., Bank, S., and Barbezat, G. O. (1976). Alkohol Pankreatitis. Aetiologie klinische Formen, Komplikatrionen. *Leber Magen Darm* 6:257-270.
46. McGuiness, E. E., Morgan, R. G., Levison, D. A., Frape, D. L., Hopwood, D., and Wormsley, K. G. (1980). The effects of long-term feeding of soya flour on the rat pancreas. *Scand. J. Gastroenterol.* 15:497-502.
47. Menguy, R. B., Hallenbeck, G. A., Bollman, J. L., and Grindlay, D. M. (1958). Intraductal pressures of sphincter resistance in canine pancreatic biliary ducts of the various stimuli. *Surg. Gynecol. Obstet.* 106:306-310.
48. Meullenet, J., Baratta, H., and Sarles, H. (1979). Alcool et anticholinergiques. Effets sur la secrétion pancréatique exocrine de l'homme. *Gastroenterol. Clin. Biol.* 3:885-892.
49. Monson, R. R., and Lyon, J. L. (1975). Proportional mortality among alcoholics' cancer. *Cancer* 36:1077-1079.
50. Morgan, R. G., and Wormsley, K. G. (1977). Cancer of the pancreas. *Gut* 18:580-596.

51. Multigner, L., Figarella, C., Sahel, J., and Sarles, H. (1980).
     Lactoferrin and albumin in human pancreatic juice, a valuable
     test for diagnosis of pancreatic diseases. *Dig. Dis. Sci. 25*:
     173-178.

51a. Multigner, L., De Caro, A., Lombardo, D., Campese, D., and
     Sarles, H. (1983). Pancreatic stone protein, a phosphoprotein
     which inhibits calcium carbonate precipitation from human pan-
     creatic juice. *Biochem. Biophys. Res. Comm. 110*:69-74.

51b. Multigner, L., De Caro, A., Campese, D., Lombardo, D., and
     Sarles, H. (1983). Measurement of stone protein in human pan-
     creatic juice during the course of chronic calcifying pancreati-
     tis. *Gastroenterology 84*:1255.

52. Nakamura, K., Sarles, H., and Payan, H. (1972). Three di-
     mensional reconstruction of the pancreatic ducts in chronic
     pancreatitis. *Gastroenterology 62*:942-949.

53. Noel-Jorand, M. C., Colomb, E., Astier, J. P., and Sarles,
     H. (1984). Compared study of pancreatic basal secretion in al-
     cohol-fed dogs and normal dogs. Submitted to *Dig. Dis. Sci.*

54. Noel-Jorand, M. C., Colomb, E., Astier, J. P., and Sarles,
     H. (1984). Persisting modifications of dogs basal exocrine pan-
     creatic secretion after repeated intravenous calcium injections.
     Accepted by *Eur. J. Clin. Invest.*

55. Payan, H., Sarles, H., Demirdjian, M., Gauthier, A. P., Cros,
     R. C., and Durbec, J. P. (1972). Study of the histological
     features of chronic pancreatitis by correspondance analysis.
     Identification of chronic calcifying pancreatitis as an entity.
     Rev. Eur. Etud. Clin. Biol. 17:663-670.

56. Perec, C. J., Celener, D., Tiscornia, O. M., and Baratti, C.
     (1979). Effects of chronic ethanol administration on the auto-
     nomic innervation of salivary glands pancreas and heart. *Am.
     J. Gastroenterol. 72*:46-59.

57. Pirola, R. C., and Davis, A. E. (1967). The role of ethyl
     alcohol in the etiology of pancreatitis. *Gut 8*:526-536.

58. Pitchumoni, C. S., Bonnenshein, M., Candido, F. M., Pan-
     chacharam, P., and Cooperman, J. M. (1980). Nutrition in the
     pathogenesis of alcoholic pancreatitis. *Am. J. Clin. Nutr. 33*:
     631-636.

59. Planche, N. E., Chau Huu, T., Lai, P. P., and Sarles, H.
     (1977). Chronic alcohol consumption does not modify cholecy-
     stokinin blood levels estimated by bioassay in the dog. *Diges-
     tion 16*:194-198.

60. Planche, N. E., Palasciano, G., Meullenet, J., Laugier, R., and
     Sarles, H. (1984). The effects of intravenous alcohol on pan-
     creatic and biliary secretion in man. In preparation.

61. Pour, P., Althoff, J., Gingell, R., and Kupper, R. (1976). A
     further pancreatic carcinogen in Syrian golden hamsters N-ni-
     trosobis(2-acetoxypropryl)amine. *Cancer Lett. 1*:197-202.

62. Pour, P., Mohr, U., Cardesa, A., Althoff, J., Kruger, F. W., and Chem, D. (1975). Pancreatic neoplasms in an animal model: morphological, biological and comparative studies. *Cancer* 36:379-389.
63. Renner, G., Rinderknecht, H., and Douglas, A. P. (1978). Profiles of pure pancreatic secretions in patients with acute pancreatitis: the possible role of proteolytic enzymes in pathogenesis. *Gastroenterology* 75:1090-1098.
64. Renner, G., Rinderknecht, H., Valenzuela, J. E., and Douglas, A. P. (1978). Abnormalities in pure pancreatic juice from human alcoholics. *Clin. Res.* 26:112.
65. Rinderknecht, H., Renner, I. G., and Koyama, H. H. (1979). Lysosomal enzymes in pure pancreatic juice from normal healthy volunteers and chronic alcoholics. *Dig. Dis. Sci.* 24:180-186.
66. Rinderknecht, H., Renner, I. G., and Carmack, C. (1979). Trypsinogen variants in pancreatic juice of healthy volunteers, chronic alcoholics and patients with pancreatitis and cancer of pancreas. *Gut* 20:886-891.
67. Sahel, J., and Sarles, H. (1979). Modifications of pure human pancreatic juice induced by chronic alcohol consumption. *Dig. Dis. Sci.* 24:897-905.
68. Sarles, H. (1973). An international survey on nutrition and pancreatitis. *Digestion* 9:389-403.
69. Sarles, H. (1976). Alcohol and the pancreas. In *Advances in Experimental Medicine and Biology Alcohol Intoxication and Withdrawal, IIIa: Biological Aspects of Ethanol*, M. M. Gross, Ed., Plenum Press, New York, pp. 429-448.
70. Sarles, H., and Figarella, C. (1967). Etude de l'action de l'ethanol et des graisses alimentaires sur le pancréas de rat. 1. Variation des enzymes pancréatiques (lipase, amylase, chymotrypsinogène, trypsinogène). *Pathol. Biol.* 15:725-731.
71. Sarles, H., Figarella, C., and Clemente, F. (1971). The interaction of ethanol dietary lipids and proteins on the rat pancreas. *Digestion* 4:1322.
72. Sarles, H., and Tiscornia, O. M. (1974). Ethanol and chronic calcifying pancreatitis. *Med. Clin. N. Am.* 58:1333-1346.
73. Sarles, H., Cros, R. C., Bidart, J. M., and the International Group for the Study of Pancreatic Diseases (1979). A multicenter inquiry into the etiology of pancreatic diseases. *Digestion* 19:110-125.
74. Sarles, H., Tiscornia, O. M., and Palasciano, G. (1977). Chronic alcoholism and canine exocrine pancreas secretion. A long-term follow-up study. *Gastroenterology* 72:238-243.
75. Sarles, H., Sahel, J., Lebreuil, G., and Tiscornia, O. M. (1975). Pancréatite alcoolique chronique expérimentale du chien. Etude anatomo-pathologique. *Biol. Gastroenterol.* 8:152-155.
76. Sarles, H., Sahel, J., Palasciano, G., Capitaine, Y., and

Meullenet, J. (1980). Alcohol consumption and the human pancreas. 1. Alcohol-induced modifications of exocrine pancreas function. In *Alcohol and Gastrointestinal Tract,* Colloques de l'INSERM, 95.

77. Sarles, H., Clemente, F., Colomb, E., De Caro, A., Figarella, C., Guy, O., Lohse, J., Multigner, L., Noel-Jorand, M. C., Ribeiro, T., and Verine, H. (1980). Alcohol consumption and the human pancreas. 2. Alcohol induced chemical and physical modifications of pancreatic juice. Formation of the lesions. In *Alcohol and Gastrointestinal Tract,* Colloques de l'INSERM 95.

78. Sarles, H., Lebreuil, G., Tasso, F., Figarella, C., Clemente, F., Devaux, M. A., Fagonde, B., and Payan, H. (1971). A comparison of alcoholic pancreatitis in rat and man. *Gut 12:* 377-388.

79. Schmidt, E., and Schmidt, F. W. (1960). Enzyme-muster menschlicher Gewebe. *Klin. Wochenschr. 38:*957-961.

80. Segi, M., Kurimara, M., and Matsuyama, T. (1969). Cancer mortality for selected sites in 24 countries, No. 5 (1964-1965). Department of Public Health. Tohoku Univ. School of Medicine, Sendai, Japan.

81. Strum, W. B., and Spiro, H. M. (1971). Chronic pancreatitis. *Ann. Intern. Med. 74:*264-277.

82. Tasso, F., and Stemmelin, N., Clop, J., Cros, R. C., Durbec, J. P., and Sarles, H. (1973). Comparative morphometric study of the human pancreas in its normal state and in primary chronic calcifying pancreatitis. *Biomedicine 19:*1-11.

83. Tiscornia, O. M., Gullo, L., and Sarles, H. (1973). The inhibition of canine exocrine pancreatic secretion by intravenous ethanol. *Digestion 9:*231-240.

84. Tiscornia, O. M., Palasciano, G., and Sarles, H. (1974). Pancreatic changes induced by chronic (2 years) ethanol treatment in the dog. *Gut 15:*839-843.

85. Tiscornia, O. M., Palasciano, G., and Sarles, H. (1974). Effect of chronic ethanol administration on canine exocrine pancreatic secretion. Further studies. *Digestion 11:*172-182.

86. Tiscornia, O. M., Palasciano, G., and Sarles, H. (1975). Atropine and exocrine pancreatic secretion in alcohol-fed dogs. *Am. J. Gastroenterol. 63:*3336.

87. Tiscornia, O. M., Singer, M., Mendes De Oliveira, J. P., and Sarles, H. (1977). Exocrine pancreatic response to a test meal in the dog. Changes induced by 3 months ethanol feedings. *Am. J. Dig. Dis. 22:*769-774.

88. Tiscornia, O. M., Hage, G., Palasciano, G., Brasca, A., Devaux, M. A., and Sarles, H. (1973). The effects of pentholinium and secretion by intravenous ethanol. *Biomedicine 18:* 159-163.

89. Treffot, M. J., Laugier, R., Bretholz, A., Voirol, M., and Sarles, H. (1980). Increased gastrin release in chronic calcifying pancreatitis and in chronic alcoholism. *Horm. Metab. Res.* 12:240-242.

90. Treffot, M. J., Tiscornia, O. M., Palasciano, G., Hage, G., and Sarles, H. (1975). Chronic alcoholism and endogenous gastrin. *Am. J. Gastroenterol.* 63:21-32.

91. Valenzuela, J. E., Taylor, I. L., and Walsh, J. H. (1979). Pancreatic polypeptide response in patients with chronic pancreatitis. *Dig. Dis. Sci.* 24:862-864.

92. Weir, J. M., and Donn, J. E. (1970). Smoking and mortality: a prospective study. *Cancer* 25:105-112.

93. Wynder, E. L., Mabuchi, K., Maruchi, N., and Fortner, J. G., (1973). A case control study of cancer of the pancreas. *Cancer* 31:641-648.

15

Risk Factors in Drug-Induced Nutritional Deficiencies

Daphne A. Roe
Cornell University, Ithaca, New York

I. IS MALNUTRITION IN DRUG RECIPIENTS DRUG-INDUCED?

It is generally accepted that drug-induced nutritional deficiencies are a subclass of adverse drug reactions. According to Stolley (1981), an adverse drug reaction may be defined as a deleterious and unwanted effect of a drug, which may be due either to an increase in the desired pharmacological action of the drug, or due to a secondary pharmacological property of the drug that is unwanted in some particular situation.

Adverse drug reactions have been grouped by Parish (1973), who suggested that these reactions include recognized but unwanted side effects of drugs which are related to high dosage, excessive side effects from drugs at therapeutic dosages occurring in groups at special risk, and idiosyncratic reactions. The Parish method of grouping adverse drug reactions is more applicable to risk assessment and can be utilized in projecting risk of adverse nutritional outcomes of drug usage. Use of this system allows the investigator to assess the relative importance of drug versus host factors in the etiology of specific cases of drug-related nutritional deficiency.

Drug-related nutritional deficiencies are commonly multifactorial, where etiological factors pertain to the host and to drug usage. Prediction of risk of drug-induced nutritional deficiencies requires knowledge of the mechanism for nutrient depletion by the drug to be administered, the dose and duration of drug usage, as well as the characteristics of the person taking the drug. From this information sig-

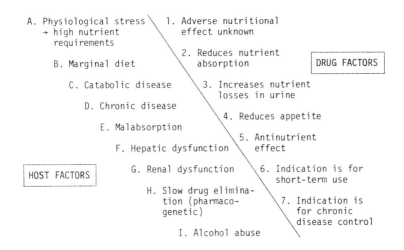

A. Physiological stress → high nutrient requirements

B. Marginal diet

C. Catabolic disease

D. Chronic disease

E. Malabsorption

F. Hepatic dysfunction

HOST FACTORS

G. Renal dysfunction

H. Slow drug elimination (pharmacogenetic)

I. Alcohol abuse

1. Adverse nutritional effect unknown

2. Reduces nutrient absorption

DRUG FACTORS

3. Increases nutrient losses in urine

4. Reduces appetite

5. Antinutrient effect

6. Indication is for short-term use

7. Indication is for chronic disease control

Prediction of Adverse Nutritional Outcome

At high dose	At normal dose	Idiosyncratic
2, 2 + 7	A + B	1
3, 3 + 7	A + B + C	
4, 4 + 7	A + B + C + D	
	A + B + C + D + E	
	A + B + C + D + E, F, G, H or I	
	5, 5 + 6, 5 + 7	

Figure 1   Risk assessment for drug-induced nutritional deficiencies.

nificant predictive factors can be computed, as indicated in Figure 1. From this diagram it can be seen that the risk of adverse nutritional outcome from drugs causing nutrient depletion is strongly influenced by dose and duration of drug administration.

Vesell (1980) has pointed out that until very recently, relationships between diet and drug response were not suspected in people, and that knowledge of these relationships has come only as an outcome of very limited investigations. He has proposed that more studies are required to establish relationships between dietary factors and specific processes of drug absorption, distribution, excretion, and receptor interaction.

Karch and Lasagna (1977) reemphasized that while the goal in assessing adverse drug reactions must be to establish a causal relationship between the suspected drug and the clinical outcome, achievement of this goal is rendered extremely difficult by the ambiguous character of the reaction or commonly by the fact that the patient is taking several drugs. A special problem is the ability of the investigator to utilize specific and sensitive cause-effect tests to establish the relationship.

Interobserver differences exist and indeed are very common in interpretation or assessment of adverse drug reactions. It seems that there are no standard guidelines to the investigator in the evaluation of reactions that are suspected to be due to the effects of drugs (Karch et al., 1976).

The following criteria have been proposed by Folb (1980) for acceptance of adverse drug reactions:

1. The association should be consistent.
2. The association should be specific.
3. There should be a reasonable temporal relationship between exposure and development of the alleged effect.
4. The association should be plausible.

In answering the question as to whether malnutrition in drug recipients is drug induced, these guidelines should be followed (Folb, 1980; Surgeon General's Advisory Committee on Smoking and Health, 1964).

II. DEFINITION OF DRUG-INDUCED NUTRITIONAL DEFICIENCY

Drug-induced nutritional deficiencies comprise symptoms, signs, or laboratory evidence of one or more micro- or macronutrient deficiencies occuring in individuals or groups while taking the drug, where impairment of nutritional status can be positively associated with drug intake per se, or with intake of the drug under special conditions. Indentification and causal attribution of drug reactions with adverse nutritional outcomes may be from single clinical observations, drug reaction reporting systems, or from case control and cohort studies.

Drug-induced malnutrition may be acute or chronic. Acute forms are usually due to effects of potent antinutrients, whereas chronic forms may develop because the drug reduces nutrient absorption, increases nutrient catabolism, increases nutrient losses via the urine, or otherwise decreases nutrient utilization.

Definite cases of drug-induced nutritional deficiency have the following characteristics:

1. There is a constant temporal relationship of drug usage and the development of a biochemical and/or clinical nutritional deficiency.
2. Drug-induced nutritional deficiency has been demonstrated in an animal model.
3. The causal mechanism is known.
4. The development of the deficiency state is retarded or reversed when the drug is discontinued.
5. The deficiency state is prevented by concurrent administration of available and utilizable nutrient supplements. (Effective treatment is by discontinuing the drug and giving a specific nutrient supplement to the patient).
6. The specific deficiency state is exacerbated by a dietary deficiency of the same nutrient in an animal model and in human subjects.

Probable drug-induced nutritional deficiencies bear the constant temporal association with administration of the drug. Their progression is halted when the drug is discontinued. Proof of association with the drug is as yet unknown; previous association has been established between the administration of pharmacologically similar drugs and the development of a specific nutritional deficiency state.

False positive cases of drug-induced nutritional deficiency are particularly common. Drug-induced nutritional deficiency may be provisionally diagnosed when a patient who is taking a particular drug develops a nutritional deficiency but confirmation must await analysis of the other characteristics of the drug user, which could explain the deficiency state. For example, the reason that people on a particular drug may develop a nutritional deficiency may be that their diet lacks a specific nutrient. Other reasons are that the person receiving this particular drug may have disease-induced malnutrition. Further explanation of false association of a particular drug with a specific nutritional deficiency state is that the same patient is taking another drug or several other drugs which have adverse nutritional effects.

Drug-induced nutritional deficiency may be missed (false negative). For example, if the drug group in a particular study has better nutritional status than the nondrug group, or when the drug group has lower nutrient requirements than the nondrug group. Other common reasons for missing drug-induced nutrient depletion are that the study is too short, so that nutrient depletion cannot be defined by available tests, or because the variation in nutritional status of the drug and nondrug group is large and overlapping. Diagnostic components which prove, suggest, or disprove drug-induced nutritional deficiency are grouped in Table 1.

Table 1 Diagnostic Criteria for Drug-Induced Nutritional Deficiency

	Proven	Suggested	Disproven
Evidence of deficiency	Clinical and biochemical signs are specific	Clinical and biochemical signs are specific	Clinical and biochemical signs are specific; biochemical signs also indicate primary disease
Drug	Is known to cause deficiency	Is suspected to cause deficiency	Is not known to cause deficiency
Diet	Contains physiological nutrient requirements	Marginal intake of nutrients	Contains physiological nutrient requirements
Disease	Is not associated with nutritional deficiency	Is associated with nutritional deficiency	Is associated with nutritional deficiency
Intervention	Progress of deficiency is halted when drug is stopped	Deficiency progresses after drug is stopped	Deficiency progresses after drug is stopped
	Cure of deficiency is with specific nutrient supplement	Cure of deficiency is with specific nutrient supplement	Cure of deficiency is by disease control

III. MECHANISMS OF DRUG-INDUCED MAL-
NUTRITION

Drug-induced malnutrition may be induced by one of four mechanisms.
These mechanisms can be categorized as follows:

1. Drug exerts an antinutrient effect (e.g., the drug is a vitamin
   or other nutrient antagonist).
2. The drug induces maldigestion and/or malabsorption.
3. The drug promotes urinary hyperexcretion of minerals, trace
   elements, or vitamins.
4. The drug causes hypercatabolism of nutrients or impairs utilization. Drugs having these separate adverse effects on nutrition
   are listed in Table 2.

Recognition that a drug has the capacity to induce malnutrition may
be obtained from semi-in vitro studies or animal studies which are carried out with the objective of defining the biochemical functions of a
particular nutrient. In screening new drugs, tests should include examination of effects on nutritional status in laboratory animals and human subjects. However, demonstration that a drug is capable of inducing an adverse nutritional effect is not synonymous with assessment
of risk. Induction of malnutrition by drugs having this capacity is not
inevitable. The highest risk is with drugs exerting a profound acute
and/or chronic antinutrient effect. In this category are drugs which
are vitamin antagonists, such as coumarin anticoagulants; antifolate
drugs; drugs which are vitamin B_6 antagonists; and nitrous oxide,
which has been found to have an antivitamin B_{12} effect. On the other
hand, drugs that induce mild absorption or a modest increase in the
urinary excretion or catabolism of nutrients may or may not cause a
clinical state of malnutrition, depending on circumstances (Roe, 1976).
   Statements in the literature suggest that it is very often unclear
which factors determine development of individual cases of drug-induced malnutrition. For example, Thompson (1979), in a textbook on
hematology, when discussing megaloblastic anemia associated with use
of anticonvulsant drugs, comments: "It is also unknown why only a few
patients develop megaloblastic anemia out of thousands taking the same
drug in the same dosages; there is no explanation for the finding that
quite a high proportion of these patients on anticonvulsants have
a mild macrocytosis without anemia or megaloblastic change." However,
our experience is that drug-induced nutritional deficiencies can be explained easily when risk factors are known. Factors that determine
risk need to be systematically assessed in all clinical situations where it
is suspected that drug-induced malnutrition is present. Risk factors
are classified by drug group in Table 3.

Table 2 Common Drugs That Cause Nutritional Deficiencies by Mode of Action

	Decreased nutrient absorption
Vitamin antagonism	
Folacin antagonists	
Methotrexate	Laxatives (mineral oil) — β-Carotene, fat-soluble vitamins
Pyrimethamine	Antibiotic (neomycin) — Fat, nitrogen, K, Ca, Fe, vitamin B_{12}
Triamterene	Hypocholesterolemic agents (cholestyramine, colestipol) — Fat, fats of vitamins, folate
Triemethoprin	Anti-inflammatory agents — Fat, carotene, Na, K, vitamin B_{12}, lactose
Sulfasalazine	Colchicine
Vitamin B_6 antagonists	*Mineral depletion by hyperexcretion*
Isoniazid	Diuretics — Potassium, calcium, magnesium, zinc
Hydrazine	Antibiotics (aminoglycoside) gentamicin — Magnesium
Cycloserine	Glucocorticoids — Potassium, calcium
L-dopa	Chelating agents (penicillamine) — Zinc, copper
Vitamin B_{12} antagonists	Cancer chemotherapeutic drugs (cisplatin)[a] — Magnesium
Nitrous oxide	
Vitamin K antagonists	
Coumarin anticoagulants	

[a]Cisplatin, cisplatin (II) dichlorodiamine.

Table 3 Risk Factors for Drug-Induced Malnutrition by Drug Group, Drug, and Deficiency State

Risk factor	Drug group	Drug[a]	Deficiency state
1. Drug characteristic. Example: vitamin antagonist	Cancer chemotherapeutic agent	MTX	Acute folate deficiency
2. Drug metabolism. Example: slow acetylation	Tuberculostat	INH	Vitamin B_6 deficiency, pellagra
3. Drug dosage. Example: chronic abuse	Laxative	Phenolphthalein	Potassium deficiency, steatorrhea
4. Duration of drug use. Example: prolonged intake	Hypocholesterolemic agent	Cholestyramine	Folate deficiency
5. Diet. Example: low potassium	Diuretic	Furosemide, thiazide	Potassium deficiency
6. Coexistent disease. Example: regional enteritis	Anti-inflammatory drug	SASP	Folate deficiency
7. Physiological stress. Example: pregnancy	Anticonvulsant	DPH	Folate deficiency mother, vitamin K deficiency infant
8. Environmental. Example: lack of UV exposure	Anticonvulsant	DPH	Rickets, osteomalacia
9. Multiple drug intake. Example: infection with two or more pathogens	Two antibiotics	Cephalothin	Magnesium deficiency
10. Multifactorial determinants. Example: marginal diet + catabolic + multiple drugs in geriatric population	Diuretic, laxative	HCT, senna	Potassium deficiency

[a]MTX, methotrexate; INH, isoniazid (isonicotinic acid hydrazide); DPH, diphenylhydantoin; SASP, sulfasalazine (salicylazosulfapyridine); HCT, hydrochlorothiazide.

IV. MISSED DIAGNOSES DUE TO ABSENCE OF DIAGNOSTIC CRITERIA

Diagnosis of drug-induced malnutrition usually requires definition of all diagnostic postulates. However, it should be recognized that true positive cases of drug-induced malnutrition can present which do not fulfill all criteria. A common barrier to the recognition of drug-induced malnutrition is that the symptoms and signs do not respond to the administration of the nutrient for which deficiency has been created. Such may be the case when acute intoxication develops following intake of a vitamin antagonist. The classical example is with methotrexate poisoning, which presents acute folacin deficiency, but in which the signs of intoxication do not respond to folic acid (Werkheiser, 1963).

It has long been recognized that methotrexate is a potent antifolate which binds firmly to the dihydrofolate reductase enzyme and displaces folacin from the enzyme, rendering exogenous sources of the vitamin nonutilizable. The antidote is folinic acid (citrovorum factor), which can be utilized as a folacin source despite the enzyme block (Sullivan et al., 1959).

Acute drug overdosage causing B_6 deficiency may not respond or may respond incompletely to administration of the vitamin (Brown, 1972). Isoniazid intoxication, when acute, is attended by convulsions. These seizures are analogous to pyridoxine-responsive convulsions of infants (Roe, 1976). Pyridoxine is generally considered to be the antidote for INH intoxication, but as pointed out by Chin et al. (1981), this B_6 vitamer does not always prevent convulsions, even when high dosage is administered. On the other hand, anticonvulsant drugs alone are also not particularly effective in seizure control. Combined treatment of INH-induced convulsions with pyridoxine and a barbiturate or diazepam controls INH convulsions in dogs and in human patients (Chin et al., 1978,1981). The convulsive effect of INH is apparently related to a reduced level of γ-aminobutyric acid (GABA) in the brain. Pyridoxine prevents inhibition of glutamic acid decarboxylase by INH and partially restores neuronal synthesis of GABA. Barbital or pentobarbital, or diazepam, potentiate postsynaptic GABA synthesis (Saad et al., 1972).

A generalization can be made that when drug-induced malnutrition is acute and is caused by a vitamin antagonist, reversal of signs may not be changed with the nutrient, which is functionally useless. Either a usable vitamer can be employed as the antidote, or it may be necessary to give massive doses of the nutrient which is complexed by the drug, and also to supply adjuvant therapy to control signs. We are not fully able to interpret the latter therapeutic necessity, but presently assume a slow reversibility of the chemical lesion.

V. COMPLEX ETIOLOGY OF DRUG-INDUCED NUTRITIONAL DEFICIENCIES

Etiological factors that determine drug-induced nutritional deficiencies may be synchronous, sequential, and/or interactive. A number of common drugs, available for self-medication, can produce adverse nutritional effects. Laxatives misuse and abuse have been shown to be a prominent cause of potassium depletion, and antacid abuse can lead to phosphate depletion (Insogna et al., 1980). Aspirin, among nonnarcotic analgesics, is a common cause of iron-deficiency anemia (Leonards et al., 1973).

Multiple factors that lead to drug-related malnutrition are presented by case histories of over-the-counter (OTC) drug abuse. Clinical malnutrition, associated with self-medication, is commonly an outcome of long-term drug excess. The observation that drug-induced nutritional deficiencies are often seen in OTC drug abusers is easier to understand when the characteristics of OTC drug abusers are examined. For example, laxative abusers include girls and occasionally boys with anorexia nervosa, neurotic middle-aged women, and the elderly of both sexes who, because of poor dietary habits and low fiber intake as well as debilitating disease, fail to obtain a daily bowel movement unless drugs are taken. A generalization is that laxative abuse is by people who have appetitive disorders or unsatisfactory diets.

The malnutrition that ensues is due to the combined effect of the laxative and dietary deficiency. Dietary deficiency is often the result of following a fad diet which eliminates foods that are rich sources of nutrients. Abuse of common laxatives, including phenolphthalein, bisacodyl, and senna, is most commonly associated with potassium depletion and sometimes associated with cachexia and hypoproteinemias.

The 64-year-old woman whose case history was reported by Levine et al. (1981) provides a classical example of laxative abuse with multiple nutritional consequences. This woman was admitted to hospital in 1980 for the investigation of chronic diarrhea and weight loss. Weight at the time of admission was 24 kg and she had lost 45% of her normal body weight. In several previous hospital admissions over the past 8 years, no cause had been found for her chronic diarrhea. During these previous admissions, she had been found to have hypokalemia and steatorrhea. Investigation during the most recent admission showed that she had hypokalemia, hypoalbuminemia, and hypogammaglobulinemia. She also presented with finger clubbing. Total body potassium measurement indicated a 25% loss of lean body mass. Her average plasma potassium level was 2.3 mmol/liter. Diarrhea was persistent, with an average daily stool weight of 700 g. Her physical and biochemical signs indicated potassium deficiency, chronic protein-energy malnutrition due to inadequate intake, and protein-losing enteropathy secondary to laxative-induced gut injury. A search was made of her locker and 200 Senokot (senna) tablets were found. After this discovery, she agreed to stop taking senna and to eat more food. She was also provided with liquid nutrient supplements. With dietary intervention and discontinuation of her laxatives, she gained weight and her signs of malnutrition were reversed.

In this woman, drug-related malnutrition was the outcome of laxative abuse and dietary inadequacy, and both we suspect were secondary to weight phobia as seen in anorexia nervosa. In laxative abusers, development of multiple nutritional deficiencies is predictable when the drug abuse is a manifestation of this disease.

VI. MULTIPLE-RISK-FACTOR MODELS DESCRIBING DRUG-INDUCED NUTRITIONAL DEFICIENCIES

In order to explain intergroup and interindividual differences in the incidence and evolution of malnutrition between users of drugs having this pharmacological potential, it has previously been stated that drug-induced nutritional deficiencies are determined not only by drug characteristics but also by coexisting host variables which singularly or collectively cause a nutritional deficiency. Conceptual models have been developed to allow prediction of the nutritional risks of other drugs to individuals and to specific patient populations.

For predictive purposes relevant information is whether etiological factors present together in a discrete time frame (synchronous or concurrent), whether risk factors make a sequential appearance, or whether risk factors are apparent at the time of initiation of drug therapy, but outcome is dependent on the total drug dosage over time. A further model (interactive) is required to explain outcomes of interaction of multiple variables at several time points. These models are illustrated in Figures 2 to 4.

A. Sequential-Event Model

When two or more drugs that impair vitamin status, such as a coumarin anticoagulant and cholestyramine or a coumarin anticoagulant and clofibrate, are given together to a patient with alcoholic liver disease, the risk of acute vitamin K deficiency with bleeding is extremely high (Dollery et al., 1974).

Drug-induced malnutrition is influenced by episodic or continuous disease-related nutrient depletion and/or interactive effects of a multiple-drug regimen with a second or third drug having the same potential for nutritional impairment as the primary drug. Thus severe magnesium and potassium depletion during gentamicin therapy is influenced by the pathophysiology of the disease for which gentamicin is received, adjunct drug therapy, and the effects of potassium depletion on genta-

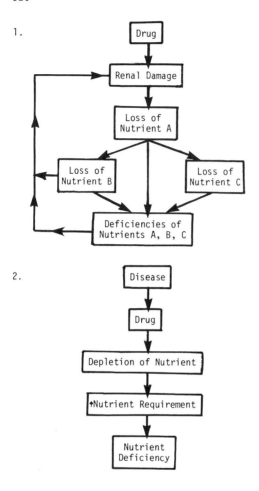

Figure 2 Sequential model.

micin nephrotoxicity, which may potentiate the magnesium wasting
(Kluft et al., 1975; Brinker et al., 1981).

Sequential drug and nondrug factors that contributed to the development of mineral deficiencies are illustrated by the case described
by Kelnar et al. (1978). A 12-year-old boy sustained severe injuries
in a traffic accident. Healing of a transverse fracture of the right fe-
mur was delayed by osteomyelitis and sepsis surrounding the bone.
A *Proteus* species, sensitive only to gentamicin, was grown. Gentamicin was administered for 4 months at a dose of 60 mg i.m. twice
daily to a total dose of 144 g. Several weeks after the drug was dis-

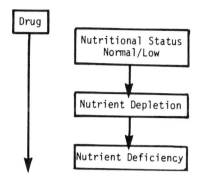

Figure 3 Continuity model.

continued, the boy became unwell and began vomiting. Investigation revealed renal tubular proteinuria and hypokalemia (plasma K^+ 1.1 mmol/liter). The boy was treated with potassium supplements. After 2 weeks, tetany developed with hypocalcemia (serum Ca 1.6 mmol/liter or 6.4 mg/100 ml) and hypomagnesemia (serum Mg 0.2 mmol/liter or 0.5 mg/100 ml). He was treated with calcium and magnesium supplements. Potassium, calcium, and magnesium levels in serum/plasma were reversed, and renal function was normalized.

In this case, gentamicin apparently caused the original renal tubular damage, with resultant hypomagnesemia due to hypermagnesuria. Magnesium depletion due to renal tubular damage may have initiated hypocalcemia and hypokalemia. Potassium depletion increased the toxic effect of the gentamycin on the kidney with increased hypermagnesemia and the clinical manifestation of tetany.

A sequence of nutritional stresses and chronic drug use provides a high-risk situation for development of drug-related malnutrition. Clinical signs of drug-induced nutritional deficiencies are more likely to occur in those whose nutrient requirements are suddenly or repeatedly increased, as for example in succeeding pregnancies. This course of events explains the development of folate-responsive megaloblastic anemia in epileptic women receiving diphenylhydantoin during succeeding pregnancies (Chanarin, 1969).

B. Continuous-Use (Continuity) Model

Drugs of choice in the management of certain chronic diseases may cause nutrient depletion or deficiency over time. Thus folacin depletion has been found in children with familial hypercholesterolemia with prolonged intake of cholestyramine. With this drug, the folacin depletion

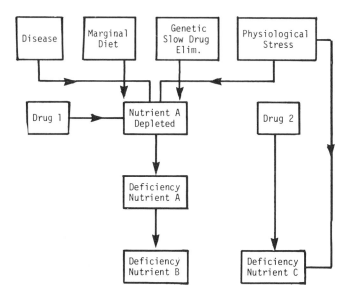

Figure 4 Interactive model.

is believed to be due to adsorption of folacin onto the drug, which is
an anion exchange resin (West and Lloyd, 1975).

A certain laissez-faire may develop in physicians who prescribe drugs
having small potential for induction of nutrient depletion. Thus if the
U.S. literature indicates that nutrient depletion induced by a drug over
time is insufficient to pose a risk of clinical malnutrition, clinicians may
be unjustifiably reassured. It is important, however, to remember that
whereas patients who start drug therapy with adequate nutritional status may be able to take the drug for long periods of time with only modest biochemical evidences of depletion, other patients who are nutri-
tionally depleted at the onset of therapy may develop nutritional deficiencies with time. Sequential chemical assessments of nutritional
status are indicated in all patients on chronic drug therapies where the
drug has shown any evidence of adverse nutritional effect. There is
particular need for such nutritional monitoring in growing children and
in others whose requirement for miconutrients is high. If nutrient depletion over time is found, appropriate management is by administration
of physiological supplements of nutrients which are not being received
at levels to meet the requirements imposed by the drug as well as by
physiological factors.

It is important to emphasize further that patients most likely to develop nutrient depletion while taking drugs that carry this potential
are those who show best compliance with the therapeutic regimen. This

has been pointed out by Schwarz et al. (1980) with respect to vitamin A depletion in patients on colestipol, and we have observed a similar phenomenon of potassium depletion being most evident in patients on long-term thiazide intake.

C. Interactive Model

The association of nutritional deficiency with drugs is now well known, but insufficient attention has been given to complex interactions of drug, diet, and disease in the etiology of drug-related malnutrition. In patients with regional enteritis and other forms of inflammatory bowel disease, Franklin and Rosenberg (1973) reported that folacin malabsorption was present, apparently due to the disease process and due to the administration of sulfasalazine for disease management (Franklin and Rosenberg, 1973).

In a subsequent study of Gerson and Cohen (1976), folic acid absorption was found to be normal in five patients with regional enteritis, in whom tests of absorptive capacity were carried out by jejunal perfusion of folic acid with a triple lumen technique. These authors suggest that in patients with regional enteritis, the prominant cause of folacin deficiency may be inadequate intake of folacin.

In reviewing cases of folacin deficiency, with or without megaloblastic anemia, which have occurred in patients with inflammatory bowel disease and which have been attributed to effects of sulfasalazine, it is clear that diet, drug, and disease are all major etiological factors. It has also been suggested by Schneider and Beeley (1977) that sulfasalazine may interfere with the microbiological assay of folacin, thus producing spuriously low plasma and erythrocyte folacin values. Sulfasalazine, the drug of choice in many cases of regional enteritis and ulcerative colitis, has antifolate actions which have been described by Baum et al. (1981).

In a study of elderly patients in an extended care facility in which patients were on multiple-drug regimens including diphenylhydantoin, glutethimide, trimethoprim, and cholestyramine, which have an adverse effect of folacin status, we found a high correlation between folacin intake and serum folacin. Within this population, patients on tranquilizers had a significantly lower folacin status as measured by erythrocyte folacin levels than those of patients not taking these drugs (Liebman, 1977). However, it appeared that in this sample, diet was more important than drugs in explaining the folacin deficiency or sufficiency.

In order to illustrate further the complexity of the interactive model, it is pertinent to analyze a case report of multiple nutritional deficiencies arising in a patient receiving a multiple-drug regimen (Meyrick Thomas et al., 1981). The patient was a vegetarian Indian woman, living in the United Kingdom. She was found to have pulmonary tuberculosis during a pregnancy. Treatment was with isoniazid and rifampicin. After the birth of her infant and while she was breast feeding, she became depressed and was additionally given amitryptyline. During the course of treatment of her tuberculosis and over the period of physiological stress related to her pregnancy and lactation, she developed multiple B vitamin deficiencies with clinical and biochemical signs of pyridoxine deficiency, pellagra, and ariboflavinosis. Her nutritional deficiencies were of complex etiology. It is likely that prior to drug administration, her intake of B vitamins was marginal because of her vegetarian diet. Further, her requirements for vitamin B_6, niacin, and riboflavin would have been increased by pregnancy and lactation. Her tuberculosis may have contributed to urinary losses of riboflavin which are increased by pyrexia and catabolic states. Isoniazid induces vitamin B_6 deficiency both because of urinary loss of the Schiff base complex of pyridoxal and isonicotinic acid hydrazine (INH) and because INH is a pyridoxal kinase inhibitor.

Further, this woman was shown to be a slow acetylator of INH, which would decrease the rate of elimination of the drug and enhance the risk of development of vitamin B_6 deficiencies. The appearance of pellagra is explained in that in circumstances where vitamin B deficiency is associated with marginal intake of niacin and tryptophan (the latter due to a low protein intake), there is insufficient preformed and tryptophan-derived niacin for metabolic needs. Finally, riboflavin deficiency, which is suggested by her glossitis, may have been precipitated by intake of amytryptyline. Amitryptyline is one of the tricyclic antidepressant drugs which has been shown to inhibit riboflavin metabolism in rat tissues, and riboflavin deficiencies could secondarily impair vitamin B_6 metabolism (Pinto et al., 1981).

It has been recorded that combined use of INH and rifampicin may result in hepatoxicity in slow INH açetylators (Lal et al., 1972). It would be pure conjecture to suggest either that this woman had any evidence of hepatotoxicity or that such hepatotoxicity could contribute to her malnutrition. However, such a possibility cannot be completely excluded. Similarly, it would be difficult to evaluate the role of the tuberculosis in the determination of her impaired nutritional status. In concluding the analysis of this complex case, the statement can be made that pharmacogenetic, dietary, physiological disease, and drugs contributed to the production of pellagra vitamin B_6 deficiency and possible ariboflavinosis in this woman.

In the first case of pellagra induced by isoniazid, described by Pegum (1952), the "burning foot" syndrome, characteristic of vitamin B_6 deficiency, was also present. However, in 30 years we have moved forward in our ability to dissect the various etiological factors contributing to the development of pellagra in patients taking INH.

VII. SUMMARY OF FACTORS OBSCURING THE DIAGNOSIS OF COM-
PLEX DRUG-INDUCED NUTRITIONAL DEFICIENCY

The case of the woman with INH-induced pellagra exemplifies the multiple etiology of drug-induced nutritional deficiency in which all variables contributing to outcome are easily defined. Once the dominant
clinical signs were recognized as signs of avitaminosis, the antinutrient
effects of the drugs could be placed in the mosaic of etiological factors.
It is, however, rare to have the opportunity to explain interrelationships with such rationality. The course of events is more completely
explained when there is failure to assess effects of physiological, diet,
and disease variables separately and together on the nutrient requirements of patients on chronic drug therapies. It cannot be too strongly
emphasized that drug-induced malnutrition occurs most in people whose
nutriture is precarious before drug therapy as initiated and in those in
whom marginal diet and active disease contribute to deficiency states
during drug therapy.

REFERENCES

Baum, C. L., Selhub, J., and Rosenberg, I. H. (1981). Antifolate
actions of sulfasalazine on intact lymphocytes. *J. Lab. Clin.
Med.* 97:779-784.
Brinker, K. R., Bulger, R. E., Dobyan, D. C., Stacy, T. R.,
Southern, P. M., Henrich, W. L., and Cronin, R. E. (1981).
Effect of potassium depletion on gentamycin nephrotoxicity. *J.
Lab. Clin. Med.* 98:292-301.
Brown, C. V. (1972). Acute isoniazid poisoning. *Am. Rev. Respir.
Dis.* 105:206-216.
Chanarin, I. (1969). *The Megaloblastic Anemias.* Blackwell Scien-
tific Publications, Oxford.
Chin, L., Sievers, M. L., Laird, H. E., Herrier, R. N., and
Picchioni, A. L. (1978). Evaluation of diazepam and pyridoxine
as antidotes to isoniazid intoxication in rats and dogs. *Toxicol.
Appl. Pharmacol.* 45:713-722.
Chin, L., Sievers, M., Herrier, R. N., and Picchioni, A. L. (1981).
Potentiation of pyridoxine by depressants and anticonvulsants in
the treatment of acute isoniazid intoxication in dogs. *Toxicol.
Appl. Pharmacol.* 58:504-509.
Dollery, C. T., George, C. F., and Orme, M. L'E. (1974). Drug
interactions affecting cardiovascular therapy. In *Clinical Effects
of Interaction Between Drugs*, L. E. Cluff, and J. C. Petrie,
Eds., American Elsevier, New York, pp. 119-130.
Folb, P. I. (1980). *The Safety of Medicines. Evaluation and Pre-
diction*, Springer-Verlag, Berlin, p. 88.

Franklin, J. L., and Rosenberg, I. H. (1973). Impaired folic acid absorption in inflammatory bowel disease: effects of salicylazosulfapyridine (Azulfidine). *Gastroenterology* 60:417-425.

Gerson, C. D., and Cohen N. (1976). Folic acid absorption in regional enteritis. *Am. J. Clin. Nutr.* 29:182-186.

Insogna, K. L., Bordley, D. R., Caro, J. F., and Lockwood, D. H. (1980). Osteomalacia and weakness from excessive antacid ingestion. *JAMA* 244:2544-2546.

Karch, F. E., and Lasagna, L. (1977). Toward the operational identification of adverse drug reactions. *Clin. Pharmacol. Ther.* 21:247-254.

Karch, F. E., Smith, C. L., Kerzner, B., Marzullo, J., Weintraub, M., and Lasagna, L. (1976). Adverse drug reactions—a matter of opinion. *Clin. Pharmacol. Ther.* 19:489-492.

Kelnar, C. J. H., Taor, W. S., Reynolds, D. J., Smith, D. R., Slavin, B. M., and Brook, C. G. D. (1978). Hypomagnesaemic hypocalcaemia and hypokalaemia caused by treatment with high dose gentamycin. *Arch. Dis. Child.* 53:817-820.

Kluft, F. C., Patel, V., Yum, M. N., Patel, B., and Kleit, S. A. (1975). Experimental aminoglycoside nephrotoxicity. *J. Lab. Clin. Med.* 86:213-220.

Lal, S., Singhal, S. N., Burley, D. N., and Crossley, G. (1972). Effect of rifampicin and isoniazid on liver function. *Br. Med. J.* 1:148-150.

Leonards, J. R., Levy, G., and Niemczura, R. (1973). Gastrointestinal blood loss during prolonged aspirin administration. *N. Engl. J. Med.* 289:1020-1021.

Levine, D., Goode, A. W., and Wingate, G. L. (1981). Purgative abuse associated with reversible cachexia, hypogammaglobulinaemia and finger clubbing. *Lancet* 1:919-920.

Liebman, B. F. (1977). Determinants of folacin status in institutionalized elderly individuals. M. S. thesis, Cornell University, Ithaca, N. Y.

Meyrick Thomas, R. H., Rowland Payne, C. M. E., and Black, M. M. (1981). Isoniazid-induced pellagra. *Br. Med. J.* 283:287-288.

Parish, P. A. (1973). Drug prescribing—the concern of all. *R. Soc. Health J.* 93:213-217.

Pegum, J. S. (1952). Nicotinic acid and burning feet. *Lancet* 2:536.

Pinto, J., Huang, Y. P., and Rivlin, R. S. (1981). Inhibition of riboflavin metabolism in rat tissues by chlorpromazine, imipramine and amitryptyline. *J. Clin. Invest.* 67:1500-1506.

Roe, D. A. (1976). *Drug-Induced Nutritional Deficiencies.* AVI, Westport, Conn.

Saad, S. F., El Masry, A. M., and Scott, P. M. (1972). Influence of certain anticonvulsants on the concentration of gamma-amino-butyric acid in the cerebral hemispheres of mice. *Eur. J. Pharmacol.* 17:386-392.

Schneider, R. E., and Beeley, L. (1977). Megaloblastic anaemia associated with sulphasalazine treatment. *Br. Med. J.* 1:1683-1639.

Schwartz, K. B., Goldstein, P. D., Witztum, J. L., and Schonfeld, G. (1980). Fat soluble vitamin concentrations in hypocholesterolemic children treated with colestipol. *Pediatrics* 65:243-250.

Stolley, P. D. (1981). Prevention of adverse effects related to drug therapy. In *Preventive and Community Medicine,* 2nd ed., D. W. Clark and B. MacMahon, Eds., Little, Brown, Boston, p. 141.

Sullivan, R. D., Miller, E., and Sikes, M. P. (1959). Antimetabolite-metabolite combination cancer therapy. Effects of intraarterial methotrexate and intramuscular citrovorum factor therapy in human cancer. *Cancer* 12:1248-1262.

Surgeon General's Advisory Committee on Smoking and Health (1964). Smoking and Health. *U.S. DHEW/PHS Publ. 1103,* Washington, D. C.

Thompson, R. B. (1979). *A Short Textbook of Haematology,* 5th ed., Pitman, Medical, London, p. 219.

Vesell, E. S. (1980). Gene-environment interactions in drug metabolism. In *Proc. First World Conf. Clin. Pharm. Ther.,* P. Turner, Ed., Macmillan, London, 1980, pp. 3-79.

Werkheiser, W. C. (1963). The biochemical, cellular and pharmacological action and effects of the folic acid antagonists. *Cancer Res.* 23:1277-1285.

West, R. J., and Lloyd, J. K. (1975). The effect of cholestyramine on intestinal absorption. *Gut* 16:93-98.

Author Index

Numbers in parentheses are reference numbers and indicate that an author's work is referred to although his name is not cited in the text. Italic numbers give the page on which the complete reference is listed.

A

Aamodt, R. L., 351, *371*
Aarons, L. J., 27(30), 34(30, 44), *45, 46*
Abbott, D. C., 357, *359*
Abbot, V., 67(82), *90*
Abbott, V., 230, *278*
Abe, T., 136(117), 149(117), *168*
Abel, E. L., 388, 389, *395*
Abel, J. G., 35(51), *47*
Abell, N. S., 183, 184, *213*
Aberg, H., 345, *366*
Ablitt, L., 151(244), *174*
Abou el Makarem, M. M., 131(54), *166*
Abraham, E. C., 150(230), *173*
Abrams, G., 320, *328*
Acari, J., 155(283), *175*
Acheson, K. J. B., 392, *395*
Adamec, J., 389, *404*
Adams, R., 388, *395*
Adams, R. N., 146(194), *172*
Adekunle, A. A., 104, 105, *113*
Adriaenssens, P. I., 181, 187, *218*

Aggeler, P. M., 452(150), *469*
Agnati, L. F., 386, *399*
Agnew, J. E., 348, *367*
Ahlborg, U. G., 106, *113*
Ahrens, E. H., 332, *365*
Airaksinen, M. M., 379, *399*
Akagi, M., 193, *223*
Akerboom, T. P. M., 180, *213*
Albert, R. E., 96, *116*
Albert, Z., 195, *213*
Aldrige, A., 354, *360*
Alexander, W. D., 348, *367*
Aleyassine, H., 308, *326*
Algeri, S., 136(114), *168*
Al-Haddad, I. K., 10, *16*
Alheid, G. F., 387, *402*
Allan, N. C., 479(50), *484*
Allan, V., 440(80), *464*
Allan, W. C., 354, *359*
Allen, C. M., 185, *213*
Allen, L., 187, 196, 197, *213*
Allen, M. G., 393, *397*
Allen, R., 381, *406*
Allen, R. P., 381, *406*
Allentuck, S., 388, *395*
Alleva, F. R., 236, *278*
Alleva, J. J., 236, *278*

Allgén, L. G., 341, *359*
Allison, R. D., 190, 196, *213*
Allonen, H., 347, *363*
Almquist, H. J., 430(5), *459*
Al-Shahristani, H., 10, *16*
Althoff, J., 495(61,62), *500*
Alvan, G., 273, *294*
Alvares, A. P., 67(76), *90*, 97, *113*
Amato, D., 345, *359*
Amdisen, A., 350, *371*
Amelotti, J. M., 432(28), 433(28), 441(89), 442(89), *461, 465*
Ames, F., 388, *395*
Amos, W. H., 226, 227, *290*
Ananth, J., *359*
Anantharaman, K., 392, *395*
Anders, M. W., 183, *213*
Andersen, B. N., 492(17), *497*
Anderson, G. H., 163(338), *178, 333, 360*
Anderson, K. E., 67(76), *90*
Anderson, M. E., 136(118), 149(118), *168*, 181, 190, 196, *213*
Anderson, M. W., 10, 11, *16, 18*
Anderson, T. L., 208, *213*
Anderson, B., 131(56,59,60), 139(56), *166*, 185, *218*
Andreana, A., 134(101), *168*
Andreasen, F., 452(143), *468*
Andreone, T. L., 84(143), *92*
Andrews, L. S., 268, *278*
Angst, J., 384, *406*
Anna, Z., 392, *407*
Ansari, A., 496(8), *497*
Ansell, J. E., 441(84), *464*
Antelman, S. M., 387, 391, *395*
Aprison, M. H., 390, *404*
Aranda, J. V., 336, 354, *359, 360, 369*
Arbesman, C. E., 339, *362*
Arcos, J. C., 56(19), *87*

Arias, I. M., 143(169), 144(169), 145(169), *171*, 191, 192, *213, 216, 217, 218*, 349, *360*
Armstrong, M., 151(246), 153 (246), 154(246), *174*
Arnaud, S. B., 415, 416, *422*
Arneson, M. A., 493(20), *497*
Arreagza-Plaza, C. A., 479(54), *484*
Artigou, J. Y., 148(214), 149 (214), *173*, 204, *221*
Aschbacher, P. W., 200, 201, 209, 210, *213*
Asghar, K., 146(199), *172*
Ashbrook, J. D., 24(14), *44*, 336, *372*
Ashkar, S., 187, 207, *213*
Ashkenazi, H., 349, *372*
Ashley, D. V. M., 163(338), *178*
Astier, J. P., 492(53,54), *500*
Atkin, S. D., 69(89), 70(89), *90*
Atkinson, S. A., 333, *360*
Auer, R., 60(55), *89*
Augenlicht, L. H., 54(18), *87*
Avanda, J. V., 97, *116*
Avenia, R. W., 245, *278*
Avigan, J., 69(90), *90*
Avioli, L. V., 411, 414, 416, 417, *422, 424, 426*
Awapara, J., 154(272), 155(272), 156(272), *175*
Axelrod, J., 227, 239, 244, 247, 259, 264, *279*
Azarnoff, D. L., 33(39), *46*, 230, *279*
Azarroff, D. L., 336, *364*
Azerad, R., 454(178), *471*

B

Baastrup, P. C., 384, *406*
Baba, S., 435(52), *462*

Babson, J. R., 146(195), *172*, 180, 183, 184, 187, 205, *213*, *222*
Bachmann, G., 392, *400*
Bachouk, P. S., 476(16), *482*
Badiani, G., 154(277), *175*
Baettig, K., 393, *395*
Baez, D. A., 378, *395*
Bagheri, S. A., 80(126), *92*
Bai, N. J., 263, *283*
Baile, C. A., 386, *395*
Baille, C. A., 386, *398*, *404*
Baird, M. B., 105, *113*
Baird, W. M., 78(118), 86(118), *91*
Baker, D. H., *177*
Baker, E. M., 227, 237, *279*, *284*, *285*
Baker, G. L., 159(300), *176*
Baker, H., 239, *279*, 477(27), *482*
Baker, J. H., 477(21), *482*
Baker, S. J., 333, *365*
Bakke, J. E., 182, 200, 201, 209, 210, *213*, *214*, *219*
Balazs, T., 236, *278*
Baldessarini, R., 137(127), 161 (127), *169*
Baldessarini, R. J., 134(82,83, 86,92), 135(86,92), 136(86, 92), 137(82,86,92,128), 159 (82,86,92), *167*, *169*
Ball, E. G., 186, *222*
Baloch, K. H., 441(85), *464*
Banerjee, S., 237, 263, *279*, *281*
Banerjee, S. K., 263, *281*
Bank, S., 488(45), 489(45), 493(1), *496*, *499*
Bansal, B. R., 75(111), *91*
Bansal, S. C., 75(111), *91*
Barabas, K., 263, *279*
Baran, D. T., 415, 417, *422*, *425*
Baratta, H., 490(48), *499*
Baratti, C., 492(56), *500*
Baratti, J., 198, *220*

Barbeau, A., 153(259), *175*
Barber, T. A., 160(310), 161 (310), *177*
Barbezat, G. O., 488(45), 489 (45), *499*
Barbin, G., 384, *399*
Barden, H. S., 421, 422, *423*
Barilla, D. E., 417, *423*
Barkhan, P., 430(9), 431(9,13), 432(9), 433(9), 434(13), 435(58), 436(9,13,58,61), 437(65,66), 438(58), 439(9, 58,61,73,74), 440(80), 442 (9,61,73), 444(66), *459*, *460*, *462*, *463*, *464*
Barlow, O. W., 261, *289*
Barnes, R. E., 163(336), *178*
Barnsley, E. A., 211, *222*
Barofsky, I., 388, *397*
Barone, F. C., 381, 392, *395*, *396*
Barr, E., 381, *406*
Barr, F., 381, *406*
Barros Mott, C., 490(12), *497*
Barrowman, J., 476(15), *481*
Barry, H. D., 389, *407*
Barsivala, V. M., 332, *360*
Bartfai, T., 444(114), *466*
Bartholomew, C., 493(2), *496*
Bartoc, R., 150(229), *173*
Bartoli, G. M., 144(181), 145 (182), *171*, 205, *214*
Bartosek, I., 134(102), 137(126), *168*, *169*, 241, *283*
Bartsch, G. E., 342, *372*
Bartwhistle, W., 198, *219*
Bass, L., 122(12), *164*
Bass, N. M., 192, *214*
Bassir, O., 104, 105, *113*
Basu, D., 6, 14, *19*
Basu, T. K., 98, *114*, 239, 254, *293*
Batalden, P., 149(221), *173*
Bates, L. B., 388, *407*
Bates, M., 416, *427*

Bath, I. S., 14, *17*
Batt, A. M., 132(70), 141(70),
    166, 204, *221*
Battig, K., 393, *404*
Baty, J. D., 343, *369*
Batzinger, R. P., 192, *214*
Bauer, J. H., 346, *360*
Baugh, C. M., 476(19), 477(21,
    36), *482, 483*
Baum, C. L., 519, *521*
Baumann, C. A., 73(102,105,
    107,108,109), *91*
Bayless, J. D., 416, *427*
Beattie, A. D., 272, 273, *279*
Beatty, P., 205, *214*
Beatty, P. W., 143(171), 144
    (171), 145(171), 146(195),
    148(171), 149(171,219),
    150(171), 160(171), 162
    (171), 163(332), *171, 172,
    173, 178*, 180, 181, 187,
    202, 205, 207, *221, 222,*
    268, *291*
Beaudoin, A. R., 307, *322*
Beaudry, P. H., 308, *329*
Bech, P., 384, 385, *408*
Beck, L. H., 413, 414, *423*
Beck, L. V., 204, 207, *214*
Becking, G. C., 98, 103, 104,
    113, 248, *279*
Beeley, L., 519, *523*
Beer, A. E., 84(140), *92*
Beermann, D., 452(140,141),
    468
Beeson, P. B., 433(42), *461*
Behm, H. L., 27(33), *46*
Belinsky, S. A., 132(72), *166*
Bell, R. A., 434(50), 435(50),
    462
Bell, R. D., 417, *423*
Bell, R. G., 435(55), 439(75),
    440(55,75), 441(89), 442
    (89,92,93,95,96), 443(75,
    92,95,96,100,102), 451(75,
    92,96,102,135,136), 452
    (102,145,151,153,154), 453
    (155,160,161), 457(155),

[Bell, R. G.]
    462, 464, 465, 468, 469, 470
Ben-Adereth, N., 311, *322*
Bend, J., 191, *214*
Bend, J. R., 97, 100, 101, 102,
    113, 115, 116, 151(252), *174,*
    182, 183, 210, 211, *217, 221,*
    223
Bending, M. R., 29(35), *46*
Benesh, F. C., 134(84), *167*
Benet, L. Z., 39(68), *48*
Benevenga, N. J., 159(294), 160
    (307,308,310), 161(308,310,
    311,312,314,315,316), 162
    (294), *176, 177*, 203, *223*
Bengtsson, C., 393, *404, 405*
Benhamou, J. P., 204, *221*
Bennett, I. L., 442(98), *465*
Bennett, P. N., 139(138), *169*
Bennun, M., 303, *322*
Benson, A. M., 192, *214*
Berg, G., 9, *17*
Berg, L. R., 265, *279*
Bergen, S. S., 383, *396*
Berger, H., 341, *360*
Berger, H. M., 151(244), *174*
Bergman, K. E., 333, *365*
Bergsteinsson, H., 354, *359*
Bergstrom, W. H., 416, *427,*
    428
Berkow, S. G., 5, *16*
Berland, T., 382, *396*
Berlin, C. M., 336, 342, 355,
    360
Berman, L., 320, *328*
Berman, R., 379, *400*
Bernard, J. C., 339, *361*
Berndt, E., 146(198), *172*
Bernhard, W. G., 312, *327*
Berry, M. N., 183, *214*
Berry, W. T. C., 6, *16*
Berthezene, P., 496(24), *498*
Bertilsson, L., 26(22), 27(22),
    29(22), *45*
Bertino, J. R., 477(26), *482*
Beuding, E., 192, *214*
Beutler, E., 180, 189, 190, *214,*

[Beutler, E.]
219, 221, 223
Bewsher, P. D., 413, 427
Beyer, K. H., 259, 279
Bhadrachari, N., 78(120), 92
Bhattacharyya, A., 257, 263,
265, 280, 281
Bhavova, P. M., 183, 218
Biale, Y., 311, 322
Bialy, G., 349, 370
Bicker, M., H., 26(19), 34(43),
45, 46
Bickers, D. R., 97, 113, 122
(14), 164
Bidart, J. M., 487(73), 488(23,
73), 496(23,24), 498, 501
Biddle, F. G., 318, 319, 322
Bieber, M. A., 208, 213
Biessmann, H., 54(18), 87
Bill, K., 351, 370
Billingham, R. E., 84(140), 92
Binder, H. J., 477(26), 482
Bingham, S. A., 6, 17
Binkiewicz, A., 353, 360
Binkley, F., 146(201), 172, 187,
193, 196, 207, 213, 214
Bircher, J., 240, 288
Birge, S. J., 416, 424
Birke, G., 9, 16
Birkett, D. J., 23(6,7), 44
Birnbaum, L. S., 105, 113
Bischoff, K. B., 10, 16
Bisdom, C. J. W., 353, 356, 360
Bissel, D. M., 241, 279
Biswas, D. K., 237, 279
Bjorkhem, I., 243, 250, 279,
415, 417, 423
Bjornsson, T. D., 35(57), 47,
434(47), 435(56,57), 441
(57), 442(47,56), 462
Bjorntorp, P., 393, 405
Bjorum, N., 385, 404
Black, C. A., 387, 391, 395
Black, M. M., 519, 522
Black, O., 495(3,4), 496
Blackburn, H., 393, 396

Blacker, K. H., 350, 360
Blackstone, S., 265, 279
Blackwell, E., 139(138), 169
Blake, D. A., 345, 368
Blakely, R., 161(318), 177
Blanchard, J., 239, 272, 273,
294
Bland, E. P., 351, 361
Blaschke, T. F., 26(25), 33(38),
34(38), 39(72), 40(72), 45,
46, 48, 434(47), 435(56,57),
441(57), 442(47,56), 462
Blau, G. E., 12, 19
Blitzer, P. H., 393, 396
Block, W. D., 160(301), 176
Blomstrand, R., 431(14), 434
(14), 460
Bloom, F. E., 387, 405
Bloom, S. R., 492(7), 497
Blumenthal, H. P., 355, 371
Blundell, J. E., 379, 383, 396
Board, P. G., 189, 214, 223
Bobek, P., 236, 238, 250, 277,
284
Bock, F. G., 84(142), 92
Bock, K. W., 130(49), 131(49,
54), 132(49), 165, 166
Bockman, D. E., 495(4), 496
Bode, H. H., 348, 361
Boeijinga, J. K., 240, 281
Bois-Joyeux, B., 160(305), 176
Boisseau, V. C., 410, 411, 412,
415, 424
Bolanowska, W., 131(55), 166
Bollag, W., 95, 97, 113
Bollman, J. L., 493(47), 499
Bolme, P., 386, 399
Bolognese, R. J., 339, 368
Bolt, M. G., 80(126), 92
Bolub, E. E., 417, 423
Bone, A. H., 134(95), 136(95,
113), 137(95), 159(95), 167,
168
Bonnenshein, M., 488(58), 493
(58), 500
Bono, V., 187, 196, 218

Bono, V. H., 196, *215*
Boobis, S. W., 27(29), 34(29),
    45
Boorner, J. W., 493(20), *497*
Booth, A. G., 197, *214, 219*
Borchardt, R., 133(74), *166*
Borchardt, R. T., 133(80), 136
    (80), *167*
Bordalo, O., 492(19), *497*
Borderon, J. C., 339, *361*
Bordier, P., 415, 418, *423*
Bordley, D. R., 514, *522*
Borek, E., 133(73), *166*
Borg, S. A., 96, *117*
Borgå, O., 26(22), 27(22), 29
    (22), 34(47,48,49), 36(61),
    45, 46, 47, 48
Borgen, L. A., 389, *396*
Borm, P. J. A., 211, *215*
Bornstein, W. A., 106, *113*
Boruchow, I. B., 479(52), *484*
Borzelleca, J. F., 11, *17*
Bos, R. P., 211, *216*
Bosch, V., 479(54), *484*
Bösterling, B., 243, *279*
Bouillon, R., 411, *423*
Bouquet, J., 390, *396*
Bourry, J., 494(5,6), *496*
Bousquet, W. F., 257, *285*
Bow, T. M., 227, *292*
Bower, S. G., 197, *224*
Bowman, K., 388, *395*
Bowmer, C. J., 27(31), 34(31),
    45
Boxenbaum, H., 121(3), 122(3),
    163
Boyd, E. M., 392, *405*
Boyd, M. R., 148(212), 150
    (238), *172, 174,* 202, 204,
    214
Boyd, S. C., 202, 204, *214*
Boyer, J. L., 80(126), *92*
Boyland, E., 147(206,208), *172,*
    181, 183, 210, *214*
Boyle, P. H., 477(37), *483*
Boyns, A. E., 85(152), *93*

Bracken, W. M., 64(64), *89*
Bradley, C., 380, *396*
Braithwaite, R., 26(22), 27(22),
    29(22), 45
Bralow, S. P., 57(24), 75(24),
    87
Brambel, C. E., 343, *361*
Brandt, R., 352, *361*
Brasca, A., 492(88), *502*
Brattsten, L., 98, *117*
Braude, M. C., 388, 389, *406,*
    407
Braun, W. H., 12, 14, *19*
Brauner, M. G., 189, *220*
Braunlich, H., 336, *361*
Brawn, W. H., 12, 14, *18*
Bray, G. A., 244, 245, 247, 256,
    257, *281*
Bray, H. G., 126(29), 140(29),
    141(29), *164*
Breckenridge, A. M., 343, *369,*
    439(73), 442(73), *463*
Breen, M., 387, *402*
Brehe, J. E., 145(190), 146(190),
    171
Breimer, D. D., 240, *281*
Breisch, S. T., 383, *396*
Bresnick, E., 106, *113,* 243,
    280
Bresnick, G., 183, *215*
Bressler, R., 154(276), *175*
Bretholz, A., 491(89), 492(7),
    497, 502
Bridges, J. W., 123(16), 126(23),
    164
Bridges, R. J., 149(217), *173,*
    181, 196, *213, 216*
Briggs, G. M., 229, *291*
Briggs, M., 303, *322*
Briggs, M. H., 303, *322*
Briggs, R. M., 313, *322*
Bright-See, E., 236, 275, *294*
Brimacombe, J. S., 495(40), *499*
Brin, H., 477(29), *483*
Brin, M., 237, *288, 289*
Brinker, K. R., 516, *521*

Brizuela, B. S., 103, 104, *115*
Brobeck, J. R., 392, *396*
Brodersen, R., 23(11), *44*
Brodie, A., 205, *214*
Brodie, A. E., 146(195), *172*, 180, 187, 205, *222*
Brodie, B. B., 204, *220*, 227, 239, 244, 247, 259, 264, *279*
Broermann, I., 389, *405*
Broitman, S. A., 77(115), *91*
Bronner, F., 417, *423*
Bronzert, D., 384, *401*
Brook, C. G. D., 516, *522*
Brophy, E. J., 188, 198, *219*
Brosseau, M., 243, *280*
Brouns, R. M. E., 211, *216*
Brown, A. K., 341, *361*
Brown, C. V., 513, *521*
Brown, G. A., 151(244), *174*
Brown, L. L., 390, *403*
Brown, M., 334, *367*
Brown, N., 477(38), *483*
Brown, R. D., 350, *373*
Brown, R. E., 342, *370*
Brown, R. F., 386, *396*
Brown, R. R., 63(63), *89*
Brown, T. C. K., 336, *361*
Broxmeyer, B., 194, 195, *216*
Brozek, J., 392, 393, *396*
Brueton, M. J., 151(244), *174*
Bruhis, S., 150(229), *173*
Brunner, R. L., 311, *328*
Brunngraber, E. G., 139(141), *169*
Brush, M. K., 227, *293*
Bryan, G., 80(131), *92*
Bryan, G. T., 61(60), *89*
Bryan, M. H., 333, *360*
Bryan, W., 312, *327*
Brzezinsky, A., 339, *371*
Büch, H., 139(137), 141(137), *169*
Buchan, R., 85(152), *93*
Buchanan, G. R., 434(46), *462*
Buchanan, N., 33(41), *46*
Buchanan, R. A., 337, *361*

Bucheler, J., 495(21), *497*
Buchthal, S. D., 453(161), *470*
Buff, E., 388, 389, *406*
Buimovici-Klein, E., 343, *361*
Bulger, R. E., 516, *521*
Bull, A. W., 78(117), *91*
Bungay, P. M., 10, 11, *16*
Burch, G. E., 496(8), *497*
Burch, H. B., 145(190), 146 (190), *171*
Burch, M. K., 134(85), *167*
Burk, R. F., 145(182), *171*, 183, *214*
Burke, M. D., 67(79), *90*, 188, *223*
Burkhart, B., 339, *364*
Burley, D. N., *522*
Burnet, F. R., 134(98), *167*
Burnett, G., 390, *402*
Burns, F. J., 96, *116*
Burns, J. J., 98, *114*, *115*, 235, 240, 241, 244, 245, 247, 250, 251, 255, 256, 257, 261, 274, *280*, *281*, *287*
Burns, R. F., 392, *407*
Burr, M. L., 238, *280*
Burse, R. L., 394, *396*
Busk, L., 106, *113*
Busse, K., 433(31), *461*
Butcher, R. E., 311, 317, 321, *325*, *328*
Butler, J. J., 442(98), *465*
Butler, V. P., 346, *367*
Butterworth, C. E. Jr., 476(19), *482*
Butterworth, C. F. Jr., 477(21), *482*
Byck, R., 386, *397*
Bynum, G. D., 394, *396*
Byrne, T., 343, *361*

C

Caballero, F. M., 434(46), *462*
Cade, J. F. J., 384, *397*

Cagen, L. M., 190, *214*
Cain, G. D., 476(10), *481*
Calcutt, G., 204, *214*
Calder, I. C., 199, *214*
Caldwell, J., 138(129a), 144
    (241,242), *169, 174*
Caldwell, P. T., 439(75), 440
    (75), 443(75), 451(75), 452
    (145,151), *464, 469*
Calloway, D. H., 159(298), 162
    (298), *176*
Cameron, E. H. D., 85(153), *93*
Cameron, J. L., 493(10), 494
    (9), *497*
Campbell, J. A., 163(335), *178*
Campbell, R., 204, *214*
Campbell, R. L., 75(110), *91*
Campbell, R. M., 334, *363*
Campbell, S. C., 105, *113*
Campbell, T. C., 51(1), 63(1),
    65(1), 84(1), *86*, 98, 105,
    113, 114
Campese, D., 489(51a,51b), *500*
Canady, W. J., 103, 104, *114*
Canales, E. S., 347, *361*
Candido, F. M., 488(58), 493
    (58), *500*
Canfield, L. M., 447(123), 450
    (123), 451(123), 454(123,
    172), 455(123), 456(123),
    467, 471
Canham, J. E., 237, *285*
Capel, C. D., 128(35), *165*
Capitaine, Y., 490(12), 491(76),
    493(11), *497, 501*
Capogrossi, M. C., 392, *397*
Capuzzi, D. M., 494(9), *497*
Cardesa, A., 261, *280*, 495(62),
    500
Carela, G., 392, *399*
Carey, D. J., 454(174), *471*
Carey, J. B., 69(91), *90*
Carl, G. F., 134(84), *167*
Carleton, A., 250, *289*
Carlini, E. A., 389, *397, 400*
Carlisle, H. J., 387, *405*

Carlisle, T. L., 447(125,126),
    450(125,126), 452(125,126),
    453(125,126), 456(126), *467*
Carlson, K., 159(293), *176*
Carmack, C., 490(66), *501*
Caro, J. F., 514, *522*
Carpenter, M. P., 245, *280*
Carpio, N. M., 132(69), *166*
Carr, R., 381, *399*
Carrell, H. L., 133(77), *167*
Carroll, K. K., 52(8), 73(106),
    81(8,106), 83(136), 84(8),
    86, 91, 92
Carruba, M. P., 379, *397*
Case, G. L., 161(312,314), *177*
Casey, C. E., 333, *361*
Casida, J. E., 192, *219*, 307,
    327
Casper, R. C., 383, *400*
Cassidy, M. K., 122(7), *163*
Castegnaro, M., 58(38), *88*
Castellano, M. A., 307, *323*
Castle, W. B., 477(23,34), *482,
    483*
Castro, J. A., 204, *215*, 240,
    280
Catto, E., 136(114), *168*
Catto, G., 413, *427*
Catz, C., 98, *114*
Cavallini, D., 133(75), 163(337),
    167, 178
Cawthorne, M. A., 69(89), 70
    (89), *90*
Ceccarelli, G., 339, *368*
Celener, D., 492(13,56), *497,
    500*
Cerven, J., 250, *284*
Cevik, N., 341, *361*
Cha, Y.-N., 192, *214*
Chadwick, R., 244, *280*
Chadwick, R. W., 227, 244, *280*
Chakraborty, D., 257, 263, 265,
    280, 281
Chalmers, J. P., 137(128), *169*
Chamberlain, J. G., 306, *323*
Chambers, H., 307, *327*

Chambers, W., 381, *400*
Chamoiseau, G., 65(72), 67(72), *89*
Chan, P. C., 81(133), 85(150, 151), *92, 93*
Chan, V., 346, *361*
Chanarin, I., 477(28), *483*, 517, *521*
Chanez, M., 160(305), *176*
Chang, A. E., 388, *397*
Chang, C. F., 134(90), 137 (90), 159(90), *167*
Chang, R. L., 56(22), *87*
Chapman, G. S., 183, *215*
Chapman, P. H., 452(144), *468*
Chartrand, L., 80(127), *92*
Charvet, J. G., 126(24), *164*
Chasseaud, L. F., 147(206,208), *172*, 181, 183, 210, *214, 215*
Chastenay, B. F., 416, *425*
Chatfield, D. H., 199, *215*
Chatterjee, A., 263, *281*
Chatterjee, G. C., 257, 263, 265, *280, 281, 292*
Chatterjee, J., 263, 265, *280, 292*
Chatterjee, K., 257, 263, 265, *280, 281*
Chatterjee, S., 257, 263, *280*
Chatterji, R., 195, 196, *216*
Chau Huu, T., 492(59), *500*
Chaudhury, R. R., 387, *406*
Chaung, A. H. L., 183, *215*
Chausseaud, L. F., 181, *214*
Chayen, J., 146(200), *172*
Chelibonova-Lorer, H., 130(46), 131(46), *165*
Chem, D., 495(62), *500*
Chen, C. B., 58(35), *88*
Chen, C. C., 57(28), *88*
Chen, S. Y., 133(80), 136(80), *167*
Chen, Z., 25(18), 33(18), *44*
Cherek, D. R., 350, *373*
Cherian, M. G., 266, *284*
Chessa, P., 386, *404*

Chesters, M., 413, *427*
Chhabra, R. S., 52(11), 67(75, 78), 72(97), *87, 90, 91, 97*, 98, 100, 101, 102, 107, 108, 110, 111, 112, *114, 116*
Chien, Y. W., 122(13), *164*
Chignell, C. F., 26(20), 27(29), 34(29), *45*
Chin, L., 513, *521*
Chiroff, R. T., 416, *427, 428*
Chiu, A., 455(187), 456(187, 196), *472, 473*
Cho, C., 150(235), *173*
Cho, E. S., 160(302), 162(326), *176, 177, 203, 215*
Cho, K., 340, *373*
Chodos, R. B., 475(1), 479(53), *480, 484*
Chomchai, C., 78(120), *92*
Chopra, G. S., 388, *397*
Chopra, R. N., 388, *397*
Chou, R. C., 35(58), *47*
Chou, T. C., 134(88), 139(88), *167*
Christensen, A. K., 183, ·*218*
Christensen, H. N., 163(339), *178*
Christensen, M. S., 410, 411, 412, 418, *426*
Christiansen, C., 410, 411, 421, 422, *423, 427*
Christiansen, G., 59(46), *88*
Christiansen, G. M., 207, *214*
Christiansen, L., 124(18), *164*
Chu, E. W., 95, *114*
Chuang, A. H. L., 106, *113*
Chubb, J., 155(283), *175*
Chvapil, M., 236, *292*
Ciaffi, G., 339, *368*
Ciaranello, R. D., 390, *397*
Cikryt, P., 145(184), *171*, 205, *224*
Cinti, D. L., 417, *423*
Claes, D. J., 476(11), *481*
Claes, J. H., 411, *423*
Claes, P., 476(12), *481*
Claeys, A. E., 441(88), *464*

Clark, A. G., 191, *215*
Clark, A. J., 160(303), *176*
Clark, D. A., 393, *397*
Clark, E., 337, *369*
Clark, E. M., 304, 305, *326*
Clark, G. F., 388, *407*
Clark, J. H., 337, *361*
Clark, M. E., 159(293), *176*
Clarkson, T. W., 9, *16*
Classen, W., 393, *395*
Clayman, C. B., 338, *361*
Clayton, C. C., 73(108), *91*
Clemente, F., 489(77), 490(14,
   77), 491(15,26), 492(71,78),
   497, 498, 501, 502
Clifford, A. J., 159(299), *176*
Clineschmidt, B. V., 379, 384,
   397
Clop, J., 488(82), 490(82), 491
   (82), *502*
Clyde, D. F., 342, *362*
Coakley, G., 161(318), *177*
Cobert, B., 204, *221*
Coble, P. A., 391, *403*
Cobo, E., 353, *362*
Coghill, G., 495(40), *499*
Cohen, B. I., 78(124), 80(124),
   92
Cohen, G. M., 72(98), *91*
Cohen, H., 477(38), *483*
Cohen, L. A., 81(133), 85(150,
   151), *92, 93*
Cohen, L. C., 52(9), 75(9),
   77(9), 78(9), 86(9), *87*
Cohen, M. H., 96, *114*
Cohen, N., 14, *17*, 519, *522*
Cohen, N. L., 321, *323, 325*
Cohen, S., 388, *397*
Cohlmia, J. B., 33(39), *46*
Cohn, V. H., 180, *215*, 433(43),
   461
Colby, H. D., 103, 104, *114*
Cole, A. P., 352, *362*
Cole, E. N., 85(152), *93*
Cole, T. J., 6, *17*
Coleman, R., 198, 199, *215*

Collinge, J. M., 354, *360*
Collins, M., 237, *281*
Colomb, E., 489(77), 490(77),
   492(53,54), *500, 501*
Coltart, D. J., 480(63), *485*
Colvin, B. T., 441(83), *464*
Comai, K., 376, 379, *407*
Cominos, D. C., 347, *362*
Comstock, G. W., 393, *397*
Comstock, T. J., 33(42), *46*
Conit, J. M., 381, *405*
Conklin, J., 433(33), *461*
Conners, C. K., 381, *397*
Conney, A. H., 56(22), 67(76,
   83), *87, 90*, 97, 98, *114, 115*,
   235, 240, 241, 242, 244, 245,
   247, 250, 251, 255, 256, 257,
   261, *281, 287, 288*, 414, *423,
   426*
Connolly, R. B., 146(202), *172*,
   204, 207, *218*
Conolly, M. E., 122(8), *164*
Conrad, G. W., 140(149), 142
   (149), *170*
Conrad, K. A., 239, 272, 273,
   294
Cook, C. E., 354, *360*
Cook, D. A., 155(281), *175*
Cook, G. W., 388, *407*
Cook, P. G., 393, *406*
Coomes, T. J., 6, *16*
Coon, R. A., 263, *286*
Cooney, D. S., 196, *215*
Cooper, B. A., 477(25), *482*
Cooper, B. R., 387, *398*
Cooper, C. W., 388, *395*
Cooper, J., 3,79, *401*
Cooper, L. Z., 343, *361*
Cooper, T. G., 455(185), *472*
Cooperman, J. M., 488(58), 493
   (58), *500*
Coper, H., 380, 389, *403, 405*
Corbett, B. D., 351, *368*
Corbin, J. E., *177*
Corcoran, G. B., 267, 269, *281*
Cornatzer, W. E., 136(112),

[Cornatzer, W. E.]
137(112), *168*
Corney, D. A., 187, 196, *218*
Cornforth, J. W., 133(77), *167*
Correa, P., 58(41), *88*
Correia, M. A., 183, *214*
Corrigan, J. J., 433(39), *461*
Corson, S. L., 339, *368*
Coryell, M. N., 333, *362*
Costantopoulos, A., 131(67), *166*
Costillo, A., 136(116), *168*
Coté, C. J., 353, *362*
Cote, M. G., 416, *424*
Cotham, R. H., 36(62), 39(74), *48, 49*
Coulter, A. W., 136(123), *169*
Cowan, J. W., 163(335), *178*
Coward, J. K., 133(80,81), 136 (80), *167*
Coward, K. H., 237, *287*
Cox, J. H., 113, *114*
Cox, R. H., 182, 210, 211, *217, 223*
Cox, V. C., 381, *408*
Coyle, P. J., 195, *218*
Craft, I., 303, *324*, 479(47), *484*
Craig, W. A., 34(46), *46*
Craing, C., 433(29), *461*
Crandon, J. H., 237, *281*
Crane, R. K., 188, *215*
Cranmer, M., 244, *280*
Cranmer, M. F., 227, 244, *280*
Craven, P. A., 72(96), *91*
Cravens, W. W., 308, *328*
Crawford, J. D., 348, *361*
Crawford, J. S., 351, *361*
Creek, M. J., 199, *214*
Creveling, C. R., 133(74), *166*
Criep, L. H., 339, *362*
Crissey, M. H., 151(250), *174*
Cronin, R. E., 516, *521*
Crooks, P. A., 133(81), *167*
Cros, R. C., 487(73), 488(55,

[Cros, R. C.]
73,82), 490(82), 491(82), *500, 501, 502*
Crossley, G., *522*
Crouch, S., 84(142), *92*
Cruz, M., 422, *427*
Cuello, C., 58(41), *88*
Curdhey, T. J., 61(57), *89*
Curthoys, N. P., 193, 195, 196, 197, 199, 205, *218, 220, 221, 224*
Curtis, C. G., 122(9), 141(152), *164, 170*
Curtis, E. M., 349, *362*
Cyr, W. H., 204, *217*
Czarnecki, S. K., 254, *287*
Czygan, P., 67(81), *90*

D

Dacaney, E. P., 383, *403*
D'Acosta, N., 204, *215*
Dahlen, P., 388, 389, *406*
Dailey, J. W., 350, *373*
Dale, G. L., 189, 190, *219*
Dally, P. J., 388, *398*
Daly, J. W., 105, *114, 115*, 208, *215*, 392, *407*
Dam, H., 429(1), *459*
Damon, A., 393, *398*
Danforth, E. R., 394, *396*
Danhof, M., 240, *281*
Daniel, C. H., 355, *360*
Daniel, V., 192, *215*
Danielson, L., 444(104,110), 445 (104,110), 446(104), 454 (110), *466*
Danielson, V., 381, *408*
Danish, M. A., 340, *364*
Dannenberg, A. M., 356, *369*
Danon, A., 25(18), 33(18), *44*
Dao, T. L., 84(142), *92*
Darby, A. J., 416, *425*
Das, M., 197, *215*
Dashman, T., 99, *114, 261, 287*

Dauterman, W. C., 191, *215,*
    220
David, D. S., 493(33), *498*
Davidson, C., 161(322), *177*
Davidson, C. S., 161(323), *177,*
    442(97), *465*
Davidson, E. D., 151(253,254),
    152(253), *174*
Davies, D. M., 452(144), *468*
Davies, D. S., 122(8), 139(138),
    164, 169
Davies, R. E., 96, *114*
Davis, A. E., 493(57), *500*
Davis,, D. C., 97, *114*
Davis, D. W., 230, *288*
Davis, J. M., 383, *400*
Davis, N., 204, *215*
Davis, N. C., 204, *215*
Davis, W. M., 389, *396*
Davison, K. L., 113, *114, 219*
Davison, S. C., 67(74), *89*
Dawber, T. R., 393, *400*
Dawson, V., 386, *408*
Day, P. A., 148(213), 149(213),
    172
Dean, V. L., *224*
DeBacker, G., 393, *402*
DeBartolo, T. F., 417, 418,
    425
DeBell, J. T., 305, *329*
Debry, G., 132(70), 141(70),
    166
DeCaro, A., 489(16,51a,51b,
    77), 490(77), *497, 501*
DeCastro, C. R., 204, *215*
Decker, K., 130(53), *166*
Decker, M. E., 351, *361*
Decottignies-LeMarechal, P.,
    454(178), *471*
Dedrick, R. L., 10, 11, *16, 18*
Deem, M. A., 381, *400*
Deering, R. H., 352, *369*
DeFenos, O. M., 204, *215*
DeFerreyra, E. C., 204, *215*
DeForest, A., 342, *362*
Defrawy, E. L., 72(98). *91*

DeGier, J. J., 27(27), *45*
Degkwitz, E., 233, 241, 245, 247,
    248, 258, *282, 284, 288, 294*
Degott, C., 148(214), 149(214),
    173, 204, *221*
Dehaven, D. L., 381, 392, *396*
Deichmann, W. B., 7, *18*
Delaney, R., 454(182,184), 455
    (187,192), 456(187,192,196),
    457(182,192), *471, 472, 473*
Delap, L. W., 195, *215*
De LaVergue, P. M., 390, *405*
DeLeenheer, A. P., 441(88), *464*
DeLiberti, J. H., 342, *362*
Delhomme, B., 160(305), *176*
Dell, A., 429(4), *459*
Della Fera, M. A., 386, *398*
DeLange, R. J., 197, *215*
Deloria, L., 67(82), *90,* 230, *278*
DeLuca, H. F., 413, 415, 416,
    423
Del Villano, B. C., 319, *323*
Delvin, E. E., 417, *423*
DeMarco, C., 163(337), *178*
Demirdjian, M., 488(55), *500*
Demol, P., 492(17), *497*
DeMoor, P., 411, *423*
Denda, A., 495(18), *497*
Dent, C. E., 410, *423*
Deodhar, A. D., 333, *362*
Derache, L., 65(72), 67(72), *89*
Deren, J. J., 480(68), *485*
DeRubertis, F. R., 72(96), *91*
Descatoire, V., 148(214), 149
    (214), *173,* 204, *221*
Deschner, E. E., 78(124), 80
    (124), *92*
Desiderio, M., 437(71), *463*
Desmond, P. V., 35(53), *47*
DeSomer, P. H., 476(13), *481*
DeSwiet, M., 343, *369*
Devarajan, L. V., 343, *365*
Devaux, M. A., 492(78,88), *502*
Devine, M. M., 240, *283*
DeVivo, D. C., 414, *425*
Dewey, W. L., 388, *398*

Dey, P. K., 261, 263, *282*
Deykin, D., 441(84), *464*
Dhar, G. J., 478(40), 479(44), *483, 484*
Dhar, J. G., 477(30), *483*
Diamond, L., 78(118), 86(118), *91*
Diaz Gomez, M. I., 204, *215*
Dickerson, J. W., 98, *114*
Dickerson, J. W. T., 239, 254, *293*
Dickinson, L. C., 380, 381, *398*
Didato, F., 85(151), *93*
Diederich, D., 317, *324*
Dietrich, J. W., 418, *423*
Dietschy, J. M., 69(92), *90*
Dietz, A., 196, *217*
DiGirolamo, M., 392, *397*
Diliberti, J. H., 342, *362*
Dill, D. B., 237, *281*
Dimant, E., 190, *215*
Dingell, J. V., 356, *366*
Dinner, M., 320, *328*
Dion, R. L., 187, 196, *218*
Disselduff, M. M., 6, *16*
Dobbins, W. O., III, 475(7), 476(7), *481*
Dobrzanski, S., 392, *398*
Dobson, R. L., 351, *373*
Dobyan, D. C., 516, *521*
Dodo, H., 72(101), *91*
Dodson, W. E., 354, *372*
Doggett, N. S., 392, *398*
Doisy, E. A., 432(25,28), 433 (28), *460, 461*
Dolder, A., 148(214), 149(214), *173*, 204, *221*
Doll, R., 72(100), *91*
Dollery, C. T., 29(35), *46*, 122 (8), *164*, 515, *521*
Dommerud, S. A., 320, *326*
Donaldson, S. S., 389, *398*
Donn, J. E., 496(92), *503*
Donohue, A. M., 243, *291*
Door, N. W., 312, *323*
Doorn, R. V., 211, *215, 216*

Dorian, R., 180, 181, *216*
Doroshow, J. H., 271, *282*
Doss, F. W., 387, *398*
Dost-Kempf, E., 204, *223*
Douglas, A. P., 490(63,64), *500, 501*
Dow, J., 247, 251, *282*
Dowling, R. H., 476(15), *481*
Dowsett, L., 491(32), *498*
Doyon, G., 80(127), *92*
Dramaix, M., 393, *402*
Dreckmann, J. G., 204, *223*
Dreiling, D. A., 492(19), *497*
Dressel, T. D., 493(20), *497*
Drew, R., 96, *117*
Drewitt, D., 85(153), *93*
Driscoll, J. M., Jr., 208, *216*
Dronamraju, K. R., 311, *323*
Druchrey, H., 495(21), *497*
Druckery, H., 54(17), 69(17), *87*
Druckrey, H., 54(15), 57(33), 59(47), *87, 88*
Druga, A., 304, *324*
Duane, W. C., 227, 239, 272, 273, 277, *285*
Dubach, R., 250, 266, *289*
Dubberstein, M., 245, 247, *282*
Dubin, A., 455(187), 456(187, 196), *472, 473*
Dubinstein, B., 381, *400*
Duchan, L., 410, *426*
Duello, T. J., 435(59), *463*
Duerre, J. A., 136(112), 137 (112), *168*
Duffield, R., 418, *423*
Dugan, E., 69(94), *90*
Duncan, B., 204, 207, *214*
Duncan, B. R., 348, *366*
Duncan, G. S., 136(120), *168*
Duncan, J. H., 345, *373*
Dunlop, N. M., 96, *117*
Dunn, G. D., 35(53), *47*
Duquette, P. H., 226, 228, 238, 239, 249, 250, 251, 252, 253, 254, 261, 272, 277, *290*

Durand, S., 491(15), *497*
Durbec, J. P., 487(22), 488(22, 23,55,82), 490(82), 491(82), 496(23,24), *498, 500, 502*
Durham, W. F., 7, *17*
Dus, K. M., 454(174), *471*
Dutta, S. K., 477(30), *483*
Dutton, G. J., 127(34), 128(36), 130(36,48), 131(36,48), 132 (34), *165, 166*
Dybing, E., 271, *283*
Dyniewicz, J. M., 350, *363*
Dziewiatkowski, D. D., 159 (296), *176*

E

Eade, N. R., 65(69), *89*
Eaton, C. J., 337, *361*
Ebaugh, F. G., 14, *19*
Eckert, E. D., 383, *400*
Eckert, T., 312, *323*
Eckstein, H. B., 343, *362*
Ecobichon, D. J., 336, *362*
Edelman, C. M., 336, *362*
Edelstein, S., 415, *427*
Eden, P., 379, *400*
Edery, H., 389, *400*
Edholm, O. G., 385, *398*
Eeade, N. R., *359*
Eeg-Olofsson, O., 338, *363*
Egan, H., 357, *363*
Egan, W., 429(2), *459*
Egeberg, K., 447(124), 450 (124), *467*
Egle, J. L., Jr., 11, *17*
Eikemeyer, J., 146(204), *172*
Einarsson, K., 84(146), *93*
Eisen, H. J., 243, 255, 257, *289*
Eisenberg, L., 381, *397*
Eisenbud, M. C., 14, *17*
Ekert, H., 309, *327*, 388, *398*
Ekman, B., 23(8), 24(8), *44*
El-Attar, A. A., 496(44), *499*
Elce, J. S., 193, 194, 195, 197, 199, 201, *216, 218*

Elders, I. C., 380, 381, *398*
Elders, J., 381, *399*
Eling, T. E., 10, 11, *18*
Elion, G. B., 136(120), *168*
Elliott, G. R., 452(137), *468*
Elliott, M. C., 432(26), *460*
Ellis, H. A., 479(51), *484*
Ellis, W. W., 146(195), 150(237), *172, 174*, 180, 181, 187, 197, 205, 207, 210, *214, 222*
Ellison, A. C., 315, *323*
Ellman, G. L., 202, *216*, 350, *360*
Ellory, J. C., 190, *224*
El Masry, A. M., 513, *522*
Elmy, T. E., 10, 11, *16*
Eloranta, T. O., 134(94), 135(94, 106), 137(94,106), 159(94), *167, 168*
Elsborg, L., 477(33), *483*
Elsmore, T. F., 389, *403*
Elson, L. A., 393, *398*
Eluyn, D. H., 189, *216*
Elvehjem, C. A., 237, *281*
Elwin, C. E., 338, *363*
Elwood, P. C., 238, *280*
Emmelot, P., 198, *216*
Encarnacion, D., 240, *283*
Encrantz, J. C., 151(248), *174*
Endicott, J., 391, *407*
Enger, S. C., 393, *398*
English, P. D., 69(89), 70(89), *90*
Engström, G. W., 195, *216*
Ensor, C., 392, *400*
Erickson, S. H., 337, 341, 350, *363*
Erikson, M., 98, *114*
Erikssen, J., 393, *398*
Eriksson, G., 131(60a), *166*
Erkkola, R., 347, *363*
Ernst, J. A., 332, 349, *366*
Ernster, L., 444(104,105,106, 110,111,112,114), 445(104, 105,110,116,117,118), 446 (104,105,116,117,118), 454 (110), *466, 467*
Erturk, E., 61(60), 80(131), *89, 92*

Ervin, F. R., 389, *399*
Eschenhof, E., 351, *363*
Eschrich, C., 139(137), 141
  (137), *169*
Esmon, C., 441(90), 443(90),
  446(90), 455(192), 456(192),
  457(192), *465, 472*
Esmon, C. T., 446(120), 450
  (131,133), 454(131,169,180,
  183), 455(131,183), 456
  (133), 457(131,183), *467,
  468, 470, 471, 472*
Esnouf, M. P., 456(200), *473*
Estabrook, R. W., 104, *117*
Esterling, R. E., 97, *113*
Estevenon, J. P., 490(25), *498*
Estival, A., 491(26), *498*
Estrela, J. M., 149(216,222),
  150(222), *173*
Evans, C., 244, 245, 247, 256,
  257, *281*
Evans, G. H., 39(73), 40(73),
  48
Evans, M. E., 121(1), *163*
Evans, R. K., 132(72), *166,*
  211, *218*
Evard, E., 475(4), 476(4), *481*
Evenson, J. K., 160(309), 161
  (309), *177*
Evenson, M. A., 34(46), *46*
Evenson, M. C., 205, *214*
Evered, D. F., 154(273), *175*
Everett, G. B., 161(316), *177*
Eyberg, C., 33(41), *46*
Eyer, P., 126(20), *164*
Eysenck, H. J., 393, *399*
Eyssen, H., 475(4), 476(4,13),
  481

F

Fagonde, B., 492(78), *502*
Fahey, R. C., 180, 181, *216*
Fahndrich, C., 380, *403*
Fahrenkrug, A., 491(27), *498*

Fainstat, T. D., 300, *323*
Fajardo, M., 392, *399*
Fales, H. M., 190, *214*
Faloon, W. W., 475(1,2,8), 476
  (8,9), 479(53,56), *480, 481,
  484*
Fang, W. F., 72(95), *90*
Fantus, B., 350, *363*
Farber, E., 136(115,116), *168*
Farooqui, A. A., 139(142), *169*
Farquhar, J. D., 343, *363*
Farr, R. F., 351, *361*
Fasco, M. J., 441(91), 444(91),
  465
Fau, D., 160(305), *176*
Fausto, A., 455(193), *473*
Fausto, A. C., 417, *422*
Fazzini, E., 78(124), 80(124),
  92
Featherston, W. R., 162(331),
  178
Fedail, S. S., 490(28), *498*
Feeney, R. E., 159(299), *176*
Feger, J., 384, *399*
Fehske, K. J., 23(10,12), 24
  (12), *44*
Feil, V. J., 182, 209, 210, *213,
  214*
Feingold, S., 477(27), *482*
Feldmann, R. J., 5, *17*
Felix, E. L., 96, *114*
Fell, B. F., 334, *363*
Felsher, B. F., 132(69), *166*
Ferguson, B. B., 356, *363*
Fernandez, M., 389, *399*
Fernandez, S. B., 11, *17*
Fernlund, P., 429(2), *459*
Fernstrom, J., 161(321,322),
  177
Fernstrom, J. D., 24(16), *44,*
  161(323), *177*, 332, *373*
Ferraro, D. P., 389, *400*
Ferrendelli, J. A., 417, 418, *423*
Ferro, A. J., 133(76), *167*
Feuerstein, S., 148(215), 149
  (215), *173*

Fiala, A. E., 150(232), *173*
Fiala, E. S., 59(46), 60(51),
　88, 89
Fiala, S., 150(232), *173*
Field, M., 480(60), *485*
Fielding, A. M., 247, *283*
Fieser, L. F., 442(94), *465*
Figarella, C., 489(51,77), 490
　(14,25,51,77), 491(51), 492
　(70,71,78), *497, 498, 500,*
　501, 502
Filer, L. J., 159(300), *176*, 333,
　365
Finch, C. A., 442(99), *465*
Finch, E., 344, *363*
Finch, W., 337, *369*
Fine, D. H., 496(30), *498*
Finean, J. B., 198, 199, *215*
Fingl, E., 433(32), *461*
Finkelstein, J. D., 134(99), 137
　(99), 150(240), 159(292),
　160(292), 161(99,319), 162
　(240), *168, 174, 176, 177*
Finley, J. P., 346, *363*
Finnan, J. L., 454(177,179),
　455(179,188), *471, 472*
Finnell, R. H., 309, *323*
Firor, W. M., 231, *284*
Fischbein, J. W., 209, *222*
Fischl, J., 340, *372*
Fiscina, B., 381, *400*
Fisher, L. J., 142(157), *170*
Fisher, R. B., 188, *216*
Fisher, S., 389, *408*
Fiskerstrand, C., 148(210), *172*
Fitzgerald, O., 493(2), *496*
Fjermestad, J., 65(68), 67(68),
　68(68), 72(68), *89*
Fleishner, G., 191, 192, *213,*
　216, 217
Fleishner, G. A., 195, *216*
Fletcher, A., 386, 387, *399*
Fletcher, B. D., 351, *370*
Fletcher, J. E., 24(14), *44,*
　336, *372*
Fletcher, J. G., 385, *398*

Flock, E. V., 436(63), 437(63,
　69), *463*
Flohe, L., 205, *222*
Flohe, L., 145(185), *171*
Florea, J., 381, *400*
Floridi, A., 135(109), *168*
Floss, H. G., 133(81), *167*
Floyd, E. P., 265, *289*
Floyd, R. A., 84(144), *93*, 446
　(122), *467*
Flynn, A., 319, *323*
Flynn, E. J., 240, 242, 245, 247,
　252, *295*
Focella, A., 199, *216*
Fogel, R., 480(58), *484*
Folb, P. I., 507, *521*
Fomon, S. J., 333, *365*, 441(87),
　464
Fonteles, M. C., 207, *216*
Fordyce, M. K., 240, *283*
Forest, A. P. M., 85(152), *93*
Forman, W. B., 151(253), 152
　(253), *174*
Forsgren, L., 431(14), 434(14),
　436(62), *460, 463*
Forsum, E., 333, 349, *367*
Forte, A. J., 268, *290*
Fortner, J. G., 496(93), *503*
Foster, D. W., 157(289), *176*
Foster, R. B., 340, *365*
Foureman, G. L., 182, *217*
Fourman, P., 493(39), *499*
Fouts, J. R., 52(11), 67(75,78),
　72(97), *87, 90, 91*, 97, *113,*
　116, 191, *214*
Fox, F. W., 238, *283*
Fox, M. R. S., 263, 266, *283,*
　291
Fraley, S., 389, *408*
Francendese, A., 392, *397*
Frank, C., 150(227), *173*
Frank, O., 239, 279, 477(27),
　482
Frankena, H., 142(155), 159
　(155), *170*
Frankenheim, J. M., 389, *404*

Franklin, A. L., 308, *323*
Franklin, J. L., 478(39), *483,*
   519, *522*
Frantz, I. D., Jr., 69(91), *90*
Frape, D. L., 495(46), *499*
Fraser, F. C., 300, 301, 302,
   306, 312, *323, 327, 328*
Fratta, W., 386, *399, 404*
Fraumeni, F. J., 496(41), *499*
Frear, D. S., 191, *216*
Frear, H. R., 191, 192, *222*
Freed, J. H., 442(97), *465*
Freedland, R. A., 163(333), *178*
Freedman, O. M., 195, 196, *216*
Freeman, J. M., 345, *368*
Frei, D., 388, *406*
French, M. R., 126(23), *164*
Freudenthal, R. I., 56(20), *87*
Frias, J. L., 309, *327*
Fricke, H. H., 267, *288*
Frieden, E., 248, *290*
Friedman, B. A., 347, *363*
Friedman, N., 381, *399*
Friedman, P., 446(119), 447
   (119), *467*
Friedman, P. A., 435(51), 440
   (78), 444(113), 446(113),
   447(51,130), 450(78,130),
   452(113), 453(162,163,164),
   454(78), 455(78,186,190,
   191), 457(78,113), *462, 464,*
   466, 467, 470, 472
Friedrich, P., 384, *399*
Friend, D. S., 183, *214*
Frisi, C., 135(109), *168*
Fristrom, S., 379, *399*
Frohlich, T., 237, *286*
Frost, D. V., 304, *324*
Fry, B. E., Jr., 263, 266, *283,*
   291
Fry, J. R., 123(16), *164*
Frymoyer, J. W., 418, *423*
Fuchs, A. R., 353, *363*
Fujii, O., 203, *219*
Fujita, K., 236, 261, 271, *283*
Fukami, J.-I., 191, *222*
Fukayama, G., 433(33), *461*

Fukushima, M., 392, *406*
Furth, J., 84(147), *93*
Fuxe, K., 386, *399*
Fyffe, J., 130(48), 131(48), *165*
Fysh, J. M., 268, *278*

G

Gailes, L., 389, *401*
Gaillard, D., 65(72, 67(72),
   89
Gainey, P. A., 129(44), *165*
Gal, I., 303, *324*
Gala, R. R., 348, *363*
Galen, M., 379, *400*
Galinsky, R. E., 139(139), *169*
Galletti, P., 133(78), 134(101),
   167, 168
Galli-Kienle, M., 134(100,103),
   168
Gallop, P. M., 453(162,165), 455
   (190), *470, 472*
Gallus, A. S., 441(81), *464*
Gandhi, G., 478(43), *484*
Gangolli, S. D., 129(43), *165,*
   255, 268, *288*
Gans, J. H., 392, *407*
Garattini, S., 241, *283*
Garbarg, M., 384, *399*
Garbutt, J. T., 154(280), *175*
Garcia, F., 237, *288, 289*
Garcia, J., 389, *399*
Gardner, E. J., 455(185,193),
   472, 473
Garg, B. D., 106, *117*
Garland, W. A., 67(76), *90*
Garle, M., 26(22), 27(22), 29
   (22), *45*
Garr, A., 416, *427*
Garrett, E. R., 334, *363*
Garrido, J. T., 347, *361*
Garro, A., 67(81), *90*
Garrow, J. S., 385, 389, *399*
Gartner, L. M., 349, *360*
Gascon-Barre, M., 416, *424*
Gatley, S. J., 151(251),

[Gatley, S. J.]
152(251), *174*
Gatmaitan, F., 191, *217*
Gatmaitan, S., 192, *213*
Gaudry, M., 454(178), *471*
Gaull, G. E., 133(75), 157(285, 286), *167, 176, 208, 219*
Gauthier, A. P., 488(55), *500*
Gay, R. J., 150(234), *173*
Gaynor, M. F., 309, *326*
Geber, W. F., 388, *399*
Gebhard, R. L., *285*
Gebhardt, O., 444(115), 446(115), *466*
Gebre-Medhin, M., 333, *367*
Gehring, P. J., 12, 13, *17, 18, 19*
Geison, R. L., 141(153), *170*
Gelenberg, A. J., 351, *364*
Gellene, R. A., 477(27), *482*
Geller, S., 141(154), *170*
Georgakopoulos, P. A., 340, *366*
George, C. F., 515, *521*
George, J. C., 227, *286*
George, S. G., 197, *219*
George, T., 263, *283*
Gerber, N., 437(71), *463*
Gergely, V., 131(56), 139(56), *166*
Gerlach, U., 142(159), *170*
Germino, N. I., 307, *323*
Gerson, C. D., 477(38), *483, 519, 522*
Gerstenecker, C., 205, *222*
Gessa, G. L., 386, *404*
Gessner, T., 131(55), *166*
Geweke, L. O., 451(134), 454(175), 455(188), 456(134), 457(175), *468, 471, 472*
Ghosh, M. N., 383, *399*
Giacomini, J. C., 26(25), *45*
Giacomini, K. M., 26(25), *45*
Gibaldi, M., 42(75), *49,* 240, *283*
Gibbs, F. A., 183, *218*
Giefer, E. E., 393, *396*

Giese, J. E., 73(108), *91*
Gigon, P. L., 240, *280*
Gilbert, J., 413, *427*
Giles, H. G., 35(51), *47*
Gillette, J. R., 37(63), 42(80), *48, 49,* 97, *114,* 121(2), 122(2), 124(17), *163, 164,* 204, 211, *218, 220,* 240, 242, 267, 268, 271, *278, 280, 283, 289, 290*
Gingell, R., 495(61), *500*
Ginter, E., 229, 236, 237, 238, 250, 252, 272, 273, 277, *284*
Giovanella, B. C., 134(90), 137(90), 159(90), *167*
Giovanoli-Jakubczak, T., 9, *17*
Girardot, J. M., 446(122), 454(182,184), 455(192), 456(192), 457(182,192), *467, 471, 472*
Gjeruldsen, S. T., 320, *326*
Glass, R. C., 351, *371*
Glass, R. L., 332, *364*
Glaumann, H., 142(158), *170, 194, 222*
Glauser, E. M., 393, 394, *399*
Glauser, S. C., 393, 394, *399*
Glazenburg, E., 162(327), 163(327), *177*
Glazer, J. P., 340, *364*
Glazer, R. I., 135(107), *168*
Glick, S. D., 389, *400*
Glickman, R. M., 479(55), *484*
Gloor, H., 434(48), 435(48), 436(48), 437(48), *462*
Glorieux, F. H., 417, *423*
Glover, E., 63(61), *89*
Gluck, J. P., 389, *400*
Glusker, J. P., 133(77), *167*
Glynne, A., 410, *424*
Go, V. L. W., 415, *422*
Godwin, H. A., 476(18), 477(23, 34), *482, 483*
Goebell, H., 488(29), *498*
Goetsch, C., 308, *324*
Goff, E. U., 496(30), *498*

Gogerty, J. H., 379, *400*
Gold, F., 339, *361*
Goldberg, A., 247, 251, *282*
Goldberg, J. A., 195, 196, *216*
Goldberg, M., 413, 414, *423*
Goldberg, N. H., 388, *397*
Goldberg, S. C., 383, *400*
Golden, N. L., 319, *323*
Goldfarb, S., 69(93), *90*
Goldman, B. F., 394, *396*
Goldsmith, R. S., 415, *422*
Goldstein, A., 21(1), 43(1), *43*
Goldstein, L., 145(183), 146
    (183), *171*, 211, *218*
Goldstein, P. D., 519, *523*
Goldstone, A. H., 479(50), *484*
Goldyne, M. E., 306, *323*
Golvano, M. P., 445(117), 446
    (117), *466*
Gongaware, R. D., 208, *216*
Gonzales, D. E., 14, *17*
Gonzales, L. J., 261, *293*
Gonzales, S. C., 389, *400*
Goodale, R. L., 493(20), *497*
Goode, A. W., 514, *522*
Goodman, D. G., 96, *116*
Goodman, H. L., 454(176,177),
    471
Goodman, S. R., 443(101), *465*
Goodwin, D., 415, *427*
Gordon, H. W., 312, *327*
Gordon, T., 393, *400*
Gori, G. B., 72(99), *91*
Gorman, W., 354, *359, 360*
Gorski, T., 495(31), *498*
Gostof, 343, *364*
Gotestam, K. G., 380, *400*
Goth, R., 54(18), *87*
Gottenborg, S., 393, *401*
Gottlieb, L. S., 77(115), *91*
Gould, L. V., 416, *427, 428*
Goulding, R., 357, *359, 363*
Goyer, R. A., 266, *284*
Graef, J. W., 309, *326*
Grafstrom, R., 126(25), 145
    (187), *164, 171*

Grafström, R., 188, 189, *216*
Grafstrom, R. C., 67(79), *90*,
    188, *223*
Graham, G. G., 39(68), *48*
Graham, J. D. P., 389, *400*
Gram, T. E., 96, 97, *113, 115*,
    117, 122(6), *163*, 235, 237,
    239, 241, 245, 247, 253,
    292
Grant, G. A., 450(132), 454
    (169,170), *468, 470*
Grant, P., 308, *324*
Grantham, F. H., 81(132), *92*
Grau, E. M., 194, *223*
Grav, H. J., 229, *284*
Graves, C. B., 452(147), *469*
Gray, P., 413, *427*
Graziano, J. H., 150(239), *174*
Greedman, B., 85(153), *93*
Greeley, G. H., 381, *400*
Green, F. E., 240, *280*
Green, H. J., 339, *364*
Green, J., 69(89), 70(89), *90*
Green, M. D., 226, 227, *290*
Green, M. R., 456(200), *473*
Green, R. M., 199, 201, *216*
Green, S., 250, *289*
Green, S. E., 386, 387, *399*
Greenberg, E., 195, *216*
Greenberg, I., 389, *408*
Greenberg, L. M., 381, *400*
Greenblatt, M., 261, *284*
Greenhalf, J. O., 349, *364*
Greenhill, L. L., 381, *400*
Greenstein, A., 492(19), *497*
Greffe, J., 126(24), *164*
Greiling, H., 141(150), *170*
Greim, H., 67(81), *90*
Greiner, J. W., 103, 104, *114*
Gretch, M., 21(3), *43*
Griciute, L., 58(38), *88*
Griep, A. E., 444(113), 446(113),
    452(113), 455(190), 457(113),
    466, 472
Griffith, O. W., 136(118,119),
    144(175), 146(191), 147(175),

[Griffith, O. W.]
149(118,175,216a,217), *168,*
171, 173, 180, 190, 194, 196,
197, *216*
Griffiths, K., 85(152), *93*
Griminger, P., 433(45), *462*
Grimshaw, W. T. R., 61(58), *89*
Grindlay, D. M., 493(47), *499*
Grisolia, S., 317, *324, 350, 364*
Groby, W. G., 153(258), *175*
Grof, P., 384, *406*
Grollman, A., 231, *284*
Gronow, M., 180, *216, 224*
Groshong, T., 346, *360*
Gross, M. D., 381, *400*
Gross, R. L., 106, *113*
Grossman, S. P., 386, 387, *402*
Grossowicz, N., 477(29), *483*
Grover, P. C., 191, *216*
Grubbs, C. J., 96, *116*
Gruboff, S. I., 379, *400*
Grunfeld, Y., 389, *400*
Guaitani, A., 134(102), 137
(126), *168, 169,* 241, *283*
Gualano, M., 134(102,103), 137
(126), *168, 169*
Guentert, T. W., 42(76,82), *49*
Guenthner, T., 230, *278*
Guenthuen, T., 67(82), *90*
Gueris, J., 415, 418, *423*
Guerri, C., 149(216), *173,* 350,
364
Gugler, R., 33(39), *46,* 336,
338, *364, 371*
Guidotto, A., 154(277), *175*
Guldberg, H. C., 135(111), 136
(111), *168*
Gullino, P. M., 81(132), *92,* 96,
115
Gullo, L., 490(12), 492(83),
497, 502
Gundermann, K., 247, *284*
Gunn, T., 354, *359*
Gunther, M., 333, 334, *364*
Gustafsson, B. E., 182, 200,
201, 209, 210, *213, 214*
Gustafsson, B. F., 84(146), *93*

Gustafsson, J.-A., 182, 200,
201, 209, 210, *213, 214*
Gustafsson, J. E., 84(146), *93*
Guthrie, H. A., 332, 333, 334,
364, 369
Gutiennez, L., 476(15), *481*
Gutmann, H. R., 57(28), *88*
Guttman, D. E., 21(2), 30(2),
31(2), *43,* 304, *328*
Guy, O., 489(77), 490(77), *501,*
502
Guzelian, P. S., 11, *17,* 241, *279*

H

Ha, L. T., 355, *365*
Habeel, A. F., 146(203), *172*
Häberle, D., 145(186), *171*
Habig, W. H., 190, 191, 192, 193,
217, 218, 220
Habs, M., 57(32), *88*
Hackman, R. M., 318, 319, *324*
Haddad, J. G., 411, 421, *423,*
427
Haddad, J. G., Jr., 410, 411,
412, 413, 415, 416, 417, 419,
422, *424, 427*
Hafeman, D. G., 98, *115*
Hafford, B., 259, *279*
Hage, G., 492(88,90), *502*
Hageman, J. M., 454(173,175),
457(175), *471*
Hagenfeldt, L., 194, *222*
Hagerman, L. M., 155(281), *175*
Hahn, B. H., 413, *424*
Hahn, P. F., 352, *370*
Hahn, R., 145(185), *171,*
Hahn, T. J., 410, 411, 412, 413,
414, 415, 416, 417, 418, 419,
421, 422, *424, 425*
Hailey, D. M., 352, *362*
Haines, K., 338, *370*
Haldi, J., 392, *400*
Hale, F., 300, *324*
Hales, B. F., 243, *291*
Hall, B., 333, *364*

Hall, J. M., 445(117), 446(117), *466*

Hallenbeck, G. A., 493(47), *499*

Hallesy, D. W., 315, *326*

Halmekoski, J., 379, *399*

Halmi, K. A., 383, *400*

Halpaap-Wood, K., 209, 210, *217*

Halpern, F., 381, *400*

Halsema, I. C. M., 129(40), 139 (40), *165*

Halstead, L. R., 410, 411, 414, 415, 416, 417, 418, 421, 422, *424, 425*

Halsted, C. H., 476(19), 477 (20), 478(42,43), 480(64), *482, 483, 484, 485*

Halver, J. E., 227, 237, *279, 284*

Halverson, J. D., 416, *427*

Ham, J. M., 441(82), *464*

Hambraeus, L., 333, 349, *367*

Hamilton, C. L., 392, *401*

Hammarström, J., 190, *221*

Hammerstrom-Wiklund, B., 161 (323), *177*

Handlogten, M. E., 163(339), *178*

Hanka, L. J., 196, *217*

Hanker, J. S., 209, *222*

Hankin, J. H., 83(138), *92*

Hänninen, O., 127(34), 132(34), *165*

Hanninen, O., 67(73), 68(73, 87), 72(87), *89, 90*

Hannum, C. H., 133(76), *167*

Hansen, S., 180, *221*

Hanson, D., 65(71), 72(71), *89*

Hanssen, I., 229, *284*

Hansten, P. D., 273, 274, *284*

Hanstrom, L., 418, *426*

Hanwell, A., 334, 335, *364*

Hard, G. C., 82(135), *92*

Hardison, W. G. M., 153(264, 266,267), 154(267,269), *175*

Harisch, G., 146(204), *172*

Harland, B. F., 6, *17*, 263, 266, *283*

Harley, J. D., 341, *364*

Harlow, H. F., 389, *401*

Haro, E. N., 475(2), *481*

Harper, M., 390, *401*

Harris, B., 390, *401*

Harris, B. J., 161(319), *177*

Harris, L. S., 388, 389, *395, 398, 404*

Harris, M., 416, 418, *425*

Harris, M. E., 333, *362*

Harris, R., 410, *426*

Harris, R. A., 129(43), *165*, 268, *288*

Harris, W. S., 247, 252, *285*

Harrison, G. G., 239, 272, 273, *294*

Harrison, H. C., 418, *425*

Harrison, H. E., 418, *425*

Hart, B. J. T., 27(27), *45*

Hart, G. W., 142(160), *170*

Hartiala, K., 97, *115*

Hartz, S. C., 309, *326*

Harvey, F., 490(28), *498*

Harvey, J. A., 383, *401*

Harvey, M. S., 154(273), *175*

Harvey, R. F., 491(32), *498*

Harvey, W. P., 442(99), *465*

Hashimoto, M., 126(22), 147 (22), 148(22), *164*, 270, *286*

Hasselblatt, A., 131(61,63), *166*

Hattori, T., 356, *365*

Hauschka, P. V., 453(162,164), *470*

Haussler, M. R., 415, 417, *425*

Hauswirth, J. W., 103, 104, *115*

Haux, N. W. H., 191, *221*

Havelka, J., 340, *364*

Haven, G. T., 261, *280*

Hawkins, C. F., 479(51), *484*

Hawkins, D. E., 334, *364*

Hawkins, R. A., 85(153), *93*

Haworth, J. C., 416, *422*

Hayden, M. T., 78(117), *91*

Hayes, J. R., 98, *114*

Hayes, K. C., 151(246), 153 (246,261), 154(246), 156 (261), *174, 175*
Hayton, W. L., 273, 274, *284*
Hazell, K., 441(85), *464*
Hazelton, G. A., 144(179), 150 (179), *171*
Head, J. F., 81(133), *92*
Hecht, S., 56(21), 57(21), 67 (21), *87*
Hecht, S. S., 58(35,36), *88*
Heinivaara, O., 480(65,66,70, 71), *485*
Heinle, H., 189, *217*
Heinonen, P. O. P., 309, *326*
Heird, W. C., 208, *216, 219*
Heizer, W. D., 162(328), *177*
Hejzlar, M., 340, *364*
Held, F., 342, *370*
Helgeland, A., 393, *401*
Helgeland, L., 447(124), 450 (124), 453(166,168), 454 (166,168), 457(166), *467, 470*
Heller, A., 383, *401*
Hemker, H. C., 430(6), *459*
Hems, R., 149(224), 150(224), 161(313), *173, 177*
Hendelberger, C., 67(80), *90*
Henderson, P. T., 126(27), 129 (42), 131(42), 132(42), *164, 165,* 211, *215, 216*
Hendin, B. A., 410, 411, 412, 413, 415, 416, 419, *424*
Henkin, R. I., 351, *371,* 384, *401*
Henrich, W. L., 516, *521*
Henriksson, B. G., 389, *402*
Hensley, W. J., 26(24), *45*
Hepner, G. W., 153(263), 154 (263), *175,* 240, *285,* 477 (38), *483*
Herbai, G., 138(130), *169*
Herbert, V., 477(38), *483*
Herbst, J. J., 480(57), *484*
Hermanson, R., 184, *224*

Hermodson, M. A., 452(148), *469*
Hernandez, L., 379, *401*
Hernandez, O., 182, 210, 211, *217, 223*
Herndon, B. J., 106, *117*
Herrero, B. A., 475(7), 476(7), *481*
Herrier, R. N., 513, *521*
Hertz, C. G., 350, *372*
Herzberg, M., 349, *372*
Herzer, C., 98, *117*
Heslin, P., 199, *216*
Hess, D. R., 480(69), *485*
Hewick, D. S., 452(142), *468*
Hibasami, H., 133(80), 136(80), *167*
Hickey, N., 393, *401*
Hietanen, E., 65(70), 67(73), 68 (73,87), 69(88), 72(87,88), 132(71), *166*
Higashi, T., 144(174,176), 149 (174,220), 150(226,228), 162 (220,228), 163(74,226), *171, 173,* 203, 204, 207, *217, 220, 223, 224*
Higginbottom, M. D., 333, *365*
Highman, B., 204, *217*
Hikita, K., 203, *224*
Hilf, J. R., 150(234), *173*
Hilf, R., 146(192), *171,* 180, *217*
Hill, C. H., 263, 265, *285*
Hill, D. L., 97, *115*
Hill, H. A. O., 456(200), *473*
Hill, P., 52(9), 75(9), 77(9), 78 (9), 86(9), *87*
Hilman, B., 350, *373*
Hilton, J. W., 227, *286*
Himmelsbach, C. K., 388, *408*
Hingtgen, J. N., 390, *404*
Hinson, J. A., 147(209), 148 (209), *172,* 267, 268, *278, 289, 290*
Hintz, K. L., 36(60), *47*
Hintze, K. L., 36(59), *47*
Hirano, I., 61(59), *89*
Hirayama, T., 496(36), *499*

Hirom, P. C., 154(268), *175*
Hiroto, N., 54(16), *87*
Hirsch, K. S., 316, *324, 328*
Hirsh, J., 332, *365*, 441(81), *464*
Hissin, P. J., 146(192), *171*, 180, *217*
Hite, R. L., 343, *361*
Hjelmeland, L. M., 243, 255, 257, *289*
Hjermann, J., 393, *401*
Hobby, G. L., 339, *364*
Hoch-Gelerent, E. L., 493(33), *498*
Hoch-Ligeti, C., 495(34), *498*
Hochli-Kaufmann, L., 247, 248, *282, 288*
Hockin, L. J., 185, *213, 221*
Hodges, H. M., 386, 387, *399*
Hodges, R. E., 237, *285*
Hodgson, E., 191, *220*
Hoebel, B. C., 378, *401*
Hoebel, B. G., 379, 383, *396, 401*
Hoekstra, W. G., 98, *115*
Hoeldtke, R., 227, *292*
Hoench, H., 188, *217*
Hoensch, H., 67(77), *90*
Hoffbrand, A. V., 309, 311, *324*, 477(24a,35), *482*
Hoffman, D. G., 257, *285*
Hoffman, J., 135(105), *168*
Hoffman, S. P., 380, 381, *408*
Hoffmann, D., 56(21), 57(21), 58(34,35), 67(21), *87, 88*
Hoffmann, D. R., 136(112), 137 (112), *168*
Hoffmann, J. L., 161(320), *177*
Hoffmeister, H., 488(29), *498*
Hofmann, A. F., 153(263), 154 (263), *175*
Högberg, J., 183, 184, 185, *217, 220, 224*
Hokfelt, T., 386, *399*
Hole, D. J., 238, *280*
Hollander, D., 431(15,16,17), 432(19,20,21,22,23,24), *460*

Hollander, P. M., 445(116), 446, (116), *466*
Hollister, L. E., 387, 388, 389, *401*
Hollman, S., 255, 256, 257, *285, 294*
Holloway, B. A., 227, 229, 231, 233, *285*
Holloway, D. E., 226, 227, 228, 229, 230, 231, 233, 234, 236, 238, 239, 249, 250, 251, 252, 253, 254, 255, 261, 272, 273, 276, 277, *285, 290*
Holm, E. E. T., 452(151), *469*
Holmberg, G., 341, *359*
Holmberg, I., 415, 417, *423*
Holme, I., 393, *401*
Holst, A., 237, *286*
Holtzman, J. L., 242, 250, 271, *290*
Homolka, 343, *364*
Honour, A. J., 351, *368*
Hood, J., 237, *285*
Hook, G. E. R., 97, *113, 115*
Hopkins, G. J., 65(66), 72(66), 82(135), 83(136,137), 84 (137), *89, 92*
Hopwood, D., 495(40,46), *499*
Horecker, H., 389, *405*
Horejsi, T., 189, *217*
Horio, F., 257, *286*
Horiuchi, S., 195, *217*
Hornady, G. J., 479(48), *484*
Hornig, D. H., 231, 235, *286*
Horning, E. C., 267, 269, *281*
Horning, M. G., 209, 210, *217*
Hornstein, S., 308, *329*
Horton, G. G., 381, *402*
Horvath, C. A., 304, *324*
Horwitt, M. K., 433(41), *461*
Hosbach, R. E., 340, *365*
Hoskin, F. C. A., 437(68), *463*
Hosokawa, Y., 203, *218, 219*
Hotz, J., 488(29), *498*
Houlihan, M., 477(37), *483*
Houlihan, W., 379, *400*

Houpt, K. A., 386, *396*
House, F. R., 338, *370*
Houser, R. M., 443(101), 454
    (174), 455(193), *465, 471,*
    473
Houston, J. B., 122(4,7), *163,*
    226, 270, 273, 274, *286*
Howard, J. B., 429(3), *459*
Howard, J. L., 387, *398*
Howard, P., 6, 14, *19*
Howard, R. B., 183, *218*
Howat, H. T., 489(35), 490
    (35), 492(35), 493(35), *498*
Howe, J. M., 159(293), *176*
Howell, D. D., 7, 10, *17*
Howell, R. W., 393, *401*
Howie, D., 181, 187, *218*
Howze, G. B., 183, *221*
Hsia, S. L., 432(25), *460*
Hsiao, K. C., 67(76), *90*
Huang, Y. P., 520, *522*
Hudecova, A., 250, 252, *284*
Hudson, J. H., 134(84), *167*
Hueper, W. C., 261, *286*
Huffman, D. H., 33(39), *46*
Hugenroth, S., 209, 210, *217*
Hughes, R. E., 233, 235, 238,
    247, 265, *279, 280, 283, 286*
Hughey, R. P., 193, 195, 197,
    199, *218*
Hukkoo, R. K., 16, *17*
Hulser, D. F., 54(18), *87*
Humphris, B. G., 126(29), 140
    (29), 141(29), *164*
Huncher, H. A., 334, *367*
Hunsz, W., *406*
Hunter, C. G., 7, 8, 9, *17, 18*
Hunter, I. P., 410, *424*
Hunter, J., 410, *425*
Hunter, R. E., 343, *361*
Hunter, W. H., 199, *215*
Hurlbert, R. B., 134(91), *167*
Hurley, L. S., 315, 316, 318,
    319, 320, 321, *323, 324,*
    325, 328

Hurley, R. J., 238, 265, *279,*
    280
Hurwitz, R., 480(57), *484*
Husted, S., 452(143), *468*
Hutson, N. J., 157(287), *176*
Hutton, S. W., 227, 239, 272,
    273, 277, *285*
Huxtable, R., 154(276), *175*
Huxtable, R. J., 153(256,259),
    155(282,283), 156(282), *174,*
    175, 355, *365*
Huy, N. D., 389, *401*
Hvidt, S., 475(3), 476(3), *481*
Hyde, C. L., 135(108), *168*
Hytten, F. E., 333, 334, *365*

I

Idle, J. R., 154(268), *175*
Ilebekk, A., *401*
Imada, I., 437(67,70), *463*
Imai, Y., 243, *286*
Ingall, D., 335, *372*
Ingebretsen, W. R., 183, *224*
Ingold, K., 387, *398*
Ingram, J., 197, *219*
Innami, S., 113, *115*
Inoue, M., 195, *217*
Insogna, K. L., 514, *522*
Insull, W., 332, *365*
Inui, A., 495(18), *497*
Ioannides, C., 201, *221*
Irreverre, F., 162(328), *177*
Irving, C. C., 127(32), *165*
Isaacs, B., 432(26), *460*
Isaacs, J., 146(201), *172*
Ishakawa, S., 72(101), *91*
Ishii, K., 496(36), *499*
Isrealstam, K., 387, *405*
Itzcovics, J., 162(325), *177*
Ivankovic, S., 57(33), *88,* 314,
    324, 495(21), *497*
Ivy, A. C., 432(26), *460*
Iyngkaran, N., 151(244), *174*

J

Jack, B., 343, *362*
Jackson, A. J., 317, *324*
Jackson, C. M., 430(11), 438
(11), *459*
Jackson, I. I. A., 333, *367*
Jackson, R. C., 189, 195, *218*
Jacob, S. T., 183, *218*
Jacobi, H. P., 73(102), *91*
Jacobs, D. R., 393, *401*
Jacobs, R. M., 266, *283*
Jacobsen, E., 233, *286*
Jacobsen, J. G., 152(255), 157
(255), *174*
Jacobsen, S., 27(32), *45*
Jacobson, E. D., 475(1,8), 476
(8), *480, 481*
Jacobson, M., 67(83), *90*
Jacquez, J. A., 11, *17*
Jadhay, M., 333, *365*
Jaeger, R. J., 146(202), *172*,
204, 207, *218*
Jaeger, V., 454(181), *471*
Jagerstad, M., 477(24), *482*
Jähnchen, E., 39(66), *48*, 452
(140), *468*
Jahns, R., 131(61,63), *166*
Jakoby, W. B., 143(169), 144
(169), 145(169), *171*, 190,
191, 192, 193, 200, *217, 218,
220, 221, 224*
Jakubovič, A., 356, *365*
James, D. F., 442(98), *465*
James, L. H., 227, *295*
James, M. O., 151(252), *174*
James, T., 332, *365*
James, W. P. T., 6, *17*
James, W. T., 389, *402*
Jamieson, D., 263, *286*
Janas, L. M., 352, *365*
Jänne, J., 133(79), 136(79), *167*
Janowitz, H. D., 477(38), *483*
Jansen, G. S. I. M., 139(145),
142(156), *170*
Janssen, L. H. M., 27(26), *45*

Jaques, L. B., 437(68), *463*
Jarbe, T. V. C., 389, *402*
Jarboe, C. H., 355, *365*
Jarrett, W. F., 61(58), *89*
Jarvick, M. E., 387, *402*
Javert, C. T., 433(30), *461*
Jayaram, H. N., 187, 196, *215,
218*
Jeffery, E., 230, *278*
Jeffrey, E., 67(82), *90*
Jenkins, J., 388, *398*
Jenkins, L. J., Jr., 263, *286*
Jenkins, M. V., 418, *425*
Jenner, A., 34(49), 35(49), *47*
Jenner, D. A., 85(153), *93*
Jenness, R., 332, *364*
Jensen, N. M., 148(211), *172*
Jensen, R. L., 333, *365*
Jensen, W. E., 188, *223*
Jequier, E., 392, *395*
Jerina, D., 56(22), *87*
Jerina, D. M., 105, *114, 115*
Jeske, A. H., 207, *216*
Jobe, P. C., 350, *373*
Jobson, K., 390, *402*
Jocelyn, P. C., 145(188), *171*
Johansen, S., 124(18), *164*
Johansson, B., 453(158), *470*
Johansson, E. D. B., 349, *368*
John, T. J., 343, *365*
John, T. M., 227, *286*
Johnels, A. G., 9, *16*
Johns, D. G., 345, *365*
Johnsen, D. O., 237, *279*
Johnson, B. C., 141(153), *170,*
446(122), 454(171,182,184),
455(187,192), 456(187,192,
196), 457(182,192), *467, 471,
472, 473*
Johnson, B. G., 154(279), *175*
Johnson, D. A., 248, *290*, 387,
402
Johnson, F. N., 384, *402*
Johnson, J. L., 162(329), *177*
Johnson, R. L., 442(93), *465*
Johnston, G. S., 351, *371*

Johnston, M. F. M., 453(159),
    470
Jolicoeur, F. B., 392, 404
Jollow, D. J., 57(29), 88, 126
    (22), 147(22), 148(22), 164,
    204, 211, 218, 220, 266, 269,
    270, 286, 291
Jolly, D. W., 433(29), 456(199),
    461, 473
Jones, A. C., 183, 215
Jones, A. E., 351, 371
Jones, A. O. L., 266, 283
Jones, C. A., 123(16), 164
Jones, D. J., 163(338), 178
Jones, D. P., 146(196), 172,
    185, 186, 187, 207, 213, 218,
    220, 221
Jones, J. P., 455(185,193), 472,
    473
Jones, P. R., 233, 235, 286
Jones, P. W., 56(20), 87
Jörnvall, H., 146(196), 172
Joyce, B. E., 237, 279
Jubiz, W., 410, 411, 414, 417,
    422, 425, 427
Jukes, T. H., 308, 323
Jundt, S., 389, 398
Jungerman, K., 183, 218
Jurand, J., 182, 219
Jurk, I. H., 388, 398
Jusko, W. J., 21(3), 43, 354,
    355, 371, 373
Juul, S., 344, 365

                        K

Kachole, M. S., 226, 255, 258,
    287
Kadis, B., 456(199), 473
Kadlec, G. J., 355, 365
Kafetzis, D. H., 340, 366
Kahn, A. J., 418, 424
Kahn, G. C., 29(35), 46
Kajander, E. O., 135(106), 137
    (106), 168

Kajitani, T., 72(101), 91
Kakolewski, J. K., 381, 408
Kalamegham, R., 103, 106, 115,
    261, 291
Kallner, A., 243, 250, 279
Kalter, H., 300, 312, 323, 325
Kamala, R., 14, 17
Kamath, P. R., 14, 17
Kamisaka, K., 192, 216, 218
Kamm, J. J., 98, 99, 114, 115,
    235, 240, 241, 247, 250, 251,
    261, 287
Kamm, M. L., 351, 373
Kampffmeyer, H. G., 126(20),
    164
Kaneko, S., 344, 366
Kannel, W. B., 393, 400
Kanolkar, V. S., 14, 17
Kanto, J., 347, 363
Kao, J., 123(16), 164
Kaplowitz, N., 145(183), 146(183,
    197), 171, 172, 211, 218
Kappas, A., 67(76), 90, 97, 113,
    248, 289
Karch, F. E., 507, 522
Karibo, J. M., 355, 365
Karl, I., 417, 422
Karlberg, B., 345, 366
Karle, J. M., 56(22), 87
Karmeli, F., 480(58,59), 484,
    485
Karniol, I. G., 389, 400
Karnofsky, D., 308, 325
Kassouny, M. E., 240, 283, 287
Kates, R. E., 33(42), 46
Katims, J. J., 392, 407
Kato, K., 61(59), 89
Kato, N., 257, 263, 277, 287
Kato, R., 240, 245, 247, 287
Katoch, D. S., 16, 17
Katona, E., 139(140), 169
Kattan, K. R., 418, 425
Katz, F. H., 348, 366
Katz, M., 342, 370
Kauffman, F. C., 132(72), 166,
    211, 218

Kaufman, L., 247, *282*
Kaufman, P. L., 393, *408*
Kautz, H. D., 339, *366*
Kawachi, T., 54(13), *87*
Kawai, K., 257, 263, 277, *287*
Kawai, M., 454(176), *471*
Keen, C. L., 320, 321, *323, 324,*
325
Keen, J. H., 191, *218*
Keen, P. M., 28(34), *46*
Kehoe, R. A., 11, *19*
Keiding, S., 124(18), *164*
Keiser, H. R., 384, *401*
Kelley, B. C., 140(147), *170*
Kelley, J. N., 192, *221*
Kello, D., 9, *17*
Kelly, H. J., 333, *367*
Kelly, J., 386, 387, *402*
Kelly, P. H., 378, *402*
Kelnar, C. J. H., 516, *522*
Kenepp, N. B., 353, *362*
Kennedy, J. S., 389, *404*
Kenny, A. J., 197, 198, *214,*
219
Kent, G. N., 417, *426*
Keppler, D., 130(53), *166*
Kerbey, A. L., 157(287), *176*
Kermack, W. O., 333, *366*
Kern, F., 493, *499*
Kerr, M. A., 197, *219*
Kerry, R. J., 384, 385, *402*
Kershaw, D., 197, *219*
Kerzner, B., 507, *522*
Kesaniemi, Y. A., 353, *366*
Kessler, K. M., 35(55), *47*
Kessler, M., 227, *292*
Ketelaars, H. C. J., 126(27),
164
Ketley, J. N., 192, *218*
Kettering, W. G., 150(232), *173*
Keulemans, K., 139(135), *169*
Keyler, D. E., 257, *291*
Keys, A., 392, 393, *396*
Khan, A. K. A., 338, *366*
Khanna, N. N., 336, 337, *366,*
372

Khor, H. T., 73(106), 81(106),
91
Khosla, T., 393, *402*
Khouw, V., 35(52), *47*
Kielb, M., 432(19), *460*
Kienholz, E. W., 265, *290*
Kilberg, M. S., 163(339), *178*
Kilgore, B. S., 380, 381, *398*
Killen, E., 85(153), *93*
Killenberg, P. G., 151(254),
174
Kilra, V., 190, *219*
Kim, H., 209, *222*
Kim, K. S., 233, 247, *282*
Kim, S., 133(78), *167*
Kim, Y. S., 188, 198, *219*
Kimmel, C. A., 316, 317, 321,
325
Kimmich, G. A., 188, *219*
Kinde, A. S., 63(61), *89*
King, C. G., 267, *288*
Kinkel, A. W., 337, *361*
Kinney, C. S., 308, *325*
Kinscherf, D. A., 417, 418, *423*
Kinsell, L. W., 433(33), *461*
Kipfer, R. K., 453(157), *469*
Kircher, C. H., 495(37), *499*
Kirksey, A., 333, *373*
Kirsch, K., 479(55), *484*
Kirsch, R., 192, *213*
Kirsh, R. E., 192, *214*
Kirskey, A., 332, 349, *366*
Kitchell, B. B., 35(57), *47*
Kitter, F., 393, *402*
Kizer, J. S., 381, *400*
Kjeldsen, K., 475(3), 476(3),
481
Klatt, T. J., 239, 244, *291*
Klausner, H. A., 356, *366*
Kleimola, T., 347, *363*
Klein, P. D., 335, *372*
Klein, R., 150(229), *173*
Kleinrock, S., 381, 392,
395
Kleit, S. A., 516, *522*
Klinck, G. H., Jr., 261, *289*

Kline, B. E., 73(107,109), 91
Klipstein, F. A., 477(31), 483
Kluft, F. C., 516, 522
Klume, S., 389, 399, 405
Knauer, G. R., 456(198), 473
Knauer, T., 447(129), 467
Knauer, T. E., 440(77), 441(89), 442(89), 447(128), 464, 465, 467
Knight, M. K., 237, 279
Knight, R. H., 181, 210, 219
Knights, R. M., 381, 402
Knopf, K., 151(246), 153(246), 154(246), 174
Knox, J. H., 182, 219
Kobayashi, M., 230, 231, 294
Kober, Å., 34(49), 35(49), 47
Kober, A., 23(8), 24(8), 34(47, 48), 35(47), 44, 46, 47
Koch, H. C., 418, 425
Koch-Weser, J., 23(5), 36(5), 38(5), 44
Kociba, R. J., 314, 325
Kodama, J., 392, 406
Koeff, S. T., 337, 361
Koelle, G. B., 393, 408
Koetsawang, S., 349, 366
Kohashi, N., 203, 218, 219
Kohl, F.-V., 106, 115
Kojuma, J., 204, 220
Kolakowska, T., 350, 373
Kolski, S. M., 159(293), 176
Konicoff, N. G., 339, 370
Konishi, T., 435(52), 462
Konishi, Y., 495(18), 497
Konz, K. H., 148(215), 149(215), 173
Koornhof, H. J., 33(41), 46
Kopin, I. J., 134(82), 137(82), 159(82), 167
Kori, Y., 203, 218, 219
Kornhauser, D. M., 126(26), 164
Kornitzer, M., 393, 402
Korsgaard, S., 387, 403
Koshakji, R. P., 317, 321, 325
Koshy, E., 14, 17

Kosinova, A., 250, 252, 284
Kosower, E. M., 144(180), 146 (205), 171, 172, 180, 181, 201, 216, 219
Kosower, N. S., 144(180), 146 (205), 171, 172, 201, 219
Koster, H., 129(40), 139(40), 165
Kosterlitz, H., 204, 214
Kostial, K., 9, 17
Kotake, A., 67(82), 90, 230, 278
Kottke, B. A., 247, 252, 285
Koup, J. R., 340, 371
Koyama, H. H., 490(65), 501
Kozak, E. M., 198, 219
Kraft, D., 418, 425
Kramer, C., 389, 397
Kramer, C. G., 12, 13, 17
Kramer, R. E., 103, 104, 114
Kratz, C. M., 384, 403
Krause, R. F., 103, 104, 114
Krauss, I. K., 379, 401
Krawitt, E. L., 416, 425
Kraybill, L. F., 386, 404
Krebs, H. A., 149(224), 150 (224), 161(313), 173, 177, 237, 287
Kredich, N. M., 136(121), 168
Krees, S. V., 346, 373
Kremmer, K. S., 202, 224
Kretchner, N., 480(57), 484
Krijgsheld, K. R., 126(21), 139 (134a,136), 141(21,151), 142 (151,155), 159(155), 162 (327), 163(327), 164, 169, 170, 177
Krishman, N., 204, 219
Krishna, G., 146(199), 172
Krishnamurthi, D., 261, 291
Krishnamurthy, S., 263, 283
Krishnaswamy, K., 33(40), 46, 103, 106, 115, 194, 222
Kristoferson, A., 183, 184, 217, 224
Kritchevsky, D., 254, 287
Krom, D. P., 240, 281
Kruger, E., 381, 408

Kruger, F. W., 495(62), *500*
Krumdieck, C. L., 477(20,21, 36), *482, 483*
Kruse, R., 409, *426*
Kuenzig, W., 98, *115*, 235, 237, 240, 241, 247, 250, 251, *287, 288, 289*
Kueter, K., 239, 244, *291*
Kuhlenkamp, J., 145(183), 146 (183,197), *171, 172*, 211, *218*
Kulakis, C., 59(46), *88*
Kulkarni, A. P., 191, *220*
Kumaoha, H., 193, *223*
Kumar, R., 415, *426*, 441(84), *464*
Kuntzman, I., 67(83), *90*
Kuntzman, R., 242, *288*
Kunze, F. M., 7, *17*
Künzel, B., 131(62,63,64), *166*
Kupfer, D. J., 391, *403*
Kupper, R., 495(61), *500*
Kurata, D., 26(23), 29(23), 35 (23), *45*
Kurimara, M., 496(80), *502*
Kurup, P. A., 142(162,163,164, 165,166), *170*
Kurz, H., 26(21), 28(21), 29 (21), *45*
Kvenzer, W., 335, *373*
Kyle, W. E., 161(319), *177*

L

Lachenmaier, C., 145(186), *171*
Lack, L., 154(280), *175*
Lacy, W. W., 384, *407*
Laerum, O. D., 54(18), *87*
Lai, P. P., 492(59), *500*
Laird, H. E., 155(282), 156 (282), *175*, 513, *521*
Laitanen, M., 67(73), 68(73,87), 69(88), 72(87,88), *89, 90*

Lake, B. G., 129(43), *165*, 255, 268, *288*
Lakshmanan, F. L., 159(295), 163(336), *176, 178*
Lakshmanan, M. R., 69(94), *90*
Lal, H., 263, *292*
Lal, S., *522*
Laliberte, R. E., 442(92), 443 (92), 451(92,136), 452(154), *465, 468, 469*
Lalich, J., 160(310), 161(310), *177*
Lalich, J. J., 160(308), 161(308), *177*
Lam, L. K. T., 63(62), *89*
Lamberg, B. A., 150(236), *174*
Lambert, L., 68(85,86), 69(85, 86), *90*
Lambert, P. W., 415, *422*
Lamden, M. P., 106, *113*
Lamoureux, G. L., 191, *219*
Landauer, N., 304, *326*
Landauer, W., 303, 304, 305, 306, *325, 326*
Landberg, E., 190, *215*
Landoldt, M., 227, *293*
Lane, M. D., 157(288), *176*
Lang, C. A., 144(179), 150(179, 230), *171, 173*
Lang, J., 348, *367*
Lang, M., 67(73), 68(73), *89*
Lang, M. A., 243, 255, 257, *289*
Langman, M. J. S., 272, 273, *292*
Lang-Sellers, M. L., 23(5), 36 (5), 38(5), *44*
Laqueur, G. C., 59(43), *88*
Larin, F., 161(321), *177*
Laron, Z., 142(167), *170*
Larranaga, A., 339, *368*
Larsen, G. L., 200, 201, 209, 210, *213, 219*
Larson, A. E., 447(123), 450 (123), 451(123), 454(123), 455(123,189), 456(123), *467, 472*

Larson, P. S., 261, *293*
Larson, R., 184, *217*
Larson, S. M., 351, *366*
Larsson, A., 194, *222*
Lasagna, L., 383, *403*, 507, *522*
Laster, L., 162(328), *177*
Latham, C. J., 379, 383, *396*
Laug, E. P., 7, *17*
Laugier, J., 339, *361*
Laugier, R., 490(60), 491(89),
    492(38), *499, 500, 502*
Laurendeau, G., 80(127), *92*
Laurer, R., 14, *17*
Lauterburg, B. H., 148(209a),
    150(231), *172, 173,* 184,
    207, 208, *219,* 240, *288*
Lauvard, D., 198, *220*
Laval, J., 491(15), *497*
Lavenstein, A. F., 383, *403*
Lavik, P. S., 73(105), *91*
Lavy, T. L., 12, 14, *18*
Law, E., 413, *427*
Lawley, P. D., 54(12), *87*
Lawrence, J. N. P., 14, *18*
Lawrence, W. W., 265, *279*
Lay, M. M., 192, *219*
Layne, D. S., 349, *370*
Layton, W. M., 315, *326*
Lazarides, C. V., 340, *366*
Leaf, D. S., 57(28), *88*
Leaf, G., 204, *219*
Leavy, C. M., 477(27), *482*
Leber, H.-W., 247, *282, 288*
Lebreuil, G., 492(75,78), *501,
    502*
Lechene de la Porte, P., 492
    (13), *497*
Leck, J. B., 343, *366*
Ledbrink, P., 386, *399*
Le Donarec, J. C., 394, *403*
Lee, C., 342, *360*
Lee, C. H., 163(334), *178*
Lee, H. K., 381, 392, *396*
Lee, J., 380, 381, *398*
Lee, M., 433(34), *461*
Lee, S., 308, *326*
Lee, S. W., 414, *426*

Leech, R. C., 35(55), *47*
Leeson, P. M., 493(39), *499*
Lefevere, M. F., 441(88), *464*
Legg, R. F., 185, *221*
Lehr, R. E., 56(22), *87*
Lehrman, S. R., 454(173,175,
    176), 455(188), 457(175),
    471, 472
Leibach, F. H., 207, *216*
Leibowitz, S. F., 390, *403*
Leighton, P. C., 345, *365*
Leijdekkers, C. M., 211, *215,
    216*
Lemberger, L., 388, *403*
Lemberle, J., 389, *398*
Leng, M. L., 12, *18*
Leonard, H. S. D., 349, *364*
Leonards, J. R., 514, *522*
Lepow, M. L., 342, *372*
Leren, P., 393, *401*
Lerner, U., 418, *426*
Lertrataninkoon, K., 209, 210,
    217
Leshem, M. B., 379, 383, *396*
Leshem, M. M., 383, *396*
Leskinen, E., 129(41), 131(41),
    165
Lesser, R. L., 393, *408*
Lester, R., 335, *372, 373*
Levander, T., 380, *400*
Level, R., 204, *221*
Levene, C. I., 307, *326*
Levesque, D., 492(7), *497*
Levi, A. S., 141(154), *170*
Levin, J., 316, *328*
Levin, W., 56(22), *87,* 97, *115,*
    243, *280,* 414, *426*
Levine, D., 514, *522*
Levine, R. A., 480(62), *485*
Levinson, J. C., 417, *426*
Levinson, R. A., 414, *425*
Levison, D. A., 495(40,46), *499*
Levitsky, D. A., 376, 380, 384,
    388, *403*
Levy, D., 138(132), *169*
Levy, G., 27(28), 35(58), 36(59,
    60), 39(66,70,71), 40(70,71),

[Levy, G.]
42(75,78,79), *45, 47, 48, 49,*
139(139), *169,* 226, 270, 274,
286, 336, 337, *366, 373,* 514,
522
Levy, L. F., 238, *283*
Levy, R. J., 453(165), *470*
Levy, W., 350, *366*
Lewander, T., 380, *403*
Lewenthal, H., 311, *322*
Lewin, I., 14, *19*
Lewis, P. J., 343, *369*
Li, D. M. F., 389, *400*
Li, L. F., 453(157), *469*
Li, F. P., 496(41), *499*
Lian, J. B., 453(163,165), *470*
Liau, M. C., 134(90,91), 137
(90), 159(90), *167*
Lickrish, G. M., 346, *363*
Liddle, G. W., 384, *407*
Liebling, L. I., 384, 385, *402*
Liebman, B. F., 519, *522*
Lifshitz, F., 411, 413, 421, *426*
Lijinsky, W., 58(39), *88*
Lin, G. W., 134(91), *167*
Lind, C., 444(111,112), 445(117,
118), 446(117,118), *466, 467*
Lindblad, B. S., 332, *367*
Lindeman, N. J., 261, 267, 269,
290
Lindeman, R. D., 261, *295*
Lindenbaum, J., 346, *367*
Lindeskog, P., 182, *214*
Lindgren, L., 410, *426*
Lindstrand, K., 477(24), *482*
Lindstrom, E., 392, *408*
Lindup, W. E., 27(31), 34(31),
45
Link, K. P., 452(148), *469*
Linke, I., 145(186), *171*
Linkswiler, H. M., 162(324), *177*
Linnoila, M., 390, *402*
Linscheer, W. G., 150(235), *173*
Linzell, J. L., 334, 335, *364*
Lipkin, M., 80(130), *92*
Lipman, R. S., *406*

Lipmann, F., 139(133,146), *169,
170*
Lippincott, S. E., 155(282), 156
(282), *175*
Lissens, W., 411, *423*
Liszewski, M. K., 453(159), *470*
Litterest, C. L., 97, *115*
Litterst, C. L., 237, 241, 245,
247, *292*
Litwach, G., 191, *223*
Litwak, G., 192, *215*
Livesey, G., 161(317), *177*
Ljungdahl, A., 386, *399*
Ljunggren, M., 444(104,110), 445
(104,110), 446(104), 454
(110), *466*
Ljungstedt-Påhlman, I., 23(8),
24(8), *44*
Lloyd, A. G., 255, *288*
Lloyd, B. J., 388, *408*
Lloyd, J. K., 433(35), *461,* 518,
523
Lloyd, M. J., 441(83), *464*
Locker, G. Y., 271, *282*
Lockwood, D. H., 514, *522*
Loeliger, E. A., 430(6), *459*
Lohse, J., 489(16,42,77), 490
(77), *497, 499, 501, 502*
Lomakina, L. Y., 54(18), *87*
Lombardini, J. B., 134(85), 153
(257), 154(278), 155(257,
284), *167, 174, 175*
Lombardo, D., 489(51a,51b),
500
Lome, C. R., 393, *402*
London, I. M., 190, *215*
Londowski, J. M., 415, *426*
Long, G. I., 336, *367*
Longenecker, H. E., 267, *288*
Longland, R. C., 129(43), *165,*
255, *288*
Longnecker, D. S., 61(57), *89*
Longstreth, J. A., 10, *16*
Lönnerdal, B., 320, 321, *323,
325*
Lönnerdal, B., 333, 349, *367*

Lopez, H., 229, *289*
Lorber, J., 344, *363*
Losito, R., 436(63), 437(63,69), *463*
Lotan, R., 96, *115*
Lotlikar, P. D., 199, *219*
Lotti, V. J., 384, *397*
Loub, W. D., 63(62), *89*, 230, *288*
Loughman, P. M., 97, *116*
Loughnan, P., 388, *398*
Loughnan, P. M., 336, 346, 354, *359, 360, 367*
Loveridge, N., 146(200), *172*
Low, L. C. K., 348, *367*
Lowenthal, J., 440(79), 454 (181), *464, 471*
Lowman, J. T., 149(221), *173*
Loy, M., 56(21), 57(21), 67(21), *87*
Loyd, B. C., 96, *114*
Lozner, E. L., 237, *291*
Lu, A. Y. H., 52(10), *87*, 97, *115*, 242, 243, *288, 291*
Lu, H. Y. H., 67(83), *90*
Luch, L. J., 154(273), *175*
Luff, R. D., 345, *368*
Luft, D., 247, 248, *282, 288*
Luginbuhl, H., 392, *408*
Lund, B., 410, 411, 412, 418, *426*
Lund, C. C., 237, *281*
Lund, M., 410, 411, *427*
Lund, P., 161(317), *177*, 411, 421, 422, *423*
Lundberg, D., 345, *366*
Lund-Larsen, P. G., 393, *401*
Lunn, G., 189, 190, *219*
Lupoli, J., 380, 388, 391, *403*
Luther, L., 343, *365*
Lutz, P. G., 332, *370*
Lutz, R. J., 10, 11, *16, 18*
Lyle, J., 180, *215*
Lyle, R. E., 58(38), *88*
Lynch, M., 240, 242, 245, 247, 252, *295*

Lyon, J. L., 496(49), *499*
Lyon, J. P., 263, *286*
Lysnes, H., 229, *284*

M

Mabuchi, K., 496(93), *503*
McAweeney, W., 421, 422, *423*
McBride, R., 456(199), *473*
McBride, W. G., 300, *326*
McBurney, A., 430(9), 431(9), 432(9), 433(9), 436(9,61), 437(66), 439(9,61,73,74), 442(9,61,73), 444(66), *459, 463, 464*
McCain, T. A., 415, 417, *425*
McCance, R. A., 385, *398*
McChesney, E. W., 261, *289*
McClelland, D. B. L., 333, *367*
McConomy, J., 136(116), *168*
McCormick, D. L., 96, *116*
McCoy, G. D., 52(9), 58(36), 75(9), 77(9), 78(9), 86(9), *87, 88*
McDermott, W., 433(42), *461*
MacDonald, H., 344, *369*, 442 (97), *465*
MacDonald, J., 63(63), *89*
McDonald, J. K., 193, 198, *220*
McDonough, J. H., 389, *403*
McGarry, J. D., 157(289), *176*
McGee, D., 393, *400*
McGeeney, K. J., 493(2), *496*
McGeer, P. L., 356, *365*
McGrath, J., 333, *367*
McGuffin, J. C., 379, *397*
McGuiness, E. E., 495(46), *499*
Machlin, L. J., 237, *288, 289*
McHugh, P. R., 387, *405*
McIntyne, T. A., 480(64), *485*
McIntyre, T. M., 196, 197, 205, *220, 221*
McIntyre, W. I. M., 61(58), *89*
Mack, D. O., 446(122), 454(182), 455(192), 456(192), 457(182,

[Mack, D. O.]
192), *467, 471, 472*
McKay, E., 413, *427*
McKenzie, S. A., 348, *367*
McKinney, J. D., 182, *217*
Maclaren, N. K., 411, 413, 421, *426*
McLaughlin, C. L., 386, *395, 398, 404*
McLean, A. E., 148(213), 149 (213), *172*
McLean, A. E. M., 65(67), *89,* 204, *220*
McLean, E. K., 204, *220*
McLeod, S. M., 65(69), *89*
Macleod, S. M., *359*
MacMahon, M., 476(12), *481*
McMahon, S., 381, *400*
McMillan, D. E., 388, 389, *395, 404*
McNamara, P. J., 42(75), *49*
McQueen, E. G., 42(77), *49*
Macri, C., 433(30), *461*
Mctigue, J. J., 455(189), *472*
Macy, I. G., 333, 334, *362, 367*
Madaric, A., 250, 252, *284*
Madsen, J. A., 410, 411, 422, *427*
Magadia, N. E., 78(121), *92*
Magdalou, J., 132(70), 141(70), *166*
Magee, P. N., 57(23,30), 58 (23), *87, 88*
Magnusson, S., 429(4), *459*
Magour, S., 380, *403*
Mahar, C. Q., 479(53), *484*
Maibach, H. I., 5, *17, 18*
Maines, M. D., 248, *289*
Mainguet, P., 383, *403*
Maiorana, A., 96, *115*
Majerus, P. W., 189, *220*
Majumdar, K., 257, 263, 265, *280, 281*
Makhija, S. J., 226, 255, 258, *287*
Mallette, L. E., 413, *426*

Mallinson, C. N., 433(34), 435 (58), 436(58), 438(58), 439 (58), *461, 462*
Mallory, A., 493, *499*
Malloy, M. H., 208, *219*
Malmgren, R. A., 95, *114*
Malmros, I., 338, *363*
Mancuso, T. F., 496(44), *499*
Mandel, H. G., 433(43), *461*
Mandelli, M., 336, *371*
Mandelstam, P., 188, *215*
Mangat, S., 77(116), 78(119), *91, 92*
Manger, W. M., 389, *404*
Manis, B., 198, *221*
Mannering, G., 67(82), *90,* 230, *278*
Mannering, G. J., 72(98), *91,* 236, 257, 275, *289, 291*
Manning, F. J., 389, *403*
Manning, J. A., 431(18), *460*
Manno, B. R., 350, *373*
Manno, J. E., 350, *373*
Manocha, S. L., 356, *372*
Mansbach, C. M., 475(7), 476 (7), *481*
Mantegazzo, P., 379, *397*
Mantel, N., 496(41), *499*
Mantyla, R., 347, *363*
Mapson, L. W., 237, *287*
Marangos, P. J., 392, *407*
Marathe, G. V., 195, *219*
March, B. E., 433(37), *461*
Marcus, A. H., 11, *18*
Marcus, C. J., 190, 192, 193, *220*
Marcus, F. I., 433(39), *461*
Maren, T. H., 315, *323, 326*
Margolis, S., 493(10), 494(9), *497*
Marie, P., 415, 418, *423*
Marini, J. L., 384, *403*
Märki, F., 444(108,109), 445 (108), 446(108), *466*
Markovs, M. E., 160(301), *176*
Marks, I. N., 488(45), 489(45),

[Marks, I. N.]
    493(1), *496, 499*
Mark-Savage, P., 320, *325*
Markulis, M. A., 227, *292*
Maroon, Y., 440(80), *464*
Maroux, S., 198, *220*
Marquardt, H., 54(16), *87*
Marsden, C. A., 135(111), 136
    (111), *168*
Marsden, C. D., 410, *426*
Marselos, M., 127(34), 132(34),
    165
Marshall, C. R., 388, *404*
Marshall, G. R., 454(174), *471*
Marshall, W. J., 65(67), *89*
Martier, S. S., 319, *323*
Martin, A. D., 444(112), *466*
Martin, C. W., 65(68), 67(68),
    68(68), 72(68), *89*
Martin, J. J., 161(319), *177*
Martin, J. R., 393, *395*
Martin, N., 204, *221*
Martin, S. L., 451(134), 456
    (134), *468*
Martin, W. G., 153(258), *175*
Martius, C., 444(107,108,109),
    445(108), 446(108), *466*
Marty, F., 192, *214*
Maruchi, N., 496(93), *503*
Maruyama, E., 204, *220*
Maruyama, S., 340, *373*
Marzullo, J., 507, *522*
Mason, H. S., 97, *116*, 185, *218*
Mason, K. E., 433(38), *460*
Mason, M., 347, *361*
Mason, M. M., 388, 389, *407*
Mason, R. P., 271, *289*
Masry, S., 72(98), *91*
Mathieu, P., 126(24), *164*
Mathur, M. S., 491(32), *498*
Matsaniotis, N., 131(67), *166*
Matschiner, J., 447(129), 452
    (146), *467, 469*
Matschiner, J. T., 432(25,28),
    433(28), 435(54,55,59), 437
    (64), 440(55,77), 441(89),

[Matschiner, J. T.]
    442(89,95,96), 443(95,96,
    100,102), 447(127,128), 450
    (127), 451(96,102,127,136),
    452(102,153), 454(127), 456
    (198), *460, 461, 462, 463,
    464, 465, 467, 468, 469, 473*
Matsumoto, N., 437(70), *463*
Matsuo, T., 230, 231, *294*
Matsushima, M., 80(131), *92*
Matsuyama, T., 496(80), *502*
Matsuzawa, T., 80(128), *92*
Matthews, H. B., 10, 11, *16,
    18, 191, 220*
Matthysse, S., 134(83), 136(124),
    137(127), 161(127), *167, 169*
Mattice, J. D., 11, *18*
Mattila, M., 480(71), *485*
Mattox, V. R., 415, *426*
Maxwell, J. D., 410, *425*
Maxwell, R. A., 387, *398*
Mayo, C. C., 353, *367*
Mazess, R. B., 421, 422, *423*
Mazur, A., 250, *289*
Mazzarese, R., 56(21), 57(21),
    67(21), *87*
Meadow, S. R., 309, *328*
Meck, R., 187, 196, 197, *213*
Meck, R. A., 150(237), *174*, 180,
    187, 205, *222*
Medina, E. V., 153(257), 155
    (257), *174*
Meffin, P., 336, *367*
Meffin, P. J., 39(72), 40(72),
    48, 434(47), 435(56,57), 441
    (57), 442(47,56), *462*
Mefford, I., 146(194), *172*
Mehler, A. H., 193, *220*
Meikle, A. W., 414, *425*
Meilman, E., 475(5), 476(5), *481*
Meister, A., 136(118,119), 143
    (172), 144(172,173,175,177),
    145(172,189), 147(175), 149
    (118,175,217,218), 155(172),
    168, 171, 173, 181, 189, 190,
    194, 195, 196, 197, 199, *213,*

[Meister, A.]
 215, 216, 220, 221, 223, 224
Meites, J., 84(149), *93*
Mellerup, E. T., 385, *404*
Mellors, A. J., 227, *289*
Melmon, K. L., 39(72), 40(72), 48
Melsen, F., 410, 411, 412, 418, *426*
Meltzer, H., 308, *326*
Mendelson, J., 317, *324*
Mendes De Oliveira, J. P., 492 (87), *502*
Menguy, R. B., 493(47), *499*
Menon, P. V. C., 142(165), *170*
Menzel, H., 205, *222*
Mercier-Parot, L., 309, 310, *326, 348, 367*
Meredith, M. J., 185, 203, 204, 205, *220*
Mereu, G. P., 386, *404*
Merkel, A. D., 392, *404*
Merkin, T., 7, *18*
Meslin, J. C., 80(129), *92*
Meullenet, J., 490(48,60), 491 (76), *499, 500, 501*
Meyer, J. G., 311, *326*
Meyer, M. C., 21(2), 30(2), 31 (2), *43*
Meyer, M. B., 356, *367*
Meyer, U. A., 183, *215*
Meynall, M. J., 477(32), *483*
Meyrick Thomas, R. H., 519, *522*
Micevova, J., 189, *217*
Michaelis, G. D., 433(33), *461*
Michelakis, A. M., 185, *220*
Midelfort, C. F., 193, *220*
Midtbøll, I., 124(18), *164*
Miettinen, T. A., 129(41), 131 (41), *165*, 476(14,17), *481, 482*
Mikus, L., 229, 250, *284*
Millburn, P., 128(35), 154(268), *165, 175*
Miller, A. B., 83(139), *92*

Miller, A. T., 376, *407*
Miller, C. C., 199, *219*
Miller, C. E., 15, *18*
Miller, D. J., 148(210), *172*
Miller, D. S., 392, *404*
Miller, E., 513, *523*
Miller, E. C., 51(4), 52(6), 54 (6), 57(6,31), 61(6,31), 63 (63), 64(6), 73(108), *86, 88, 89, 91*, 255, *281*
Miller, H., 351, *368*
Miller, J. A., 51(4), 57(31), 61 (31), 63(63), 73(107,109), *86, 88, 89, 91*, 199, *219, 255, 281*, 454(182), 457(182), *471*
Miller, J. J., 122(9), *164*
Miller, J. K., 351, *368*
Miller, J. R., 300, *328*
Miller, L. L., 453(156), *469*
Miller, N. E., *401*
Miller, R., 442(99), *465*
Miller, R. A., 333, *366, 367*
Miller, R. P., 142(157), *170*
Miller, R. W., 496(41), *499*
Miller, S., 333, *362*
Miller, S. I., 319, *323*
Milli, U., 61(60), *89*
Millichap, J. C., 381, *404*
Millichap, M., 381, *404*
Milloy, S., 389, *400*
Mills, I. H., 390, *404*
Mills, J. N., 336, *368*
Mills, L. R., 495(4), *496*
Milne, D. B., 247, 248, *289*
Milunsky, A. J., 309, *326*
Mimnaugh, E. G., 235, 237, 239, 241, 245, 247, 253, *292*
Minnhaugh, E. G., 97, *115*
Minnich, V., 189, *220*
Mintz, R., 392, *404*
Miranda, C. L., 100, 101, 102, 107, 108, 110, 111, 112, *116*
Miravet, L., 415, 418, *423*
Mirkin, B. L., 344, *368*
Mirkin, J. N., 359, *368*

Mirvish, S. S., 58(40), *88*, 261, *280*
Mischler, T. W., 339, *368*
Mishkin, S., 192, *213*
Mitchell, A. D., 161(311,315, 316), *177*
Mitchell, J. R., 42(81), *49*, 126 (22), 147(22,209), 148(22, 209,209a), 150(231), *164, 172, 173*, 184, 204, 207, 208, 211, *218, 219, 220,* 266, 267, 268, 269, 270, *281, 283, 286, 290, 291*
Mitchell, W. G., 265, *289*
Miya, T. S., 257, *285*
Miyazaki, M., 113, *115*
Mjølnerød, O. K., 320, *326*
Mjos, O. D., *401*
Mobilia, J., 388, *398*
Mochizuki, S., 257, *287*
Mohamad, H. A., 383, *406*
Mohan, P. S., 142(168), *170*
Mohindru, A., 150(232), *173*
Mohr, U., 495(62), *500*
Moiel, R. H., 348, *368*
Moldeus, P., 126(25), 131(56, 59,60), 139(56), 142(158), 146(196), 149(223), 150 (223), *164, 166, 170, 172, 173*, 183, 184, 185, 186, 187, 188, 189, 194, 205, 207, *216, 220, 222, 224*
Moldoveanu, E., 150(229), *173*
Molla, M. A. R., 14, *18*
Mondovi, B., 163(337), *178*
Monson, R. R., 309, *326,* 496 (49), *499*
Montesano, R., 57(23), 58(23), *87*, 96, *117*
Montgomery-Bissell, D., 183, *215*
Moon, R. C., 96, *116*
Moore, C. V., 250, 266, *289*
Moore, D. C., 390, *404*
Moore, K., 189, *223*

Moore, R. Y., 383, *401*
Moran, D., 58(41), *88*
Moreland, T. A., 452(142), *468*
Morgan, B., 69(89), 70(89), *90*
Morgan, H. E., 134(96), *167*
Morgan, J. R., 341, *371*
Morgan, J. W., 122(8), *164*
Morgan, R. G., 495(46,50), 496 (50), *499*
Morgan, R. G. H., 495(40), *499*
Morganti, G., 339, *368*
Mori, H., 54(16), 61(59), *87, 89*
Morimoto, H., 437(67,70), *463*
Morino, Y., 195, *217*
Morre, D. J. D., 435(54), *462*
Morris, E. R., 238, *292*
Morris, H. P., 150(232), *173*
Morris, H. R., 429(4), *459*
Morse, L. M., 308, *325*
Morselli, P. C., 335, 336, *368*
Morselli, P. L., 335, 336, *368, 371*
Mortimer, E. A., 345, *368*
Mosbach, E. H., 274, *280*
Moscioni, A. D., 307, *327*
Mosekilde, L., 410, 411, 412, 418, *426*
Moser, U., 231, 235, *286*
Moss, D. W., 211, *224*
Moss, J., 157(288), 160(302), *176*
Motooka, I., 230, 231, *294*
Motoyama, N., 191, *220*
Motzok, I., 157(290), *176*
Mould, J. J., 347, *368*
Mozzi, R., 135(109), *168*
Mucklow, J. C., 29(35), *46*
Mudd, S. H., 159(292), 160(292), 162(328), *176, 177*
Mueller, P. S., 390, *405*
Muir, C., 72(100), *91*
Mukhtar, H., 100, 101, 102, *116,* 183, *215*
Mulcahy, R., 393, *401*
Mulder, G. J., 125(19), 126(19,

[Mulder, G. J.]
21,30), 129(40), 131(19),
138(129,129a,131), 139(19,
40,129,134a,135,136), 141
(19,21,129,151), 142(129,
151,155), 159(155,297), 162
(327), 163(327), *164, 165,
169, 170, 176, 177*, 267, 268,
289
Mulherkar, L., 312, *328*
Muller, W. E., 23(9,10,12), 24
(12), *44*
Muller-Oerlinghausen, B., 131
(61,62,63,64,65,66), *166*
Mulley, B. A., 347, *368*
Multigner, L., 489(51a,51b,77),
490(51,77), 491(51), *500,
501, 502*
Munns, T. W., 453(159), *470*
Munro, H., 161(322), *177*
Munro, H. N., 161(323), *177*
Munson, P. J., 30(36), 31(36),
46
Munster, G., 393, *404*
Muralidhara, K. S., 431(16),
432(22), *460*
Murchison, L. E., 413, *427*
Murphy, G. M., 335, *368*
Murphy, J. J., 493(2), *496*
Murphy, S. D., 146(202), 147
(207), 148(207), *172*, 190,
204, 207, *218, 222*
Muth, O. H., 157(291), 159
(291), 162(291), *176*
Muttart, C., 208, *213*
Myant, N. B., 351, *368*
Myers, C. E., 271, *282*
Myoga, K., 236, *290*

N

Nachlas, M. M., 198, *221*
NcNeil, P. E., 61(58), *89*
Nagatsu, T., 236, 261, 271, *283*
Nagayama, H., 390, *404*

Nagayama, S., 113, *115*
Nagubandi, S., 415, *426*
Nahas, G. G., 389, *404*
Nahrwold, D. L., 227, *289*
Naidu, A. N., 33(40), *46*
Nakamura, A., 113, *115*
Nakamura, K., 488(52), 496(36),
499, 500
Nakamura, T., 383, *405*
Nakashima, K., 144(174), 149
(174), 150(228), 162(228),
163(174), *171, 173*
Nakashimo, K., 203, *223*
Nakatsu, K., 209, 210, *217*
Nambison, B., 142(163), *170*
Nankin, H., 475(2), *481*
Naranjo, C. A., 35(51,52), *47*
Nariai, H., 230, 231, *294*
Narisawa, T., 54(14), 59(48,
50), 77(113), 78(121,122),
*87, 88, 89, 91, 92, 96,
116*
Naruse, A., 144(174,176), 149
(174,220), 162(220), 163
(174), *171, 173*, 203, 204,
207, *217, 223, 224*
Naschemeyer, R. H., 195, *219*
Nash, G., 195, *219*
Nathanson, M. H., 376, *404*
Navazio, F., 444(106), *466*
Navia, J. M., 229, *289*
Naylor, A., 300, *328*
Naylor, J. N., 386, *398*
Neal, R. A., 204, *224*
Neale, G., 211, *224*, 415, 416,
427
Nebert, D. W., 148(211), *172*,
243, 255, 257, *289, 290*, 311,
327
Necheles, R. F., 477(35), *483*
Necheles, T. F., 309, 311, *324*,
479(46), *484*
Needleman, H. L., 390, *404*
Negishi, M., 243, 255, 257, *289,
290*
Neil, G., 187, 196, *218*

Neims, A. H., 97, *116*, 336, 354, 356, *359, 360, 369*
Neiss, E. S., 339, *368*
Nelsestuen, G. L., 429(3), *459*
Nelson, M. N., 306, *323*
Nelson, S. D., 147(209), 148 (209), *172*, 268, 271, *283, 290*
Nelson, T. E., 433(29), 456 (199), *461, 473*
Nemec, R., 250, *284*
Nepokeroeff, C. M., 69(94), *90*
Nerland, D., 67(82), *90*, 230, *278*
Ness, G. C., 69(94), *90*
Nestel, P., 332, *370*
Nettesheim, P., 95, 96, *116*
Netzloff, M. L., 309, *327*
Neuberger, A., 204, *219*
Neumann, H., 477(22), *482*
Neven, C., 394, *403*
Nevo, Z., 142(167), *170*
Newberg, A., 387, *402*
Newberne, P. M., 60(52), 75 (112), *89, 91*, 96, 106, *113, 116, 117*
Newman, D. A., 194, *222*
Newman, M. W., 10, *18*
Newman, W. F., 10, *18*
Newton, D., 14, *18*
Newton, D. L., 96, *117*
Newton, G. L., 180, 181, *216*
Niblett, J. S., 345, *359*
Nicholas, D. J. D., 140(147), *170*
Nicholson, J. A., 188, 198, *219*
Nicholson, J. F., 208, *213*
Niebyl, J. R., 345, *368*
Nielsen, C. T., 411, 421, *423*
Nielsen, S. W., 495(37), *499*
Niemczura, R., 514, *522*
Nies, A. S., 39(73), 40(73), *48*
Niewoehner, D. E., 261, 267, 268, 270, 271, *291*
Nigro, N. D., 75(110), 78(117, 120), *91, 92*

Niimi, H., 236, 261, 271, *283*
Nikkila, E., 150(236), *174*
Nilsen, O. G., 27(32), 36(61), *45, 48*
Nilsson, B. E., 410, *426*
Nilsson, S., 349, *368*
Nims, B., 334, *367*
Nishide, E., 113, *115*
Nishikimi, M., 271, *290*
Nishino, Y., 456(197), *473*
Nishizuka, Y., 82(134), *92*
Nitzsche, C., 254, *287*
Noble, R. E., 383, *404*
Noda, K., 160(306), *177*
Noel-Jorand, M. C., 489(77), 490 (77), 492(53,54), *500, 501, 502*
Noff, D., 415, *427*
Noppa, H., 393, *404, 405*
Norling, A., 131(59,60), *166*
Norman, A. W., 416, *427*
Norred, W. P., 64(65), 68(84), 72(84), *89, 90*, 98, *116*
Norris, D. L., 387, *405*
Norvin, E., 480(67), *485*
Notis, W. M., 480(60), *485*
Notten, W. R. F., 129(42), 131 (42), 132(42), *165*
Nurre, C., 379, *408*
Nygren, K. G., 349, *368*
Nyhan, W. L., 333, *365*
Nyquist, S. E., 435(54), *462*

O

Oates, J. A., 42(81), *49*
O'Brien, J. R., 337, *369*
O'Brien, T. G., 78(118), 86 (118), *91*
Ockner, R. K., 431(18), *460*
O'Connel, R. A., 384, *405*
Odam, E. M., 452(137), *468*
Odar-Cederlöf, I., 34(47,48,49), 35(47,49), *46, 47*
Odashima, S., 58(42), *88*
O'Dell, B. L., 238, *292*, 317, *327*

Odell, G. B., 336, *369*
Oeriu, I., 150(229), *173*
Oeriu, S., 150(229), *173*
Oesch, F., 452(140,141), *468*
Ogren, S. O., 386, *399*
Ohanian, C., 307, *323*
Ohlin, G., 386, *405*
Ohmori, T., 57(27), 77(27), *88*
Ohno, T., 236, *290*
Øie, S., 38(65), 42(76,78,79, 82), *48, 49*
Okada, G., 136(117), 149(117), *168*
Okada, T., 263, *287*
Okey, A. B., 243, 255, 257, *289*
Okita, T., 160(306), *177*
Okoye, Z. S. C., 104, 105, *113*
Olavesen, A. H., 122(9), 127 (31), *164, 165*
Oldfield, J. E., 157(291), 159 (291), 162(291), *176*
Olinger, E. J., 477(26), *482*
Oliva, A., 133(78), *167*
Olsen, J. P., 453(156), *469*
Olson, J. D., 265, *290*
Olson, R. E., 430(8), 443(101), 452(147), 453(8,157,159), 454(174), 455(185,193), 457 (8), *459, 465, 469, 470, 471, 472, 473*
Olszyna-Marzys, A. E., 357, *369*
Omaye, S. T., 226, 227, 239, 247, 248, *289, 290, 294*
Ono, T., 383, *405*
Oomwa, Y., 383, *405*
Opitz, K., 384, 385, *405*
Oppenheim, G. L., 337, 341, 350, *363*
Oppenoorth, F. J., 191, *221*
Ordonez, L., 134(89), 135(89), 136(89), *167*
Ordonez, L. A., 134(97), 137 (97), 161(97), *167*
O'Reilly, R. A., 435(60), 452 (150), 457(60), *463, 469*

Orellana, S. A., 480(60), *485*
Orlando, J., 194, *223*
Orlowski, J., *213*
Orlowski, M., 195, *213*
Orme, M. L., 343, *369*, 515, *521*
Ormstad, K., 126(25), 131(60), 146(196), *164, 166, 172*, 185, 186, 187, 188, 189, 205, 207, *216, 220, 221*
Örning, L., 190, *221*
Ornoy, A., 415, *427*
O'Rourke, T., 388, *398*
Orr, M. W., 350, *373*
Orrenius, S., 67(79), *90*, 126 (25), 145(187), 146(196), 149 (223), 150(223,225), *164, 171, 172, 173*, 183, 184, 185, 186, 187, 188, 189, *216, 217, 218, 220, 221, 222, 223, 224*
Orsulak, P. J., 350, *371*
Osaki, S., 248, *290*
O'Shaughnessy, W. B., 388, *405*
Oshima, T., 245, 247, *287*
Oshinsky, R. J., 72(95), *90*
Otagiri, M., 27(25), *45*
Otani, G., 131(54), *166*
Otaysek, M. A., 479(54), *484*
Ou, S.-Y. L., 192, *214*
Outerbridge, E. W., 354, *360*
Ovecka, M., 236, 238, 250, *284*
Overall, J. E., *406*
Owen, C. A., 436(63), 437(63, 69), *463*
Owen, G., 384, 385, *402*
Owen, T. C., 154(279), *175*

P

Pabst, M. J., 191, 192, *217*
Pace, H. B., 389, *396*
Paes, I. C., 475(2), 476(9), 479 (56), *481, 484*
Pagano, J. S., 342, *370*
Paik, W. K., 133(78), *167*

Paine, A. J., 185, *213, 221*
Painter, M. J., 344, *369*
Pak, C. Y. C., 417, *423*
Pak, M. S., 75(110), *91*
Palasciano, G., 490(60), 491(76),
    492(74,84,85,86,88,90),
    500, 501, 502
Palekar, A. G., 149(218), *173*
Palmer, G. D., 69(89), 70(89),
    90
Palmer, K. E., 352, *369*
Palmer, R. H., 80(126), *92*
Palmerini, C. A., 135(109), *168*
Palva, I. P., 480(65,66,70,71),
    485
Pamukcu, A. M., 61(60), *89*
Pan, F., 134(87), *167*
Panchacharam, P., 488(58), 493
    (58), *500*
Pandolf, K. B., 394, *396*
Pang, K. S., 39(69), *48*, 121
    (2), 122(2), 124(17), 126
    (28), 129(40), 139(40), *163,
    164, 165*
Paniagua, M., 349, *370*
Pantuck, E. L., 67(76), *90*
Paoby, P., 480(67), *485*
Papadatos, C. J., 340, *366*
Pape, B., 346, *360*
Papeu, G., 154(277), *175*
Papsin, F. R., 341, *371*
Pardi, G., 336, *371*
Parikh, H. C., 189, *216*
Parish, P. A., 505, *522*
Park, B. K., 343, *366*
Park, Y. K., 6, *17*
Parke, D. V., 98, *114*, 201, *221*
Parker, C. M., 261, *293*
Parker, P. B., 342, *362*
Parkinson, C. E., 303, *324*
Parr, G. D., 347, *368*
Parsons, D. S., 188, *216*
Parsons, L. G., 237, *287*
Parsons, V., 410, *425, 426*
Parsons, W. B., 354, *369*
Parsons, W. D., 336, 354, 356,
    359, 369

Parvathy, S., 383, *399*
Passey, R. D., 393, *398*
Patel, B., 516, *522*
Patel, J. M., 99, *116*
Patel, V., 516, *522*
Paterson, J. W., 121(1), 122(8),
    163, 164
Patrick, M. J., 352, *369*
Patrick, R. L., 390, *397*
Patterson, M., 476(10), *481*
Patterson, P., 308, *325*
Pau, W. K., 347, *368*
Paul, S. M., 392, *407*
Pauling, L., 239, 253, *279, 290*
Pawar, S. S., 99, *116*, 226,
    255, 258, *287*
Pawlowski, G. J., 383, *405*
Payan, H., 488(52,55), 492(78),
    500, 502
Paykel, E. S., 390, *405*
Peaker, M., 334, *369*
Peale, A. L., 135(107), *168*
Pearson, O. H., 84(148), *93*
Peck, G. C., 312, *327*
Peer, L. A., 312, *327*
Pegg, A. E., 133(80), 136(80),
    167
Pegum, J. S., 520, *522*
Pelchar, A. G., 189, *221*
Penberthy, C., 379, *400*
Peneda, E. P., 195, 196, *216*
Peng, Y. S., 160(309), 161(309),
    177
Penney, J. R., 231, 233, 237,
    290
Pennings, E. J. M., 140(148),
    170
Peoples, A., 244, *280*
Peoples, A. J., 227, 244, *280*
Perec, C. J., 492(56), *500*
Perera, W. D. A., 159(295), *176*
Peret, J., 160(305), *176*
Perez de la Mora, M., 386, *399*
Perkins, E. G., 160(303a), *176*
Perlman, H. H., 344, 352, 356,
    369, 372
Perraudin, M. L., 356, *369*

Perrier, D., 240, *283*
Perris, A. D., 188, *221*
Perrotto, J. L., 479(55), *484*
Perry, J., 477(28), *483*
Perry, M. A., 141(152), *170*
Perry, T. L., 180, *221*
Persson, B., 341, *359*
Pesch, L. A., 183, *218*
Pessayre, D., 148(214), 149
   (214), *173*, 204, *221*
Peters, J., 479(47), *484*
Peters, J. M., 392, *405*
Peters, R. A., 237, *287*
Peters, T. J., 477(24a), *482*
Petersen, T. E., 429(4), *459*
Peterson, F. J., 226, 227, 228,
   229, 230, 236, 238, 239,
   242, 249, 250, 251, 252,
   253, 254, 261, 268, 269,
   270, 271, 272, 273, 277,
   285, *290*, *291*
Peterson, P., 413, *427*
Pettigrew, H. M., 81(132), *92*
Pezzoli, C., 134(100), 137
   (126), *168*, *169*
Pfaff, E., 134(100), *168*
Pfaff, G., 432(27), *460*
Pfeiffer, U., 247, *282*
Pfleger, K., 139(137), 141
   (137), *169*
Pflueger, A. B., 379, *397*
Phelps, C. F., 129(44), *165*
Phil, D., *359*
Phillips, F. S., 308, *328*
Phillips, J. C., 268, *288*
Philpot, R. M., 97, *116*
Piafsky, K. M., 24(17), 25(17),
   33(17), 36(17,61), *44*, *48*
Picchioni, A. L., 513, *521*
Picciano, M. F., 332, 333, 334,
   352, *364*, *365*, *369*
Pichanick, G. G., 148(210), *172*
Pickett, C. B., 243, *291*
Picotti, G. B., 379, *397*
Pijoan, M., 237, *291*
Pikkarainen, P. H., 353, *370*

Pillion, D. J., 207, *216*
Pincus, G., 349, *370*
Pineo, G. F., 441(81), *464*
Ping-Antich, J., 381, *400*
Pinkus, L. M., 192, *221*
Pinto, J., 520, *522*
Piper, W. N., 12, *18*
Pippenger, C., 344, *369*
Pirola, R. C., 493(57), *500*
Pisano, J. J., 190, *214*
Pisciotto, P. T., 150(239), *174*
Pitchumoni, C. S., 488(58), 493
   (58), *500*
Pitlick, W., 344, *369*
Pitot, H. C., 69(93), *90*, 185,
   222
Pittard, W. B., 351, *370*
Pittel, P., 392, *395*
Planche, N. E., 490(60), 492
   (59), *500*
Platt, B. S., 237, *287*
Plotkin, S. A., 340, 342, *364*,
   370
Plummer, J. L., 183, *221*
Pochin, E. E., 351, *368*
Pohl, E., 14, *18*
Pohl, R. J., 67(75), *90*, 97, *116*
Pohl-Ruling, J., 14, *18*
Poirier, L. A., 135(108), *168*
Polakis, S. E., 157(288), *176*
Poland, A., 63(61), *89*
Poley, J. R., 480(69), *485*
Pollard, D. R., 306, *327*, *328*
Polizos, P., 380, 381, *408*
Pommerenke, W. T., 352, *370*
Pool, J. G., 452(150), *469*
Poole, C. J. F., 433(36), *461*
Popov, V., 340, *364*
Popper, H., 67(81), *90*
Porcellati, G., 135(109), *168*
Porcelli, M., 134(101), *168*
Porter, J. A., 69(94), *90*
Poschel, B. P. H., 386, *405*
Posner, A. C., 339, *370*
Pösö, H., 133(79), 136(79), *167*
Postgate, J. R., 139(143), *169*

Potter, D. W., 146(195), *172,*
180, 187, 205, *222*
Potter, J., 205, *214*
Potter, J. M., 332, *370*
Potter, W. Z., 126(22), 147(22),
148(22), *164,* 204, *220,* 266,
269, 270, *286, 291*
Poullain, B., 132(70), 141(70),
166
Pounder, R. E., 211, *224*
Pour, P., 495(61,62), *500*
Powell, G. M., 122(9), 127(31),
141(152), *164, 165, 170*
Powell, H. R., 309, *327*
Powell, J. R., 356, *370*
Pratt, R., 477(25), *482*
Prchal, J., 190, *221*
Prescott, L. F., 181, 187, *218*
Preuss, U., 204, *223*
Preussman, R., 495(21), *497*
Preussmann, R., 57(23,33), 58
(23,37), *87, 88,* 314, *324*
Price, C. E., 182, 200, *213*
Price, J. A., 455(192), 456
(192), 457(192), *472*
Prickett, C. S., 7, *17*
Prigge, W. F., *285*
Prigot, A., 339, *370*
Principe, L. M., 441(91), 444
(91), *465*
Principi, N., 336, *371*
Printen, K. J., 160(302), *176*
Prior, J. T., 475(8), 476(8),
481
Pritchard, J. A., 311, *327,*
341, *371*
Procházka, J., 340, *364*
Proctor, N. H., 307, *327*
Proffitt, J. H., 153(266,267),
154(267), *175*
Prosky, L., 6, *18*
Prusiner, S., 196, *221*
Prydz, H., 444(115), 446(115),
453(158,167), 454(167), 455
(167), *466, 470*
Puigserver, A. J., 159(299),
176

Purdy, S., 227, *292*
Pütter, J., 342, *370*
Pynnönen, S., 344, *370*

Q

Quinn, P. O., 381, *405*
Quiring, K., 432(27), *460*

R

Rabenstein, D. L., 146(193), *172*
Rabøl, A., 124(18), *164*
Race, T. F., 479(56), *484*
Rachlis, A. R., 341, *371*
Rachmilewitz, D., 480(58,59),
484, 485
Radhakrishnan, H. N., 197, *215*
Radomski, J. L., 7, *18*
Rafaelsen, O. J., 384, 385, *404,
408*
Raffin, S. B., 67(77), *90*
Rafter, J., 182, 200, 201, 209,
210, *213, 214*
Raghuram, T. C., 261, *291*
Ragni, N., 336, *360*
Raheja, K. L., 150(235), *173*
Rahimtoola, R. J., 332, *367*
Raiband, P., 80(129), *92*
Raicht, R. F., 78(124), 80(124),
92
Raiha, N. C. R., 353, *370*
Raina, A., 133(79), 136(79), *167*
Raina, A. M., 135(106), 137
(106), *168*
Raja, Z., 383, *406*
Rajagopalan, K. V., 162(329),
177
Rajalakshmi, R., 333, *362*
Rajewsky, M. F., 54(18), *87*
Rama, F., 307, *323*
Rama, P. B. R., 142(161), *170*
Ramakreshan, C. V., 333, *362*
Ramsey, J. D., 12, 14, *18, 19*
Rand, W., 58(41), *88,* 161

[Rand, W.]
(322), *177*
Rand, W. M., 161(323), *177*
Randall, L. O., 386, *405*
Randle, P. J., 157(287), *176*
Rane, A., 142(158), *170*, 194, *222*, 344, *370*
Rankin, B. B., 193, 197, 199, *218*, *221*
Rao, A. V., 236, 275, *294*
Rao, G. H., 433(38), *461*
Rao, K. S. J., 142(168), *170*
Rapoport, J. C., 381, *405*
Rapoport, J. L., 381, *405*
Rase, B., 444(111,112,114), 445 (117), 446(117), *466*
Rasmussen, F., 334, 339, *370*
Rasmussen, H., 185, *221*, 415, 418, *423*
Rasmussen, K., 320, *326*
Rassin, D. K., 157(286), *176*, 208, *219*
Rathburn, W. B., 189, *221*
Rating, D., 389, *399*, *405*
Rawlings, M. D., 452(144), *468*
Rawlings, V., 83(138), *92*
Ray, J. R., *221*
Rayner, P. H. W., 381, *405*
Read, A. E., 491(32), *498*
Read, W. W. C., 332, *370*
Reavey, P., 352, *369*
Reddy, B. G., 146(199), *172*
Reddy, B. S., 52(9), 57(26,27), 59(45,48,50), 65(68,71), 67 (68), 68(68), 72(68,71), 75 (9), 77(9,27,113,114,116), 78(9,119,122), 80(125), 86 (9), *87*, *88*, *89*, *91*, *92*, 96, *116*
Reddy, T. V., 113, *116*
Redetzki, H. M., 350, *373*
Reed, D. J., 143(171), 144 (171), 145(171), 146(195), 148(171), 149(171,219), 150 (171,225,237), 160(171),

[Reed, D. J.]
162(171), 163(332), *171*, *172*, *173*, *174*, *178*, 180, 181, 183, 184, 185, 186, 187, 197, 202, 203, 204, 205, 207, 210, *213*, *214*, *220*, *221*, *222*, *224*, 268, *291*
Reed, D. L., 184, *224*
Reed, P. I., 338, *370*
Reed, S. B., 353, *362*
Reed, S. C., 299, *327*
Rees, J. A., 351, *371*
Reeve, J., 145(183), 146(183, 197), *171*, *172*, 211, *218*
Reeves, P. G., 317, *327*
Regan, W. O., 238, *292*
Reichard, S. A., 133(77), *167*
Reid, M. E., 229, *291*
Reidenberg, M. M., 34(45), *46*, 393, 394, *399*
Reigh, D. L., 84(144), *93*
Reik, L., 243, *280*
Reilly, R. W., 188, *223*
Reiner, E. B., 476(10), *481*
Reinke, L. A., 132(72), *166*, 211, *218*
Reisenauer, A. M., 477(20), 478 (42), *482*, *483*
Remmer, H., 97, 104, *117*
Ren, P., 439(75), 440(75), 442 (92,93), 443(75,92), 451(75, 92), 452(154), *464*, *465*, *469*
Renner, G., 490(63,64), *500*, *501*
Renner, I. G., 490(65,66), *501*
Rennert, O. M., 309, *327*
Renton, K. W., 65(69), *89*, 257, *291*, *359*
Resman, B. H., 355, *371*
Retallack, R. W., 417, *426*
Rettger, L. F., 227, *295*
Reuvers, J., 211, *215*
Revel, J. P., 186, *222*
Rey, A. A., 7, *18*
Reynaert, J., 411, *423*
Reynolds, D. J., 516, *522*

Reynolds, E. H., 311, *327*, 410,
    426
Reynolds, G., 317, *327*
Reynolds, R. W., 387, *405*
Rhoads, J. E., Jr., 75(111), *91*
Rhodes, M. B., 304, *326*
Ribeiro, R., 490(14), *497*
Ribeiro, T., 489(77), 490(77),
    501, 502
Ribelles, M., 350, *364*
Ribet, A., 491(15,26), *497, 498*
Rich, D. H., 454(173,176), *471*
Rich, D. M., 454(175), 457
    (175), *471*
Richards, A. J., 121(1), *163*
Richards, D. R., 355, *365*
Richards, R. K., 239, 244, *291*
Richardson, C. A., 418, *424*
Richardson, M. E., 263, *291*
Richardson, R. J., 147(207),
    148(207), *172*, 190, *222*
Richens, A., 309, *327*, 410, 411,
    413, *423, 427*
Richert, D. A., 437(72), *463*
Richman, P., 144(173), *171*
Richter, C. B., 237, *288*
Ricour, C., 389, *398*
Ridgeway, L., 308, *325*
Riecls, V. D., 204, 207, *214*
Rieder, J., 351, *363*
Riegelman, S., 356, *370*
Rikans, L. E., 235, 242, 247,
    248, 250, *291*
Rikong-Adie, H., 454(178),
    471
Rim, E., 431(16,17), 432(19,
    20,21,22), *460*
Rimm, A. A., 393, *396*
Rinderknecht, H., 490(63,64,
    65,66), *500, 501*
Rinehimer, D. A., 261, *293*
Ringdahl, I., 381, *399*
Ringdahl, J. C., 380, 381, *398*
Rivera, G. M. V., 440(79), *464*
Rivers, J. M., 226, 227, 229,
    230, 231, 236, 238, 239,
    240, 249, 250, 251, 252,

[Rivers, J. M.]
    253, 254, 261, 272, 277,
    283, 285, 287, 290
Rivest, M. R., 80(127), *92*
Rivlin, R. S., 520, *522*
Roach, J. A. G., 154(279), *175*
Robbins, F. C., 342, *372*
Robbins, P. W., 139(133), *169*
Robbins, R. W., 139(146), *170*
Roberts, D. C., 57(25), *87*
Roberts, M. L., 417, *422*
Roberts, R. J., 142(157), 150
    (227), *170, 173*
Roberts, R. K., 35(53), *47*
Robertson, D., 35(56), *47*
Robertson, R. M., 35(56), *47*
Robin, H., 341, *364*
Robins, E., 391, *407*
Robinson, D. A., 103, 104, *114*
Robinson, J., 7, 8, 9, *17, 18*
Robinson, M. J., 353, *360*
Robinson, R., 33(41), *46*
Robinson, R. G., 387, *405*
Roburn, J., 357, *363*
Roche, A., 381, *399*
Roche, A. F., *406*
Rodbard, D., 30(36) 31(36), *46*
Rodbro, P., 410, 411, 421, 422,
    423, 427
Rodgers, W. E., 141(153), *170*
Roe, D. A., 154(274), *175*, 510,
    513, *522*
Roepke, J. L., 332, 349, *366*
Roepke, J. L. B., 349, *366*
Roepstorff, P., 429(2), *459*
Rogers, A. E., 75(112), *91*, 106,
    117
Rogers, A. L., 476(16), *482*
Rogers, J. C., 307, *327*
Rogler, J. C., 162(331), *178*
Rokosova, B., 236, *292*
Rollins, D., 194, *222*
Rollins, D. E., 142(158), *170*
Romano, F. A., 416, *428*
Romer, J., 34(43), *46*
Romero, F. J., 149(216,222), 150
    (222), *173*

Roor, D. M., 141(154), *170*
Rosa, F. W., 348, *371*
Rosalki, S. B., 209, *222*
Rose, C. M., 137(127), 161
   (127), *169*
Rose, J. Q., 12, 13, *17, 18*
Rose, P. G., 421, 422, *423*
Rose, R. C., 227, *289*
Rose, W. C., 202, *224*
Rosekrantz, H., 388, 389, *406,*
   407
Rosen, J. E., 14, *17*
Rosenberg, H. C., 386, *406*
Rosenberg, I., 478(40), *483*
Rosenberg, I. H., 476(18), 477
   (22,23,30,34), 478(39,41),
   479(44), *482, 483, 484,* 519,
   521, 522
Rosenberg, L., 309, *326*
Rosenblatt, D., 198, *221*
Rosenburg, S. A., 388, *397*
Rosenthal, H. E., 31(37), *46*
Rosoff, B., 14, *19*
Ross, H. S., 413, *427*
Ross, J. F., 14, *19*
Ross, J. G., 389, *406*
Ross, L. L., 194, 195, 199, *220*
Ross, S., 389, *406*
Rothstein, J., 387, *402*
Round, J. M., 411, 421, *427*
Routledge, P. A., 35(57), *47,*
   122(10), 123(10), *164,* 452
   (144), *468*
Rowe, D. J. F., 410, 411, 413,
   416, 421, *423, 425, 427*
Row, V. K., 12, 13, *17*
Rowe, L., 98, *117*
Rowland, M., 34(44), 39(67,68,
   69,72), 40(72), *46, 48,* 126
   (28), *164*
Rowland, N. E., 387, 391, *395*
Rowland Payne, C. M. E., 519,
   522
Rowson, A., 479(51), *484*
Roy, A. B., 139(144), *169*
Roy, C. C., 80(127), *92*

Roy, P. E., 389, *401*
Rozansky, R., 339, *371*
Rubert, M. W., 476(9), *481*
Rubin, R. A., 134(97), 137(97),
   161(97), *167*
Rubinstein, D., 391, *403*
Ruble, P. C., 388, *408*
Ruble, P. E., 432(20), *460*
Rüdiger, H. W., 106, *115*
Rudra Pal, D., 263, 265, *281,*
   292
Ruggiero, G., 134(101), *168*
Rugstad, H. E., 453(158), *470*
Rumble, W. F., 351, *371*
Rummel, W., 139(137), 141(137),
   169
Rund, D. G., 346, *367*
Runner, M. N., 300, *328*
Rusch, H. P., 73(107,109), *91*
Russel, R. M., 477(30), *483*
Russell, J., 414, *426*
Rustage, J. S., 11, *19*
Rusten, R., 135(108), *168*
Rustin, R. M., 393, *402*
Rusy, B. F., 393, 394, *399*
Rutenburg, A. M., 195, 196,
   209, *216, 222*
Rutherford, L. D., 345, *365*
Ryan, D. E., 243, *280*
Ryan, J. A., 187, 196, *215, 218*
Ryan, J. R., 348, *368*
Ryckwaert, A., 415, 418, *423*
Rydell, R. E., 57(28), *88*
Rye, R. M., 347, *368*
Rýznar, J., 350, *372*

S

Saad, S. F., 513, *522*
Sabry, Z. I., 163(335), *178*
Sacher, E. J., 381, *400*
Sack, C. M., 340, *371*
Sacquet, E., 80(129), *92*
Sadowski, J., 441(90), 443(90),
   446(90), *465*

Sadowski, J. A., 439(76), 442
    (76,96), 443(76,96), 444
    (103), 446(120), 447(103),
    450(103,131,133), 451(76,96,
    103), 452(139), 454(131,
    180), 455(131), 456(133),
    457(131,180), *464, 465, 466,
    467, 468, 471*
Saetre, R., 146(193), *172*
Safer, D., 381, *406*
Safer, D. J., 381, *406*
Saffiotti, U., 96, *117*
Saha, J. R., 346, *367*
Sahel, J., 489(51), 490(51,67),
    491(51,76), 492(75), *500,
    501*
Sahyoun, N., 203, *215*
Sakai, S., 268, *293*
Sakamoto, Y., 144(174,176), 149
    (174,220), 150(228), 162
    (220,228), 163(174), *171,
    173,* 203, 204, 207, *217,
    220, 223, 224*
Sakata, T., 392, *406*
Salam, N., 306, *326*
Salas, M., 106, *117*
Sallan, S. E., 388, *406*
Saller, C., 389, *403*
Salvatore, E., 133(73), *166*
Salvatore, F., 135(104), 136
    (104), 137(104), 159(104),
    168
Samachson, J., 14, *19*
Sampson, D., 26(24), *45*
Sampson, W. L., 442(94), *465*
Samson, R. R., 333, *367*
Samuel, P., 475(5,6), 476(5),
    481
Samuelsson, B., 190, *221*
Sanchez, A., 160(303), *176*
Sandler, R., 122(8), *164*
Sannella, J. J., 410, 411, 422,
    427
Sansom, L., 356, *370*
Santodonato, J., 6, 14, *19*
Santos, E. C., 24(14), *44,* 336,
    372

Santos, I., 317, *324*
Sanzgiri, R. R., 383, *406*
Sapico-Ohl, V., 191, *223*
Sargant, W., 388, *398*
Sarles, H., 487(22,68,73), 488
    (22,23,52,55,68,73,82), 489
    (16,35,42,51a,51b,77), 490
    (12,14,25,35,48,51,60,67,
    77,82), 491(51,69,76,82,89),
    492(7,13,17,35,38,53,54,59,
    69,70,71,72,74,75,78,83,
    84,85,86,87,88,90), 493(11,
    35), 494(5,6), 496(23,24),
    *496, 497, 498, 499, 500, 501,
    502, 503*
Sarrazin, D., 389, *398*
Sarver, K. P., 34(46), *46*
Sarwal, A. N., 78(124), 80(124),
    92
Sasame, H., 240, *280*
Sasame, H. A., 97, *114,* 150
    (238), *174,* 271, *283*
Sasaoka, I., 61(59), *89*
Sasse, D., 183, *218*
Sato, M., 191, *222*
Sato, P., 98, *117*
Sato, P. H., 242, 245, 247, 248,
    253, *292*
Sato, T., 236, 261, 271, *283,*
    344, *366*
Sauberlich, H. E., 226, 227, 237,
    285, 290
Sauerhoff, M. W., 12, *19*
Saunders, S. J., 148(210), *172,*
    192, *214*
Saville, B., 180, *222*
Sawatzhi, G., 189, *217*
Schaefer-Ridder, M., 56(22), *87*
Schaeppi, V. H., 388, 389, *407*
Schafer, G., 384, 385, *405*
Schaffalitzky de Muckadell,
    O. B., 491(27), *498*
Schaffner, W., 356, *363*
Schall, G. L., 351, *366*
Scharp, C. R., 410, 411, 412,
    413, 415, 416, 417, 418, 419,
    422. *424*

Schary, W. I., 34(44), *46*
Schattner, F., 67(81), *90*
Schatz, R. A., 134(93), 136(93), 137(93), 159(93), *167*, 263, *292*
Schearer, H. L., 162(325), *177*
Schechter, M. D., 393, *406*
Scheckel, C. L., 388, 389, *406*
Schedewie, H. K., 380, 381, *398*
Scheinberg, H. I., 320, *328*
Scheinberg, P., 442(98), *465*
Schenker, S., 35(53), *47*
Schenkman, J. B., 104, *117*
Schersten, T., 151(243), *174*
Schertel, M. E., 263, 266, *283*
Schichi, H., 148(211), *172*
Schiff, B. B., 389, *395*
Schinke, G., 131(66), *166*
Schlenk, F., 133(73,76), *166, 167*
Schmahl, D., 314, *324*
Schmähl, D., 57(32,33), *88*
Schmahl, D., 60(55), *89*
Schmeltz, I., 58(34), *88*
Schmid, R., 188, *217*
Schmidt, E., 491(79), *502*
Schmidt, F. W., 491(79), *502*
Schmidt, R., 67(77), *90*
Schmidt, W., 452(140), *468*
Schneider, D. L., 153(265), 154(265), 155(281), *175*
Schneider, P. B., 351, *372*
Schneider, R. E., 519, *523*
Schnoes, H. K., 444(103), 447(103), 450(103), 451(103), *466*
Schoental, R., 60(54), *89*
Schole, J., 146(204), *172*
Scholtens, E., 126(30), 129(40), 138(131), 139(40,134a,136), 141(151), 142(151,155), 159(155), 162(327), 163(327), *165, 169, 170, 177*
Schonfeld, G., 519, *523*
Schou, M., 350, *371*, 384, *406*
Schrader, R. E., 316, *328*

Schraffenberger, E., 300, *329*
Schramm, L. C., 388, *399*
Schrogie, J. J., 433(40), *461*
Schwartz, K. B., 519, *523*
Schryver, H. F., 386, *396*
Schticke, C. P., 353, *367*
Schulder, B., 141(150), *170*
Schulenberg, S., 274, *280*
Schulert, A. R., 317, 321, *325*
Schullinger, J. N., 208, *216*
Schulze, H.-U., 247, *292*
Schumacher, H. J., 317, 321, *324, 325*
Schütt, A., 204, *222*
Schuyler, D., 383, *407*
Schwabe, C., 193, 198, *220*
Schwartz, A., 349, *372*
Schwartz, I. W., 389, *404*
Schwartz, J., 384, *399*
Schwartz, N. B., 128(37), 131(37), 142(37), *165*
Schwarz, L. R., 130(51), 131(57,58), 132(58), 139(58), *165, 166*
Schwersguth, O., 389, *398*
Schwetz, B. A., 12, 13, *17*
Scott, D. E., 311, *327*
Scott, G. C., 386, *404*
Scott, J. M., 477(37), *483*
Scott, P. M., 513, *522*
Scott, R. B., 433(34), *461*
Scribner, J. D., 199, *219*
Scrimshaw, N. S., 159(295), *176*
Searcey, M. T., 452(147), *469*
Searl, P., 476(9), *481*
Searle, C. E., 51(3), *86*
Segi, M., 496(80), *502*
Seglen, P. O., 183, *222*
Seibert, R. A., 437(71), *463*
Seibert, S., 456(199), *473*
Seipp, C. A., 388, *397*
Seiving, B., 23(8), 24(8), *44*
Sekura, R., 144(177), *171*
Selhub, J., 477(29), 478(40), 479(44), *483, 484*, 519, *521*
Seligman, A. M., 198, 209, *221, 222*

Sellakumar, R. R., 96, *117*
Sellers, E. M., 23(5), 35(50,51, 52), 36(5), 38(5), *44, 47*
Selley, J. A., 348, *367*
Sellinger, O. Z., 134(93), 136 (93), 137(93), 159(93), *167*
Selman, T. E., 61(58), *89*
Seltzer, C., *406*
Semenza, G., 227, *292, 293*
Sen, A., 257, 263, *280*
Sen, L. C., 159(299), *176*
Senior, B., 353, *360*
Sereni, F., 336, *371*
Serlin, M. J., 343, *369*
Sesame, H. A., 202, 204, *214*
Sethi, G., 190, 198, *219*
Severn, B. J., 129(43), *165*
Shadarevian, S. B., 163(335), *178*
Shah, D. K., 387, *406*
Shah, D. V., 447(126), 450 (126), 452(126,149), 453 (126), 454(172), 456(126, 194,195), 457(201), *467, 469, 471, 473*
Shamberger, R. J., 84(143), *92*
Shamoto, M., 236, 261, 271, *283*
Shand, D. G., 35(54,57), 36 (62), 37(64), 39(64,73,74), 40(64,73), 42(81), *47, 48, 49*, 122(10), 123(10), 126 (26), *164*
Shank, F. R., 6, *18*
Shannon, B. M., 159(293), 162 (325), *176, 177*
Shapiro, R. E., 9, *16*
Shapiro, S., 309, *326*
Shapiro, S. K., 135(104), 136 (104), 137(104), 159(104), *168*
Shaw, L. M., 194, *222*
Sheard, M. H., 384, *403*
Shearer, M. J., 430(9), 431(9, 13), 432(9), 433(9,34), 434 (13), 435(58), 436(9,13,58,

[Shearer, M. J.] 61), 437(65,66), 438(58), 439(9,58,61,73,74), 440(80), 442(9,61,73), 444(66), *459, 460, 461, 462, 463, 464*
Sheehe, D., 332, *364*
Sheehe, D. M., 333, 334, *369*
Sheep, W. L., 388, *407*
Sheiff, R. R., 477(23), *482*
Sheinfil, A., 78(119), *92*
Sheldon, J. M., 339, *362*
Shemer, M., 160(303a), *176*
Shen, D. D., 349, *372*
Shepard, J. S., *11, 18*
Shepherd, A. M. M., 452(142), *468*
Sherk, H. H., 422, *427*
Sherlock, J. C., 6, *16*
Sherlock, S., 272, 273, *279*
Sherratt, H. S. A., 151(251), 152(251), *174*
Shia, M., 440(78), 446(119), 447(119), 450(78), 454(78), 455(78), 457(78), *464, 467*
Shia, M. A., 453(164), 455(186, 190), *470, 472*
Shih, T.-W., 97, *115*
Shihab, K., 10, *16*
Shiling, D. J., 388, *397*
Shimabukuro, R. H., 191, 192, *219, 222*
Shimizu, H., 194, 196, 200, *223*
Shimizu, T., 340, *373*
Shin, H. K., 162(324), *177*
Shinpo, K., 236, 261, 271, *283*
Shinya, S., 149(220), 162(220), *173*, 204, *223*
Shiozaki, H., 144(174), 149(174), 163(174), *171*, 203, *223*
Shires, R. A., 417, *425*
Shirkey, H. C., 335, *371*
Shishido, T., 191, *222*
Shochet, S. B., 340, *372*
Shoemaker, W. C., 189, *216*
Shoeman, D. W., 33(39), *46*, 336, *364*

Shojania, A. M., 479(48), *484*
Shrader, E. A., 344, 352, *372*
Shubik, P., 261, *280*
Shugart, L., 135(110), *168*
Shull, K. H., 136(115,116), *168*
Shute, G. T., 342, *362*
Siafas, C. A., 340, *366*
Sibcon, R., 343, *369*
Sibinga, M. S., 342, *362*
Siddik, Z. H., 96, *117*
Siddle, N. C., 347, *368*
Siegel, B. B., 339, *362*
Siegel, J., 263, *286*
Siegers, C.-P., 204, *222, 223*
Siegfried, C., 440(77), 447 (129), *464, 467*
Siegfried, C. M., 452(138), 456 (198), 457(138), *468, 473*
Siemens, A. J., 389, *406*
Sies, H., 143(170), 144(170, 181), 145(170,182,186), *171*, 180, 183, 205, 213, *214, 221, 222*
Siest, G., 132(70), 141(70), *166*
Sievers, M., 513, *521*
Sievers, M. L., 513, *521*
Sikes, M. P., 513, *523*
Sikic, B. I., 235, 237, 239, 241, 245, 247, 253, *292*
Sikka, S. C., 190, *219*
Siler, J. F., 388, *407*
Siliprandi, L., 227, *292*
Sillanpaa, M., 344, *370*
Silver, J., 415, 416, *427*
Silverman, H. I., 379, *400*
Silverstone, H., 73(104), 84 (141), *91, 92*
Silverstone, T., 383, *407*
Simon, R. M., 388, *397*
Simons, P. *224*
Simpson, R. C., 163(333), *178*, 238, *292*
Sims, E. A. H., 394, *396*
Sims, P., 191, 210, *214, 216*

Sinaiko, A. R., 357, *371*
Singer, E., 335, *368*
Singer, M., 492(87), *502*
Singh, D. V., 75(110), *91*
Singh, H. D., 237, *279*
Singh, J., 130(51), 131(57), *165, 166*
Singh, K. D., 238, *292*
Singhal, S. N., *522*
Singstake, C. B., 389, *408*
Siperstein, M. D., 69(92), *90*
Sirica, A. E., 185, *222*
Sitar, D. S., 336, 354, *359*
Sjödin, T., 23(8,11), 24(8), *44*
Sjöholm, I., 23(8,11), 24(8,13), 34(47,48,49), 35(47,49), *44, 46, 47*
Sjoqvist, F., 273, *294*
Sjoqvist, F., 273, *294*
Sjostom, L., 385, *407*
Sjövall, J. J., 151(247,248), *174*
Skausig, O. B., 387, *403*
Sklan, N. M., 211, *222*
Skolnick, P., 392, *407*
Slaga, T., 64(64), *89*
Slattery, J. T., 36(59,60), *47*, 139(139), *169*
Slavin, B. M., 516, *522*
Sleight, S. S., 314, *325*
Slinger, S. J., 227, *286*
Sloan, C. S., 316, *325*
Sloan, R. E., 333, *367*
Slone, D., 309, *326*
Smalley, T. K., 480(69), *485*
Smart, T., 388, 389, *406*
Smiciklas-Wright, H., 162(325), *177*
Smith, A. L., 340, *371*
Smith, B. R., 182, 183, 210, 211, *217, 221, 223*
Smith, C. A., 335, *371*
Smith, C. L., 507, *522*
Smith, C. R., 235, 242, 247, 248, 250, *291*
Smith, D. R., 516, *522*

Smith, D. S., 342, *362*
Smith, E. E., 195, 196, *216*
Smith, E. L., 197, *215*
Smith, G. G., 261, *293*
Smith, G. H., 341, *363*
Smith, G. J., 192, *215*
Smith, G. L., 191, *223*
Smith, J. A., 341, *371*
Smith, J. E., 189, 190, *214,*
   222, 223
Smith, J. M., 96, *117*
Smith, J. N., 191, *215*
Smith, J. T., 154(271), 156
   (271), *175*
Smith, K. A., 334, *363*
Smith, L. H., 152(255), 157
   (255), *174*
Smith, M. B., 189, *220*
Smith, M. T., 146(200), *172*
Smith, M. W., 435(51), 447
   (51,130), 450(130), *462,*
   467
Smith, N. J., 150(235), *173*
Smith, P. B., 245, 247, *294*
Smith, P. G., 479(49), *484*
Smith, P. L. R., 338, *370*
Smith, R. L., 126(23), 127(33),
   164, 165
Smith, R. R., 227, *284*
Smith, U., 393, *405*
Smith, W. H., 388, *407*
Smithard, D. J., 272, 273, *292*
Smith-Barbaro, P., 65(68,71),
   67(68), 68(68), 72(68,71),
   89
Snell, E. S., 308, *328*
Sobotka, H., 477(27), *482*
Soda, D. M., 337, *366*
Soderberg, U., 386, *405*
Sodetz, F. J., 389, *403*
Sofia, R. D., 389, *407*
Sokofoff, N., 356, *369*
Sokol, R. J., 319, *323*
Sokoloski, T. D., 33(42), *46*
Solari, M. E., 154(273), *175*
Söling, H. D., 183, *223*

Soloman, L., 320, *328*
Solomonraj, G., 199, *224*
Somogyi, A., 338, *371*
Soong, L. M., 84(144), *93*
Soper, W. Y., 386, *407*
Sopher, D., 313, *326*
Sörbo, B., 341, *359*
Sorbö, B., 154(275), *175*
Sorensen, O. H., 410, 411, 412,
   418, *426*
Soria, J., 347, *361*
Sorin, M., 356, *369*
Soroko, F., 387, *398*
Sottrup-Jensen, L., 429(4), *459*
Soullier, B. K., 78(117), *91*
Sourkes, T. L., 130(50), *165*
Southern, P. M., 516, *521*
Soutoul, J. H., 339, *361*
Sovner, R., 350, *371*
Spaeth, D. G., 153(265), 154
   (265), *175*
Spann, J. F., 35(55), *47*
Sparr, R. A., 341, *371*
Spector, A. A., 24(14,15), *44,*
   336, *372*
Spector, R., 161(318), *177*
Speidel, B. D., 309, *328*
Speier, J. L., 63(62), *89*
Speir, T. W., 191, *215*
Spencer, H., 14, *19*
Spencer, R. P., 227, *292*
Spengler, F., 5, *19*
Spiegel, H. E., 237, *288*
Spinks, J. W. T., 437(68), *463*
Spiro, H. M., 493(81), *502*
Spitzer, A., 336, *362*
Spitzer, R. L., 391, *407*
Sporn, M. B., 96, *116, 117*
Sporne, G. H., 351, *371*
Sprince, H., 261, *293*
Srinavas, L., 142(161), *170*
Srivastava, S. K., 190, *221, 223*
Stacy, T. R., 516, *521*
Stadtman, E. R., 196, *221*
Stafford, L. E., 191, *219*
Stamburgh, J., 422, *427*

Stamp, T. C. B., 410, 411, 421, *423, 427*

Stanbury, S. W., 336, *372*

Stancier, J. E., 333, *364*

Stanley, P. E., 140(147), *170*

Stark, P., 451(135), *468*

Stark, P. Y., 442(93), *465*

Staudinger, H., 241, 245, 247, 248, 258, *282, 284, 288, 292*

Stead, A. H., 145(187), 146 (196), *171, 172,* 186, 188, *216*

Steele, B. F., 160(301), *176*

Steele, J. W., 210, 211, *223*

Steele, R. D., 160(310), 161 (310), *177*

Steen, B., 194, *222,* 338, *363*

Steen, J. B., 229, *284*

Stegink, L. D., 159(300), 160 (302), 162(326), *176, 177,* 203, *215*

Stein, E. H., 195, 196, *216*

Steinberg, D., 69(90), *90*

Steinmetz, D., 132(70), 141(70), *166*

Stemmelin, N., 488(82), 490 (82), 491(82), *502*

Stenflo, J., 429(2), 430(12), *459, 460*

Stenger, R. J., 204, *219*

Stephens, D. S., 336, *362*

Stephens, M. E. M., 479(47), *484*

Stephenson, J., 137(127), 161 (127), *169*

Sterling, T. D., 11, *19*

Stern, B. K., 188, *223*

Stern, L., 336, 337, *366, 372*

Sternberg, S. S., 59(44), *88*

Sternlieb, I., 320, *328*

Stetson, P., 197, *223*

Stevenson, I. H., 452(142), *468*

Stevenson, N. R., 227, *293*

Stewart, D. A., 410, *425*

Stewart, J. J., 350, *373*

Stickler, G. B., 416, *422*

Stiel, J. N., 384, *407*

Stillman, R. C., 388, *397*

Stillwell, W. G., 150(231), *173,* 184, 207, 208, 209, 210, *217, 219*

Stipanuk, M. H., 159(294), 160 (304), 162(294,304), 163 (304), *176,* 203, *223*

Stock, M. J., 392, *404*

Stockings, G. T., 388, *407*

Stohs, S., 67(79), *90*

Stohs, S. J., 188, *223*

Stokstad, E. L. R., 308, *323*

Stolerman, I. P., 387, 388, *407*

Stolley, P. D., 505, *523*

Stone, C. L., 266, *283*

Stone, H., 435(52), *462*

Stone, R. W., 393, *397*

Story, J. A., 254, *287*

Stowe, F. R., 376, *407*

Stramentinoli, G., 134(100,102, 103), 136(114), 137(126), *168, 169*

Strath, D., 131(60a), *166*

Strauss, R. G., 441(87), *464*

Strean, L. P., 312, *327*

Street, J. C., 243, *294*

Streett, R. P., Jr., 204, *217*

Streiff, R., 479(45), *484*

Streiff, R. P., 309, *327*

Streiff, R. R., 477(34), *483*

Strobel, G. E., 353, *362*

Strobel, H. W., 72(95), *90*

Strombeck, D. R., 480(61), *485*

Strother, A., 98, *117*

Strubelt, O., 204, *222, 223*

Strufe, R., 444(107), *466*

Strum, W. B., 493(81), *502*

Strupp, B. J., 376, 380, 388, *403*

Stuart, J. A., 392, *404*

Stuart, M. A., 84(144), *93*

Sturman, J. A., 151(246), 153 (246,261,262,263), 154(246, 263), 156(261), 157(285, 286), *174, 176*

Stutzman, J. W., 259, *279*

Subbiah, M. T. R., 247, 252, *285*

Sudlow, G., 23(6,7), *44*
Suen, E., 455(192), 456(192),
    457(192), *472*
Suen, E. T., 454(182), 455
    (187), 456(187,196), 457
    (182), *471, 472, 473*
Sufrin, J. R., 136(123), *169*
Suga, T., 193, *223*
Sugahara, K., 128(37), 131(37),
    142(37), *165*
Sugimori, M., 383, *405*
Sugimura, T., 54(13), *87*
Sullivan, A. C., 376, 379, *407*
Sullivan, R. D., 513, *523*
Sunagawa, M., 495(18), *497*
Sunshine, P., 480(57), *484*
Suojanen, J. N., 150(234), *173*
Suphakaran, V., 96, *116*
Sushama, D. C. S., 142(164),
    170
Suttie, J., 441(90), 443(90),
    446(90), *465*
Suttie, J. W., 430(7,8,10,11),
    431(7), 434(7,49), 435(7,
    49,53), 437(53), 438(10,11),
    439(76), 440(7,49), 442(76),
    443(76), 444(103), 446(120,
    123,125,126), 447(103,123,
    125,126), 450(103,123,125,
    126,131,132,133), 451(76,
    103,123,134), 452(125,126,
    139,148,149,152), 453(8,10,
    125,126), 454(123,131,169,
    170,172,173,175,176,177,
    179,180,183), 455(123,131,
    179,183,188,189), 456(123,
    126,133,134,194,195), 457
    (8,10,131,175,180,183,201),
    *459, 462, 464, 466, 467,
    468, 469, 470, 471, 472, 473*
Sutton, J. L., 239, 254, *293*
Suveges, G., 263, *279*
Suzuki, K., 344, *366*
Suzuki, S., 194, 196, 200, *223*
Suzuki, T., 265, *293*

Swain, W. R., 149(221), *173*
Swanson, E. W., 351, *368*
Swanson, H. R., 191, 192, *216,
    222*
Sweetman, L., 333, *365*
Swenerton, H., 315, 316, *328*
Swenseid, M. E., 160(303), *176*
Swezey, S. E., 26(25), *45,* 435
    (56,57), 441(57), 442(56),
    462
Synder, L. M., 479(46), *484*
Synder, S. H., 392, *407*
Szczepanik, P., 335, *372*
Szefler, S. J., 349, *372*
Szewczuk, A., 195, *213*

T

Taber, R. I., 261, *293*
Tager, J. M., 183, *223*
Taggart, W. V., 437(64), *463*
Tait, R. M., 356, *365*
Takahashi, A., 240, *287*
Takahashi, M., 78(124), 80(124),
    92
Takahashi, S., 495(18), *497*
Takanaka, A., 245, 247, *287*
Takano, A., 72(101), *91*
Takano, S., 80(131), *92*
Takenaka, Y., 263, *287*
Takeuchi, T., 236, 261, 271,
    283, 496(36), *499*
Takimoto, M., 340, *373*
Talahay, P., 192, *214*
Talalay, P., 133(77), 134(85,
    88), 136(123), 139(88), *167,
    169*
Talbot, T. R., 14, *19*
Tallarid, R. J., 393, 394, *399,
    400*
Tamura, T., 478(43), *484*
Tanaka, M., 148(211), *172,* 209,
    223
Tani, T., 257, *287*

Tannenbaum, A., 73(103,104),
    84(141), *91, 92*
Tannenbaum, S. R., 58(41), *88*
Taor, W. S., 516, *522*
Tarka, S. M., Jr., 392, *407*
Tarver, H., 134(87), *167*
Tashjian, A., 332, *370*
Tasso, F., 488(82), 490(82), 491
    (82), 492(78), *502*
Tate, S. S., 149(218), *173, 189,*
    194, 195, 196, 197, 198, 199,
    215, 216, 219, 220, 221, 223
Tateishi, N., 144(174,176), 149
    (174,220), 150(226,228),
    162(220,228), 163(174,226),
    171, 173, 194, 196, 200, 203,
    204, 207, *217, 223, 224*
Tatton, J. O., 357, *359, 363*
Taufek, H. R., 134(95), 136
    (95,113), 137(95), 159(95),
    167, 168
Taylor, H. L., 393, *396*
Taylor, I. L., 491(91), *503*
Taylor, J. F., 150(230), *173*
Teeter, R. G., *177*
Teitel, S., 199, *216*
Teitelbaum, S. L., 416, 418,
    424, 427
Telakowski-Hopkins, C. A.,
    243, *291*
Telang, N. T., 312, *328*
Ten Cate, A. R., 236, 275, *294*
Texter, N., 139(137), 141(137),
    169
Thakur, A. K., 30(36), 31(36),
    46
Thakker, D. R., 56(22), *87*
Thiercelin, J. F., 356, *370*
Thierry,M. J., 434(49), 435(49,
    53), 437(53), 440(49), *462*
Thiersch, J. B., 308, *328*
Thiessen, J. J., 39(67), *48*
Thoma, K., 432(27), *460*
Thomas, B. H., 199, *224*
Thomas, C., 60(55), *89,* 495
    (21), *497, 498*

Thomas, J., 14, *17,* 336, *367,*
    381, *399*
Thomas, L. N., 333, *365*
Thomas, P. E., 243, *280*
Thomas, P. J., 153(263), 154
    (263), *175*
Thompson, D. E., 154(270), *175*
Thompson, G. A., 196, *224*
Thompson, G. R., 388, 389, *407,*
    415, 416, *427,* 476(12,15), *481*
Thompson, J. B., 480(69), *485*
Thompson, R. B., 510, *523*
Thompson, R. D., 379, *401*
Thompson, R. M., 437(71), *463*
Thomson, A. E., 336, *372*
Thomson, H. G., 385, *404*
Thomson, J. A., 410, *424*
Thor, H., 149(223), 150(223),
    173, 184, 185, *218, 224*
Thorgeirsson, S. S., 126(22),
    147(22), 148(22), 150(233),
    164, 173, 266, 268, 269, 270,
    286, 291, 293
Thorpe, W. V., 126(29), 140
    (29), 141(29), *164*
Thouvenot, J. P., 491(15), *497*
Throckmorton, J. K., 98, *117*
Thurman, R. G., 132(72), *166,*
    211, *218*
Tibblin, E., 393, *405*
Tietze, F., 144(178), 145(178),
    146(178), *171,* 179, *224*
Tilstone, W. J., 352, *369*
Ting, M., 204, *214*
Tiscornia, O. M., 492(7,13,56,
    72,74,75,83,84,85,86,87,88,
    90), *497, 500, 501, 502*
Tisdale, M. J., 136(122), *168*
Tishler, M., 442(94), *465*
Tiwari, R., 263, *281*
Tjaczevski, V., 98, *115*
Tkaczevski, V., 235, 240, 241,
    247, 250, 251, *287*
Toaff, R., 349, *372*
Tobin, R. E., 351, *372*
Todd, P., 180, *216, 224*

Toggenburger, G. , 227, *293*
Toghill, F. J. , 479(49), *484*
Tognoni, G. , 336, *371*
Tolbert, B. M. , 227, 237, *279,*
284
Tolman, K. G. , 410, 411, 413,
417, 422, *425, 427*
Toothaker, R. D. , 122(5), *163*
Tortora, J. L. , 307, *323*
Tosheva, R. , 130(52), 131(52),
165
Toskes, P. P. , 480(68), *485*
Totaro, J. A. , 379, *397*
Touster, O. , 255, 256, 257, *285,*
294
Townsend, M. G. , 444(112), 452
(137), *466, 468*
Toyoda, M. , 437(67), *463*
Tozer, N. , 126(28), *164*
Tozer, T. N. , 38(65), 42(76),
48, 49
Trahair, R. C. S. , 393, *408*
Trang, J. M. , 239, 272, 273,
294
Trasler, D. G. , 300, *328*
Traverso, H. P. , 453(162), *470*
Tredger, J. M. , 97, 98, *114*
Treffot, M. J. , 491(89), 492
(90), *502*
Trenk, D. , 452(141), *468*
Troolin, H. A. , 332, *364*
Troup, S. B. , 453(156), *469*
Trudell, J. R. , 243, *279*
Trudinger, P. A. , 139(144),
169
Truelove, S. C. , 338, *366*
Truex, C. R. , 98, *117*
Trunk, H. , 26(21), 28(21), 29
(21), *45*
Truscott, T. C. , 432(23,24),
460
Try, G. P. , 6, *16*
Tsai, H. C. , 416, *427*
Tsai, M. D. , 133(81), *167*
Tsai, T.-L. , 332, 349, *366*
Tsai, W. H. , 381, 392, *396*

Tsao, B. , 195, 197, *224*
Tse, T. F. , 346, *361*
Tse-Eng, D. , 346, *367*
Tso, J. Y. , 197, *224*
Tsubaki, T. , 9, *19*
Tsuhako, M. , 230, 231, *294*
Tsukuda, K. , 136(117), 149(117),
168
Tsuzuki, O. , 337, *366*
Tuchmann-Duplessis, H. , 309,
310, *326*
Tuchweber, B. , 106, *117*
Tuff, S. A. , 192, *214*
Tulinius, H. , 6, *19*
Tunnessen, W. W. , 350, *372*
Tuovinen, O. H. , 140(147), *170*
Turnbull, J. D. , 226, 227, 239,
247, 248, *290, 294*
Tybring, G. , 26(22), 27(22),
29(22), *45*
Tyenger, M. A. R. , 14, *17*
Tyler, B. , 161(313), *177*
Tyor, M. P. , 154(280), *175*
Tyrala, E. E. , 354, *372*
Tyson, R. M. , 344, 352, *372*

                                    U

Udall, J. A. , 39(71), 40(71),
48, 433(44), *461*
Udenfriend, S. , 227, 239, 244,
247, 259, 264, *279*
Ueda, I. , 203, *218, 219*
Uhlíř, F. , 350, *372*
Umezawa, C. , 160(303), *176*
Umezawa, H. , 236, 261, 271,
283
Uraguchi, K. , 60(56), *89*
Urbanek, R. , 335, *373*
Usdin, E. , 133(74), *166*
Ushasri, V. , 33(40), *46*
Ushimaru, Y. , 61(59), *89*
Usui, K. , 191, *222*
Utili, R. , 135(104), 136(104),
137(104), 159(104), *168*

V

Vadi, H. V., 204, 224
Vainio, H., 68(87), 72(87), 90
Vaishnav, Y., 150(231), 173,
    268, 290
Vaishnav, Y. N., 267, 269, 281
Vaishnava, S., 333, 365
Vaishnov, Y., 184, 207, 208, 219
Valenstein, E. S., 381, 408
Valenzuela, J. E., 490(64), 491
    (91), 501, 503
Vallner, J. J., 21(4), 44
Van Bergen, T. J., 211, 215
Van Boxtel, C. J., 240, 273,
    281, 294
Van Couvering, K., 132(69),
    166
Van den Bosch, J. F., 476(11),
    481
Van den Brenk, H. A. S., 263,
    286
Van der Giesen, W. F., 27(26),
    45
Vanderhaegre, H., 475(4), 476
    (4,13), 481
Vander Jagt, D. L., 224
Vander Meer, J., 430(6), 459
Van der Pas, L. J. T., 191, 211
Van der Walt, A., 347, 362
Van de Walle, C., 348, 363
Vandeween, J. E., 6, 17
Van Elk, R., 142(156), 170
van Ginnekan, C. A. M., 126
    (27), 164
Vanjonack, W. J., 348, 361
Van Kempen, G. M. J., 140
    (148), 170
Van Kempen, G. M. J., 138
    (129a), 139(145), 142(156),
    169, 170
Van Metre, T. E., 383, 403
Vanni, P., 227, 292
Van Rooyen, A. J. L., 347, 362
Van Rossum, J. M., 126(27),
    164

Vargova, D., 277, 284
Varpela, E., 307, 328
Varsano, I., 340, 372
Vasko, M., 417, 423
Vaughan, D. A., 163(336), 178
Vavrousek-Jakuba, E., 77(115),
    91
Veen-Baigent, M. J., 236, 275,
    294
Vejmolova, J., 272, 273, 284
Vendsborg, P. B., 384, 385,
    408
Vennart, J., 15, 19
Verbeek, R., 240, 281
Vergnaud, R., 339, 361
Verine, H., 489(42,77), 490(77),
    499, 501, 502
Verma, R. S., 157(290), 176
Verrusio, A. C., 306, 328
Vesell, E. S., 240, 285, 506, 523
Vessey, D. A., 151(245,249,250),
    174
Vest, M. F., 336, 372
Viallet, A., 477(25), 482
Vidal, C., 392, 399
Viherkoski, M., 150(236), 174
Vijay, K. K., 356, 372
Vijayakumar, S. T., 142(162),
    170
Vijayammal, P. L., 142(166), 170
Vijayarathnam, P., 343, 365
Viktorinová, D., 340, 364
Villa, P., 134(102), 137(126),
    168, 169
Villareale, M., 416, 427
Villareale, M. E., 416, 428
Villa-Trevino, S., 136(115), 168
Vina, J., 149(216,222,224), 150
    (222,224), 173
Vina, J. R., 149(222), 150(222),
    173
Virkar, K. D., 332, 360
Visek, W. J., 98, 117
Visintine, R. E., 433(33), 461
Visser, A., 198, 216
Visser, C. M., 274, 294

Vitale, J. J., 77(115), *91*
Vivian, V. M., 154(270), *175*
Vogel, C. L., 345, *365*
Vogt, M., 134(83), 136(116), *167, 168*
Voirol, M., 491(89), 492(7), *497, 502*
Volle, R. L., 393, *408*
Volpe, J. J., 354, *359*
Völpel, M., 204, *223*
Von Bahr, C., 142(158), *170, 194, 222*
Von Dippe, P., 138(132), *169*
Von Herrath, D., 418, *425*
Vonk, R. J., 138(129a), *169*
Vorhees, C. V., 311, 321, *325, 328*
Vorherr, H., 348, *372*
Vozeh, S., 356, *370*
Vree, T. B., 126(27), *164*
Vuataz, L., 392, *408*
Vukovich, R. A., 339, *368*
Vukusich, D., 59(50), 77(113), *89, 91*
Vuopio, P., 150(236), *174*

W

Waber, D., 390, *404*
Wade, A. E., 64(65), 68(84), 72(84), *89, 90, 98, 116,* 245, 247, *294*
Wade, D. N., 23(6,7), *44*
Wagle, S. R., 183, *224*
Wagner, G., 353, *363*
Wagner, J. G., 27(33), *46,* 122 (15), *164*
Wagnild, J. P., 34(46), *46*
Wagstaff, D. J., 243, *294*
Wahlländer, A., 145(186), *171*
Waingankar, U. S., 14, *17*
Waizer, J., 380, 381, *408*
Walgate, J., 415, *424*
Walker, B. E., 300, *323*
Walker, E. A., 58(38), *88*

Walker, J. C., 312, *327*
Walker, M., 182, *217*
Walker, S. R., 121(1), *163*
Wallace, J. K., 453(164), *470*
Wallace, K., 475(2), *481*
Wallin, R., 444(115), 446(115, 121), 451(121), 453(167), 454(167), 455(167), *467, 466, 470*
Walloe, A., 410, *426*
Walloeger, E. E., 195, *216*
Walpole, A. L., 57(25), *87*
Walsch, S., 245, 247, *282, 294*
Walsh, J. H., 491(91), *503*
Walsh, W. C., 191, 192, *222*
Walshe, J. M., 320, *328*
Walters, B., 6, *16*
Walters, C. L., 338, *370*
Walters, S. J., 456(200), *473*
Wandscheer, J.-C., 148(214), 149(214), *173,* 204, *221*
Warburton, D., 300, 312, *323, 328*
Ward, J. M., 59(49), *88*
Wardell, W. M., 42(77), *49*
Warkany, J., 299, 300, 308, *328, 329*
Warner, M., 97, *116*
Warren, R. J., 342, *372*
Warwick, G. P., 52(7), *86*
Wasserkrug, H. L., 209, *222*
Wasserman, R. H., 416, *427, 428*
Watanabe, K., 57(26), 59(45), 78 (123), 80(125), *87, 88, 92*
Watanabe, M., 437(67,70), *463*
Waterhouse, J., 72(100), *91*
Waters, K. D., 388, *398*
Watkins, C. A., 134(96), *167*
Watkins, J. B., 335, *372*
Wattenberg, L. W., 52(5), 63(5, 62), 64(5), *86, 89,* 230, *288, 294*
Watters, G., 354, *360*
Waxman, M. B., 346, *363*
Waydhas, C., 145(182), *171*
Wayner, M. J., 381, 389, 392,

[Wayner, M. J.]
  395, 396, 404, 408
Weaver, J. C., 351, 373
Webb, D. I., 479(53), 484
Webb, J. K. G., 333, 365
Weber, W. W., 128(38), 165
Webster, G. R., 431(13), 434
  (13), 435(58), 436(13,58),
  438(58), 439(58), 460, 462
Webster, L. T., 151(253,254),
  152(253), 174
Webster, P. D., 495(3,4), 496
Weeks, C. E., 263, 266, 283
Weetch, R. S., 351, 368
Weideman, M. M., 27(26), 45
Weiner, R., 153(264), 175
Weinshilboum, R. M., 128(39),
  165
Weinstein, B. J., 350, 360
Weinstein, H. I., 339, 362
Weintraub, M., 507, 522
Weir, D. B., 477(37), 483
Weir, J. M., 496(92), 503
Weis, P., 384, 406
Weisburger, E. K., 113, 116
Weisburger, J. H., 52(9), 54
  (14,16), 57(24), 59(45,46,
  48,50), 75(9,24), 77(9,113,
  114,116), 78(9,119,121,122,
  123), 84(145), 86(9), 87,
  88, 89, 91, 92, 93, 96, 116
Weisburger, J. W., 51(2), 53
  (2), 57(2), 61(2), 62(2),
  86
Weisiger, R. A., 200, 224
Weisner, M. M., 188, 224
Weiss, G., 381, 408
Weitering, J. G., 126(21), 141
  (21), 164
Weitz, B., 26(21), 28(21), 29
  (21), 45
Welch, R. M., 414, 426
Welling, P. G., 122(5), 163
Welsh, J. D., 480(69), 485
Wendel, A., 143(170), 144(170),
  145(170,184,185), 148(215),

[Wendel, A.]
  149(215), 171, 173, 189, 205,
  217, 224
Werkheiser, W. C., 513, 523
Werthman, M. W., 346, 373
West, C., 180, 214
West, C. E., 65(66), 72(66), 82
  (135), 83(137), 84(137), 89,
  92
West, I., 357, 373
West, J., 433(35), 461
West, K. D., 333, 373
West, R. J., 518, 523
West, S., 67(83), 90
West, S. B., 242, 243, 288
Westesson, A. K., 477(24), 482
Weston, W. O., 154(274), 175
Wetle, T., 389, 408
Whalley, P. J., 311, 327
Wharton, B. A., 151(244), 174
Whipple, C., 204, 215
Whitaker, J. R., 159(299), 176
White, H. L., 387, 398
White, I. N. H., 130(49), 131
  (49), 132(49), 165, 202, 224
White, K., 126(29), 140(29), 141
  (29), 164
Whitehead, V. M., 477(25), 482
Whitfield, J. B., 211, 224
Whitlon, D. S., 452(139), 468
Whittle, B., 154(271), 156(271),
  175
Whittle, B. A., 163(334), 178
Whyley, G. A., 334, 364
Widdowson, E. M., 385, 398, 408
Wiebel, F. J., 130(51), 165
Wiegand, U. W., 36(59,60), 47
Wiernik, P. H., 345, 373
Wig, N. N., 387, 406
Wikler, A., 388, 408
Wiklund, B., 161(322), 177
Wilbraham, A. C., 154(279), 175
Wiles, D. H., 350, 373
Wilkinson, G. R., 26(23), 29
  (23), 35(23,53,56), 37(64),
  39(64,74), 40(64), 45, 47,

[Wilkinson, G. R.]
 48, 49, 122(11), 126(26),
 164
Willard, D., 379, *401*
Williams, B. S., 379, *408*
Williams, E. G., 388, *408*
Williams, G., 51(2), 53(2), 57
 (2), 61(2), 62(2), *86*
Williams, G. M., 54(16), 84(145),
 87, 93
Williams, H. H., 333, *362*
Williams, K. I. H., 349, *370*
Williams, M. H., 57(25), *87*
Williams, M. L., 95, *116*
Williams, P. J., 199, *214*
Williams, R., 410, *425*
Williams, R. L., 39(72), 40(72),
 48
Williams, R. T., 126(23), 128
 (35), 154(268), *164, 165,*
 175
Williams, S. P., 384, *403*
Williams-Ashman, H. G., 133
 (73), *166*
Williamson, D., 268, *294*
Williamson, J. R., 183, *223*
Willingham, A., 447(129), *467*
Willingham, A. K., 440(77), 447
 (127,128), 450(127), 451
 (127,134,136), 454(127),
 456(134), *464, 467, 468*
Willis, C. E., 84(143), *92*
Willis, E. D., 98, *117*
Wills, E. D., 67(74), 68(85,86),
 69(85,86), *89, 90,* 146(200),
 172
Wills, M. R., 418, *425*
Wilson, D. J., 356, *363*
Wilson, F. H., 393, *397*
Wilson, J. G., 299, 302, 309,
 329
Wilson, J. T., 273, *294,* 350,
 373
Wilson, P. S., 78(117), *91*
Wilson, R., 80(128), *92*
Wilson, S. P., *224*

Wilson, W. G., 337, *361*
Wilting, J., 27(26,27), *45*
Windorfer, A., Jr., 335, *373*
Wingard, L. B., 39(66), *48*
Wingate, G. L., 514, *522*
Winter, J., 245, 247, *282*
Winterbourn, C. C., 268, *294*
Winters, R. W., 208, *216*
Wirth, P. J., 268, *293*
Wise, L., 416, *427*
Wise, R. A., 386, *407, 408*
Wisniewski, K., 350, *366*
Wiss, O., 434(48), 435(48), 436
 (48), 437(48), *462*
With, P. J., 150(233), *173*
Witkop, B., 105, *114*
Witztum, J. L., 519, *523*
Wogan, G. N., 60(53), *89*
Wolberg, G., 136(120), *168*
Wolf, G., 141(154), *170*
Wolfe, H. R., 4, 7, *17, 19*
Wolfensberger, M. R., 455(192),
 456(192), 457(192), *472*
Wollert, U., 23(9,10,12), 24(12),
 44
Womack, M., 202, *224*
Wong, C.-Q., 96, *116*
Wong, G. B., 35(50), *47*
Wong, K. P., 130(47,50), 139
 (134), 140(134,149a), *165,*
 169, 170
Wong, L. T., 199, *224*
Wong, P. Y., 346, *363*
Wong, V., 346, *361*
Wong, Y. K., 349, *373*
Woo, C. H., 67(77), *90,* 188,
 217
Woo, M. L., 140(149), 142(149),
 170
Wood, A. J. J., 35(53,54,56),
 47
Wood, A. W., 56(22), *87*
Wood, B. S., 349, *373*
Wood, C. A., 153(266), *175*
Wood, E. J., 197, *219*
Wood, J. K., 479(50), *484*

Wood, M., 35(54,56), 47
Wood, P. B., 126(29), 140(29), 141(29), 164
Wood, S. G., 122(4), 163
Woodson, W., Jr., 381, 392, 396
Woodward, B., 433(37), 461
Woodward, G. W., 133(81), 167
Wooley, O. W., 379, 408
Wooley, S. C., 379, 408
Woolfolk, D., 475(2), 481
Wormsley, K. G., 495(40,46,50), 496(50), 499
Worth, G. K., 417, 426
Wright, P., 59(50), 89
Wright, P. C., 190, 224
Wu, B., 245, 247, 294
Wu, F., 207, 214
Wurtman, R., 161(322), 177
Wurtman, R. J., 134(89,97), 135(89), 136(89), 137(97, 125,127,128), 161(97,127, 321,323), 167, 169, 177
Wurzner, H. P., 392, 408
Wusteman, F. S., 141(152), 170
Wynder, E. L., 52(9), 58(36), 59(48,50), 72(99,101), 75 (9), 77(9,113,116), 78(9, 119,121,122,123), 81(133), 86(9), 87, 88, 89, 91, 92, 393, 408, 496(93), 503
Wyngaarden, J. B., 433(42), 461
Wynn, W., 392, 400
Wurtman, J. J., 332, 373
Wurtman, R. J., 24(16), 44
Wyburn, J. R., 352, 373

Y

Yacobi, A., 27(28), 39(70,71), 40(70,71), 45, 48
Yaffe, S., 336, 372
Yaffe, S. J., 98, 114, 336, 340, 360, 364
Yagen, B., 182, 210, 211, 217, 223

Yagi, H., 56(22), 87
Yalciner, S., 61(60), 89
Yam, J., 150(227), 173
Yamada, K., 236, 261, 271, 283
Yamaguchi, K., 203, 218, 219
Yamano, H., 136(117), 149(117), 168
Yamazaki, M., 60(56), 89
Yates, H. T., 342, 362
Yeh, M. H., 160(308), 161(308), 177
Yeo, T., 139(134), 140(134), 169
Yerkes, R. M., 389, 408
Yew, M. S., 236, 276, 295
Yoshida, A., 257, 263, 265, 277, 286, 287, 293
Yoshioka, H., 340, 373
Yost, Y., 57(28), 88
Younes, M., 204, 223
Young, A. R., 197, 219
Young, J. D., 190, 224
Young, J. D., 12, 19
Young, L., 181, 210, 219
Young, R. M., 227, 295
Young, V. R., 159(295), 176
Yum, M. N., 516, 522
Yunice, A. A., 261, 295
Yunis, A., 187, 196, 197, 213
Yurchak, A. M., 354, 373

Z

Zaharko, D. S., 10, 16
Zahorska-Morkiewic, Y., 392, 395
Zajicek, J., 346, 360
Zakim, D., 151(249,250), 174
Zalkin, H., 197, 224
Zambotti, F., 379, 397
Zampaglione, N., 211, 218
Zannoni, V. G., 98, 117, 235, 240, 242, 245, 247, 248, 250, 252, 253, 291, 292, 295
Zappia, V., 133(73,75,78), 134 (101), 135(104), 136(104),

[Zappia, V.]
   137(104), 159(104), *166,*
   167, 168
Zárate, A., 347, *361*
Zaylishie, R. G., 191, *219*
Zedeck, M. S., 59(44), *88*
Zeisel, S. H., 137(125), *169*
Zelenka, 343, *364*
Zeller, J., 314, *324*
Zemlan, F. P., 383, *396*
Zerwekh, J., 417, *423*
Zezulke, A. Y., 159(298), 162
   (298), *176*
Zhivkov, V., 130(45,46,52),
   131(46,52), *165*
Zhivkova, Y., 130(52), 131(52),
   165

Ziller, H., 477(27), *482*
Zilva, S. S., 231, 233, 236, 237,
   290, 295
Zimmerman, A., 443(102), 451
   (102), 452(102,146,153),
   465, 469
Zimmerman, T. P., 136(120),
   168
Zinberg, N. E., 388, *406*
Zinman, R., 354, *360*
Zoumas, B. L., 392, *407*
Zuideman, G. D., 493(10), 494
   (9), *497*
Zweens, J., 142(155), 159(155),
   170
Zwilling, E., 305, *329*
Zytkovicz, T. H., 429(3), *459*

Subject Index

A

Acetaminophen
  conjugate, 186
  glutathione conjugate, 187
  in human milk, 336
Acetazolamide
  accelerates drug osteomalacia, 413
  inhibits carbonic anhydrase, 315
  interaction with potassium, 319
  interaction with zinc, 319
  phosphaturic action of, 413
  potassium-retaining agent, 315
  produces systemic acidosis, 414
  teratogenicity, 315
Acetazolamide, potassium depletion, 315
Acetyl-CoA, cosubstrate acetylation, 157
Acetylpyridine, 3-AP, 305
Adenocarcinoma, exocrine, 495
Adenosine 3',5'-biphosphate (PAP), 138
Adenosine 3'-phosphate 5'-sulfatosphosphate (PAPS), 125
Adenosyl 3'-phosphate 5'-sulfatophosphate (PAPS), 137
Adriamycin, cardiotoxic effect, 271

Aflatoxin B2, cardiotoxic effect, 60
Aflatoxin B1, carcinogenic, 60
Aflatoxin G1, 60
Aflatoxin M1, 60
Aflatoxins, *Aspergillus flavus*, 60
Alanine 3-sulfinate (syn. cysteine sulfinate), 162
Albumin
  binds anions, cations, drugs, 23
  catabolic half-life, 23
  colloid osmotic pressure, 23
  human, binding sites, 23
  liver synthesis, 22
  source of amino acids/protein, 23
Alcohol, toxicity to pancreas, 488
Alcohol consumption and gastrin release, 491
  and secretin release, 492
  and zinc in plasma, 319
Aldrin (HEOD), 7
Alkylnitrosoureas, All-trans-retinoic acid, benzo[A]pyrene metabolism, 106
Alpha$_1$-acid glycoprotein
  acute-phase protein, 24
  drugs binding to, 25
  inflammation, 24
  orosomucoid, 24

Amines
  carcinogenic, aromatic, 57
  carcinogenic, heterocyclic, 57
Amino acid transport, erythrocyte, 190
Amino-1,3-4-thiadiazole (ATDA),
  306
Aminonicotinamide (6-AN), 305
Aminopeptidase M, 197, 198
Aminopterin, (4-aminopteroyl-
  glutamic acid), 308
  abortion, 308
  embryo DNA levels, 308
  folic acid antagonist, 308
  malformations, 308
  rat litter resorption, 308
Aminopyrine breath test, para-
  aminosalicylic acid
  in tuberculosis, 480
  steatorrhea with, 480
  vitamin B_{12} malabsorption
    with, 480
Amphetamine
  antinarcoleptic, 376
  CNS stimulation, 376
  delays hunger, 379
  potentiates catecholamines,
    378
Amphetamines, in children, 380
Anti-inflammatory drugs, in
  human milk, 337
Antibiotics, tumor induction, 60
Anticoagulants, in human milk,
  343
Anticonvulsant drug dosage,
  and seizure frequency, 410
Anticonvulsant drugs
  biological effect and vitamin
    D, 416
  dihydroxyvitamin D and, 417
  direct effect on mineral metab-
    olism, 418
  disorder of mineral metabol-
    ism, 411
  disorder of vitamin D metabol-
    ism, 411

[Anticonvulsant drugs]
  hypocalcemia with, 409
  increase hepatic MFO activity,
    414
  vitamin D disorders and, 409
  reduce effect of vitamin D, 416
Anticonvulsant osteomalacia, 409
Anticonvulsants
  clinical spectrum, 410
  subtle clinical effects, 410
  in human milk, 344
Antioxidants
  and weight gain, 391
Appetite
  block fat effect on tumors, 75
    brain histamine and, 384
  drug effect on, 376
  loss, as general reaction, 375
Appetite suppressants, phenyl-
  ethylamines as, 378
Aromatic amines, 56, 57
Aryl-hydrocarbon hydroxylase
  effect of diet on, 52
Ascorbate
  absorption and age, 233
  alterations in MFO system, 241
  as antiteratogen, 313
  deficiency, acute, and cyt
    P-450, 252
  detoxification, 268
  detoxification agent for nitro-
    samine, 266
  excess and aminolevulinic acid
    synthetase, 254
  excess and cholesterol hy-
    droxylase, 254
  excess and drug metabolism,
    252
  excess and heme oxygenase,
    254
  function in cyt P-450 reactions,
    226
  hepatic, 227
  minimizes lipid peroxidation,
    278
  parenteral, 236

[Ascorbate]
  resupplementation and MFO
    activity, 245
  stability, 231
  synthesis and drug adminis-
    tration, 257
  synthesis, drug acceleration
    of, 226
  teratogenic with insulin, 313
Ascorbic acid
  absorption, 227
  administration, 231, 233
    antipyrine metabolism, 273
    bile acid metabolism, 230
    cancer prevention, 275
    cholesterol metabolism,
      250
    drug metabolism rates,
      274
    drugs, 225
    L-gulonolactone oxidase,
      255
    synthesis nitroso com-
      pound, 314
    biosynthesis, function,
    and drugs, 258
    cadmium and dietary iron,
      266
    chronic deficiency and
      drug metabolism, 272
    deficiency
      adrenal function, 240
      chronic, guinea pig,
        238
      drug metabolism, 244,
        245
      drug metabolism en-
        zymes, 242
      ferrous iron, 248
      guinea pig, 226, 237
      heme biosynthesis,
        250
      in trout, 227
      MFO components, 243
      plasma cholesterol,
        227

[Ascorbic acid]
  thyroid function, 240
  deficient microsomes, 250
  depletion and MFO system,
    250
  destruction, 230
  in diet, 235
    drug-induced cell dam-
      age, 268
  effect on nitrite toxicosis,
    314
  essential nutrient, 225
  excess, 238
  excess and drug conjuga-
    tion, 239
  excess and drug metabol-
    ism, 253
  hepatic damage protection,
    269
  inhibition covalent binding,
    269
  interaction toxic metabolite,
    270
  protection adriamycin toxi-
    city, 271
  protection from reactive
    metabolism, 266
  protective against drugs,
    278
  reducing agent, 225
  requirement, 275
  requirements and xenobio-
    tics, 277
  restriction and monooxy-
    genase, 244
  role in drug metabolism,
    226
  scavenger superoxide, 271
  supplement and antipyrine
    metabolism, 272
  synthesis and chemicals,
    257
  synthesis and drugs, 255
  synthesized from glucose,
    256
  tissue levels, 231

[Ascorbic acid]
    in xenobiotic metabol-
        ism/toxicology,
        274
Aspirin, in milk, 337
ATP sulfurylase, starvation ef-
    fect, 141
Avian riboflavinuria, 304
Azaserine, 60
    as carcinogen, 495
    effect and pancreatic hyper-
        trophy, 495
Azauridine (6-AZUR), 314
    bone calcium effect, (see 6-
        AZUR), 314
    teratogenic, 314
Azo dye (4-dimethylaminoazoben-
    zene), 51
    carcinogenic, 51
    dietary riboflavin, 51
Azoxymethane (AOM), analog
    cycasin, 59
    carcinogen, 59
    large-bowel cancer, 73

B

Benzodiazepine receptors and
    GABA, 386
Benzoflavone inhibitors, MFO
    activity, 64
Benzpyrene, extrahepatic meta-
    bolism, 72
Benzpyrene-induced carcinomas,
    96
    dyskeratosis, 96
    papillomas, 96
Birth defects, 299
Bisacodyl, 433
Body burden, chemical, 3
    in nuclear environment, 14
    indices, 7
    mathematical models for deter-
        mination of, 10-14
    pesticide, 8

Body weight, drug-induced
    change, 376
Bone formation, and physical
    activity, 413
Bone loss, and ketogenic diet,
    414
Bone mass
    decrease with immobilization,
        413
    in epileptic populations, 411
Bracken fern, and bladder can-
    cer, 61
Breast carcinogenesis, adipose
    tissue in, 83
Breast cancer, and lipid peroxi-
    dation, 84
Breast carcinogenesis, dietary
    fat as promoter of,
    fat effect on promotional phase,
        83
    high-fat effect, 82
British "total diet" study, 6
Bromobenzene-induced cytotoxi-
    city, 211
Butylated hydroxyanisole (BHA),
    64

C

Caffeine, anorectic effect, mech-
    anism, 392
    as anorectic, 392
    as psychoactive drug, 391
    increases metabolic rate, 392
Cannabis
    transport into milk, 354
    as antiemetic, 388
    antiemetic effect and cancer,
        389
    and feeding behavior, 389
    in glaucoma, 388
    hallucinogenic effect, 389
Carcinogenesis
    high-fat diet and, 52
    inhibition, 63

[Carcinogenesis]
inhibition by inducers, 63
and lipid peroxidation, 84
promotional phase, 78, 86
Carcinogens
chemical, 52
direct-acting, 54
epigenetic, 86
food additives/contaminants as,
72
genotoxic, 86
ultimate, 52
Cell proliferation, bile acids, in,
80
Cephalosporin antibiotics in human milk, 340
Ceruloplasmin and iron oxidation, 248
Chemical exposure, measurement
of human, 4
Chloramphenicol in human milk,
340
Chloro-K, 451
Chlorpromazine and body weight,
387
in human milk, 350
Cigarette smoking, cessation
and weight gain, 393
Cimetidine in human milk, 338
Cleft lip/palate, vitamin supplement effect, 313
Cleft palate, cortisone-induced
and B_6, 312
cortisone-induced and folic
acid, 312
and lack of prenatal vitamin
supplementation, 312
Clindamycin in milk, 341
CNS depressants, appetite increase, 382
CNS stimulants, as appetite depressants, 380
in children, 381
in reduction of body weight/
growth, 381
Cocarcinogens, food additives/
contaminants as, 72

Colchicine
alters cell generation, 479
alters water transport, 480
cyanocobalamin absorption
with, 479
diarrhea with, 479
in gouty arthritis, 479
megaloblastic anemia with, 479
Colon carcinogenesis, bile acids
and, 78
bile acids in, 80
experimental studies, 73-82
Conjugate elimination, 127
Conjugates
glucuronide, 127
primary, 127
sulfate, 127
Conjugation
competing pathways, 126-127
enzyme kinetics and, 123
with glucuronic acid, 123
with glycine, 123
lungs, 122
pharmacokinetic profile, 124
species difference, 123
sulfur-containing substrates,
157
Conjugation rates, 119
Cosubstrate, 119
for conjugation, 125
sulfation, 125
Cycad meal, and tumors, 59
Cycad plant (Cycas circinalis),
59
Cycasin
carcinogenic, 59
glucoside, methylazoxymethanol, 59
large-bowel cancer, rats, 73
Cyclophosphamide, in milk, 345
Cyproheptadine
as antihistaminergic, 383
as antiserotonergic, 383
and appetite, 382
appetite-stimulating effects,
383
Cyst(e)ine reservoirs, liver/

[Cyst(e)ine reservoirs]
  intestine glutathione as, 203
Cystathionase, common proper-
    ties, cysteine conjugate B-
    lyase, 200
Cystathionine pathway, 202
Cystathionine pathway
  methionine effect, 203
  need for cysteine biosynthe-
    sis, 203
Cysteine
  availability, cysteine and, 162
  dioxygenase, 162
  pool, 208
  source, food protein, 162
  utilization, liver, 207
Cysteine conjugate B-lyase,
    199,200
  kidney, 201
Cysteine dioxygenase, 203
Cysteine sulfinate, 162
Cysteinyl-S-acetaminophen, 187
Cytochrome P-450, 97
  inducers, 148
  vitamin A deficiency, 104

                    D

D-glucuronic acid, 320
D-penicillamine
  dimethylcysteine, 320
  effect on copper/zinc levels,
    320
  teratogenicity, 320
DDT residues, in blood/fat, 7
Dehydrocholesterol, conversion
    to vitamin D3, 413
Dermal exposure, from chemi-
    cals, 5-6
Desulfhydration, 163
Developmental interactions
  additive effect, 301
  nonadditive effect, 301
  protection effect, 301
  synergistic effect, 301
  threshold effect, 301

Dialkylhydrazines, 59
Diazepam, in milk, 352
Diet, and tumor development, 52
Dietary cholesterol and hepatic
    cyt P-450, 69
  endocrine control systems, 84
  mixed-function oxidases, 84
Dietary fat
  bile acid pattern, 78
  breast cancer, 85
  colon cancer, 77
  colon carcinogenesis, 75
  extrahepatic MFO system, 72
  lower to lessen cancer risk, 85
  mammary tumor growth, 84
  not carcinogenic, 77
  tumorigenesis, 73
Dietary fiber, and hepatic chol-
    esterol, 69
Digoxin in milk, 346
Dihydromercapturic acids, 210
Dimethylbenzanthracene (DMBA),
    cancer induced by, 56, 96
Dimethylhydrazine
  analog cycasin, 59
  large-bowel carcinogen, 73
Dimethylnitrosamine, 58
Dipeptidyl peptidase III, 197
Diphenylhydantoin
  folate absorption, 477
  folate deficiency with, 477
  megaloblastic anemia with, 477
Direct-acting carcinogens, of
    type alkylnitrosoureas, 73
Disulfide mixed, analysis of, 180
DMH (see Dimethylhydrazine),
    59
Doxycycline in human milk, 339
Drug-induced deficiencies, nut-
    ritional, definition, 507
Drug metabolism
  indices, 239
  methods, cellular level, 241
  methods, molecular level, 243
  methods, organismal level, 239
  methods, organ level, 241
  methods, subcellular level, 241

[Drug metabolism]
methods, system level, 240
Drug-metabolizing enzymes
dietary fat, 67
fatty-acid-induced changes, 68
hypervitaminosis A, 106, 109
kinetics of, 242
membrane structure, 68
protein deficiency, 98
vitamin A, 99, 112
vitamin C deficiency, 98
vitamin E, 99
Drug-induced deficiencies
continuity model, 517-519
interactive model, 519-521
nutritional, as ADR,
nutritional, complex etiology, 514
nutritional, mechanisms, 510
nutritional, risk, 505, 508
sequential event model, 515, 516, 517
Drug-induced osteomalacia
24-hr urinary calcium in, 420
diagnosis, 419
treatment, 421-422
vitamin D_3 for, 421
Drug-metabolizing enzymes
hepatic, 98
microsomal, 97
role of carbohydrates, 98
role of lipids, 98
vitamin A, 99
Drugs
anorectic in obesity, 382
extrahepatic metabolism, 122
psychoactive and appetite, 394
teratogenic effects and nutrients, 322
tuberculostatic and malformations, 307
DT-diaphorase
distribution, 444
flavoprotein, 444
induction, 445
role and inhibitors, 446

E

EDTA, teratogenicity and zinc, 315
Embryonic system, insulin lesion in, 305
Endopeptidase, neutral, 197
Enterohepatic recirculation, 127
Environmental contaminants, excreted in milk, 357
Epilepsy, adjuvant therapy, 413
Epileptics, fracture treatment, 422
Epoxide formation, 104
Equilibrium dialysis, 26
Ergot derivatives, in human milk, 347-348
Ethanol
inhibits milk ejection, 353
metabolism in pancreas, 491
Ethionine, methionine analog, 136
Exogenous hormones in milk, 348
Experimental carcinogenesis, dietary factors, 51

F

Fenfluramine
anorectic, 378
causes CNS serotonin release, 379
enhances satiety, 379
mild CNS depressant, 378
Fetal development, drugs, nutrition, and genetics in, 300
Fetal outcome
genetic background, 299
genetic factors, niacin and 6-AN, 306
First-pass effects, 119
First-pass metabolism, 122, 123
Flavoprotein reductase system, 65
Fluoride exposure, 10
Folate
absorption, 477

[Folate]
  conjugase, 477
  deficiency, 477
  in nature, 476
Folate supplementation, women
  on anticonvulsants, 312
Folic acid, convulsant properties, 311
Food contaminants, monitoring
  intake, 6

                  G

Gastric cancer, food nitrate, 54
Gastric emptying in the neonate,
  335
Glucuronic acid, synthesis and
  chemicals, 257
Glucuronidation
  cat, deficient, 126, 128
  effect of carbohydrate-rich
    diet, 132
  ethanol inhibition, 130-131
  harmol, 131
  1-naphthol, 131, 129
  paracetamol, 131
  UDP-glucuronate, 128
  xenobiotics, 129
Glutamyl transpeptidase
  AT-125, inhibitor, 196
  human liver, 194
  metabolic role, 196
Glutamyltranspeptidase, in kidney, 195
Glutathione
  assay, 145, 146
  AT-125 effect, 150
  availability and drugs, 147
  biosynthesis and cysteine, 149
  catabolism, 145
  cellular protection from, 267
  conjugate degradation, 193
  conjugate isolation HPLC, 181
  conjugate metabolism, 182
  conjugates, 179

[Glutathione]
  conjugates hepatocyte, 210
  conjugates of styrene oxide,
    210
  conjugation in cell/organ sys-
    tem, 182
  depletion, 148
  depletion, hepatocyte, 184
  diets decrease, 148
  distribution, 146
  drug depletion, 148
  feedback inhibitor, 144
  in fetal liver, 150
  fluorometric assays, 180
  formation and metal salts, 150
  functions, 145
  glycylglycine effect, 149
  in hepatomas, 150
  liver, carcinogen effect, 150
  liver, diet reduction, 149
  metabolism, 143
  metabolism, inborn errors, 144
  metabolism, AT-125 effect on,
    187
  mitochondrial pool, 203
  nonprotein sulfhydryl, 144
  in organs, 201
  oxidase, 207
  oxidized form, 144
  plasma, 145
  reduced form, 144
  reduced, diurnal variation, 146
  reductase cleavage, 179
  release, liver, 205
  S-transferase, 191
  salicylate depletion, 145
  synthesis, 143
  synthesis, methionine sulfox-
    ime and, 149
  synthetase, 190
  transpeptidation, 198
  turnover, 144
Glutathione disulfide (GSSG), 180
GSH
  S-transferases, 208
  acetaminophen depletion,

[GSH]
    kidney, 186
    biosynthesis and starvation, 207
    biosynthetic capacity, kidney, cell, 186
    complement of hepatocytes, 183
    content stomach and carcinogen resistance, 202
    cytosol pool, 204
    cytosolic, depletion of, 212
    depletion and hepatotoxicity, 184
    during bromobenzene metabolism, 211
    efflux liver, 205
    enzymic assay, 179
    hepatic, diurnal variation, 204
    interorgan maintenance, 212
    intracellular, cyt P-450 nutrition, 185
    levels and Adriamycin, 184
    mitochondrial pool, 204
    plasma, metabolism, 205
    red cell half-life, 190
    S-transferase, liver, 187
    synthesis and GSH conjugate, 202
    synthesis fetal liver, 194
    synthesis, erythrocyte, 189
    turnover, hepatocyte, rat, 183
GSH S-transferase levels, mammalian, 192
    plant, 191
GSSG, efflux erythrocytes, 190
Gunn rat, 128

H

Hair, as record of heavy metal intake, 9
Halogenated hydrocarbons in tissues, 10

Halothane transport into milk, 353
HEOD residues in blood/fat, 7-9
Hepatic cyt P-450, dietary lipid effect, 65
Hepatic drug metabolism, riboflavin deficiency, 99
Hepatocytes, isolated, 183
Hepatotoxicity, fasting and, 204
Hippuric acid synthesis, 123
Human milk
    composition, 331-332
    composition and stage of lactation, 333
    diurnal variations, 333
    drugs detected in, 336
    effect of maternal diet, 332
    feeding and antibody response, 342-343
    pH and drug transport, 334
    route of drug excretion, 331
    variation within feedings, 334
Hydrazine teratogenicity, 312
Hydroxyvitamin D (see 25OHD), 409
Hyperparathyroidism, CP and, 489
Hypervitaminosis A, cyt P-450, 109
    teratogenic, 302
Hypocalcemia, drug-induced, 410
Hypoprothrombinemia and laxative abuse, 433
Hypotaurine, 162

I

Infant intoxication, with maternal alcohol excess, 353
Intestinal cells, citrate dissociation, 188
    from chickens, 188
    oxidize GSH/GSSG, 188
Isoniazid in human milk, 341
    intoxication, antidote, 513

Isonicotinic acid hydrazide
(INH), 307

K

Kwashiorkor, chronic pancreatitis with, 487

L

L-gulonolactone oxidase absence
liability, 256
Laxative-induced diarrhea in infants, 349
Leukotriene A4, GSH conjugation, 190
Linoleic acid, and tumor growth,
83
Lipid peroxides, 83
Lithium
in milk, 350
and obesity, 385
and overfeeding, 385
thirst and weight gain, 385
and thyroxine inhibition, 386
usage and appetite, 385
and weight gain, 384
Liver cell culture, 185

M

Macronutrient intake, cancer
risk, 72-73
Major tranquilizers
and body weight, 388
hyperphagic effect, 387
Malabsorption, drug-induced,
475
Maldigestion, drug-induced, 475
Malformations
drugs and vitamins in, 302
result of interactions, 300
Mammary adipose tissue, storage
for hydrocarbons, 84

Mammary carcinogenesis, fat in-
take, prolactin and, 85
Mandelic acid, in milk, 341
Marijuana
and nursing, 356
and appetite, 388
Market-basket studies, to study
chemicals consumption, 6
Mazindol, anorectic drug, 379
Mediterranean fever, colchicine
prevention, 479
Menadiol diphosphate, 436
Menadione
absorption, rats, 432
sulfate conjugates, rats, 437
Menaquinone absorption, rats,
432
Menaquinone-4, 435
Mercaptopurine (6-MP), 316
Mercapturic acid, 187
Mercury, in hair, 9-10
Methenamine, in milk, 341
Methionine
high-dose toxicity, 160
in protein food, 159
requirement, sparing effect of
cystine, 202
serum, diurnal variation, 161
toxic effect, protection, 161
Methionine adenosyltransferase,
132,133
Methionine adenosyltransferase,
cyclic amino acids and, 136
Methionine sulfoxime, 136
Methophenazine, malformation response, 304
Methotrexate
folic acid antagonist, 308
and malformations, 309
methyl derivative aminopterin,
309
in milk, 345
poisoning, antidote, 513
Methyl chloride, workers, 211
Methylazoxymethanol (MAM), analogs and cancer in rats, 73
Methylmercaptan, 211

Methylphenidate, in children, 380
Methyltetrahydrofolate, 134
Methylthiolation pathway, 200
MFO activity, dieldrin induction and diet, 243
MFO system
  components of, 241-242
  dietary lipid effect, 64
Micromelia
  insulin-induced and nicotinamide, 304
  sulfanilamide-produced, 305
Mineral oil, 433
Minor tranquilizers
  appetite-stimulating effects, 387
  enhance appetite, 386
Mixed-function oxidases (MFO), 52, 97
Mutagenesis, retinol inhibition, 105

[Neonatal period]
  hyperacidity during, 335
Nicotinamide
  teratogenicity of 6-AN, 306
  ATDA as antagonist, 306
Nicotine
  anorectic effect, 393
  in milk, 356
  weight-suppressing effect, 393
Nitrofurantoin
  cause of hemolysis, 340
  in human milk, 340
Nitrosamine, in beer, 496
Nitrosamines
  asymmetric, 58
  cyclic, 58
  from nitrate/ite + amines/ides, 58
Nitrosonornicotine, tobacco smoke, 58
Nutrient deficiencies, alter neoplastic processes, 72

N

N-acetyltransferase, reaction of mercapturic acid, 199
N-hydroxy-2-acetylaminofluorene, 127
N-methyl-N'-nitro-N-nitrosguanide (MNNG), 96
N-Nitrosodimethylamine (DMH), 96
NADPH-cytochrome C reductase, 97
Neomycin
  antibiotic, 475
  for bowel surgery, 475
  cholesterol-lowering effect, 476
  in hepatic encephalopathy, 475
  induced intestinal changes, 476
  lipid malabsorption, 476
Neonatal period
  reduced drug metabolism, 336

O

O-xylene
  metabolism, 211
  metabolite reacts GSH, 211
ODC induction, bile acids in, 80
Oral contraceptives
  effect on lactation, 348-349
  folate deficiency with, 479
  low serum folate, 479
  megaloblastic anemia with, 479
Oral exposure, from chemicals, 6
Organotropism, 57
Ornithine conjugation, birds, 150-151
Ornithine decarboxylase (ODC), 80
Osmotic minipump, 123
Osteopenia, in anticonvulsant patients, 413

P

Pancreatic adenocarcinomas in
    hamsters, 495
Pancreatic cancer
    beer consumption, 496
    high fat intake, 496
    smoking, 496
Pancreatic secretion, alcohol-in-
    duced modifications, 490
Pancreatic stones, 489
Pancreatitis
    ACP lesions, 488
    acute alcoholic, 493
    alcoholic, 487
    alcoholic chronic (ACP), 487
    azathioprine-induced, 494
    chlorothiazide-induced, 494
    chronic calcifying, 488
    chronic (CP), 487
    drugs probably associated,
        494-495
    estrogen-induced, 493
    evolution, 489
    furosemide-induced, 494
    high fat/protein and ACP, 488
    sulfonamide-induced, 494
    tetracycline-induced, 494
PAPS
    assay, 139
    biosynthesis, 137
    purification, 140
    sulfate availability, 140
    sulfate conjugation, 138
    sulfate-donating cosubstrate,
        139
Paracetamol (acetaminophen),
    188
    -S-cysteine, 189
    -S-glutathione, 189
    conjugates, isolated liver, 188
    glutathione conjugate, 189
Parathion, skin penetration, 6
Penicillin, transfer into milk,
    339
Pentothal sodium, in milk, 352

Pharmacokinetic model, Ramsey's,
    12-13
Pharmacokinetics
    infant, 335-336
    maternal, 334-335
Phenobarbital, and vitamin D-
    hydroxylase system, 417
Phenolphthalein, conjugate in
    milk, 349
Phenylpropylethylamine, OTC
    anorectic, 379
Phenytoin
    accelerates fracture healing,
        418
    action and folic acid, 311
    and epilepsy, 309
    inhibitory effect of collagen,
        418
    inhibits bone resorptive re-
        sponse, 418
    lysosomal enzyme release, 418
    PTH-stimulated cyclic AMP, 418
    teratogenicity, 309
Photon absorption, in bone mass
    measurement, 411
Phylloquinone
    absorption, normal subjects,
        431
    absorption, rats, 431
    biliary/fecal metabolites, 438
    cyt P-450 in metabolism of, 440
    distribution, 434
    effects on metabolism, 439
    elimination, 436
    epoxidase activity and warfar-
        in, 450
    epoxidase induction, 450
    epoxidase inhibition, 451
    -2,3-epoxide, 439
    -2,3-epoxide (vitamin K_1 epox-
        ide), 442
    epoxide, warfarin-induced, 442
    glucuronide conjugates, 437
    in liver, 435
    in mitochondria, 435
    requirement, 440

[Phylloquinone]
trans and cis isomers, 440
transport, 434
turnover kinetics, 435
water-soluble metabolites, 436
Plasma binding, with acute viral
hepatitis, 34
Plasma 25OHD
in summer, 413
in winter, 413
Plasma albumin
aging and decrease, 22
diseases decreasing, 22
as transport protein, 23
Plasma binding
artifacts in, 36
cirrhosis effects, 34
competitive inhibitors, 35
consequences of displacement,
42
decreased hypoalbuminemia,
33
decreased in kwashiorkor, 33
of drugs, 21
effects on drug disposition,
36, 37, 38, 39
effects on drug elimination, 40
endogenous displacers and, 34
equilibrium dialysis method,
27, 28
factors affecting, 26-36
impaired in uremia, 34
independent of drug concentration, 41
interpretation of data, 29-31
measurement of, 26
perspectives, 43
sites, 22
C proteins, 25
ultracentrifugation method,
28, 29
ultrafiltration method, 28
Plasma lipoproteins
classified, 25
drug binding, 25
protein content, 25

Plasma proteins, in drug bind-
ing, 22
Pleiotypic response, 255, 257,
258
Polycyclic aromatic hydrocarbons,
56
Promoters, 77
Praziquantel
as anthelmintic, 342
in human milk, 342
Prednisolone, in human milk, 348
Premercapturate intermediates,
209
Procarcinogens, metabolic activa-
tion, 54
Propachlor, methylthiol glucuro-
nides, 200
Propranolol, in milk, 345
Prostaglandin synthesis, 83
Pulmonary carcinogenesis, 3-
methylcholanthrene, 95
Pyridoxal
complex with INH, 307
toxicity, 307
Pyridoxine, and hydrazine toxi-
city, 308
Pyrimethamine, in human milk,
342
Pyruvate dehydrogenase, 157

R

Radiation hazards, internal, 15
Radioactivity monitors, shadow
shield, 15
shielded chair, 15
Radionuclide
assessment methods, 15, 16
internal contamination, 15
Radiopharmaceuticals, exposure
via milk, 351
Renal riboflavinuria, 304
Reserpine, and body weight, 387
Respiratory exposure, from
chemicals, 4-5

Retinoids, 95
  anticarcinogenic effect, 105
  antineoplastic effect, 97
  carcinogenic protection, 112
  cellular immune responses,
    96
  DNA synthesis, 96
  drug-metabolizing enzymes,
    113
Retinol, inhibits mutagenicity
  AFB1, 106
Retinol-binding protein, oral
  contraceptives and, 303
Riboflavin, complex with boric
  acid, 303
Rickets, in epileptic population,
  409

                        S

S-adenosyl-L-methionine (SAM),
  132
S-adenosyl-L-methionine decarboxylase (SAMD), 80
S-adenosylhomocysteine, inhibitor transmethylation, 134
S-methyl-3-thiopropionate, 160
S-methylglutathione, 187
Salicylate, teratogenicity and
  manganese, 321
SAM
  age effect, 137
  assay, 134
  circadian rhythm, 137
  dietary methionine and, 137
  effect of fasting, 137
  HPLC separation, 135
  methionine availability for,
    133
  methylation, 133
  methylation and neurotrans-
    mitters, 134
  polyamine synthesis, 133
  pyrogallol, 135
SAMD induction, bile acids in,
  80

Scatchard plot, nonlinearity of,
  30-31
Scurvy
  monkey, human subjects, 237
  ptarmigan, 229
Sodium nitrite, fetotoxicity and
  sodium nitrite, 314
Substrate concentration, 123,
  124
Sulfamethoxypyridazine, cause
  of hemolysis, 341
Sulfapyridine, 478
Sulfasalazine
  in human milk, 338
  inhibits folic acid absorption,
    478
  macrocytosis with, 478
  metabolites, 478
  serum folate levels with, 478
Sulfate
  activation in brachymorphic
    mice, 142
  depletion, 140
  inorganic, serum concentra-
    tion, 139
  serum decrease with diet, 141
Sulfate, labeled, 138
Sulfation, 126
  at birth, 142
  brachymorphic mice, deficient,
    128
  inorganic sulfate in, 159
  rate, 125
Sulfite oxidase, deficiency, 162
Sulfotransferase, 125
  phenol, 126

                        T

Taurine
  availability, diet effects, 155-
    156
  conjugated cholate, cat, 151
  conjugation, 154
  developmental aspects, 157
  drug effects, 155

[Taurine]
effect, bile salt conjugates,
151
essential amino acid, cat, 153
increase fasting effect, 155
roles, 153
substrates for conjugation,
152
synthesis, 152, 153
Taurocholate, 154
Teratogenesis
bidrin, 307
boric acid and riboflavin, 303
insulin-induced, 303
maternal dietary deficiencies
in, 300
methyl carbamate compounds
and, 307
nutrient deficiencies in, 300
organophosphorous com-
pounds and, 307
reduction by NAD precursors,
307
Test diets
aryl hydrocarbon hydroxylase,
230
scorbutigenic, 229
TETA, and zinc, 321
Tetrahydrocannabinol (THC),
388
Thalidomide, 300
teratogenic effect and folate,
312
and zinc, 316
Theobromine, in milk, 354, 355
Thiols
HPLC, 180
separation, HPLC, 181
Tolbutamide, releases insulin,
348
Trans-retinoic acid, 95
Trans-retinol, 95
Trans-vitamin A, 95
Transsulfurylation, pyridoxal
phosphate cofactor, 161
Tricyclic antidepressants, in
milk, 350-351

Triethylenetetramine (TETA),
320
Tumor promoter, cholesterol as,
80
Tumor promoters, bile acids as,
78

U

Ubiquinone, 437
UDP-glucuronic acid (UDPGA),
128
UDP-glucuronosyltransferase,
68, 126
UDPG-dehydrogenase, 132
UDPGA
diethylether narcosis, 131
hepatic, 131
intracellular concentration, 130
liver, drug effects, 132
liver, fasting, 132
liver, fetus, 131
liver, hormonal effects, 131
liver, phenobarbital effect,
132
liver, tolbutamide effect, 131
tissue concentrations, 130
UDP glucose, 130
Ultimate carcinogens, covalent
binding, 61

V

Vitamin A
aflatoxin-induced toxicity, 104
aflatoxin-induced tumors, 104
and Trypan Blue as teratogens,
302
anticarcinogenic activity, 95
deficiency and sulfation, 142
differentiated epithelia, 95
excess, 112
glycoprotein production, 95
hepatic and toxic chemicals,
113

[Vitamin A]
  N-nitrosodimethylamine-in-
      duced colon tumors, 96
  night blindness, prevention,
      95
  plasma and oral contracep-
      tives, 303
  provitamin β-carotene, 95
Vitamin A analogs, antineo-
    plastic, 96
Vitamin A acid (see Trans-retin-
    oic acid, 95
Vitamin A aldehyde (see Trans-
    retinol), 95
Vitamin A deficiency
  aflatoxin B₁ liver tumors, 96
  cancer incidence, 95
  chemical toxicity, 96
  rat colon carcinogenesis, 96
  susceptibility carcinogenesis,
      106
Vitamin A palmitate, benzo[A]
    pyrene metabolism, 106
Vitamin C
  biologic functions, 276
  deficiency and drug metabol-
      ism, 237
  deficiency and MFO activity,
      264
  deficiency, relative, ham-
      sters, 229
  deprivation and monooxygen-
      ase, 252
  different requirement of sys-
      tems, 277
  dosage, 235
  and human health, 275
  overdose and drug conjuga-
      tion, 226
  MFO system, 248
  pharmacologic effects, 236
  pharmacokinetic studies, 240
Vitamin D
  -25-hydroxylase enzyme sys-
      tem, 415
  1,25(OH)D₂ as metabolite, 415

[Vitamin D]
  activity and sunlight, 413
  drug effects on metabolism,
      409
  enterohepatic circulation, 415
  excess, anti-vitamin K effect,
      433
  hepatic catabolism and drugs,
      416
  intake and 25OHD in epileptics,
      412
  intake and serum 25OHD levels,
      411
  metabolite-binding protein, 415
  prohormone, 415
  prophylaxis in epileptics, 422
  requirement, 415
  response to large doses, 417
  sources, 414
  sterols, 416
Vitamin D₂ (ergocalciferol), 414
Vitamin E, anti-vitamin K effect,
      433
Vitamin K
  absorption, 430
  absorption and estrogen, 433
  absorption and vitamin A, 433
  absorption, summary, 433
  antagonists, 429
  and blood coagulation, 429
  deficiency, 440-441
  deficiency and abetalipopro-
      teinemia, 434
  deficiency and malabsorption,
      441
  deficiency and biliary disease,
      441
  deficiency and prothrombin,
      429
  deficiency, chemical assays
      for, 441
  dependent clotting factors,
      steroids, 456
  dependent carboxylase, 454
  dependent carboxylase inhibi-
      tors, 456

[Vitamin K]
dependent carboxylase, location, 457
dependent carboxylation, 429
dependent protein, osteocalcin, 453
dietary deficiency, 441
discovery, 429
diseases causing malabsorption, 433
epoxidase, characteristics, 447
epoxidase, distribution, 447
epoxidase, role and inhibitors, 450
epoxide reductase, 451
epoxide reductase and warfarin, 452
epoxide reductase in endothelial reticulum, 452
epoxide, functions, 441
high content in vegetables, 440
hydroperoxide, 455
hydroquinone, functions, 441
K-deficient diets and mineral oil, 432
K-deficient diets and squalene, 432
oxidoreductase, 444
oxidoreductase (DT-diaphorase), 457
Vitamin K$_1$
epoxide, inhibitor vitamin K, 443
epoxide, warfarin effect, 442
in formula/milk, 440
hydroquinone, 443

[Vitamin K$_1$]
hydroquinone, substrate epoxide, 444
phylloquinone, 429
Vitamin K$_2$, menaquinone-7, 429

W

Warfarin-resistant rats, vitamin K epoxide reductase in, 452
Weber-Christian syndrome, 490
Weighed food records, to study chemical consumption, 6

X

Xenobiotics, and cytosolic receptor, 243
and UDP-glucose dehydrogenase, 257

Z

Zinc
6-MP teratogenic effect, 316
acetazolamide teratogenicity, 318
salicylate teratogenicity, 317
thalidomide analog, 317
deficiency and aspirin toxicity, 317
interaction with EDTA, 316
salicylate and genetic background, 318